Female Pelvic Reconstructive Surgery

Springer
London
Berlin
Heidelberg
New York
Barcelona
Hong Kong
Milan
Paris
Singapore
Tokyo

Stuart L. Stanton and Philippe E. Zimmern (Eds)

Female Pelvic Reconstructive Surgery

With 241 Figures
including 5 Colour Plates

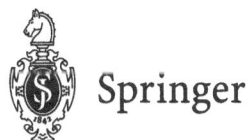 Springer

Stuart L. Stanton, FRCS, FRCOG, FRANZCOG (Hon)
Department of Obstetrics and Gynaecology, St. George's Hospital Medical School,
London, UK

Philippe E. Zimmern, MD, FACS
Department of Urology, Southwestern Medical Center at Dallas,
Dallas, Texas, USA

Cover illustration: Chapter 8, Figure 5.

British Library Cataloguing in Publication Data
Female pelvic reconstructive surgery
    1. Pelvis – Surgery   2. Surgery, Plastic
    I. Stanton, Stuart L., 1938 –   II. Zimmern, Philippe E.
    617.5′5′0592
ISBN-13:978-1-4471-1172-6   e-ISBN-13: 978-1-4471-0659-3
DOI: 10.1007/978-1-4471-0659-3
Library of Congress Cataloging-in-Publication Data
Female pelvic reconstructive surgery / Stuart L. Stanton and Philippe Zimmern (eds).
    p.;   cm.
    Includes bibliographical references and index.
    ISBN 978-1-4471-1172-6 (alk. paper)
    1. Urogynecologic surgery.   2. Pelvis – Surgery. I. Stanton, Stuart L. II. Zimmern, Philippe E.
    [DNLM: 1. Pelvis – surgery.   2. Reconstructive Surgical Procedures.   3. Women's
Health. WP 155 F3295 2002]
RG484. F457   2002
618.1′059–dc21
                                                         2001042968

ISBN 978-1-4471-1172-6 Springer-Verlag London Berlin Heidelberg
a member of BertelsmannSpringer Science+Business Media GmbH
http://www.springer.co.uk

Typeset by EXPO Holdings, Malaysia

28/3830-543210 Printed on acid-free paper SPIN 10729397

To Julia, my wife, and my children, Claire, Talia, Jo, Tamara and Noah
for their support and encouragement.
Stuart L. Stanton

To all those who have supported and encouraged my vocation,
with special gratitude to my wife Sabine and my children Segolene,
Vincent, Delphine, and Arnaud.
Philippe E. Zimmern

Foreword

Urogynecology is a complex and expanding field that has grown beyond the scope of urology or gynecology alone. This admirably comprehensive volume acknowledges this fact and includes the expertise of specialists in neurological and reconstructive surgery as well.

After two preliminary chapters on surgical anatomy and the pathophysiology of urinary incontinence, the book concentrates on surgical management in four main categories: sphincteric surgery, prolapse, urinary diversion, and fistula repair. Special emphasis is given to urinary incontinence in all its variations, of course, but the inclusion of uterine prolapse, enteroceles, anorectal anomalies, and recto- and urethrovaginal fistulas will be welcome to the busy clinician. Urinary diversion, for those unfortunate patients in whom rehabilitation is not feasible, is also covered, as is the emerging option of neuromodulation – an exciting possibility for some of these patients with intractable voiding dysfunction.

This volume should be a core holding in the library of the many physicians concerned with the multiple aspects of female pelvic reconstruction.

Emil A. Tanagho, MD
San Francisco, California

Preface

The pelvic floor, formerly the province of the gynaecologist, is now of major interest to urologists and colorectal surgeons as well. The old historical and anatomical division of the pelvis into compartments 'belonging to' one or other of these three disciplines is beginning to be abandoned in favour of a single specialist or team of specialists who recognise that the pelvic floor is a single physiological unit and approaches its disorders and their treatment with this multi-disciplinary philosophy.

It is, therefore, no surprise that a gynaecologist and urologist, together with significant input from colorectal colleagues, combine to produce a textbook which exemplifies this principle. We noted the lack of a unified and practical book on the surgery of pelvic floor reconstruction, and are grateful to all our contributors for having agreed to take part and for their contributions.

We are conscious of the emphasis now placed on evidence-based medicine, audit and clinical governance, to ensure that the patient is managed by modern and tried techniques and that surgeons are suitably trained to carry them out. At no other time have surgeons been under such close scrutiny by patients, hospital, governmental health agencies and lawyers, and the need for an up to date text, setting out clear and practical approaches to treatment, is important. In choosing our contributors, we encouraged discussion on innovative as well as conventional techniques and emphasised the importance of clinical and objective patient assessment, both before and after surgery. With a multitude of operative techniques, in the last section we put forward the views of five experienced surgeons from different disciplines, to discuss their indications and choice of operations for a variety of clinical situations.

We are indebted to the stimulus and constructive criticism from our research fellows and trainees and particularly to our secretaries, Wendy Nash and Susan Brewer, who have worked assiduously and patiently to bring this book to completion. We thank particularly Nick Mowat (former Medical Editor), Nick Wilson (current Senior Production Controller), Melissa Morton and Eva Senior of Springer-Verlag, for their professionalism and wisdom in all stages of the production of this book.

Above all, we continue to learn from our patients, whose well-being is paramount.

Stuart L. Stanton
London

Philippe E. Zimmern
Dallas

July 2002

Contents

PART III SPHINCTER SURGERY

PART V DIVERSION AND BLADDER NECK CLOSURE

PART VI FISTULAE

PART VII NEUROMODULATION

PART VIII POSTOPERATIVE MANAGEMENT

PART IX OUTCOME MEASURES

Contributors

Menachem Alcalay Head of Urogynecology Service, Department of Obstetrics and Gynecology, Chaim Seba Medical Center, Tel Aviv University, Tel Aviv, Israel

Kaven Baessler Urogynaecology Unit, St George's Hospital, London, UK

Cornelius Baeten Academic Hospital Maastricht, Maastricht, The Netherlands

J. Thomas Benson Director of Female Pelvic Medicine and Reconstructive Surgery, Division of Obstetrics and Gynecology, Indiana University, Indianapolis, USA

Alfred E. Bent Department of Obstetrics and Gynecology, Baltimore, USA

Genady Bitman Department of Obstetrics and Gynaecology, The Chaim Sheba Medical Centre, Tel Aviv, Israel

Daniel S. Blander Department of Urology, University of Texas, Southwestern Medical School, Dallas, USA

Tim B. Boone Baylor College of Medicine, Scott Dept of Urology/Scurlock, Houston, USA

Karen D. Bradshaw Department of Obstetrics and Gynecology, UT Southwestern Medical Center, Dallas, USA

Calin Ciofu Hôpital Tenon, Department of Urologie, Paris, France

Craig V. Comiter Division of Urology, University of Arizona Health Science Center, Tucson, USA

Amir A. Darakhshan Kent and Canterbury Hospital, East Kent Hospitals NHS Trust, Canterbury, UK

Ananias C. Diokno Urology Department, William Beaumont Hospital, USA

Peter L. Dwyer Department of Urogynaecology, Royal Women & Mercy Hospital for Women, Melbourne, Australia

Daniel S. Elliott Baylor College of Medicine, Scott Department of Urology/Scurlock, Houston, USA

Brigitte Fatton Hotel Dieu Maternité, University Hospital of Clérmont Ferrand, Clérmont Ferrand, France

Elizabeth Ann Gormley Section of Urology, Dartmouth-Hitchcock Medical Center, Lebanon, USA

Sharon G. Gregorcyk UT Southwestern Medical Center I, Dept of Surgery, Dallas, USA

François Haab Hôpital Tenon, Department of Urologie, Paris, France

Sender Herschorn Division of Urology, Department of Surgery, Sunnybrook Health Science Centre, North York, Ontario, Canada

Paul Hilton Department of Obstetrics and Gynaecology, Royal Victoria Infirmary, Newcastle upon Tyne, UK

Keith Holmes Department of Paediatric Surgery, St George's Hospital Medical School, London, UK

Philip J. Huber Jr Department of Surgery, St Paul Hospital, Dallas, USA

Tracy L. Hull Department of Colorectal Surgery, Cleveland Clinic Foundation, Cleveland, USA

Bernard Jacquetin Hotel Dieu Maternité, University Hospital of Clérmont Ferrand, Clérmont Ferrand, France

Saad Juma Incontinence Research Foundation, Encinitas, California, USA

Margie A. Kahn Department of Obstetrics & Gynecology, University of Texas Medical Branch, Galveston, USA

Mickey Karram Department of Obstetrics and Gynecology, Good Samaritan Hospital, Seton Center, Cincinnati, USA

Carl G. Klutke Division of Urologic Surgery, Washington University School of Medicine, St. Louis, USA

John J. Klutke Division of Urologic Surgery, Washington University School of Medicine, St. Louis, USA

Kathleen C. Kobashi Virginia Mason Medical Center, Department of Surgery, Section of Urology and Renal Transplantation, Seattle, USA

Devinder Kumar Department of Obstetrics and Gynaecology, St George's Hospital Medical School, London, UK

Richard Labasky Division of Urology, University of Utah Medical Center, Salt Lake City, USA

Gary E. Leach Tower Urology Institute for Continence, Los Angeles, USA

Gary E. Lemack Department of Urology, University of Texas, Southwestern Medical School, Dallas, USA

Elad Leron Urogynaecology Unit, St George's Hospital, London, UK

Scott E. Littwiller Urologic Specialists of Oklahoma, Tulsa, USA

Ann C. Lowry Division of Colon and Rectal Surgery, University of Minnesota, St Paul, USA

Liam McCarthy Department of Paediatric Surgery, St George's Hospital Medical School, London, UK

Tony Mundy Institute of Urology, London, UK

Victor W. Nitti NYU Urology Associates, New York, USA

Mouad Nouri Hôpital Tenon, Department of Urologie, Paris, France

Thomas M. Rashid Urology Department, William Beaumont Hospital, Royal Oak, USA

Schlomo Raz Department of Urology, University of California, Los Angeles School of Medicine, Los Angeles, USA

Feza H. Remzi Department of Colorectal Surgery, Cleveland Clinic Foundation, Cleveland, Ohio, USA

Anthony M.K. Rickwood Regional Department of Paediatric Urology, Royal Liverpool Children's NHS Trust, Alder Hey Children's Hospital, Liverpool, UK

Madan Samuel Department of Paediatric Surgery, St George's Hospital Medical School, London, UK

Bob L. Shull Department of Obstetrics and Gynecology, Scott and White Clinic and Hospital, Texas A&M University Health Science Center, Temple, Texas, USA

Mark C. Slack Department of Obstetrics and Gynaecology, Hinchingbrooke Hospital, Cambridgeshire, UK

Tony Smith St Mary's Hospital, Manchester, UK

Stuart L. Stanton Department of Obstetrics and Gynaecology, Pelvic Reconstruction and Urogynaecology Unit, St George's Hospital Medical School, London, UK

Andrew C. Steele Department of Obstetrics and Gynaecology, Good Samaritan Hospital, Seton Center, Cincinnati, Ohio, USA

Steven Straffordt Department of Gynaecology, Eemland Hospital, Amersfoot, The Netherlands

Abdul H. Sultan Department of Obstetrics and Gynaecology, Mayday University Hospital, Thornton Heath, UK

William H. Turner Department of Urology, Addenbrooke's Hospital, Cambridge, UK

Ulf Ulmsten Uppsala University, Dept of Women's and Children's Health, Section for Obstetrics and Gynaecology, Akademiska Sjukhuset, Uppsala, Sweden

Sandip Vasavada Urology Institute, Cleveland Clinic Foundation, Cleveland, USA

Suzie Venn Department of Urology, St. Richard's Hospital, Chichester, W. Sussex, UK

Ashish Wakhlu Vivek Khand, Gomti Nagar, Lucknow, India

Lewis Wall Department of Obstetrics and Gynecology, Division of Gynecology, Urogynecology and Reconstructive Pelvic Surgery, Cedars-Sinai Medical Center, Los Angeles, USA

Christopher J. Walshe Pelvic Reconstructive Surgery and Urogynecology, Tripler Army Medical Center, Department of Obstetrics and Gynecology, Honolulu, USA

Norman S. Williams Academic Department of Surgery, The Royal London Hospital, London, UK

Howard Winfield Department of Urology, University of Iowa, Iowa City, USA

Aileen M.K. Yee Department of Obstetrics and Gynecology, Baltimore, USA

Philippe E. Zimmern Department of Urology, University of Texas, Southwestern Medical School, Dallas, USA

Part I

Surgical Anatomy

1 Anatomy for the Pelvic Reconstructive Surgeon

John James Klutke and Carl Georg Klutke

Pelvic Anatomy by Structure
  Vagina
  Urethra
  Levator Ani
  Urogenital Diaphragm
  Endopelvic Fascia

Landmarks for the Reconstructive Pelvic Surgeon
  Bony Landmarks
  Retropubic Dissection
  Vaginal Surgical Relationships

This chapter describes the functional anatomy of the pelvis for the reconstructive surgeon. We anticipate that many of our readers will have a strong clinical and surgical background, and we include clinical observations to illustrate anatomic concepts. Our bias is toward clinical relevance, and the chapter is not meant as an exhaustive anatomic treatment.

Any functional description of the pelvic anatomy made today would be incomplete without a word about magnetic resonance imaging. MRI contributes importantly to this description because it illustrates anatomic relationships in the living state. The striated muscles of the pelvis, with their constant tone, behave uniquely in life. Dissection has been the gold standard for establishing anatomic truth for nearly a millennium, but is limited by its potential to misrepresent the anatomic state of the living pelvic musculature. MR images made in a living individual are unaffected by the artifact associated with cell death and tissue preparation. Other imaging modalities have advanced technologically, but none offer the exquisite resolution of soft tissue anatomy of MRI.

Studies by Strohbehn et al.[1,2] have validated MRI as a diagnostic tool, proving the close correlation between MRI findings, anatomic dissection, and histology. The state of the art in MRI technology has since improved exponentially. MRI was once limited to supine studies, but it is now possible to make MR images in other positions.[3] Important improvements have also been made in image resolution. In an MR image, signal degradation depends on the distance of the coil (signal transducer) from the tissue being imaged. The closer the coil is to the tissue, the better the signal. MRI coils can now be placed directly inside a hollow viscus,[4-6] giving maximal signal intensity. These endoluminal coils are currently available for the vagina and rectum. To further improve resolution, the signals of two or more coils, each in close contact with a different part of the pelvis, are combined into one high resolution image (multicoil phased array technique[7]). MRI can also demonstrate anatomic features dynamically, e.g., during voiding, straining or activities that precipitate urinary leakage. These "fast freeze" images are made without exposing the patient to ionizing radiation and are equal or superior to fluoroscopy in their diagnostic value.[8] MRI is, moreover, a global study in the sense that the urinary, genital and gastrointestinal systems are illustrated at the same time, allowing us to make inference about their interaction. This chapter is illustrated with MR images and we would suggest that this will increasingly become a modality of importance to the reconstructive pelvic surgeon.

Pelvic Anatomy by Structure

Vagina

The vagina is an expandable fibromuscular sheath containing large amounts of collagen, elastin and smooth muscle. It contains estrogen receptors in high concentration, and is a target organ for estrogen. Collagen is the body's premier supportive connective tissue, and estrogen deficiency of menopause has a profound effect on vaginal support and urinary continence. Collagen is secreted by fibroblasts. These cells have estrogen receptors and are influenced by estrogen. This is why the quantity and

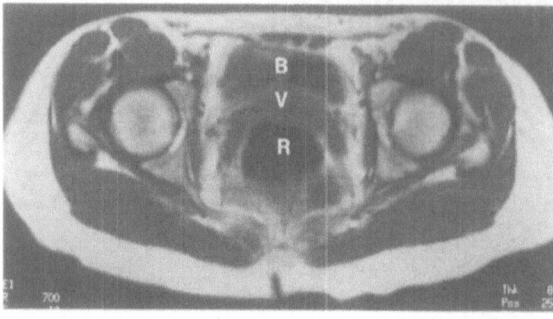

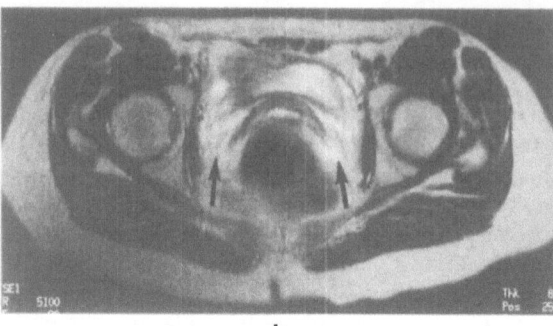

Figure 1.1 a T1 weighted image at the level of the vagina depicting surrounding vascularity. **b** T2 weighted image reveals the vaginal lumen with intravaginal fluid. Note physiologic fluid is dark on T1 weighted image, bright on T2 weighted image. B, bladder; R, rectum; V, vagina. Reprinted with permission from Klutke CG and Raz S, Evaluation and treatment of the incontinent female patient, *Urologic Clinics of North America* 1995; 22; 489–496.

quality of collagen produced in the vagina depends on estrogen. The vagina also contains elastin in high proportion, and it can stretch tremendously during childbirth and later return to normal dimensions. A

highly developed venous plexus surrounds the vagina's inner mucous membrane, which is under autonomic and estrogenic control (Fig. 1.1). The vagina itself has no glands except for a few specialized structures, and vaginal lubrication during sexual arousal results from transudation of fluid through this rich vascular layer.

The vagina attaches to the pelvis at three levels. The uterosacral and cardinal ligament complex attaches the upper (proximal) vagina posteriorly to the sacrum (Figs 1.2, 1.3). Its midportion is attached laterally to the arcus tendineus by the pubocervical fascia, a tough, fibromuscular sheet of tissue that is continuous with the endopelvic fascia. The vagina is firmly fixed at its distal end by the pubourethral ligaments anteriorly and the perineal body posteriorly. Because of its predominantly lateral attachments, the vagina is H-shaped in cross section, and is normally a potential space. Its anterior wall is like a hammock that slings underneath and supports the urethra.[9] The urethra is closely associated with the anterior vaginal wall, and the two structures rotate as a unit with increases of intraabdominal pressure. The attachments of the vagina to the pelvic bone are only a part of its support. The tone of the underlying levator ani, a striated muscle, stabilizes the anterior vaginal wall, and the urethra by extension, during straining and against the constant downward force of gravity.

Distally, the vagina, urethra and rectum traverse the levator diaphragm, the muscular floor of the pelvis. Fibers of the pubococcygeus and puborectalis muscles, constituent muscles of the levator ani, loop around these structures and pull them anteriorly toward the pubic bones like a sling. This orients the lower third of the vagina almost vertically. Above the

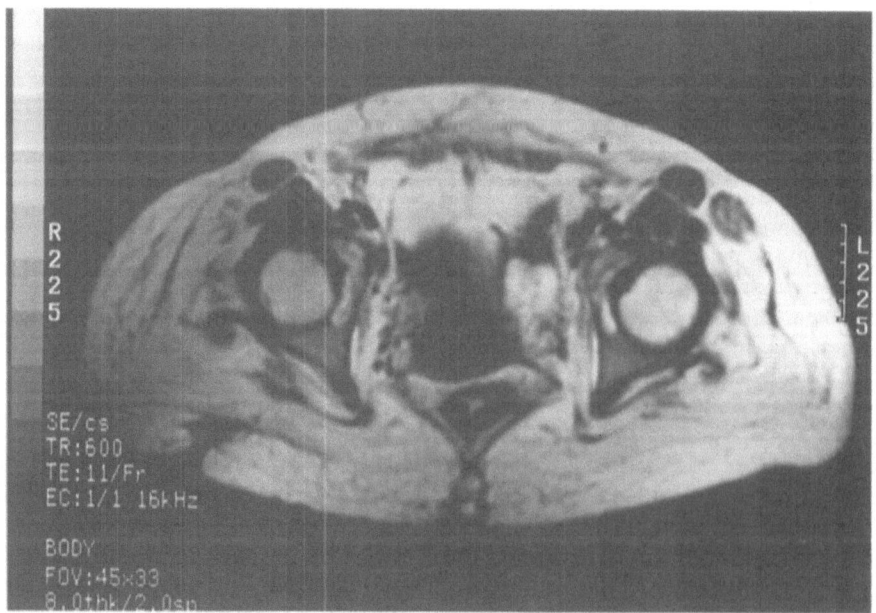

Figure 1.2 T2 weighted axial image at the level of the cervix showing the horizontally oriented cardinal ligament (arrow) passing laterally to pelvic side wall. Reprinted with permission from Klutke CG and Raz S, Evaluation and treatment of the incontinent female patient, *Urologic Clinics of North America* 1995; 22; 489–496.

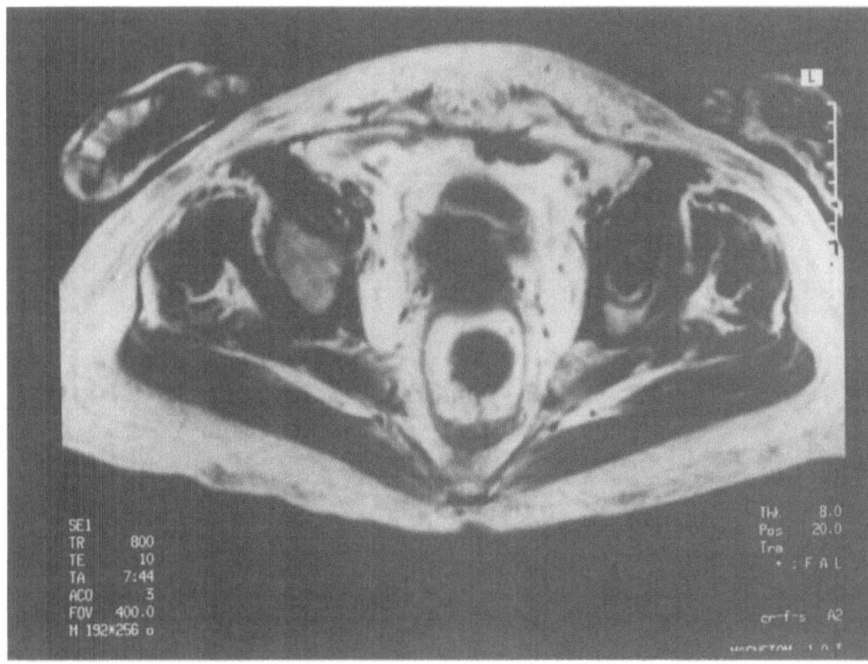

Figure 1.3 Axial section at the level of the cervix delineating the uterosacral ligaments passing from cervix posteriorly to the sacrum. Reprinted with permission from Klutke CG and Raz S, Evaluation and treatment of the incontinent female patient, *Urologic Clinics of North America* 1995; 22;489–496.

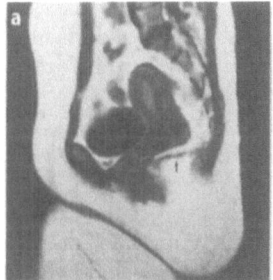
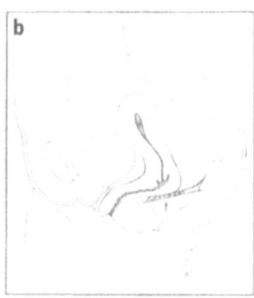
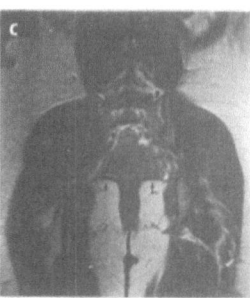

Figure 1.4 a,b Sagittal section through normal female pelvis revealing uterus and proximal 2/3 of the vagina resting posteriorly on the levator base plate. Note the change in axis between the distal vagina and proximal part due to orientation of levator muscle. **c** Coronal view of pelvic floor. Note levator base plate (arrows). Reprinted with permission from Klutke CG and Raz S, Evaluation and treatment of the incontinent female patient, *Urologic Clinics of North America* 1995; 22; 489–496.

level of the pelvic floor, the vagina is oriented horizontally by its upper attachments to lie on the base plate of the levator (Fig. 1.4). The upper vagina's horizontal orientation is important in dispersing downward acting forces to the supporting levator ani muscle. When this orientation is altered after vaginal childbirth or hysterectomy, prolapse of the vaginal apex can occur.

Urethra

The female urethra is 2–4 cm in its total length. A woman's urethra is short in comparison to a man's, and it is relatively uncommon for female outlet obstruction to occur. The urethra has several glands, concentrated distally on its dorsal surface.[10] These may become pathologically dilated as urethral diverticulae.

The urethra and vagina share a common origin. Like its sister structure the vagina, the urethra contains high concentrations of nuclear estrogen binding sites,[11] and is a target organ for estrogen. The urethra is surrounded by a plexus of thin walled veins. There is also a rich submucosal vascular layer (Fig. 1.5). Under the influence of estrogen, the lush epithelial lining of the urethra acts much like a seal, passively resisting the escape of urine.[12]

There are other passive properties relevant to continence, including the contractility of the urethra's smooth muscle and the inherent elasticity of the periurethral connective tissue. The urethra has its own fascial attachment, the urethropelvic

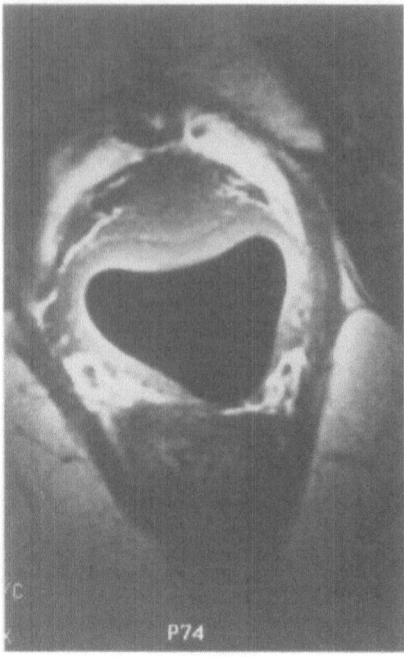

a

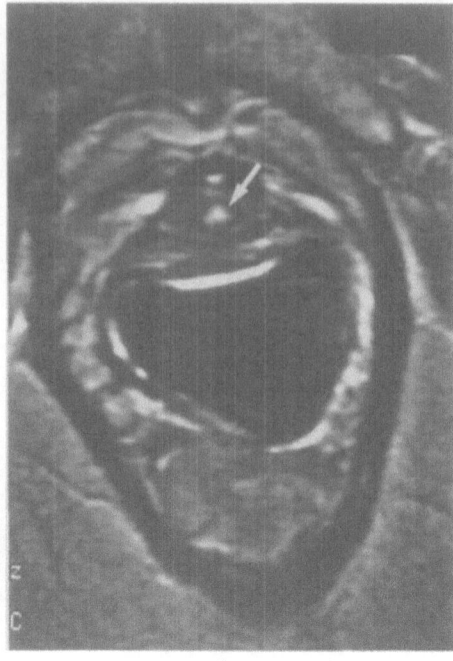

b

Figure 1.5 T1 (**a**) and T2 (**b**) weighted images illustrating the urethra. Note the bright signal intensity within the urethra on the T2 weighted image (**b**) representing the vascular plexus within the urethral submucosa. Reprinted with permission from Klutke CG and Raz S, Evaluation and treatment of the incontinent female patient, *Urologic Clinics of North America* 1995; 22; 489–496.

ligament, which attaches it laterally to the arcus tendineus.[13] It is supported throughout its length by the underlying vaginal wall, with which it forms an integral structure. A stable anterior vaginal wall, against which the urethra is compressed during increases in intraabdominal pressure, is another passive component of the urinary continence mechanism.

The greatest increase in urethral pressure is located in the midurethra. A pressure rise here actually exceeds the pressure increase produced by a cough or Valsalva maneuver.[14] This is explained by an active component of the urinary continence mechanism, contributed by the striated muscle of the urogenital diaphragm and levator ani. Both muscles maintain constant tone, and reflexively contract in response to increases in intraabdominal pressure.

Excessive mobility of the proximal urethra is a sign frequently seen with stress incontinence. Anti-incontinence surgery is effective at correcting bladder neck mobility, but it is not clear whether this is its mechanism in increasing outlet resistance. Other factors may explain why different operations for stress incontinence, with a similar anatomic effect, will result in both a different cure rate and a different incidence of de novo bladder instability.

Levator Ani

The major structural component of the pelvic floor is the levator ani muscle group. The levator is dome-shaped, not basin-shaped.[15] It is more massive than the urogenital diaphragm and its muscle fibers predominantly orient anterior to posterior. The muscle fibers, moreover, include both type I (slow twitch) and type II (fast twitch) fibers.[16] Fast twitch fibers are metabolically suited more for rapid, forceful contraction, and slow twitch fibers for providing sustained muscular tone.

The urogenital or levator hiatus is a large anterior midline opening that breaks the continuity of the levator ani. It is U-shaped, with its open end directed anteriorly. Through this opening pass the vagina, the rectum, and the urethra with its associated sleeve-like urogenital diaphragm.

Four muscles make up the levator ani: pubococcygeus, iliococcygeus, puborectalis and coccygeus muscles. The most anteromedial of the muscles are the pubococcygeus and puborectalis. These arise from the inner surface of the pelvic bones. The puborectalis forms a sling around the rectum and the pubococcygeus passes posteriorly to insert on the anococcygeal raphe and coccyx. The anococcygeal raphe is the base plate of the levator ani, providing support to the majority of the vagina. The iliococcygeus muscle arises from the arcus tendineus levator ani and inserts in the anococcygeal raphe and coccyx.

Urogenital Diaphragm

The urogenital diaphragm is a funnel-shaped sleeve of striated muscle that is closely associated with the

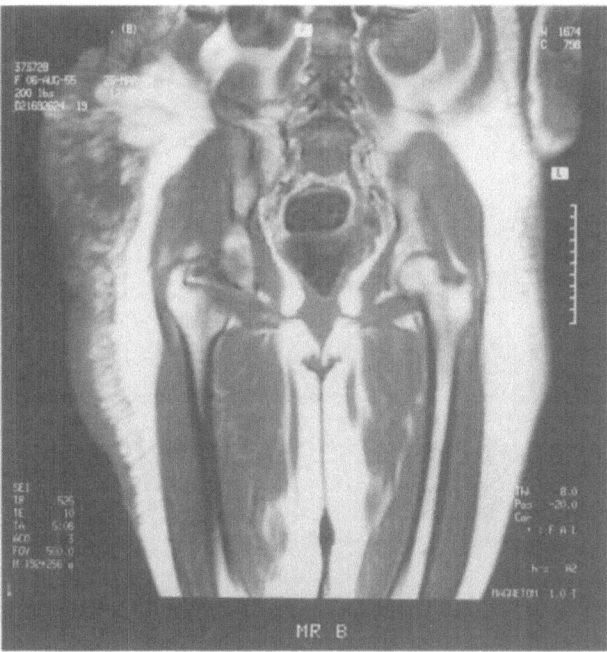

Figure 1.6 Coronal T1 weighted image. Urogenital diaphragm is seen extending laterally at the level of the vagina.

urethra as it passes through the levator's urogenital hiatus.[17] At its narrow, apical end, the urogenital diaphragm completely encircles the proximal urethra, forming an external sphincter. More distally, the sleeve like muscle inserts on the vagina and finally surrounds it near the introitus, where it joins the bulbospongiosus muscle (Fig. 1.6). Although it is closely associated with the urethra throughout its entire length, the urogenital diaphragm is anatomically and histologically distinct from both the urethra and the levator ani. The urogenital diaphragm is composed almost exclusively of slow twitch type I fibers,[16] adapted to maintain tone over long periods of time. Since it is a striated muscle, the urogenital diaphragm is under voluntary control, and has been functionally referred to as the external sphincter muscle.

The importance of the external sphincter is in its control on the voiding mechanism. The bladder itself is a visceral organ and cannot be made to contract and empty at will. It is subject to the control of its striated (voluntary) sphincter. The external sphincter is under voluntary control, and closure of the bladder neck both interrupts the stream during voiding and causes inhibition of the bladder contraction. This also explains why voiding in the normal woman is preceded by urethral relaxation, an effect that can be demonstrated urodynamically. The control exerted by the striated sphincter over voiding is the basis for using electrical sti-

mulation and biofeedback in women with voiding disorders.[18]

Endopelvic Fascia

The endopelvic fascia is a fibromuscular layer that invests the pelvic viscera. Although its local condensations are referred to as ligaments, the endopelvic fascia is composed of significant amounts of smooth muscle and elastin. In this sense, these ligaments differ from other ligaments in the body that contain dense concentrations of regularly arrayed collagen fibrils.

How much these ligaments normally contribute to the support of the pelvic organs is open to question. However, individual condensations are named and identified because they are the basis of many time-honored operations for prolapse. The upper vagina, cervix and uterus are anchored firmly over the base plate by the cardinal and uterosacral ligament complex (Fig. 1.2). The cardinal ligaments join the lower uterus, cervix, and upper vagina to the pelvic sidewall laterally. They contain fascial fibers that course along with the hypogastric vessels and their anterior branches. The uterosacral ligaments are a more medial segment of the endopelvic fascia, and serve to attach the cervix and upper vagina posteriorly toward the sacrum (Fig. 1.3).

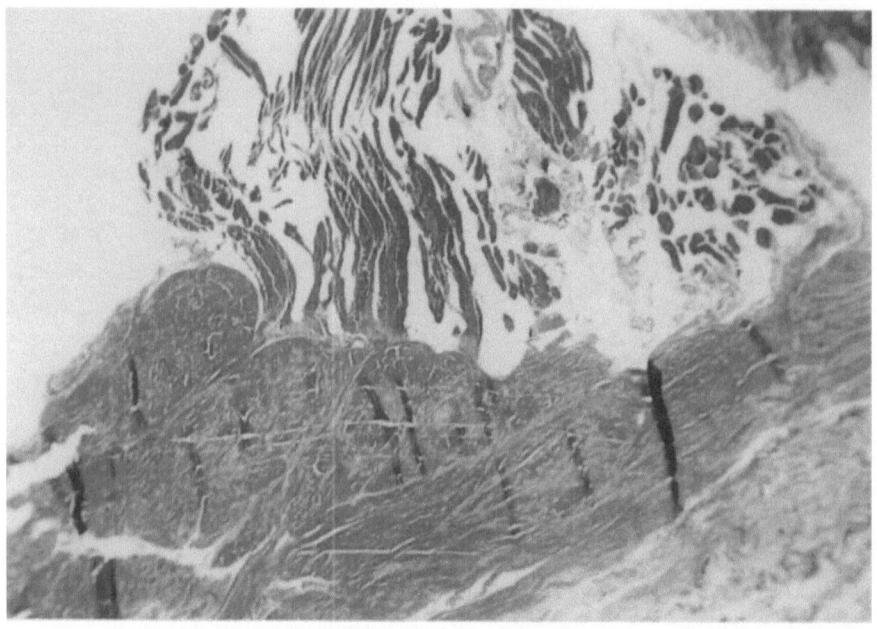

a

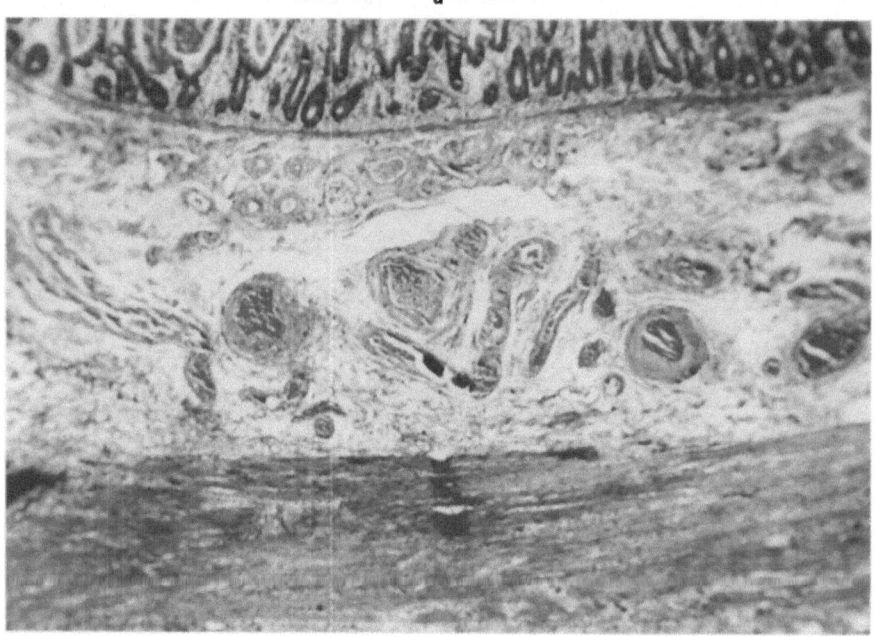

b

Figure 1.7 a Histologic section of ileopectineal (Cooper's) ligament stained with trichrome. **b** Control section of bowel illustrating staining pattern of trichrome; deep blue stained tissue is collagen. Compare with (**a**), which shows predominantly dense bundles of collagen.

The pubocervical and rectovaginal fasciae are downward continuations of the endopelvic fascia that originate laterally at the arcus tendineus. The proximal urethra and bladder neck are attached laterally by the urethropelvic ligaments. These ligaments originate in the arcus tendineus and pubis and insert on to the proximal urethra. It is important to point out that, although subdivisions of the fascia are named for surgical reference, all of the ligaments mentioned are continuous with one connective tissue structure, the endopelvic fascia.

Landmarks for the Reconstructive Pelvic Surgeon

Bony Landmarks

The goals in pelvic reconstruction differ from extirpative surgery. A precise knowledge of spatial relationships in the pelvis is especially important to restore normal anatomy. Many landmarks are easily

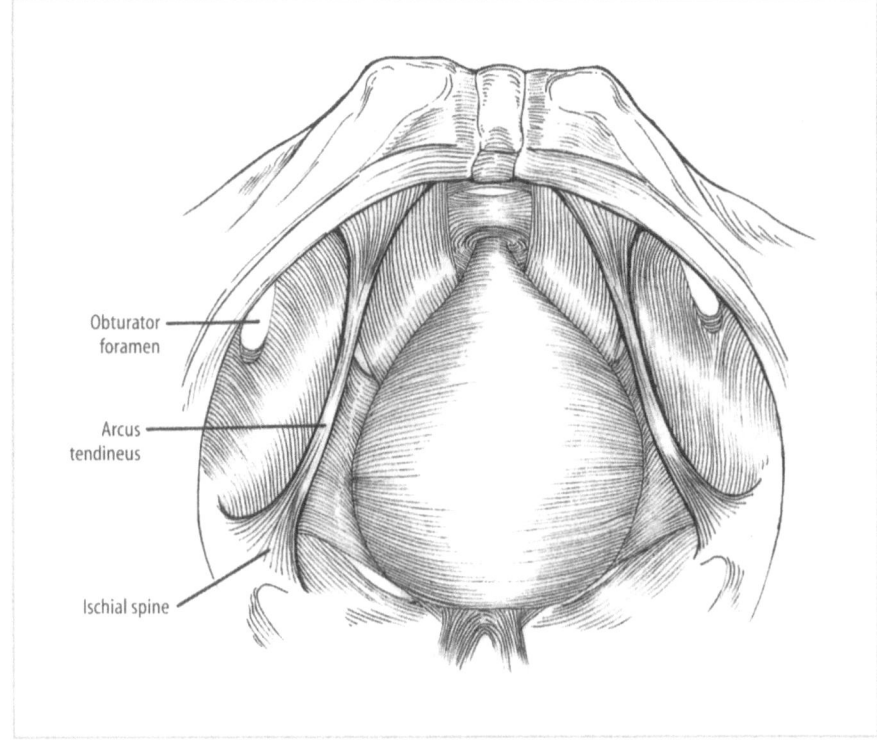

Obturator
foramen

Arcus
tendineus

Ischial spine

Figure 1.8 Abdominal view of the pelvic floor with levator muscle attached laterally to the arcus tendineus.

palpated before incision and will help map out important anatomic relationships in the pelvis.

The pelvis is an aggregate of four individual bones: the pubis, ilium, ischium and sacrum. The pubic symphysis is easily palpated in the midline, and lateral palpation will determine the location of the ileopectineal (Cooper's) ligament, palpated as the hard edge of the pelvic bone. With the patient lying prone, the crest of the ilium can be palpated from the anterior superior iliac spine to the posterior surface of the sacrum. A line drawn between a palpable lumbar spinous process and the coccyx will determine the midline on the sacrum. The sacrum has four pairs of foramina that allow transcutaneous access to the spinal nerve roots. With deep palpation, the greater sciatic notches can be defined. The intersection of a line connecting the uppermost crest of each notch with the midline will pinpoint the location of S3, which is one fingerbreadth lateral from the midline. This is the access point of the corresponding spinal nerve root and fibers of the pudendal nerve, which supply the somatic innervation to the levator ani muscle and the primary autonomic innervation to the detrusor muscle.

The inferior ramus of the pubic bone is easily palpated on digital vaginal examination. The levator ani originates on the medial surface of the pubis and the arcus tendineus, which spans from the medial surface of the pubis to the ischial spine. Having the

patient squeeze around the examiner's fingers during vaginal examination assesses muscular contraction of the levator ani. Posterolaterally, a prominence marks the location of the ischial spine. The sacrospinous ligament, embedded in the coccygeus muscle, bridges from the ischial spine to the lower part of the sacrum. The internal pudendal artery branches from the internal iliac artery, leaves the pelvis with the pudendal nerve through the greater sciatic notch, and wraps around the ischial spine and sacrospinous ligament to reenter the pelvis through the lesser sciatic notch. The nerve and artery course along the inferior surface of the levator muscle, fixed in place in Alcock's canal, a tough connective tissue sheath.

Retropubic Dissection

It is not necessary to incise the anterior peritoneum if retropubic urethropexy is performed alone. A low transverse incision is ideal for dissection of the retropubic space. Mobilizing the rectus muscle from the peritoneum and bladder allows lateral retraction of the muscle bellies for a good view caudally. The muscle is gently separated from the peritoneum with blunt dissection, and the dissection is continued laterally until the inferior epigastric vessels are identified. These vessels run longitudinally just deep to the abdominal musculature along the lateral edge of the rectus muscle. The pubic symphysis can be palpated at the inferior margin of the incision, and is a useful landmark in dissecting the retropubic space. The space should be developed cautiously, under direct visualization, with the bladder retracted downward away from the symphysis to avoid bleeding from the thin-walled veins surrounding the bladder neck and urethra (paraurethral venous plexus). Dissecting the retropubic space allows identification of the ileopectineal ligament and the obturator vessels. The ileopectineal ligament is the periosteum overlying the pectin pubis. This is a true ligament in that it contains dense concentrations of collagen, with little intervening fat, vasculature, or muscle (Fig. 1.7). The obturator foramen can be identified by gently palpating a small indentation on the inner surface of the pelvic sidewall. The lateral edge of the bladder can be defined by lifting the anterior vaginal wall laterally with a finger in the vagina and sweeping the bladder and urethra medially from above. This brings the tough, white, relatively avascular endopelvic fascia with its lateral insertion at the arcus tendineus ("white line") into view (Fig. 1.8).

Vaginal Surgical Relationships

With a Foley catheter placed to delineate the bladder neck, the anterior vaginal epithelium can be incised and mobilized from the bladder, exposing the pubocervical fascia. The dissection can be continued laterally until the inferior pubic rami can be palpated through the incision. Plication of the pubocervical fascia in the midline with "U stitches" or a purse-string suture line is often performed in the so-called anterior repair of a cystocele. In the percutaneous bladder neck suspensions, the blunt penetration of the urogenital diaphragm near the inferior pubic ramus allows entry into the retropubic space and access to the detached supportive urethropelvic ligaments. The posterior vaginal wall epithelium can be incised and reflected laterally, developing the rectovaginal space. The pararectal fascia is identified and can be drawn together in the midline to cover a bulging rectocele. The rectal pillars separate the rectovaginal space from the pararectal space. Penetration into the pararectal space allows visualization of the sacrospinous ligament so that the

ligament can be used as a fixation point for the vaginal apex.

References

1. Strohbehn K, Quint LE, Prince MR, Wojno KJ, DeLancey JOL (1996) Magnetic resonance imaging anatomy of the female urethra: a direct histologic comparison. Obstet Gynecol 88: 750–6.
2. Strohbehn K, Ellis JH, Strohbehn JA, DeLancey JOL (1996) Magnetic resonance imaging of the levator ani with anatomic correlation. Obstet Gynecol 87: 277–85.
3. Fielding JR, Versi E, Mulkern RV et al. (1996) MR imaging of the female pelvic floor in the supine and upright positions. J Magn Reson Imaging 6: 961–3.
4. Tan IL, Stoker J, Zwamborn AW et al. (1998) Female pelvic floor: endovaginal MR imaging of normal anatomy. Radiology 206: 777–83.
5. Hussain SM, Stoker J, Lameris JS (1995) Anal sphincter complex: endoanal MR imaging of normal anatomy. Radiology 197: 671–77.
6. DeSouza NM, Puni R, Gilderdale DJ, Byder GM (1995) Magnetic resonance imaging of the anal sphincter using an internal coil. Magn Reso Q 11: 45–56.
7. Siegelman ES, Banner MP, Ramchandani P, Schnall MD (1997) Multicoil MR imaging of symptomatic female urethral and periurethral disease. Radiographics 17: 349–65.
8. Lienemann A, Anthuber CJ, Baron A, Reiser M (1996) Dynamische MR-Kolpozystorektographie. Ein neues verfahren zur beurteilung von deszensus und prolaps genitalis. Aktuel Radiol 6: 182–6.
9. DeLancey JOL (1994) Structural support of the urethra as it relates to stress urinary continence: the hammock hypothesis. Amer J Obstet Gynecol 170: 1713–20.
10. Huffman J (1948) Detailed anatomy of the paraurethral ducts in the adult human female. Am J Obstet Gynecol 55: 86–101.
11. Iosif S, Batra S, Ek A, Astedt B (1981) Estrogen receptors in the human female lower urinary tract. Am J Obstet Gynecol 141: 817.
12. Zinner NR, Sterling AM, Ritter RC (1980) Role of inner urethral softness in urinary continence. Urology 16: 115–17.
13. Klutke C, Golomb J, Barbaric Z, Raz S (1990) The anatomy of stress incontinence: Magnetic Resonance Imaging of the female bladder neck and urethra. J Urol 143: 563–66.
14. Hilton P, Stanton SL (1983) Urethral pressure measurement by microtransducer: the results in symptom free women and in those with genuine stress incontinence. Br J Obstet Gynaecol 90: 919–933.
15. Hjartardottir S, Nilsson J, Petersen C, Lingman G (1997) The female pelvic floor: a dome, not a basin. Acta Obstet Gynecol Scand 76: 567–71.
16. Gosling JA, Dixon JS, Critchley HOD, Thompson SA (1981) A comparative study of the human external sphincter and periurethral levator ani muscles. Br J Urol 53: 35–41.
17. Oelrich TM (1983) The striated urogenital sphincter muscle in the female. Anat Rec 205: 223–232.
18. Schmidt RA (1986) Advances in genitourinary neurostimulation. Neurosurgery 18: 1041.

Part II

Causes and Investigations

2 Etiology and Pathophysiology

Urinary Incontinence and Prolapse

Daniel S. Blander and Philippe E. Zimmern

Pelvic prolapse and stress urinary incontinence, common conditions among aging women, account for 400 000 corrective surgical procedures every year.[1] Studies of comparative anatomy have found that these pelvic floor disorders are, with few exceptions, unique to bipeds. Among four-legged animals, the abdominal wall provides primary support for the abdominal and pelvic contents. In humans, tendon and fascia replace many muscle groups of the pelvic floor, countering effects of erect posture on the support of the pelvic viscera. Also, the bony structure of the human pelvis is such that the bones themselves impede prolapse.[2] This section discusses the specialized mechanisms of pelvic support in women and etiologies of their failure. Future studies to improve understanding of the pathophysiology of incontinence and prolapse are essential to help identify populations at risk and better repair their symptomatic defects.

Mechanisms of Continence and Support

Compartments

The specifics of pelvic anatomy are detailed elsewhere in this text, but it is important here to define the anterior, posterior, and middle compartments of the female pelvis, because prolapse of the contents of these compartments produces different clinical symptoms. The anterior compartment consists of the bladder, the urethra, and the retropubic space. The middle compartment contains the uterus and vagina, and the posterior compartment includes the pouch of Douglas and the rectum.

Bladder Neck

The most proximal continence mechanism is the internal urinary sphincter. The internal sphincter mechanism, located at the level of the bladder neck, is comprised of two structures. The deep detrusor muscle, which is continuous with Waldeyer's sheath, travels under the trigone and forms a ring which encircles the proximal urethra. This region of the bladder is rich in alpha-adrenergic receptors, which likely play a role in closing the trigonal ring with sympathetic stimulation.[3] There are also two U-shaped loops of detrusor muscle in the region of the bladder neck (Fig. 2.1). Proximally, under the trigone, is a loop which opens anteriorly, and anterior to the internal meatus is a loop which opens posteriorly. These opposing loops have been hypothesized to form a sphincteric mechanism, but this is very unlikely since, during micturition, these loops tend to contract rather than relax.

Urethra

The urethra's outermost layer is composed of the rhabdosphincter or external urinary sphincter, which has two different regions. The first region is the proximal sphincteric portion in which the striated muscle does not form a complete circle around the urethra, but rather forms an anterior "sling" which inserts posteriorly on the trigonal plate. In the distal half of the urethra, the rhabdosphincter takes the form of two bands of striated muscle, the compressor urethrae and the urethro-

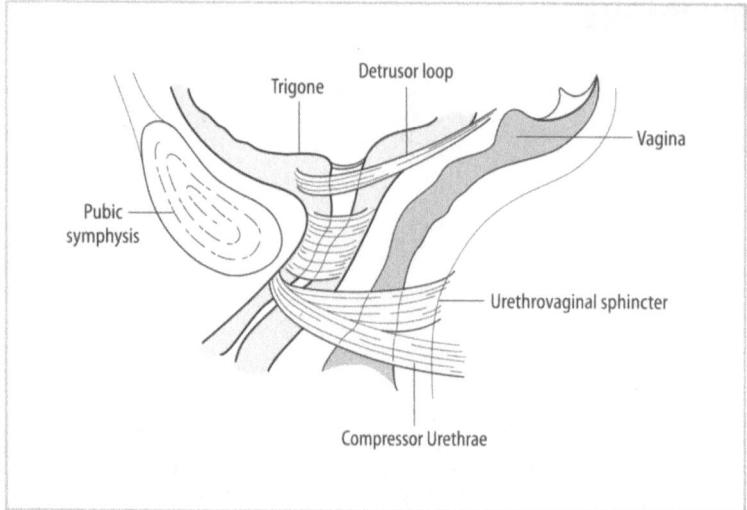

Figure 2.1 Muscular components of the internal and external urethral sphincter mechanisms.

vaginal sphincter. Although innervation of these two regions is complex, the different portions of the external sphincter are part of the same muscle group and function as a single unit.[4]

Underneath the striated muscle fibers lies a circular layer of smooth muscle, surrounding a longitudinal layer of smooth muscle (Fig. 2.2). This circular layer presumably provides urethral bulk, while the longitudinal layer shortens the urethra during voiding. A well-developed vascular submucosal layer lies between the smooth muscle and the epithelial lining of the urethra. This layer aids urethral bulking and helps provide a good mucosal seal during contraction of the sphincteric elements.

The urethra is lined with stratified squamous epithelium in its distal aspect and transitional epithelium more proximally. Depending upon the hormonal status of the patient,[4] the change between these two types of epithelium occurs somewhere in the mid-urethra.

The pubourethral ligaments and the urethropelvic ligaments, both of which are condensations of the

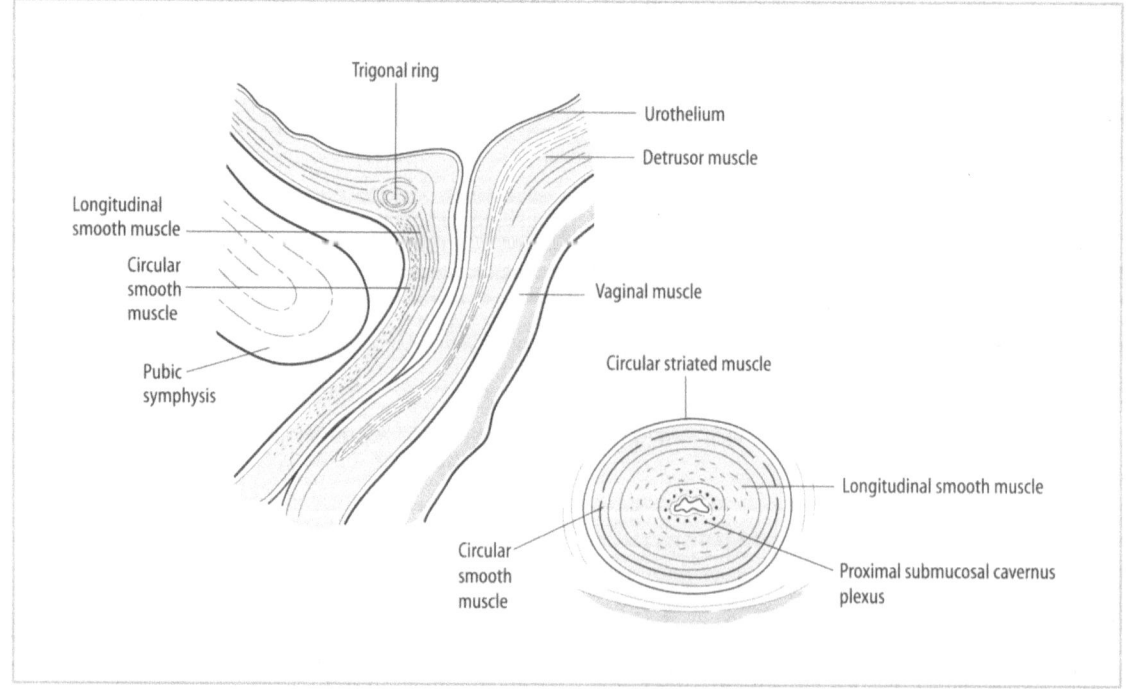

Figure 2.2 Longitudinal and cross-sectional views of the urethra demonstrating muscular, vascular, and epithelial layers.

endopelvic fascia, support the urethra. The pubourethral ligaments support the distal 2/3 of the urethra by attaching it to the pubic bone. These structures are important in both micturition and continence. By anchoring the urethra, these ligaments may allow a detrusor contraction to squeeze urine through the urethra, much as the cardinal and uterosacral complexes permit the contracting uterus to push the fetus through the cervix during parturition.[5]

Vagina

The bladder is not attached to any fixed structures in the pelvis. It derives support from its attachment to the vagina, which is connected to the pelvic sidewall.[5] The urethra and bladder are attached to the vagina at the distal urethra and at the vesicocervicouterine junction, respectively. Potential space between the vagina and bladder is filled with loose areolar tissue and smooth muscle (Fig. 2.3).

The vagina is supported by its connections to the pelvic sidewall via the levator ani complex. The arcus tendinaeus musculi levatori ani, which is covered by the arcus tendinaeus fascia pelvis, inserts on the lateral aspect of the vagina. These fibers primarily originate from the pubococcygeus muscle. The pubococcygeus, along with the rest of the levator ani complex, attaches to the pelvic sidewall directly or indirectly via the arcus tendineus. The levator complex therefore indirectly supports the bladder neck. Prolapse or increased mobility of the bladder neck with straining or increases in abdominal pressure, by definition, must be accompanied by a defect in anterior vaginal wall support.[5]

The lateral attachments of the pelvic floor muscles form a ring composed of several bony structures.

Anteriorly, the pubic bones and symphysis provide support. Anterolaterally, the arcus tendineus is suspended from the pubic bone to the ischial spine. Posterolaterally, the piriformis muscle and coccygeus complete the ring, which is closed posteriorly by the sacrum.

The upper vagina, uterus, and cervix are primarily supported by condensations of the endopelvic fascia, which connect them to the pelvic sidewall. The cardinal and uterosacral ligaments are actually only part of the broad ligamentous complex spanning to the mid-vagina. This condensation of endopelvic fascia forms a broad sheet upon which the bladder rests.

Perineum

The perineum provides additional support to the pelvic contents. The perineal membrane, also known as the urogenital diaphragm, is a musculofacial layer just inferior to the lowest portion of the levator complex. It primarily functions to connect the lateral vagina and the perineal body to the ischiopubic rami.[4] The perineal body is the fibrous condensation of tissue between the vagina and the anus. It receives contributions from the bulbocavernosus, and superficial and transverse perinei muscles, the perineal membrane, and fuses with the posterior vaginal wall.

Pathophysiology of Urinary Incontinence

Urinary Continence

Urinary continence is produced by the interaction among several structural and functional factors. In

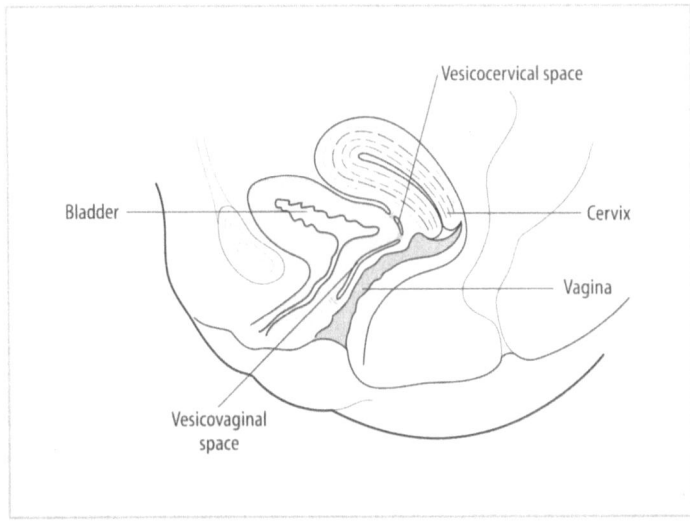

Figure 2.3 Sagittal section of the female pelvis. The bladder is connected to the uterus, cervix, and distal vagina, by fusions of adventitial tissues. The vesicovaginal and vesicocervical spaces are separated by these fusions.

order to maintain continence, urethral closing pressure must remain higher than intravesical pressure. Passive urethral pressure is sustained through the compression of healthy urethral mucosal and submucosal tissues, which are coapted by the sphincteric mechanism. Actual urethral length is not as important for the maintenance of continence as the pressure maintained in the mid-urethral continence zone. This zone functions as a secondary continence mechanism which is distal to the internal sphincter. Incontinence is not created by resection of the distal urethra or destruction of the bladder neck continence mechanism in the presence of a well-supported urethra with normal mucosal and submucosal tissues.[6]

Another contributor to continence is the maintenance of the bladder neck and urethra in a high retropubic position. The benefits of this position are twofold. First, stress induced increases in intra-abdominal pressure are transmitted to the proximal urethra, creating a functional valvular mechanism.[7] Additionally, an anatomic valvular mechanism is created by urethral kinking caused by rotation of the bladder base in the presence of a fixed bladder neck and urethra.[8]

Response of the pelvic floor musculature to stress plays an important role in preventing incontinence. Stress promotes reflex contractions of the levator and obturator groups which leads to increased tension on the urethropelvic ligaments and stabilization of the bladder neck. When this occurs, the urethra becomes functionally compressed against the "backboard" of the pelvic floor.

Urinary Incontinence

Anatomic Incontinence

Anatomic incontinence (AI) is stress incontinence resulting from defects in pelvic support which cause increased mobility of the urethra and bladder neck.

Table 2.1. Theories of stress urinary incontinence

Author	Pathophysiology
Einhorning[9]	Proximal urethral hypermobility prevents transmission of intraabdominal pressure increases to urethra causing negative pressure gradient
Snooks et al.[12]	Trauma due to vaginal childbirth causes damage to efferent branches of the pudendal nerve which innervate the sphincteric mechanism
Petros and Ulmsten[11]	Muscles and ligaments acting in multiple vectors create tension in the suburethral vaginal wall. Failure of any of these components leads to loss of tension and subsequent incontinence
DeLancey[30]	Hammock of suburethral support allows abdominal pressure increases to be transmitted to the urethra, leading to urethral closure

Many theories explain the etiology of AI (Table 2.1). Einhorning studied the relationship between intravesical and intraurethral pressures in patients with and without stress incontinence. He demonstrated that the maintenance of urethral pressures that exceeded intravesical pressures during stress was essential to maintain continence. The intrapelvic position of the proximal urethra and bladder neck during stress maneuvers allows transmission of pressure to the proximal urethra and obviates the need for a muscular internal sphincter. Failure of the anatomic support of the bladder neck and urethra leads to failure of this mechanism and subsequent stress incontinence.[9]

The observation that some patients with an extrapelvic proximal urethra may be continent (patients with large cystourethroceles) has led some researchers to believe that the Einhorning hypothesis could not completely explain AI. The "hammock theory" explains continence as the result of good suburethral support. A hammock of support is created by the endopelvic fascia and anterior vaginal wall by their connections with the arcus tendineus fasciae pelvis and levator ani muscles. During stress, the urethra is compressed between abdominal pressure from above and endopelvic fascia from below (Fig. 2.4). Failure of this suburethral support leads to inefficient compression of the urethra and subsequent stress incontinence. As long as this hammock exists, the position of the urethra and bladder neck relative to the pubic symphysis is unimportant.[10]

Similarly, the integral theory[11] states that tension in the vaginal wall is created by a number of structures including the pubourethral ligaments, the uterosacral ligaments, the arcus tendineus, the pubococcygeus muscle, the longitudinal muscles of the anus, and the levator plate (Fig. 2.5). Failure of any of these structures may produce laxity in the suburethral vaginal wall causing stress incontinence, or inability to close the bladder neck, leading to urgency or urge incontinence.

Stress incontinence has also been explained as the result of nerve damage. Snooks and co-workers[12] demonstrated abnormal motor latency in the urethral striated sphincter musculature after lumbar nerve root stimulation in women with stress incontinence. They hypothesize that abnormal motor latency resulted from traumatic pudendal nerve damage which occurred at the time of delivery. This neuropathy could contribute significantly to the immediate or later development of stress incontinence.

Intrinsic Sphincteric Deficiency

Because the urethra plays an important role in continence, stress incontinence can also be created by

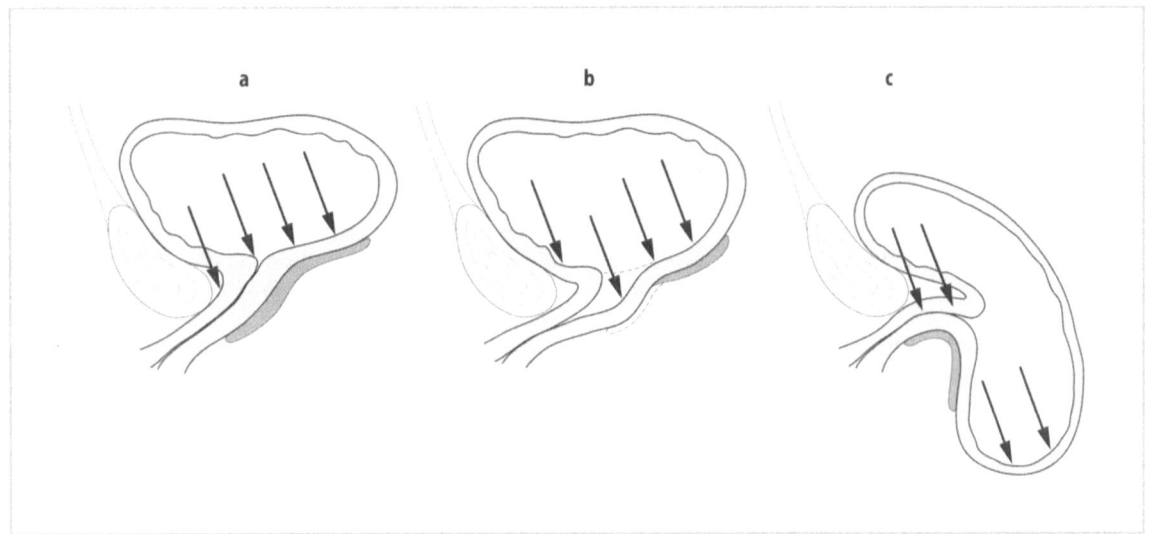

Figure 2.4 DeLancey's "hammock" hypothesis. **a** Abdominal pressure (arrows) forces the urethra against stable supportive layer (black) and compresses the urethra closed. **b** Unstable supportive layer (shaded) is ineffective in providing resistant backstop against which the urethra can be compressed. **c** In spite of low, extraabdominal position of the urethra and presence of a cystourethrocele, the supportive layer is firm and provides an adequate backstop against which the urethra may be compressed closed.

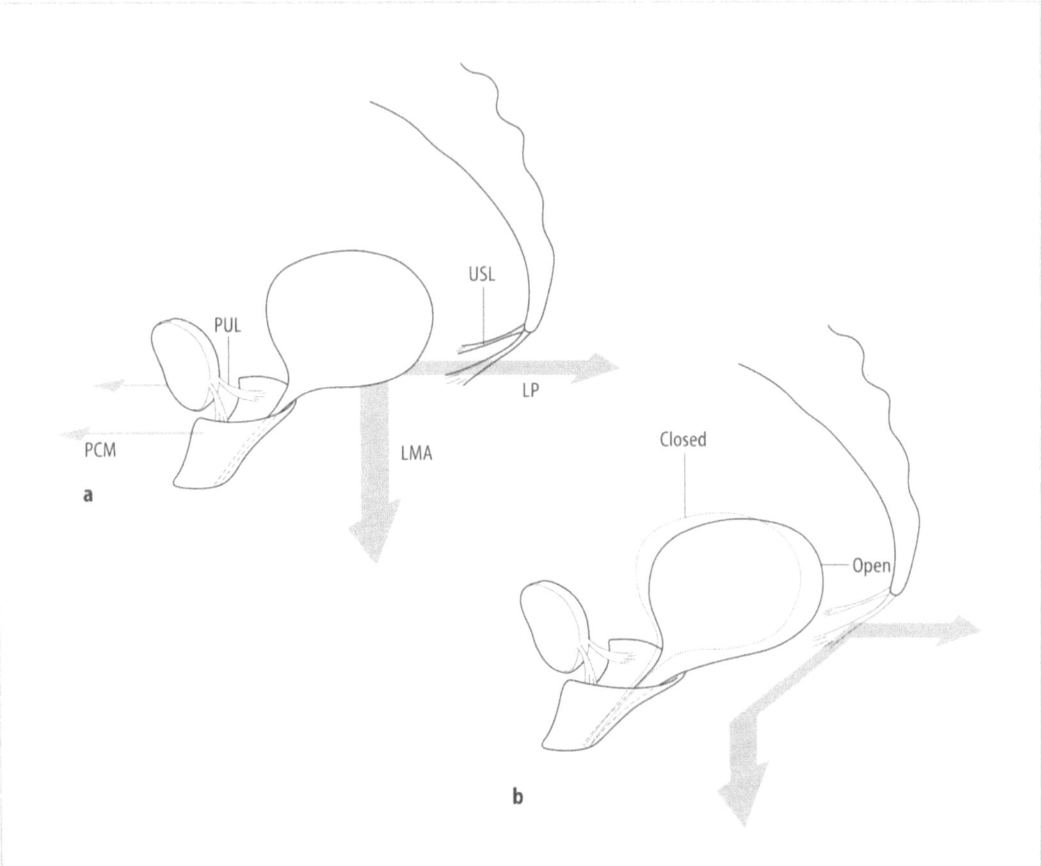

Figure 2.5 The integral theory. Tension in the vaginal wall supporting the bladder neck and urethra is created by the action of the pubococcygeus muscle (PCM), longitudinal muscles of the anus (LMA) and levator plate (LP). For these muscles to be effective, there must be no laxity in the pubourethral ligaments (PUL) or uterosacral ligaments (USL). These forces are all balanced in the resting closed position (**a**). When there is laxity in one or more of these elements, deficient closure forces are generated, allowing the bladder neck to remain open (**b**). Dotted lines represent normal resting closed position of the bladder.

conditions which effect the quality of urethral tissues, or urethral function. Insufficiency of the external sphincteric unit, as evidenced by low leak point pressure on urodynamic studies, is termed intrinsic sphincteric deficiency (ISD). ISD can result from intrinsic urethral damage (organic ISD) or anatomic factors (anterior vaginal wall laxity resulting in functional ISD).

Maturational changes in the urethral mucosa have been demonstrated in postmenopausal women. These changes appear to be caused by estrogenic stimulation. Additionally, decreases in vaginal blood flow, which can be reversed with estrogen administration, have been demonstrated in postmenopausal women. Conceivably, these hormonal changes could also effect the submucosal layer of the urethra and contribute to organic ISD in postmenopausal women.[13] Pelvic surgery or trauma can produce neuromuscular changes of the urethral continence zone, which also leads to poor mucosal coaptation.[3] These conditions will not be corrected with treatments aimed at good anatomic support of the bladder neck and urethra.[8] Radiation therapy can also adversely affect the quality of the urethral mucosa and sphincteric mechanism.[14]

Functional ISD is a result of urethral hypermobility. Using ultrasound and dynamic MRI studies, Mostwin and co-workers[15] demonstrated that rotational descent of the posterior wall of the urethra actually opens the proximal urethra and bladder neck leading to incontinence (Fig. 2.6). This supports the theory that an element of ISD exists in all patients with AI.

The number of theories regarding the etiology of stress incontinence suggests that it is a multifactorial condition. Urethral hypermobility, deficiency of suburethral support, poor urethral mucosal apposition, and neurologic factors all contribute. But, in any given patient, the relative contribution of each factor varies. Therefore adequately defining a patient's anatomic and functional defects prior to surgical repair is essential.

Pathophysiology of Pelvic Prolapse

The primary culprit in the genesis of pelvic prolapse is thought to be vaginal childbirth. Anatomic and functional analysis of the pubococcygeus muscle and pubocervical fascia have demonstrated greater evidence of denervation in women with than without prolapse, and it appears that these changes are the result of vaginal delivery. In addition, prolapse is significantly more common in women who

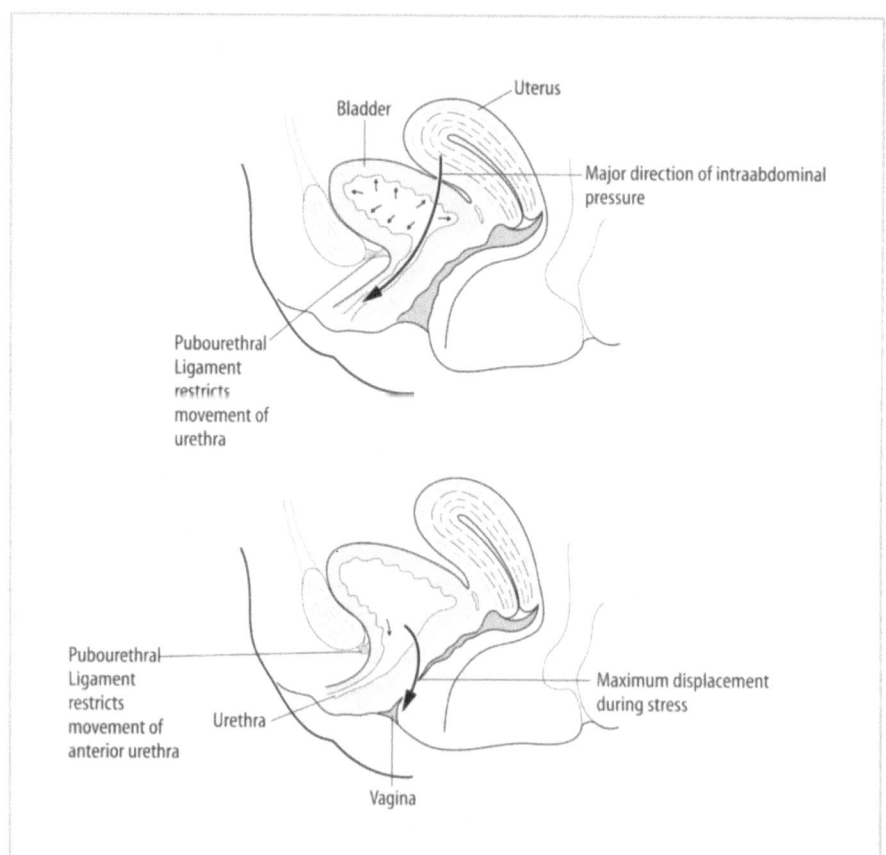

Figure 2.6 Resting (top) and straining (bottom) views demonstrating rotational descent of the bladder neck resulting in functional ISD. Motion of the anterior portion of the urethra is arrested by the pubourethral ligaments, while deficient suburethral support allows descent of the posterior wall of the urethra and poor coaptation of the urethra. Restoration of urethral support (vaginal wall sling, Burch) stabilizes the proximal urethra and bladder neck thus correcting the incontinence.

are multiparous than in women who have had only one vaginal delivery.[16]

The mechanism by which vaginal delivery leads to prolapse is not clearly elucidated, but there appear to be two major contributing factors: direct traumatic injury to the soft tissues, and neurologic injury, which leads to delayed pelvic floor dysfunction. Direct trauma to the pelvic soft tissues which occurs during normal vaginal delivery can lead to support defects. Recent evidence, however, demonstrates complete strength recovery of pelvic floor muscles within 2 months of vaginal delivery.[17] DeLancey[18] suggests that endopelvic fascial defects cause prolapse. Such defects may include lateral detachment of the fascia from the pelvic sidewall, as described by Richardson and co-workers.[19]

Because the structural and biochemical integrity of the endopelvic connective tissue plays an important role in the prevention of pelvic prolapse, factors which influence the quality of pelvic connective tissue will adversely affect pelvic support. Norton and co-workers[20] found that pelvic prolapse was significantly more common in individuals with joint hypermobility. They concluded that the same connective tissue defect might be responsible for both disorders. However, Chaliha and co-workers[21] found no association between joint hypermobility and stress incontinence, suggesting that prolapse and stress incontinence may not result from the same underlying pathophysiologic process.

Norton and co-workers[22] demonstrated an abnormally high ratio of weaker type III collagen to stronger type I collagen in women with genitourinary prolapse compared to normal women. Many investigators have correlated changes in collagen subtype and content with pelvic prolapse.[23] Recent reports linked increases in serum elastase and collagenase activity in women with stress urinary incontinence[24,25] The cervical ripening process during delivery is mediated by collagen breakdown. Because of the proximity of the cervix to the cardinal and uterosacral ligaments, this localized process may have long-term effects on the ligamentous support of the vaginal vault.[1]

Since acute traumatic damage to the endopelvic fascial support system and pelvic muscles does not produce prolapse immediately, and appears to be at least partly reversible, it is likely that secondary effects of this trauma play an important role in the genesis of prolapse. Electrophysiologic studies in primiparous and multiparous women demonstrate that cumulative nerve damage occurs as a result of childbirth.[26] The relationship between this nerve damage and the changes in pelvic muscular function has been questioned by Barnick and others.[27] Pudendal neuropathy leads to pelvic floor muscular

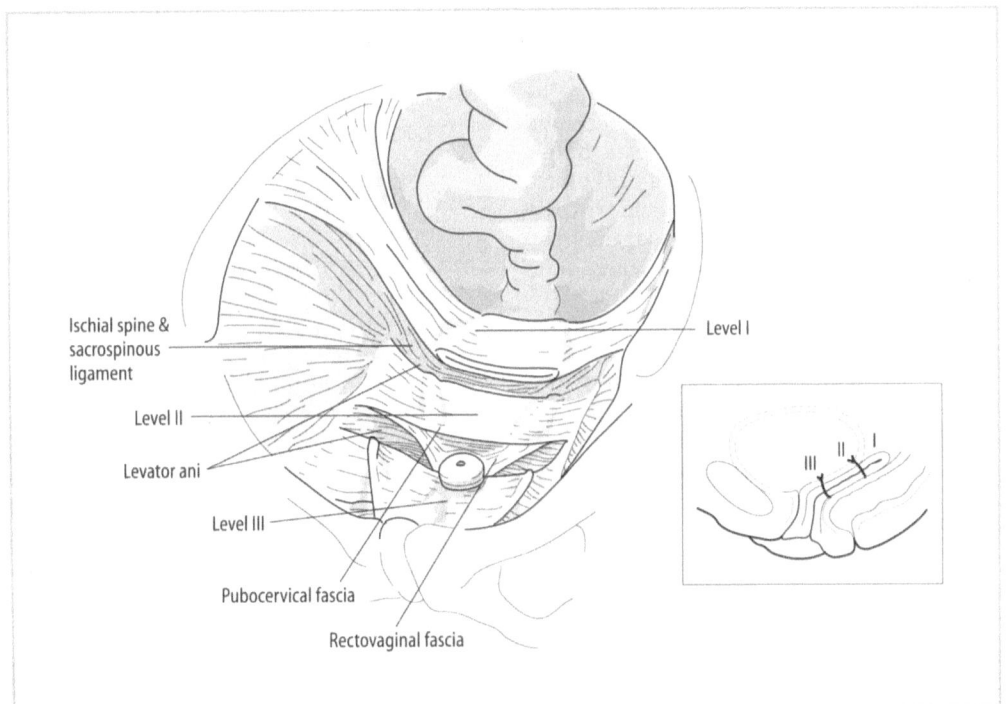

Figure 2.7 DeLancey's levels of vaginal support. Level I suspends the upper vagina and cervix from the pelvic sidewall via the cardinal and uterosacral ligaments. Level II support is created by the vaginal attachments to the arcus tendineus and fascia of the levator ani. Level III support is created by the urethropelvic ligaments. Adapted from DeLancey JOL (1993) Anatomy and biomechanics of genital prolapse. Clin Ob Gyn 36: 897–909.

dysfunction, and it is conceivable that absence of muscular support of the ligamentous structures of the pelvis ultimately leads to stretching of the supportive ligaments.[27]

Other neurologic conditions, such as spina bifida, have been associated with prolapse. Activities which cause chronic and repetitive increases in intraabdominal pressure also appear to be major contributors to prolapse. Obesity, chronic cough, and even repetitive skydiving have been associated with the development of pelvic prolapse or stress incontinence.[23]

Different defects in pelvic support lead to the different manifestations of pelvic prolapse. In an effort to clarify these defects, Delancey[29] describes three levels of vaginal support (Fig. 2.7). Failure in level I support leads to vaginal and uterine prolapse; failure of level II support leads to cystocele and rectocele. Isolated level III defects may cause intrinsic sphincteric deficiency. The importance of this classification lies in its therapeutic implications. Each level of support should be thoroughly evaluated during a patient's preoperative examination so the proper reconstructive procedure is performed.

Presentation

The presentation of urinary incontinence is usually straightforward, but pelvic prolapse can present in a multitude of ways. The main factor influencing the presentation of prolapse is the position of the originating defect. In general, once vaginal prolapse is severe enough that the vagina protrudes from the introitus, the patient will develop low backache and perineal pressure, and will complain of a bulge. These symptoms are caused by traction of the prolapsing organs on the uterosacral ligaments.[30] Once the vaginal walls or cervix are exposed, they can become ulcerated, causing pain and bleeding. Rare cases of evisceration have been reported.[31]

Few symptoms are specific to prolapse of the middle compartment. Patients with this defect may present with mass, pelvic pressure, or voiding dysfunction. The most common symptom of posterior compartment prolapse is difficulty in evacuating the rectum. If this symptom is severe enough, patients may have learned to reduce the rectocele manually in order to help with defecation. Systematic search for these symptoms during patient interview can help the clinician assess the complexity and extent of the underlying anatomic defects.

Large cystoceles can present as a vaginal mass, but smaller defects can present with voiding dysfunction as well. If there is enough distortion of the bladder base and urethra, partial or complete urinary retention may ensue. Patients may also present with stress incontinence secondary to hypermobility of the bladder neck and proximal urethra, although the incontinence is usually masked by the cystocele acting as a venting mechanism. Additionally, patients with cystocele may report urge incontinence or urgency which is felt to be the result of stretching of the bladder base, obstruction, or incomplete emptying. Rarely, patients present with significant hydronephrosis or renal failure.

Conclusions

The structure and function of the pelvic floor are quite complex. Urinary continence and pelvic support are the result of many interacting parts. Failure of any of these parts can lead to incontinence or prolapse. Failure of pelvic support mechanisms appears to cause AI and prolapse. This failure is produced by a combination of poor tissue quality, trauma, aging, and neuromuscular dysfunction. The relative contribution of each of these factors differs with each patient. Given our current understanding of these defects, we must make every effort to precisely diagnose the existing anatomic defects prior to attempting repair. We must also recognize the limitations of our current repair techniques which primarily involve the reapproximation of tissues themselves at risk for subsequent failure. Better understanding of the neuromuscular and structural defects that produce pelvic floor dysfunction should help us to create better methods of repair, and perhaps develop means to prevent these debilitating problems.

Fecal Incontinence

Amir A. Darakhshan and Norman S. Williams

Fecal Incontinence (FI) is a devastating symptom, with a psychological and social impact on the patient. It results from failure of the normal mechanisms that ensure the maintenance of continence. Often several factors are involved. Stool consistency, the rate of fecal entry into the rectum, rectal sensation, capacitance and compliance of the rectum, and the effective function of the anal sphincters and pelvic floor muscles all play a part in maintaining continence.[32,33]

The severity of the incontinence needs to be established, because this has implications on the type of treatment to be employed and ultimately will allow assessment of outcomes. Determining the severity, however, is not easy. Numerous scoring systems are in use but often they are too complicated to allow them to be widely used. Many insti-

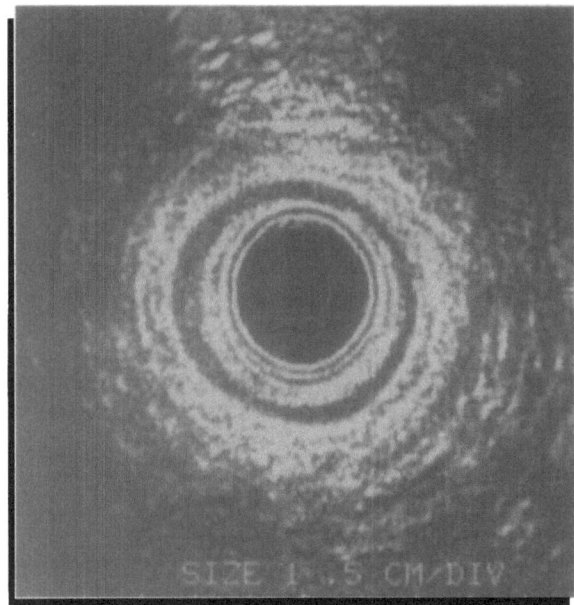

Figure 2.8 Normal anal sphincters at the level of the mid-anal canal.

Table 2.4. Fecal incontinence score as described by Jorge and Wexner[37]

Type of incontinence	Frequency				
	Never	Rarely	Sometimes	Usually	Always
Solid	0	1	2	3	4
Liquid	0	1	2	3	4
Gas	0	1	2	3	4
Wear pads	0	1	2	3	4
Lifestyle alteration	0	1	2	3	4

0 = perfect continence, 20 = complete incontinence.
Never = 0; rarely =<once per month; sometimes =<once per week,
•once per month; usually =<once per day, •once per week; always
=•once per day.

tutions have their own scoring systems, which often makes comparison of treatment modalities and outcomes difficult. Examples of different scoring systems in common use are shown in Tables 2.2–2.4.

Fecal incontinence may be broadly subdivided, depending on whether there is a sensory or a motor defect that is responsible for the incontinence. Often both defects co-exist to varying degrees. In fact, an underlying defect does not necessarily need to be present. The rate at which colonic contents are introduced to the rectum also plays a major part, as is demonstrated by the strain placed on even the healthiest of anal sphincters during bouts of diarrhea. Approximately one-third of patients with fecal incontinence are incontinent to solids, more than 50% to liquids and two-thirds to flatus.[37]

Table 2.2. Fecal incontinence score as described in Keikhley and Williams[34]

	Flatus	Fluid	Solid
Incontinence less than once a month	1	4	7
Incontinence once between a week and a month	2	5	8
Incontinence more than once a week	3	6	9

Table 2.3. Fecal incontinence score as described by Williams et al.[136]

Score	Severity
1	Continent to solids, liquids and flatus
2	Continent to solids and liquids but not to flatus
3	Continent to solids but occasionally incontinent to liquids
4	Occasionally incontinent to solids
5	Frequently incontinent to solids and liquids

Incidence

It is hard to know the incidence of fecal incontinence exactly, largely because of a combination of failure on the part of patients to report the problem to their medical practitioner and a failure on the part of medical practitioners to enquire about it. Both shortcomings no doubt stem from a reluctance to broach a socially taboo subject.

Although fecal incontinence is seen in all age groups and both sexes, it is more common in certain groups. In one population-based study 2.2% of the population were reported to suffer from fecal incontinence.[37] Of these 30% were older than 65 years and 63% were women. Other authorities have reported a community prevalence of FI ranging between 0.5% and 2% of the population.[38] One UK-based study suggested a community prevalence of 4.2 and 1.7 per 1000 people in men and women respectively, below the age of 65 years, increasing to 10.9 and 13.3 per 1000 people respectively above the age of 65 years.[33,39] Although all reports agree that fecal incontinence is much more common in the elderly, the incidence appears disproportionately high for those that are institutionalized: 7% of people over 65 year who are otherwise healthy suffer from fecal incontinence, compared to one-third of those within an institution.[37,40,41] Others have subdivided this group even further into those residing in psychogeriatric wards, with a prevalence of 56%, and those in geriatric wards, with a prevalence of 32%.[39] The incidence of fecal incontinence in nursing homes is reported to be 10–39% and that in hospitals 13–47%.[37] The cost of managing fecal incontinence is vast and difficult to calculate, but the cost of incontinence pads alone is thought to exceed $400 million per year in the USA.[38]

Pathophysiology

As mentioned above, fecal continence depends on a number of factors. The most obvious of these is a normally functioning anorectal complex. In addition to this, the compliance and capacity of the rectum, the state of rectal wall sensitivity and the volume, consistency and rate of stool entry into the rectum all play a part.

The anorectal complex consists of the internal and external anal sphincters and the puborectalis muscle plus the rectum with its associated group of receptors located within the rectal wall and the surrounding pelvic structures. These receptors not only allow rectal filling to be appreciated but also give information about the nature of the contents and the rate of entry of these contents into the rectum. They also make up part of the local and spinal reflexes which help to coordinate the normal sequence of events involving the smooth and skeletal muscles of the anal sphincters, pelvic floor muscles, and rectal wall which ultimately results in evacuation of the rectum. Higher cerebral input allows the urge to evacuate the rectum to be overridden until a more socially convenient time. Disruption of this complex mechanism may result in a failure to maintain continence. The causes of fecal incontinence are summarized in Table 2.5.

Etiology

Congenital Anomalies

Congenital abnormalities usually present soon after birth and as such are an important cause of incontinence in childhood. Their effects, however, often carry on into adolescence and adulthood and in

Table 2.5. Common causes of faecal incontinence

Aetiology	Examples
Congenital anomalies	Anorectal atresia
	Spina bifida
	Neuromuscular bowel disorders
Trauma to anal sphincters	Obstetric
	Surgical/iatrogenic
	Other trauma
Injury to nerves supplying sphincter complex	Idiopathic pelvic floor neuropathy
	Obstetric trauma
Descending perineum syndrome	
Neurological disorders	MS
	Spinal injuries
	Diabetes
	Cerebral dysfunction
Anal sphincter dysfunction	Fecal impaction
	Age related
Decreased rectal capacitance/ compliance	Inflammatory bowel disease
	Diarrhea
	Radiation proctitis
	Anterior resection syndrome
Rate of rectal filling	Diarrhea

some instances will require several operations spanning several years of the patient's life.

Anorectal atresia occurs in 1 out of every 4000 live births. It may be either a high, intermediate, or low type deformity. The low type deformity is often easily treatable and does not usually cause continence problems. The high type deformity is often more complex and may involve the urogenital system and pelvic floor muscles.[42] This group of patients often develops continence problems despite attempts at surgical correction.

Myelomeningocele is the severest form of neural tube defect affecting the vertebral column and occurs in about 1 in 1000 live births. The cause is unknown but is likely to be multifactorial. The lumbosacral region is involved in 75% of cases. If confined to the low sacral region, bowel and bladder incontinence together with perineal anaesthesia results but in the absence of other motor dysfunction.[42]

Traumatic Sphincter Disruption

Traumatic disruption of the anal sphincter complex is one of the commonest causes of fecal incontinence. Disruption of the external and internal anal sphincters is seen in 85% and 39% of cases respectively.[43] This group includes disruption following surgical treatment, obstetric trauma, and other non-iatrogenic trauma.

Obstetric Trauma

This group of patients makes up a large number of those with fecal incontinence that have not had previous surgery to their anal region. Seven per cent of women who have sustained a third-degree perineal tear (perineal lacerations that involve the anal sphincter and may also include the anorectal mucosa) following vaginal delivery suffer from fecal incontinence, with a further 12% being incontinent to flatus.[44] There is increasing evidence to suggest the damage resulting from obstetric trauma is twofold, comprising not only disruption to the anal sphincter complex but also damage to the nerves supplying the sphincters. The severity of perineal damage following vaginal delivery ranges from the less significant primary tears, to the more severe third-degree tears and the horrific fourth-degree cloacal-type injuries (Fig. 2.9). Up to 23.9% of perineal lacerations fall into the latter two groups.[45-47] It is difficult to be certain of the incidence of all sphincteric injury following vaginal delivery because the figures quoted depend on whether clinical or ultrasonographic methods of detection have been used. Clinically, 0.5–1% of women develop a

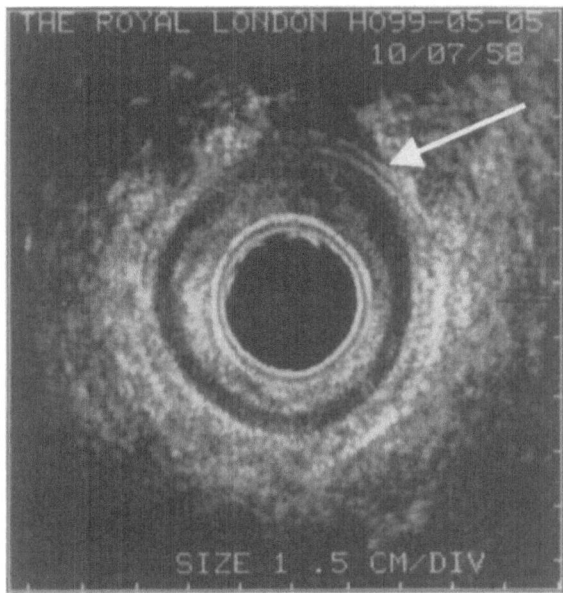

Figure 2.9 Injury to the internal and external anal sphincters caused by obstetric trauma.

third-degree tear; 85% of these will have residual sphincter damage despite a primary repair at the time of delivery (Fig. 2.10) and half of these will be symptomatic.[48] With the use of endoanal ultrasonography it has been shown that about 30% of women have some degree of sphincter damage after their first vaginal delivery and one-third of these will become incontinent (most commonly to flatus) and suffer from urgency of stool.[49,50] Of those who become incontinent after delivery, endoanal ultra-

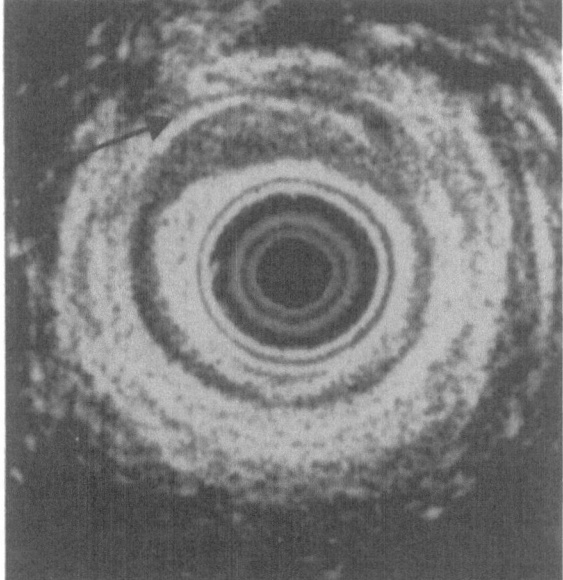

Figure 2.10 Scan showing the overlap of the external anal sphincter following an anal sphincter plication.

sonography demonstrates a defect in the external anal sphincter in 90% of cases, and disruption of the internal anal sphincter and perineal body in 65% and 44% of cases respectively.[51] The risk factors for sphincter damage as a result of vaginal delivery are: primiparous delivery, prolonged second stage of labor, high birth weight (greater than 4.0 kg), cephalopelvic disproportion, forceps assistance and occipitoposterior presentation.[36,38,52–54]

It is a matter of debate as to how effective an episiotomy is in preventing a third-degree tear, with reports that up to 74% of women with a tear have had an episiotomy.[55] In fact recent reports suggest the benefits afforded by an episiotomy are far outweighed by the risks.[56] This view, however, is not supported by other studies where it is suggested the factors responsible for a severe perineal laceration and the indications for episiotomy are the same.[57] Some workers advocate the use of mediolateral episiotomies in preference to midline episiotomies because of reports of a lower incidence of anal sphincter damage.[58,59]

As previously mentioned, the maintenance of continence is dependent on an intact anorectal sphincter complex. There is evidence of lowered resting anal tone and squeeze pressures immediately after vaginal deliveries.[44,60–63] Decreased anal sensation has also been noted[64] irrespective of forceps assistance, but this appears to be a transient abnormality, unlike the abnormal perineal descent that often accompanies these changes.[44,60] These changes are highly suggestive of pudendal nerve trauma, and the finding of prolonged pudendal nerve terminal motor latencies supports this. Again this is a transient finding in all except multiparous women who have had forceps-assisted vaginal delivery.[65]

Pudendal neuropathy and anal sphincter damage will coexist in many cases of obstetric trauma induced fecal incontinence.[45,66–68]

Surgical or Iatrogenic Sphincter Trauma

Surgical trauma to the anal sphincters is a major cause of fecal incontinence, second only to obstetric injuries.[38] The operations commonly associated with a high risk of resultant fecal incontinence include sphincterotomy, haemorrhoidectomy, anal dilation, and excision of anal fissures.

The treatment of chronic anal fissures with *lateral sphincterotomy* of the internal anal sphincter is aimed at lowering an abnormally high anal pressure to one that is more normal. Unfortunately this is associated with incontinence to solids in up to 5% of patients and incontinence to flatus in up to 35%.[69] The amount of residual sphincter and the quality of its contraction are important factors maintaining continence[70] (Fig. 2.11). The use of open lateral

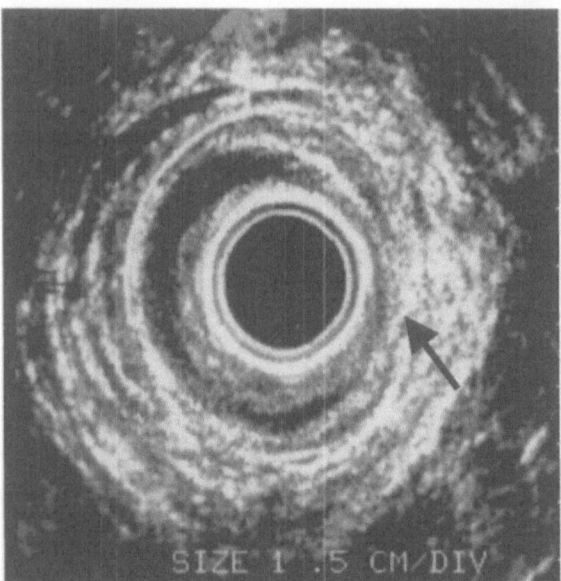

Figure 2.11 Typical appearance following a lateral sphincterotomy.

sphincterotomy as opposed to subcutaneous sphincterotomy is associated with a lower rate of fecal incontinence.[71] The functional state of the sphincters preoperatively is important in all sphincter surgery no more so than in sphincterotomy, since the aim of the operation is to partially divide the internal anal sphincter. Therefore such procedures should be used judiciously in multiparous women, those with obvious perineal descent, or prolonged pudendal nerve terminal motor latencies.

The worry with *haemorrhoidectomy* is excision of a segment of the underlying internal anal sphincter together with the specimen, or if too much stretch is applied to the sphincters during the operation (Fig. 2.12). A 10% incidence of incontinence is reported after such operations.[72] Some have suggested interference with anal sensation as a cause for the incontinence after haemorrhoidectomy[73,74] but there does not appear to be a difference in incidence with the use of submucosal haemorrhoidectomy that restores the integrity of the anal mucosa.[75]

Surgery for *fistula in ano* (Fig. 2.13) is the operation most likely to cause fecal incontinence,[33] and often this is an unavoidable complication, as with complex fistulae.[76-79] Even with surgery for low fistulae, fecal soiling may occur in up to 34% of cases.[77,80,81]

Therapeutic anal dilatation is another major cause of fecal incontinence. 12.5% of patients undergoing manual dilation will suffer from a minor degree of fecal incontinence and in 65% of cases a defect is seen on endoanal ultrasonography even in the absence of symptoms.[82] A persistent fall in anal pressures is seen with forceful anal dilatation, and if repeated or if performed in the presence of underlying anal sphincter dysfunction will result in fecal incontinence.[83-86] Internal sphincter damage has been demonstrated endosonographically in 92% of cases, and in 25% of cases there was injury to the external anal sphincter.[87] For these reasons, anal dilation should no longer be performed.

The treatment of *chronic anal fissures* by excision of the fissure is subject to the same hazards as with haemorrhoidectomy, namely excision of the underlying anal sphincter and inadvertent anal dilatation, and is associated with fecal incontinence in up to 25% of cases.[88]

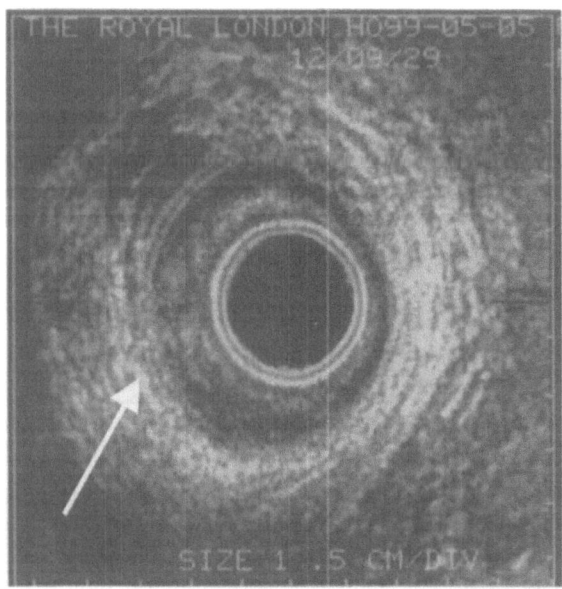

Figure 2.12 Complication of haemorrhoidectomy – the internal anal sphincter is deficient at the 9 o'clock position where it was excised with the specimen.

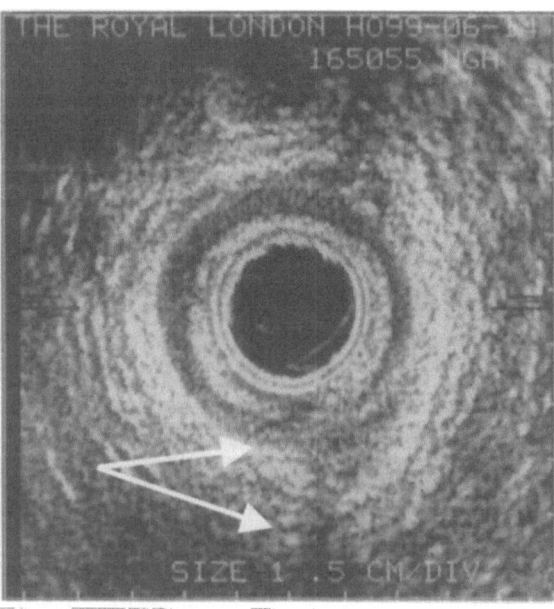

Figure 2.13 Scan showing a fistula in ano.

Disruption of the anal sphincters is also seen in patients with pelvic trauma such as occurs following a road traffic accident, or those with direct sphincter injury resulting from impalement or from forced anal penetration.[89]

Idiopathic Fecal Incontinence

The vast majority of patients in this group are multiparous women and in many cases there is a history of a prolonged or traumatic delivery. Often there is a history of defecatory problems prior to the onset of incontinence. In about 80% of patients there is evidence of denervation of the puborectalis and external anal sphincter muscles both electromyographically and histopathologically.[90-94] Often the levator ani, periurethral muscle and internal anal sphincter are also affected. The cause of this denervation is not known for certain, but the descending perineum syndrome is a likely candidate.[91,95,96] It is thought prolonged straining at stool subjects the pudendal nerves to traction forces, which ultimately results in neuropathy. The resulting weakness of the pelvic floor muscles will demand further straining in order to defecate which will lead to greater traction being applied to the nerves; eventually, damage to the pudendal nerves will occur. The end result of all this is denervation of the puborectalis and external anal sphincter leading to fecal incontinence.[92,97]

Neurological Disorders

Fecal incontinence is commonly seen in association with many neurological disorders.

Multiple sclerosis (MS) is a potentially physically disabling disease affecting the central nervous system (CNS) and often presents in younger patients (typically between ages of 20 and 40 years). Plaques of demyelination occur within the CNS, classically described as being spread over time and space. If the spinal cord is affected, upper motor neuron, posterior column, spinothalamic and autonomic symptoms and signs below the level of the lesion may result. Although sensorimotor function of the limbs is most commonly affected, bowel, bladder, and sexual function can also be disrupted.[98,99] A reduced resting anal pressure and maximal squeeze pressure is seen in MS patients with fecal incontinence.[100] Approximately 50% of patients with MS are affected by FI and in up to 25% of cases it occurs at least once per week.[101]

Spinal injuries result in FI in over 60% of patients.[102] Severe spinal injuries will in the initial stages result in spinal shock, which is associated with constipation and urinary retention. After this acute stage, symptoms and signs according to the level and severity of the injury will be manifest.[103] Cauda equina compression, surgery to the sacral outflow and tumours involving the sacrum and sacral outflow can result in lower motor neurone lesions, which cause paralysis of the anal sphincters and lead to fecal incontinence.[104] Complete transection of the spinal cord above the level of the sacral outflow is associated with "automatic defecation". The only indication the patient may have of rectal filling is autonomic effects (part of the visceral distension syndrome that includes sweating, piloerection and cardiovascular effects secondary to vasoconstriction in the zone of paralysis). The higher the lesion is, the less powerful the force of evacuation will be, but this is due to involvement of a greater proportion of the respiratory and abdominal muscles.[103] Patients with an upper motor neuron lesion have a well-preserved anal tone and are usually troubled with constipation rather than fecal incontinence.[105] In general, those who have high spinal lesions will have a better sphincter function than those with low lesions.[106]

Diabetic neuropathy affecting the gastrointestinal system is usually part of a wider autonomic neuropathy involving other systems.[107] Fecal incontinence is seen in such patients, possibly as a result of rectal hyposensation together with internal and external anal sphincter dysfunction.[108,109] When the gastrointestinal system is involved, the neuropathy usually affects the entire tract, resulting in diarrhea and urgency that often leads to incontinence in the presence of poorly functioning anal sphincters.[107]

Fecal Impaction

This is a condition that is commonly seen in elderly and infirm people who are more likely to be confined to bed or inactive. They may be suffering from confusional states or depressive illnesses requiring antipsychotic medications, or may be taking other medication predisposing to diminished colonic motility and constipation.[110] Fecal impaction is reported to be present in up to 42% of admissions to a geriatric ward, and is thought to be responsible for the admission in 18% of acute cases and in over 26% of chronic admissions.[111] Fecal impaction may be seen in children, and in most cases will resolve spontaneously. In the cases where it persists, an underlying neuromuscular disorder of the hindgut may be responsible.[38] Incontinence may occur as a result of fecal impaction due to a reflex inhibition of the internal anal sphincter (IAS) by the fecal bolus in the rectum, thus allowing liquid stool from higher up in the colon to leak from the anus.[36] An alternative mechanism for the incontinence is stretching of the anal canal by the fecal bolus.[36]

Fecal incontinence may afflict elderly people in the absence of fecal impaction. A reduction in the anal pressures and rectal compliance has been demonstrated in such cases.[112,113] This may be a result of muscle atrophy or increasing sclerosis of the IAS as demonstrated by ultrasonography and histopathology.[114,115] Furthermore, there is evidence of re-innervation of the EAS and pelvic floor muscles in older patients[93] associated with decreased squeeze pressures, increased perineal descent, and prolonged pudendal nerve latencies.[116] Such changes can be found in elderly people even in the absence of incontinence that only becomes apparent in association with another factor such as diarrhoea.[117]

Descending Perineum Syndrome

When measured with a perineometer, descending perineum syndrome (DPS) is defined as the descent of the anocutaneous junction by more than 3 cm relative to the ischial tuberosity during a maximum straining effort. If measured using radiographic means, it is defined as the downward movement of the anorectal junction from a starting position below a line drawn between the lower border of the symphysis pubis and the coccyx (pubococcygeal line). This is in comparison to the normal starting position above the pubococcygeal line.[36] Radiological means is probably the more accurate of the two, because the extent of perineal descent is underestimated by the perineometer.[118] The underlying cause for the descent of the perineum is likely to be chronic straining at stool resulting in damage to the nerves supplying the pelvic floor muscles.[119–121] There is evidence that the pudendal nerve terminal motor latencies are prolonged in such patients and this appears to increase in direct proportion to the degree of descent.[96,122] More recent studies have cast a doubt over an association between pudendal neuropathy and perineal descent.[123] An alternative theory is direct injury to the sacral nerves, pelvic floor muscles, and puborectalis during vaginal delivery.[44] That perineal descent is more common in women is in all probability due not only to obstetric-induced neuropathy but also due to the greater incidence of constipation amongst women together with the resultant straining.[124,125]

Rectal Prolapse

Rectal prolapse is a condition more commonly seen in women, and in over 60% of cases it is associated with fecal incontinence.[33,126–128] The cause for this is likely to be multifactorial. Once again, denervation of the pelvic floor muscles resulting from persistent

straining is a probable factor,[119,129] and support is given to this by the absence of neuropathy in patients with rectal prolapse who are continent to stool.[90] Other possible causes include stretching of the anal sphincters by the prolapse,[130] relaxation of the internal anal sphincter as a result of instigation of the recto-anal inhibitory reflex,[131,132] and abnormal rectal sensation.[133] It is believed that in over half of patients, surgery to correct the prolapse also corrects the incontinence.[32,134,135] In cases in whom incontinence persists, there is likely to be irreversible nerve injury resulting in persistent IAS weakness[38] and persistent rectal sensory dysfunction.[36]

Acknowledgment

The scans in Figs 2.8–2.13 were used with the kind permission of the GI Physiology Unit, The Royal London Hospital, Whitechapel.

References

1. Norton PA (1993) Pelvic floor disorders: the role of fascia and ligaments. Clin Obstet Gynecol 36: 926–38.
2. Zacharin RF (1985) Pelvic Floor Anatomy and the Surgery of Pulsion Enterocele. Springer, New York, N.Y.
3. Wahle GR, Young GPH, Raz S (1996) Anatomy and pathophysiology of pelvic support. In: Raz S (ed) Female Urology, 2nd edition. W.B. Saunders, Philadelphia.
4. Wall LL, Norton PA, DeLancey JOL (1993) Pelvic anatomy and the physiology of the lower urinary tract. In: Wall LL, Norton PA, DeLancey JOL (eds) Practical Urogynecology. Williams & Wilkins, Baltimore.
5. Mostwin JL (1991) Current concepts of female pelvic anatomy and physiology. Urol Clin North Am 18: 175–195.
6. Penson DF, Raz S (1996) Why anti-incontinence surgery succeeds or fails. In: Raz S (ed) Female Urology, 2nd edition. W. B.Saunders, Philadelphia, Pa., pp. 435–42.
7. Raz S, Little NA, Juma S (1992) Female urology In Walsh PC. In: Retik AB, Stamey TA, Vaughan ED (eds) Campbell's Urology, 6th edn. WB Saunders Philadelphia.
8. Staskin DR, Zimmern PE, Hadley HR, Raz S (1985) The pathophysiology of stress incontinence. Urol Clin North Am 12: 271–8.
9. Einhorning G (1961) Simultaneous recording of intravesical and intra-urethral pressure. Acta Chir Scand 276: 1–67.
10. DeLancey JOL (1994) Relationship of prolapse syndromes to symptoms. In: Kursh ED, McGuire EJ (eds) Female Urology. J.B. Lippincott, Philadelphia.
11. Petros PEP, Ulmsten U (1993) An integral theory and its method for the diagnosis and management of female urinary incontinence. Scand J Urol Nephrol Suppl 153: 1–93.
12. Snooks SJ, Badenoch DF, Tiptaft RC, Swash M (1985) Perineal nerve damage in genuine stress urinary incontinence. Br J Urol 57: 422–6.
13. Klutke JJ, Bergman A (1995) Hormonal influence on the urinary tract. Urol Clin North Am 22: 629–40.
14. Haab F, Zimmern PE, Leach GE (1996) Female stress urinary incontinence due to intrinsic sphincteric deficiency: recognition and management. J Urol 156: 3–17.

15. Mostwin JL, Yang A, Sanders R, Genadry R (1995) Radiography, sonography, and magnetic resonance imaging for stress incontinence. Urol Clin North Am 22: 539–549.

16. Sultan AH, Monga AK, Stanton SL (1996) The pelvic floor sequelae of childbirth. Br J Hosp Med 55: 575–9.

17. Peschers UM, Schaer GN, DeLancey JOL, Schuessler B (1997) Levator ani function before and after childbirth. Br J Obstet Gynecol 104: 1004–8.

18. DeLancey JOL (1992) Anatomic aspects of vaginal eversion after hysterectomy. Am J Obstet Gynecol 166: 1717–28.

19. Richardson AC, Lyon JB, Williams NL (1976) A new look at pelvic relaxation. Am J Obstet Gynecol 126: 568–73.

20. Norton PA, Baker JE, Sharp HC, Warenski JC (1995) Genitourinary prolapse and joint hypermobility in women. Obstet Gynecol 85: 225–8.

21. Chaliha C, Kalia V, Sultan A, Monga A, Stanton SL (1999) Joint mobility – is it a marker for stress incontinence? (abstract). Neurourol Urodynamics 18: 331.

22. Norton P, Boyd C, Deak S (1992) Collagen synthesis in women with genital prolapse or stress urinary incontinence. Neurol Urodyn 11: 300–1.

23 Gill EJ, Hurt WG (1998) Pathophysiology of pelvic organ prolapse. Obstet Gynecol Clin North Am 25: 757–69.

24. Mathrubutham M, Aybek Z, Fogarty J et al. (1999) Plasma elastase regulation in stress urinary incontinence (abstract). Neurourology Urodynamics 18: 281–2.

25. Kushner L, Chen Y, Desautel M et al. (1999) Collagenase activity is elevated in conditioned media from fibroblasts of women with pelvic floor weakening (abstract). Neurourol Urodynamics 18: 282–3.

26. Snooks SJ, Swash M, Setcdhell M, Henry MM (1984) Injury to innervation of pelvic floor sphincter musculature in childbirth. Lancet 2: 546–50.

27. Barnick CGW, Cardozo LD (1993) Denervation and re-innervation of the urethral sphincter in the aetiology of genuine stress incontinence: and electromyographic study. Br J Obstet Gynaecol 100: 750–3.

28. Wall LL, DeLancey JOL (1991) The politics of prolapse: a revisionist approach to disorders of the pelvic floor in women. Perspect Biol Med 34: 486–96.

29. DeLancey JOL (1993) Anatomy and biomechanics of genital prolapse. Clin Ob Gyn 36: 897–909.

30. DeLancey JOL (1994) Structural support of the urethra as it relates to stress urinary incontinence: the hammock hypothesis. Am J Obstet Gynecol 170: 1713–23.

31. Ginsberg DA, Rovner ES, Raz S (1998) Vaginal evisceration. Urology 51: 128–9.

32. Jorge JM, Wexner SD (1993) Etiology and management of fecal incontinence. Dis Colon Rectum 36(1): 77–97.

33. Madoff RD, Williams JG, Caushaj PF (1992) Fecal incontinence. N Engl J Med 326(15): 1002–7.

34. Keikhley MRB, Williams NS (1993) Prospective study of conservative and operative treatment for faecal incontinence. In: Surgery of the Anus, Rectum and Colon, WB Saunders, 517.

35. Baeten CG, Geerdes BP, Adang EM et al. (1995) Anal dynamic graciloplasty in the treatment of intractable fecal incontinence. N Engl J Med 332(24): 1600–5.

36. Keighley MRB, Williams NS (1993) Surgery of the Anus, Rectum and Colon. WB Saunders, London.

37. Nelson R, Norton N, Cautley E, Furner S (1995) Community-based prevalence of anal incontinence. JAMA 274(7): 559–61.

38. Kamm MA (1998) Faecal incontinence [see comments]. BMJ 316(7130): 528–32.

39. Thomas TM, Egan M, Walgrove A, Meade TW (1984) The prevalence of faecal and double incontinence. Community Med 6(3): 216–20.

40. Talley NJ, O'Keefe EA, Zinsmeister AR (1992) Melton LJd. Prevalence of gastrointestinal symptoms in the elderly: a population-based study. Gastroenterology 102(3): 895–901.

41. Johanson JF, Lafferty J (1996) Epidemiology of fecal incontinence: the silent affliction. Am J Gastroenterol 91(1): 33–6.

42. Nelson W (1996) Textbook of Pediatrics, 15th ed. WB Saunders , Phildephia, PA.

43. Law PJ, Kamm MA, Bartram CI (1991) Anal endosonography in the investigation of faecal incontinence. Br J Surg 78(3): 312–4.

44. Snooks SJ, Setchell M, Swash M, Henry MM (1984) Injury to innervation of pelvic floor sphincter musculature in childbirth. Lancet 2(8402): 546–50.

45. Thacker SB, Banta HD (1983) Benefits and risks of episiotomy: an interpretative review of the English language literature, 1860–1980. Obstet Gynecol Surv 38(6): 322–38.

46. Haadem K, Dahlstrom JA, Ling L, Ohrlander S (1987) Anal sphincter function after delivery rupture. Obstet Gynecol 70(1): 53–6.

47. Venkatesh KS, Ramanujam PS, Larson DM, Haywood MA (1989) Anorectal complications of vaginal delivery. Dis Colon Rectum 32(12): 1039–41.

48. Sultan AH, Kamm MA, Hudson CN, Bartram CI (1994) Third degree obstetric anal sphincter tears: risk factors and outcome of primary repair. Bmj 308(6933): 887–91.

49. Sultan AH, Kamm MA, Hudson CN, Thomas JM, Bartram CI (1993) Anal-sphincter disruption during vaginal delivery [see comments]. N Engl J Med 329(26): 1905–11.

50. Kamm MA (1994) Obstetric damage and faecal incontinence [see comments]. Lancet 344(8924): 730–3.

51. Burnett SJ, Spence-Jones C, Speakman CT et al. (1991) Unsuspected sphincter damage following childbirth revealed by anal endosonography. Br J Radiol 64(759): 225–7.

52. Cook TA, Mortensen NJ (1998) Management of faecal incontinence following obstetric injury. Br J Surg 85(3): 293–9.

53. Wood J, Amos L, Rieger N (1998) Third degree anal sphincter tears: risk factors and outcome. Aust N Z J Obstet Gynaecol 38(4): 414–7.

54. Sultan AH, Kamm MA, Bartram CI, Hudson CN (1993) Anal sphincter trauma during instrumental delivery. Int J Gynaecol Obstet 43(3): 263–70.

55. Walsh CJ, Mooney EF, Upton GJ, Motson RW (1996) Incidence of third-degree perineal tears in labour and outcome after primary repair [see comments]. Br J Surg 83(2): 218–21.

56. Woolley RJ (1995) Benefits and risks of episiotomy: a review of the English-language literature since 1980 Part I. Obstet Gynecol Surv 50(11): 806–20.

57. Shiono P, Klebanoff MA, Carey JC (1990) Midline episiotomies: more harm than good? [see comments]. Obstet Gynecol 75(5): 765–70.

58. Coats PM, Chan KK, Wilkins M, Beard RJ (1980) A comparison between midline and mediolateral episiotomies. Br J Obstet Gynaecol 87(5): 408–12.

59. Woolley RJ (1995) Benefits and risks of episiotomy: a review of the English-language literature since 1980 Part II. Obstet Gynecol Surv 50(11): 821–35.

60. Snooks SJ, Swash M, Henry MM, Setchell M (1986) Risk factors in childbirth causing damage to the pelvic floor innervation. Int J Colorectal Dis 1(1): 20–4.

61. Haadem K, Dahlstrom JA, Lingman G (1990) Anal sphincter function after delivery: a prospective study in women with sphincter rupture and controls. Eur J Obstet Gynecol Reprod Biol 35(1): 7–13.

62. Wynne JM, Myles JL, Jones I et al. (1996) Disturbed anal sphincter function following vaginal delivery. Gut 39(1): 120–4.

63. Rieger N, Schloithe A, Saccone G, Wattchow D (1997) The effect of a normal vaginal delivery on anal function. Acta Obstet Gynecol Scand 76(8): 769–72.

64. Cornes H, Bartolo DC, Stirrat GM (1991) Changes in anal canal sensation after childbirth. Br J Surg 78(1): 74–7.

65. Sultan AH, Kamm MA, Hudson CN (1994) Pudendal nerve damage during labour: prospective study before and after childbirth. Br J Obstet Gynaecol 101(1): 22–8.

66. Snooks SJ, Swash M, Mathers SE, Henry MM (1990) Effect of vaginal delivery on the pelvic floor: a 5-year follow-up. Br J Surg 77(12): 1358–60.

67. Snooks SJ, Henry MM, Swash M (1985) Faecal incontinence due to external anal sphincter division in childbirth is associated with damage to the innervation of the pelvic floor musculature: a double pathology. Br J Obstet Gynaecol 92(8): 824–8.

68. Jacobs PP, Scheuer M, Kuijpers JH, Vingerhoets MH (1990) Obstetric fecal incontinence. Role of pelvic floor denervation and results of delayed sphincter repair. Dis Colon Rectum 33(6): 494–7.

69. Khubchandani IT, Reed JF (1989) Sequelae of internal sphincterotomy for chronic fissure in ano. Br J Surg 76(5): 431–4.

70. Sultan AH, Kamm MA, Nicholls RJ, Bartram CI (1994) Prospective study of the extent of internal anal sphincter division during lateral sphincterotomy. Dis Colon Rectum 37(10): 1031–3.

71. Boulos PB, Araujo JG (1984) Adequate internal sphincterotomy for chronic anal fissure: subcutaneous or open technique? Br J Surg 71(5): 360–2.

72. Read MG, Read NW, Haynes WG, Donnelly TC, Johnson AG (1982) A prospective study of the effect of haemorrhoidectomy on sphincter function and faecal continence. Br J Surg 69(7): 396–8.

73. Deutsch AA, Moshkovitz M, Nudelman I, Dinari G, Reiss R (1987) Anal pressure measurements in the study of hemorrhoid etiology and their relation to treatment. Dis Colon Rectum 30(11): 855–7.

74. el-Gendi MA (1986) Abdel-Baky N. Anorectal pressure in patients with symptomatic hemorrhoids. Dis Colon Rectum 29(6): 388–91.

75. Roe AM, Bartolo DC, Vellacott KD, Locke-Edmunds J, Mortensen NJ (1987) Submucosal versus ligation excision haemorrhoidectomy: a comparison of anal sensation, anal sphincter manometry and postoperative pain and function. Br J Surg 74(10): 948–51.

76. Parks AG, Gordon PH, Hardcastle JD (1976) A classification of fistula-in-ano. Br J Surg 63(1): 1–12.

77. Lunniss PJ, Kamm MA, Phillips RK (1994) Factors affecting continence after surgery for anal fistula. Br J Surg 81(9): 1382–5.

78. Sainio P, Husa A (1985) A prospective manometric study of the effect of anal fistula surgery on anorectal function. Acta Chir Scand 151(3): 279–88.

79. Engel AF, Lunniss PJ, Kamm MA, Phillips RK (1997) Sphincteroplasty for incontinence after surgery for idiopathic fistula in ano. Int J Colorectal Dis 12(6): 323–5.

80. Sainio P, Husa A (1985) Fistula-in-ano. Clinical features and long-term results of surgery in 199 adults. Acta Chir Scand 151(2): 169–76.

81. Sainio P (1985) A manometric study of anorectal function after surgery for anal fistula, with special reference to incontinence. Acta Chir Scand 151(8): 695–700.

82. Nielsen MB, Rasmussen OO, Pedersen JF, Christiansen J (1993) Risk of sphincter damage and anal incontinence after anal dilatation for fissure-in-ano. An endosonographic study. Dis Colon Rectum 36(7): 677–80.

83. MacDonald A, Smith A, McNeill AD, Finlay IG (1992) Manual dilatation of the anus. Br J Surg 79(12): 1381–2.

84. Hancock BD (1981) Lord's procedure for haemorrhoids: a prospective anal pressure study. Br J Surg 68(10): 729–30.

85. Snooks S, Henry MM, Swash M (1984) Faecal incontinence after anal dilatation. Br J Surg 71(8): 617–8.

86. Jensen SL, Lund F, Nielsen OV, Tange G (1984) Lateral subcutaneous sphincterotomy versus anal dilatation in the treatment of fissure in ano in outpatients: a prospective randomised study. Br Med J (Clin Res Ed) 289(6444): 528–30.

87. Speakman CT, Burnett SJ, Kamm MA, Bartram CI (1991) Sphincter injury after anal dilatation demonstrated by anal endosonography. Br J Surg 78(12): 1429–30.

88. Bode WE, Culp CE, Spencer RJ, Beart RW (1984) Jr. Fissurectomy with superficial midline sphincterotomy. A viable alternative for the surgical correction of chronic fissure/ulcer-in-ano. Dis Colon Rectum 27(2): 93–5.

89. Engel AF, Kamm MA, Bartram CI (1995) Unwanted anal penetration as a physical cause of faecal incontinence. Eur J Gastroenterol Hepatol 7(1): 65–7.

90. Neill ME, Parks AG, Swash M (1981) Physiological studies of the anal sphincter musculature in faecal incontinence and rectal prolapse. Br J Surg 68(8): 531–6.

91. Henry MM, Parks AG, Swash M (1982) The pelvic floor musculature in the descending perineum syndrome. Br J Surg 69(8): 470–2.

92. Bartolo DC, Jarratt JA, Read MG, Donnelly TC, Read NW (1983) The role of partial denervation of the puborectalis in idiopathic faecal incontinence. Br J Surg 70(11): 664–7.

93. Neill ME, Swash M (1980) Increased motor unit fibre density in the external anal sphincter muscle in ano-rectal incontinence: a single fibre EMG study. J Neurol Neurosurg Psychiatry 43(4): 343–7.

94. Henry MM, Parks AG, Swash M (1980) The anal reflex in idiopathic faecal incontinence: an electrophysiological study. Br J Surg 67(11): 781–3.

95. Miller R, Bartolo DC, Cervero F, Mortensen NJ (1989) Differences in anal sensation in continent and incontinent patients with perineal descent. Int J Colorectal Dis 4(1): 45–9.

96. Jones PN, Lubowski DZ, Swash M, Henry MM (1987) Relation between perineal descent and pudendal nerve damage in idiopathic faecal incontinence. Int J Colorectal Dis 2(2): 93–5.

97. Kiff ES, Barnes PR, Swash M (1984) Evidence of pudendal neuropathy in patients with perineal descent and chronic straining at stool. Gut 25(11): 1279–82.

98. Wilkinson I (1989) Essential Neurology. Blackwell Scientific Publications, Oxford.

99. Victor RAaM (1989) Principles of Neurology. 4th ed. McGraw-Hill, Singapore.

100. Jameson JS, Rogers J, Chia YW et al. (1994) Pelvic floor function in multiple sclerosis. Gut 35(3): 388–90.

101. Hinds JP, Eidelman BH, Wald A (1990) Prevalence of bowel dysfunction in multiple sclerosis. A population survey. Gastroenterology 98(6): 1538–42.

102. Glickman S, Kamm MA (1996) Bowel dysfunction in spinal-cord-injury patients. Lancet 347(9016): 1651–3.

103. Truelove SC (1966) Movements of the large intestine. Physiol Rev 46(3): 457–512.

104. MacDonagh R, Sun WM, Thomas DG, Smallwood R, Read NW (1992) Anorectal function in patients with complete supraconal spinal cord lesions. Gut 33(11): 1532–8.

105. Frenckner B (1975) Function of the anal sphincters in spinal man. Gut 16(8): 638–44.

106. Sun WM, Read NW, Donnelly TC (1990) Anorectal function in incontinent patients with cerebrospinal disease. Gastroenterology 99(5): 1372–9.

107. Schiller LR, Santa Ana CA, Schmulen AC et al. (1982) Pathogenesis of fecal incontinence in diabetes mellitus: evidence for internal-anal-sphincter dysfunction. N Engl J Med 307(27): 1666–71.

108. Wald A, Tunuguntla AK (1984) Anorectal sensorimotor dysfunction in fecal incontinence and diabetes mellitus. Modification with biofeedback therapy. N Engl J Med 310(20): 1282–7.

109. Caruana BJ, Wald A, Hinds JP, Eidelman BH (1991) Anorectal sensory and motor function in neurogenic fecal incontinence. Comparison between multiple sclerosis and diabetes mellitus. Gastroenterology 100(2): 465–70.

110. Read NW, Abouzekry L, Read MG et al. (1985) Anorectal function in elderly patients with fecal impaction. Gastroenterology 89(5): 959–66.

111. Geboes K, Bossaert H (1977) Gastrointestinal disorders in old age. Age Ageing 6(4): 197–200.

112. McHugh SM, Diamant NE (1987) Effect of age, gender, and parity on anal canal pressures. Contribution of impaired anal sphincter function to fecal incontinence. Dig Dis Sci 32(7): 726–36.

113. Bannister JJ, Abouzekry L, Read NW (1987) Effect of aging on anorectal function. Gut 28(3): 353–7.

114. Burnett SJ, Bartram CI (1991) Endosonographic variations in the normal internal anal sphincter. Int J Colorectal Dis 6(1): 2–4.

115. Klosterhalfen B, Offner F, Topf N, Vogel P, Mittermayer C (1990) Sclerosis of the internal anal sphincter–a process of aging [see comments]. Dis Colon Rectum 33(7): 606–9.

116. Laurberg S, Swash M (1989) Effects of aging on the anorectal sphincters and their innervation. Dis Colon Rectum 32(9): 737–42.

117. Percy JP, Neill ME, Kandiah TK, Swash M (1982) A neurogenic factor in faecal incontinence in the elderly. Age Ageing 11(3): 175–9.

118. Oettle GJ, Roe AM, Bartolo DC, Mortensen NJ (1985) What is the best way of measuring perineal descent? A comparison of radiographic and clinical methods. Br J Surg 72(12): 999–1001.

119. Parks AG, Swash M, Urich H (1977) Sphincter denervation in anorectal incontinence and rectal prolapse. Gut 18(8): 656–65.

120. Lubowski DZ, Jones PN, Swash M, Henry MM (1988) Asymmetrical pudendal nerve damage in pelvic floor disorders. Int J Colorectal Dis 3(3): 158–60.

121. Lubowski DZ, Swash M, Nicholls RJ, Henry MM (1988) Increase in pudendal nerve terminal motor latency with defaecation straining. Br J Surg 75(11): 1095–7.

122. Laurberg S, Swash M, Snooks SJ, Henry MM (1988) Neurologic cause of idiopathic incontinence. Arch Neurol 45(11): 1250–3.

123. Jorge JM, Wexner SD, Ehrenpreis ED, Nogueras JJ, Jagelman DG (1993) Does perineal descent correlate with pudendal neuropathy? Dis Colon Rectum 36(5): 475–83.

124. Constipation M-GV (1984) what does the patient mean? J R Soc Med 77(2): 108–10.

125. Drossman DA, Sandler RS, McKee DC, Lovitz AJ (1982) Bowel patterns among subjects not seeking health care. Use of a questionnaire to identify a population with bowel dysfunction. Gastroenterology 83(3): 529–34.

126. Broden G, Dolk A, Holmstrom B (1988) Recovery of the internal anal sphincter following rectopexy: a possible explanation for continence improvement. Int J Colorectal Dis 3(1): 23–8.

127. Yoshioka K, Heyen F, Keighley MR (1989) Functional results after posterior abdominal rectopexy for rectal prolapse. Dis Colon Rectum 32(10): 835–8.

128. Williams JG, Wong WD, Jensen L, Rothenberger DA, Goldberg SM (1991) Incontinence and rectal prolapse: a prospective manometric study. Dis Colon Rectum 34(3): 209–16.

129. Snooks SJ, Henry MM, Swash M (1985) Anorectal incontinence and rectal prolapse: differential assessment of the innervation to puborectalis and external anal sphincter muscles. Gut 26(5): 470–6.

130. Frenckner B, Ihre T (1976) Function of the anal sphincters in patients with intussusception. Gut 17(2): 147–51.

131. Holmstrom B, Broden G, Dolk A, Frenckner B (1986) Increased anal resting pressure following the Ripstein operation. A contribution to continence? Dis Colon Rectum 29(8): 485–7.

132. Keighley MR, Makuria T, Alexander-Williams J, Arabi Y (1980) Clinical and manometric evaluation of rectal prolapse and incontinence. Br J Surg 67(1): 54–6.

133. Ihre T, Seligson U (1975) Intussusception of the rectum-internal procidentia: treatment and results in 90 patients. Dis Colon Rectum 18(5): 391–6.

134. Lazorthes F, Gamagami R, Cabarrot P, Muhammad S (1998) Is rectal intussusception a cause of idiopathic incontinence? Dis Colon Rectum 41(5): 602–5.

135. Madden MV, Kamm MA, Nicholls RJ et al. (1992) Abdominal rectopexy for complete prolapse: prospective study evaluating changes in symptoms and anorectal function. Dis Colon Rectum 35(1): 48–55.

136. Williams NS, Patel J, George B et al. (1991) Development of an electrically stimulated neoanal sphincter. Lancet 338: 1166–9.

3 Investigations

Urinary Incontinence and the Pelvic Floor

Richard F. Labasky

Accurate diagnosis of a woman's incontinence and prolapse is essential to guide treatment decisions, and because these problems may merely be indicators of more serious processes such as neoplasm, obstruction, or neurological diseases.[1] The evaluation process should lead to accurate diagnoses, and use appropriate diagnostic tests, while avoiding unnecessary ones. The evaluation should also provide an understanding of the patient's health and personal status to facilitate wise counseling about what treatments will be successful and safe for her. The evaluation includes noting details of the patient's *symptoms* of incontinence and prolapse, confirming the *signs* of urinary loss and prolapse, and possibly performing tests to isolate specifically the pathophysiological causes of the *conditions*.[2-4] The basic evaluation with all three steps – history, examination, basic tests, and an optional simple "bedside CMG" (see later) – leads to accurate diagnoses that correlate with the patient's problems of incontinence and prolapse in about 80% of patients, especially for those with stress incontinence.[5-12] If the basic evaluation fails to provide an adequate diagnosis, imaging studies, cystourethroscopy, and formal urodynamics – detailed neurophysiologic tests of the lower urinary tract – are used to confirm diagnoses. To be considered accurate and useful, it is essential that the final diagnoses correlate with the patient's primary complaints and symptoms.

Basic Evaluation

History

As discussed in Chapter 2, a simple and functional method of describing incontinence based upon symptoms is proposed by the International Continence Society.[2,3] Prolapse is defined on the basis of what vaginal compartments are out of normal anatomic position.[13,14]

Chief Complaint and Symptoms

A detailed history will allow the clinician to focus upon the probable etiologies of the incontinence and prolapse. The nature of the problems, when and how they began, their progression, and what seems to prevent, minimize, precipitate or worsen them, and when, is important. Severity of incontinence is noted as the number of incontinence episodes day and night, and the number of clothes changes or pads used per day. An incontinence grading system (Table 3.1)[15] and pad weighing tests provide some grading and objectivity to such data.[2,3,16-19] Prolapse is often described as a vaginal pressure, heaviness or mass; "sitting on a ball"; or pressure or pain in the pelvis, perineum, lower back, or abdomen. Prolapse severity is often reflected in levels of discomfort; difficulty with or needing to reduce or splint prolapse to permit voiding, defecation, or sexual intercourse.[20] Lifestyle changes are significant severity indicators for both problems. Prior treatments

Table 3.1. Incontinence severity based upon history[15]

Grade	Severity of incontinence
0	No incontinence
1	Incontinence with coughing and straining
2	Incontinence with change in position or walking
3	Total incontinence at all times of day

attempted are indicators of the patient's efforts to correct her problems, and what therapies were not successful.

Irritative symptoms – frequency, nocturia, urgency, dysuria and pelvic pain – or obstructive symptoms – intermittent or weak urinary stream, hesitancy to start; straining, or a feeling of incomplete emptying – should also be understood and related to the incontinence and prolapse descriptions. Fluid intakes and outputs are best measured with diaries.[21] Hematuria or recurrent infections are serious problems that should be evaluated separately. Paresthesias, numbness, weakness, pain, or changes in sexual response may indicate a neurologic disease process affecting the sacral nerves (S2–4) serving the lower urinary tract and pelvic organs. In the gastrointestinal system diarrhea, constipation, discomfort or pain with defecation, fecal soiling or incontinence of gas, liquid, or solid stool may be present.

Standardized questionnaires and scoresheets for many of these incontinence and prolapse symptoms can be useful, but none has been universally accepted. Such issues are thoroughly discussed in Chapters 26 and 27.

Medical History

The medical, surgical, gynecological, menstrual, hormonal, and obstetric histories, radiation therapy, and medications used[22] must be noted. These factors may point to etiologic or contributing factors for the incontinence and prolapse symptoms as they may challenge or change the continence and pelvic support mechanisms, or alter urinary or stool output. Some of these factors may also modify therapy options, or raise the possibility of other serious diseases such as tumors. Incontinence persisting since childhood raises the question of an ectopic ureter.

Physical Examination

The physical examination should help correlate the patient's history with her anatomic findings. The examination specifically helps to exclude fistulas and neurologic causes for incontinence, to confirm the presence of stress incontinence, and to confirm the type and severity of prolapse present.

The abdomen and back should be examined for scars of prior surgery or trauma, a palpable bladder or tumor mass, hernias, and pain. Defects over the lumbar and sacral spine may indicate subtle spinal cord abnormalities such as spina bifida occulta.

The vaginal/pelvic examination is the heart of the examination for incontinence and prolapse. Examine the external genitalia for skin breakdown or other changes, tenderness, and masses. Examine the vagina visually and with palpation, with the patient at rest and with straining, in lithotomy and standing positions. Look and feel from the urethral meatus, and along the anterior (bladder and urethra), middle (vault, cervix) and posterior (rectum) compartments. Document the compartments' mobility and prolapse; tenderness or masses; vaginal capacity, elasticity and atrophy; and fistulas. A lateral cystocele defect is often eliminated by an opened clamp or tongue blades placed at the anterolateral vaginal sulci; usually, this maneuver will not correct a midline defect.[23] I think the vagina is best examined with the rigid lower half of an appropriately sized speculum placed to push the posterior compartment away from the anterior compartment, and then vice versa. Confirm an enterocele versus a high rectocele with the patient straining while standing, with the index finger in the rectum, and the thumb in the vagina (Fig. 3.1).[13] Test the strength of pelvic floor and anal muscle contractions.[24]

Any prolapse can be graded as shown in Table 3.2,[14] or with the International Continence Society's recently devised prolapse staging system which uses measurements of specific sites of the vaginal wall from a fixed reference point (the hymen). (Table 3.3)[13,25] Compare examination findings with what the patient herself notes to confirm that you have found the problems significant to her.

During the vaginal examination, the patient should strain or cough with a comfortably full bladder to produce stress incontinence (SUI). With type II SUI, the urethra is descended at rest; with straining it descends more than 2 cm away from the symphysis as leakage occurs. Type I SUI displays normal resting position with less mobility than type II SUI.[26] The Marshall, Bonney, and Q-tip tests do not provide unique information, though the Q-tip test can reinforce the examiner's impression of bladder neck and urethral resting position and mobility.[24,10] With type III SUI, incontinence occurs without any urethral mobility. Such type III patients have intrinsic sphincteric deficiency (ISD) rather than poor urethral and bladder neck support as the cause of their incontinence. They usually suffer from severe incontinence, even at rest and when supine, with histories of urethral, bladder, pelvic or neurological surgery or injury, or congenital

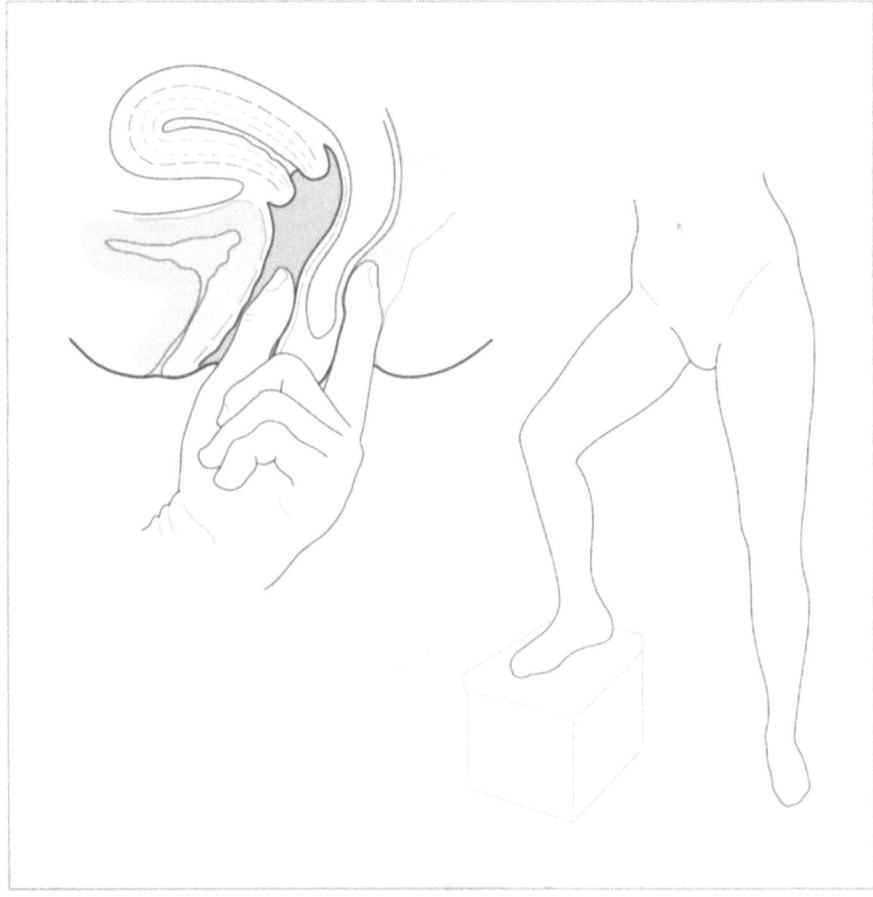

Figure 3.1 Examination for an enterocele. The patient stands with one foot on a stool. The examiner's thumb is inserted in the vagina and the index finger in the rectum, to feel the impulse of the enterocele at the vaginal apex distinct from the rectum.

Table 3.2. Prolapse grading by physical examination[14].

Grade	Descriptive	Finding
I	Mild	Minimal organ descensus with strain
II	Moderate	Organ reaching introitus with strain
III	Moderate	Organ reaching introitus at rest
IV	Severe	Organ outside introitus at rest or with strain

Table 3.3. International Continence Society prolapse staging.[13] Staging is assigned on the basis of the most severe portion of the prolapse when the full extent of the protrusion has been demonstrated

Stage	Description
0	No prolapse
I	Most distal prolapse >1 cm above the hymenal plane
II	Most distal prolapse <1 cm distal or proximal to the hymenal plane
III	Most distal prolapse is >1 cm below the hymenal plane but protrudes not farther than 2 cm less than the total vaginal length
IV	Complete eversion of the total length of the genital tract; the leading edge is usually the cervix or vaginal cuff scar

abnormalities.[12,26-28] Since any prolapse may affect the results of the stress testing, the prolapse should be reduced to accurately assess urethral response to stress maneuvers.[29]

If leakage occurs several moments after the straining maneuver, or with a sudden sense of urgency by the patient, it is probably due to an involuntary bladder contraction; this abnormality is confirmed with urodynamics. If the leakage is continuous during the examination, regardless of patient sensation or straining, continuous incontinence must be considered.

The directed neurological examination focuses upon the motor and sensory distribution of sacral roots 2,3 and 4 – the perianal and perineal areas, including the rectal sphincter.[30]

Basic Diagnostic Tests

Several simple tests can be of great value in the evaluation for incontinence (Table 3.4). If the postvoid residual urine volume (PVR) is less than 100 ml, inadequate bladder emptying is virtually ruled out as a cause for incontinence or a consequence of

Table 3.4. Use of basic laboratory tests

Test	When indicated	To detect
Urinalysis	All patients	Infection; hematuria; glucosuria; proteinuria (renal disease)
Urine culture and sensitivity	Abnormal urinalysis	Infection
Urine cytology	Hematuria; severe and rapidly increasing urgency, frequency or bladder pain	Neoplasm
Serum creatinine or blood urea nitrogen	Urinary tract obstruction; proteinuria; urinary concentration defect	Renal disease
Post void residual urine volume	All patients	Incomplete bladder emptying

prolapse. Oral medications such as phenazopyridine hydrochloride color the urine a distinct yellow-orange; vaginal discharge will not be colored. Intravesical or intravenous methylene blue or indigo carmine will stain the urine blue. With tampons and pads placed in the vagina, the nature of their staining with these agents will demonstrate non-urinary and non-urethral leakage.

Imaging Studies

There are several specific situations when imaging studies are useful, but for most patients with incontinence and prolapse they provide no unique information not already gained from other studies.[31-33] Intravenous pyelograms (IVP) and voiding cystourethrograms (VCUG) diagnose fistulas, ectopic ureters, hydronephrosis, urethral diverticula, vaginal voiding, or spina bifida occulta. An open bladder neck on a cystogram may be an involuntary bladder contraction, a normal variant, or type III SUI; this confusion can be resolved by using videourodynamics, as discussed below. The standing cystogram is useful, but not essential, in grading cystoceles and urethral position and mobility (Table 3.5).

The general usefulness of ultrasonography (especially transperineal),[34,35] computed tomography (CT) and magnetic resonance imaging (MRI) in diagnosis of incontinence and prolapse is still being examined.[36-38] The studies are primarily research

Table 3.5. Cystocele grading based upon cystogram

Cystocele grade	Inferior pubis to inferior bladder distance
I	<2 cm
II	2–5 cm
III	>5 cm

tools, or complement other findings when a diagnosis is in doubt. Defecography is very useful for stool incontinence and for distinguishing types of posterior and middle compartment prolapses.[39,40] Whatever study is used, it is essential that its results correlate with the patient's history and examination.

Cystourethroscopy

Cystourethroscopy provides an internal examination of the urethra and bladder. Urethroscopy is best performed with a blunt ended, non-beaked sheath and a 0° or 5° angle lens to permit undistorted, full distention of the urethra by fluid at the point of visualization. Despite the theoretical value of cystourethroscopy, studies have consistently shown that it provides no unique information for the general evaluation of incontinence or prolapse when compared with other less invasive tests such as the history, physical examination and urodynamics.[41-43] However, there are special situations when it is indicated (Table 3.6).

Urodynamics

Urodynamic evaluations are sophisticated neurophysiologic tests of the lower urinary tract that specifically and objectively identify lower urinary tract abnormalities causing incontinence. The International Continence Society (ICS) has provided the terminology which should be used to describe the urodynamics procedures and data.[2,3] The most important rule governing urodynamic tests is that the tests must be selected, conducted, and interpreted with the patient's clinical situation in mind,

Table 3.6. Indications for cystourethroscopy for incontinence and prolapse

- Urethral trauma, foreshortening, possible diverticulum, or before periurethral injection of bulking agents
- Continuous incontinence, with vaginoscopy, to rule out ectopic ureter, fistula, or total urethral sphincteric incompetence
- Severe or rapidly escalating irritative voiding symptoms
- After recent bladder or urethral surgery with new irritative or obstructive symptoms, or incontinence surgery with failure unexplained by other tests, to rule out bladder and urethral abnormalities
- When the basic evaluation (history, physical examination, and basic tests) and urodynamics do not diagnose the cause of the incontinence
- Cystourethroscopy may be useful with prolapse to assess the following if in doubt after other tests for prolapse:

  Bladder neck mobility

  Thin midline fascia in a central defect cystocele, using transillumination

  Cephalad extent of a cystocele versus the caudal extent of an enterocele, using transillumination

Table 3.7. Indications for multichannel urodynamic evaluations for incontinence

- After failed medical or surgical therapies
- Known or potential neurologic diseases
- Lower urinary tract altered by medications, disease, surgery, trauma
- Complex or combined types and causes of incontinence
- Contradictory, confusing or noncontributory basic evaluation steps
- Incontinence with elevated post void residual urine volumes
- Total incontinence

and that they accurately replicate the patient's symptoms.

A patient's urinary flow characteristics measured with *uroflowmetry* may correlate with her obstructive voiding symptoms, or confirm an abnormal flow pattern associated with an elevated PVR. Otherwise, the test is of little value in the evaluation of the patient with incontinence[44,45] or prolapse.[46]

The *cystometrogram* (CMG) is the most useful of the urodynamics tests in patients with incontinence because it provides objective data on the lower urinary tract during bladder filling and storage. Indications for the complex CMG yielding several channels of data (multichannel CMG) are listed in Table 3.7. The multichannel cystometrogram measures volumes and pressures within the bladder (intravesical), and often in the abdomen (intraabdominal) with a rectal or vaginal catheter. True detrusor pressure is calculated as intravesical pressure minus intraabdominal pressure. The patient's sensations and any fluid leakage (incontinence) are observed. Filling the bladder with a liquid (saline or water) facilitates seeing the leakage. Testing details and technical issues are discussed thoroughly in other references.[5,45,47,48] The most important CMG data related to incontinence are bladder pressures and observed leakage; these are the only CMG details discussed here.

For the normal patient, true detrusor pressure rises less than 15 cm water during filling to normal capacity of about 400–500 ml (Fig. 3.2) . A higher, linear pressure rise is abnormal compliance; leakage occurring with low compliance might correlate with urge, overflow, continuous, or stress incontinence. Phasic pressure increases above 15 cm water are unihibited detrusor contractions and are always abnormal; when associated with urgency or leakage replicating the patient's clinical situation, with any pressure increase, they are clinically significant. The contractions are termed detrusor hyperreflexia (DH) with a known neurological abnormality as their cause, and detrusor instability (DI) otherwise.[2,3] DI and DH are usually associated with urge incontinence. *Ambulatory urodynamics* can often demonstrate DI not found on a standard CMG or help

make a diagnosis not made with the standard CMG.[2,3,45,49–52]

The normal urethra remains closed (competent) during filling. If leakage occurs with stress maneuvers such as coughing or straining, without an increase in true detrusor pressure the diagnosis of genuine stress urinary incontinence (GSUI) is confirmed,[2,3] and urethral incompetence (underactivity) (type I, II, or III SUI) is the cause.[26] With GSUI, the patient usually reports SUI. Combinations of GSUI and DI (mixed incontinence) are not unusual. Some patients will demonstrate DI and leakage after a stress maneuver (stress-induced DI); such patients mistakenly believe they have stress incontinence.

The Valsalva leak point pressure (VLPP) is the intravesical or intraabdominal pressure at which leakage occurs with a Valsalva or stress maneuver.[53] The normal woman's leak point pressure is infinite since she does not leak. The definition of high or low VLPPs is not standardized, though a VLPP above 90–100 cm water is generally considered high, and one below 50–60 cm water is considered low.[27,28,53–55] VLPP may vary with bladder fullness, patient position, and catheter size and number. A standard method of obtaining a VLPP has not yet been accepted.[54,56–59] These variables make comparisons among studies using VLPP impossible as yet. However, the VLPP is clinically useful since it is a continuous variable that correlates inversely with severity of incontinence.[28,54–56,61–64] Also, VLPP is independent of the degree of bladder neck mobility, so any VLPP can occur with any degree of bladder neck mobility. Thus, the VLPP is a more precise and less subjective indicator of the degree of ISD than the Type III SUI criteria of history plus cystogram findings.[28,54,59–64]

Incontinence can occur with spontaneous drops in urethral closure pressure, an uncommon condition called urethral instability. The patient's symptoms may be of stress, urge, or unconscious incontinence. The diagnosis is made with intraurethral pressure measurements and sphincter electromyography.[45] Finally, overflow incontinence may result from reduced or absent sensation which results in bladder overfilling. Discomfort or pain from increased sensation may lead to urge incontinence, frequency or nocturia.

A large cystocele or other pelvic prolapse may alter urethral function by increasing VLPP or impairing voiding by compression, or dampening the force of a Valsalva maneuver. Reduce these effects by reducing the prolapse with a sponge, pessary, or other instrument and repeating the tests.[29,65] Some patients will not demonstrate DI that correlates with their symptoms of urge incontinence. These patients may benefit from provocative maneuvers to reveal the instability.[66]

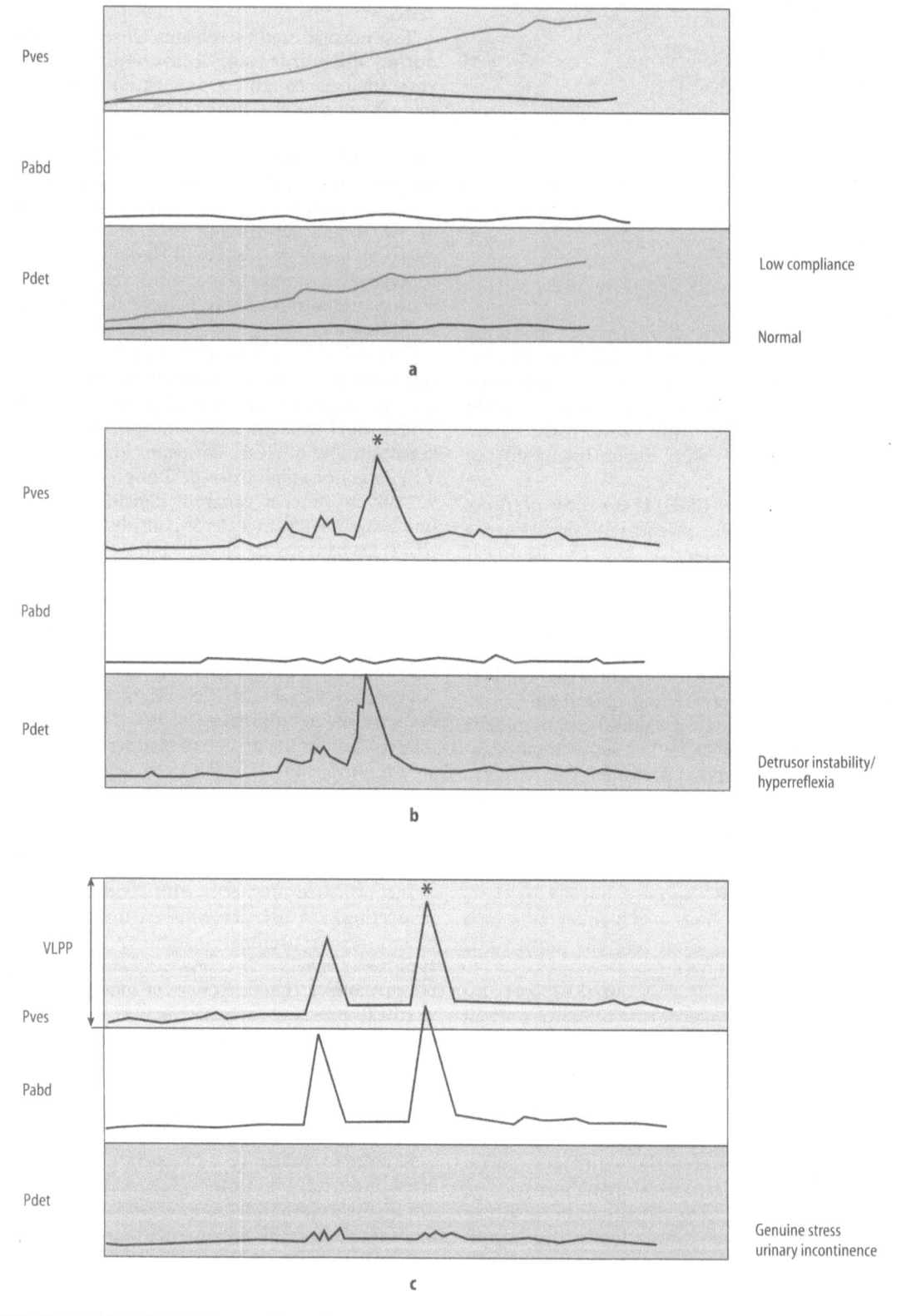

Figure 3.2 **a** Cystometrogram showing a normal bladder and one with low bladder compliance. Note that with low compliance vesical pressure changes but abdominal pressure does not. **b** Detrusor pressure rise associated with an uninhibited bladder contraction with leak at *. **c** Genuine stress urinary incontinence. Note that both vesical and abdominal pressure rise, but detrusor pressure does not. Leak occurs at *, with the vesical pressure rise above resting, empty bladder pressure to the leak point pressure equal to the VLPP. abd, abdominal; det, detrusor; P, pressure; ves, vesical; VLPP, Valsalva leak point pressure.

Simultaneous measurement of the true detrusor pressure and the urine flow rate during voiding is voiding cystometry, a *pressure/flow (PF) study*.[2,3] The test is not indicated for a patient with incontinence or prolapse unless she has an elevated PVR, obstructive voiding symptoms, or an abnormal uroflowmetry.[45,67,68] *Electromyography (EMG)* of the periurethral and perirectal muscles assesses neurologic function in these muscles. Use needle electrodes in patients with neurologic diseases.[2,3] EMG is rarely useful in neurologically normal patients. *Intraurethral pressures* [2,3] can be measured with the patient at rest, performing stress maneuvers, or voiding. A maximum resting urethral pressure below 20 cm water is considered diagnostic of an incompetent urethra or ISD. Urethral pressures are technically difficult to obtain, and because of relatively poor correlation between urethral pressure data and patients' continence status, urethral pressures are less useful clinically than the VLPP.[28,55,64,70] *Videourodynamics (VUD)*, the combination of fluoroscopy and urodynamics, allows simultaneous assessment of anatomy and function. VUD is not routinely necessary in the evaluation of incontinence or prolapse, unless the other steps in the evaluation have not led to a clear diagnosis of the incontinence.[70] Its primary use is to confirm the suspicion of a totally incompetent urethra (type III GSUI) as the study shows a bladder neck that is open without detrusor activity or straining, is not mobile, and leaks with straining. Measurement of the VLPP is usually more useful than the finding of a type III urethra with VUD. If needed for other purposes, the VUD images can replace those of a VCUG.[25,70]

Simple "Bedside" Urodynamics

A *"bedside CMG"* ("eyeball" urodynamics) can be very useful.[5,71–73] For a bedside CMG, check the PVR with a catheter, and fill the bladder via gravity with sterile saline or water. Note volumes of first sensation, urgency, and capacity. The height of the water column above the bladder is a measure of the intravesical pressure. Low compliance may cause slow filling; DI or DH may reverse the filling. At capacity, remove the catheter and test the patient for stress incontinence. A bedside CMG that correlates with the patient's clinical status often precludes the need for multichannel urodynamics.

Anal Manometry

Application of anal manometry to patients with fecal incontinence is useful, though variations in technique and terminology limits widespread

sharing of information.[47] This technique is discussed further in the next section.

Summary

The appropriate and successful evaluation of incontinence and prolapse requires a thorough, systematic approach built upon the history, physical examination and basic tests, and possibly a bedside CMG to yield adequate, accurate diagnoses. Imaging studies, cystourethroscopy and urodynamics tests are used when the basic evaluation does not yield an adequate or accurate diagnosis. Above all, to be considered worthwhile, the diagnoses should correlate with the patient's primary complaints and symptoms.

Anorectal Investigations

Devinder Kumar

History

All patients presenting with bowel symptoms as part of a pelvic floor disorder should have a careful history taken. Special attention should be paid to stool frequency, consistency, history of straining, digitation, perineal or vaginal splinting, and a previous history of difficult vaginal delivery with or without the use of forceps. Neurologic symptoms should also be recorded. Attention should be paid to symptoms suggestive of colonic or rectal disease such as the presence of diarrhea and the leakage of mucus or blood in patients with inflammatory bowel disease. Any history of previous pelvic or anal surgery, especially anal dilation, fistula surgery, prolapse repairs, and hysterectomy should be documented. History of associated urinary incontinence or uterovaginal prolapse should also be recorded.

Physical Examination

After an abdominal examination, the perineum, anus, and rectum should be examined with the patient in the left lateral position. The anus and the perineum should be inspected for any signs of scarring, fecal leakage, external openings of a fistula, a patulous anus, and a mucosal or full thickness rectal prolapse. Abnormal perineal descent both at rest and on straining is associated with pudendal neuropathy. Gaping of the anal canal at rest or on traction of the perianal skin suggests reduced resting tone. The anocutaneous reflex should be tested by stroking the perianal skin. This causes a transient contraction of the external anal sphincter and tests the integrity of the pudendal nerve and sacral plexus. It may be absent in patients with fecal incontinence.

Digital examination of the anorectum should be performed to assess the resting anal tone and changes during voluntary contractions and coughing. The presence of a fecal bolus, palpable tumors, or areas of tenderness in the rectum should be recorded. All patients should undergo procto-sigmoidoscopy to exclude neoplastic lesions, inflammatory bowel disease, fistulae, mucosal prolapse, and hemorrhoids.

Investigations

Anal Manometry

A range of pressure measurement equipment is commercially available. These include perfused tube systems, air- or water-filled balloons or micro-transducer catheters. Using these devices, the function of both internal and external anal sphincters is assessed by measuring anal canal pressures. The manometry assembly is inserted into the rectum and then gradually withdrawn. When the high pressure zone is reached, the distance from the anal verge is recorded and the pressure in the anal canal measured at 1 cm intervals as the catheter is withdrawn further. This records the resting pressure produced mainly by the internal anal sphincter. The resting sphincter length is also recorded. Manometry is the only method of measuring resting tone in the anal canal. The internal anal sphincter is responsible for approximately 70–80% of the resting tone.[74] Measurement of the resting tone therefore provides an assessment of the internal anal sphincter function. The procedure is repeated, but this time the patient is asked to voluntarily squeeze the external anal sphincter so that the maximum squeeze pressure produced by the external sphincter can be recorded. Voluntary squeeze pressure is the greatest pressure achieved above resting pressure during a maximal voluntary contraction. It is mainly an expression of the external anal sphincter function. The patient should be instructed not to use the gluteal muscles during voluntary squeeze as this will result in an erroneous recording of the squeeze pressure. In the majority of patients with incontinence the resting and squeeze pressures are significantly lower than in normal subjects.[75,76] Patients who are incontinent to liquid and solid stool have lower squeeze pressures than those who are incontinent to liquid stool alone. The length of the high pressure zone is shorter in patients with incontinence than in normal subjects.[77] In normal subjects, basal pressure is not less than 80 cm H_2O and squeeze pressure not less than 120 cm H_2O.

Rectal Volume Sensation

Rectal volume sensation can be measured by using a latex balloon tied to a rubber tube which is attached to a three-way tap and a syringe (Fig. 3.3). The balloon assembly is inserted into the rectum and known aliquots of air are injected into the balloon. The volume of air at first perception is the threshold volume. The volume at which the patient can perceive the presence of an inflated balloon inside the rectum determines the volume at constant sensation and volume at which the patient has an uncontrollable desire to defecate is the maximum tolerated volume. In patients with fecal incontinence due to rectal factors, the volume at constant sensation is often below normal. The maximum tolerable volume may also be impaired in patients with fecal incontinence. In some patients constant sensation or maximum tolerability at a low volume may be the only abnormality. These patients often have symptoms of severe urgency associated with fecal incontinence. In some patients with constipation and those with a megarectum, the volume at constant sensation is above normal and the maximum tolerable volume may not be reached.

Normal values for rectal volume are: threshold, 10–60 ml; constant, 140–160 ml; maximum, 220–250 ml.

Mucosal Electrosensitivity

In addition to measuring rectal sensation, it is useful to test and quantify anal sensation as well.

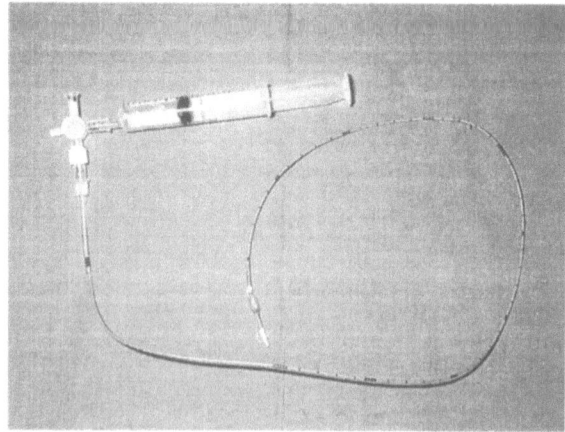

Figure 3.3 Assembly to test rectal volume sensation. The 60 ml syringe is connected to a three-way tap which is then connected to a latex balloon via a plastic tubing.

This is achieved by measuring anal mucosal electro-sensitivity.[78] (Roe et al 1986). The technique involves application of a constant current of increasing strength between two electrodes mounted on a catheter. The catheter is placed in the anal canal with the patient in the left lateral position. The level at which a tingling or tapping sensation is first perceived is recorded. Separate measurements are made for the upper, middle and lower anal canal. Anal sensation may be impaired in patients with fecal incontinence as well as those with constipation.

Normal values for anal mucosal electrosensitivity are: upper, ≤ 16 mA; mid, ≤ 16 mA; lower, ≤ 16 mA.

Electromyography

Electromyograpy is used to assess denervation or reinnervation in patients with fecal incontinence. It is commonly performed by using a concentric or single fiber needle electrode. The concentric needle electrode has a relatively large uptake area and records the activity of several motor units. It allows quantification of the activity in different muscles and within different parts of a muscle. The EMG activity will be reduced where the number of functioning fibers is reduced. This is seen when there has been denervation of muscle fibers due to neuropathy or in the presence of fibrosis due to direct muscle trauma. Patients with neuropathic fecal incontinence have reduced activity in both puborectalis and external anal sphincter muscles. EMG can be used for sphincter mapping in patients who are suspected of having a sphincter defect.[79]. It is particularly helpful in patients in whom a direct sphincter injury is suspected; in such cases the damaged muscle area is electrically silent. By contrast, the single-fiber EMG allows analysis of changes in single muscle fibers. It demonstrates reinnervation of previously denervated muscle fibers by surrounding neurons and is expressed as fiber density. It is increased in patients with neurogenic fecal incontinence and is said to be a sensitive and specific marker of neuropathy.[80]

Pudendal Nerve Terminal Motor Latency

Pudendal nerve terminal motor latency measures conduction in the terminal part of the pudendal nerve. The pudendal nerve is stimulated as it crosses the ischial spine while the evoked potential in the external anal sphincter is recorded (Fig. 3.4). This is studied using a specifically designed glove.[81] A stimulating electrode is mounted at the tip of the index finger and the recording electrode is located at the

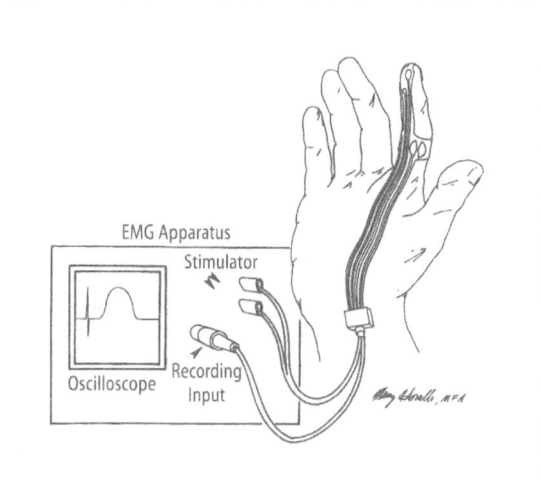

Figure 3.4 Glove electrode, showing the stimulating and recording electrodes mounted on the index finger.

base of the index finger. The contraction produced by the stimulating electrode is recorded by the electrode placed at the base of the index finger. Recordings are made from both sides of the pelvis as pudendal nerve damage may be asymmetrical in some patients. Pudendal nerve terminal motor latency is prolonged in patients with idiopathic fecal incontinence. However, it must be remembered that pudendal nerve terminal motor latency and fiber density increase with age and this should be considered when interpreting the data.[82]

Endoanal Ultrasound

Endoanal ultrasound provides high-resolution images of both the internal and external anal sphincter and the puborectalis muscles. The examination is performed with the patient in the left lateral position and serial images are obtained at rest and during squeeze in the lower, mid and upper anal canal. The normal ultrasound (Fig. 3.5) consists of a complete ring of internal sphincter muscle surrounded by the mixed echogenic uninterrupted external sphincter. In patients with a direct sphincter injury or obstetric trauma, a sphincter defect is seen in the internal and/or external anal sphincter (Fig. 3.6). Endoanal ultrasound also provides a dynamic assessment of the sphincter muscles on voluntary contraction. We have found an excellent correlation between anal ultrasonography and defects in the internal and external anal sphincters as displayed during surgical dissection.[83] This is one of the most useful investigations in the assessment of fecal incontinence. It is relatively non-invasive and delineates sphincter defects and other

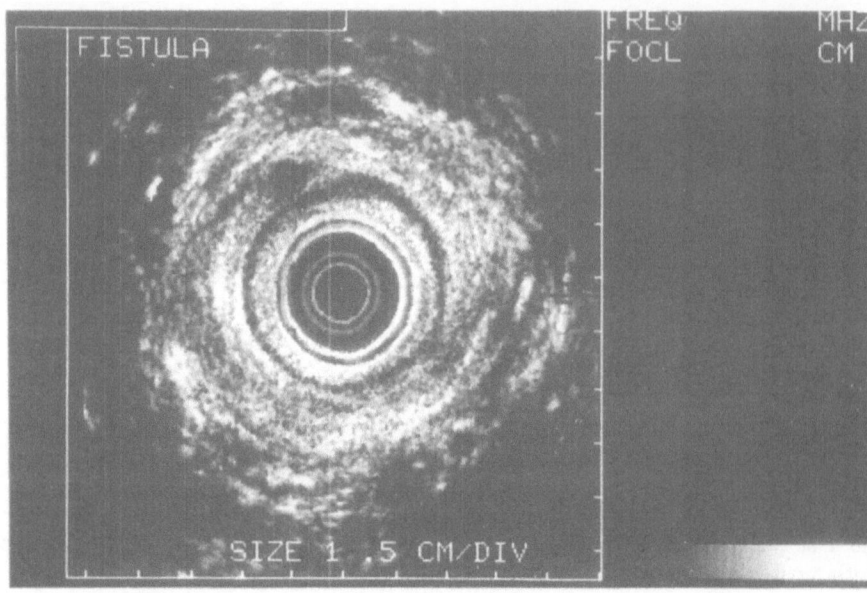

Figure 3.5 Example of a normal anal sphincter complex showing a complete ring of internal and external anal sphincters.

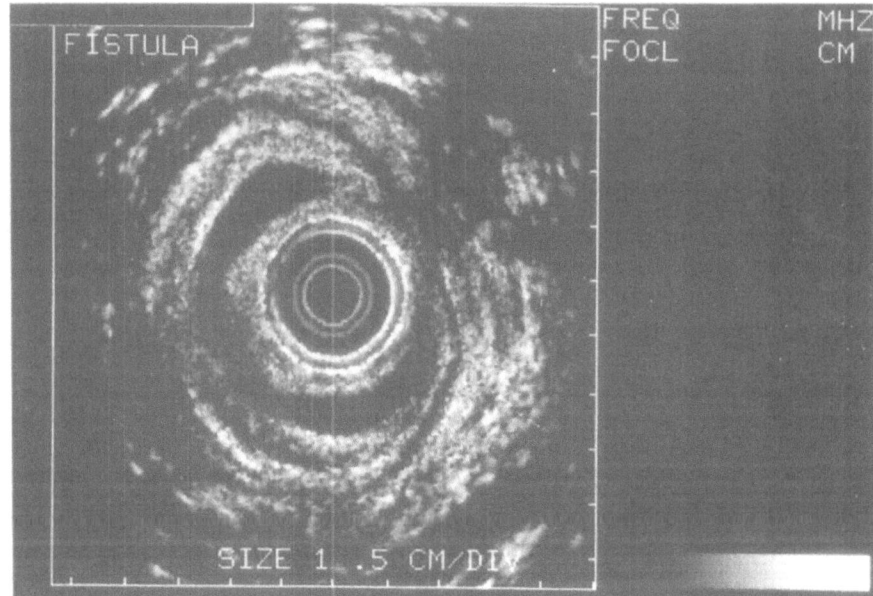

Figure 3.6 An internal and external anal sphincter defect on endoanal ultrasonography.

anatomical abnormalities such as prolapse and rectocele with precision.

Barium Proctography

Conventional assessment of anorectal function with barium proctography involves evacuation of a barium-labeled artificial stool. Barium proctography is widely used for assessment of anorectal angle, pelvic floor descent, rectocele, and mucosal pro-lapse. However, the clinical usefulness of measuring these parameters is debatable. The anorectal angle in constipated patients and in controls is similar, and there is no relationship between symptoms and the anorectal angle. Pelvic floor descent, rectocele, and mucosal prolapse are probably the result rather than the cause of impaired rectal evacuation. The most important parameter assessed by barium proctography is the efficiency of rectal evacuation. The information obtained is qualitative rather than quantitative. Another drawback with barium proctography is safety. A typical investigation involves 1–2 minutes of fluoroscopy and two or three radiographs. The radiation dose used is of particular concern in women of childbearing potential who have the highest incidence of chronic idiopathic constipation and in whom barium proctography is likely to be performed.

Scintigraphic (Isotope) Defecography

Scintigraphic defecography is a quantitative method of assessing defecation. It involves evacuation of a radiolabeled artificial stool. Radioactive markers, each containing 1 MBq activity, are placed over the subjects pubis, lumbosacral junction, and coccyx to promote alignment of images. With the subject in the left lateral position, 100 ml of an oat porridge and water mixture containing 100 MBq technetium is introduced intra-rectally. The subject is imaged while seated on a commode with a gamma camera head against the left hip. Dynamic images are acquired during defecation for up to 10 minutes. Digital images are stored on computer and replayed for analysis.

The images are replayed and a rectal region of interest is drawn around the bolus of scintigraphic activity in the rectum. Rectal emptying curves are obtained. Rectal percentage of evacuation time and evacuation rate are easily calculated. Anorectal angle, pelvic floor descent and rectocele (Figs 3.7, 3.8) can all be measured with reference to the markers and the anal canal. The advantage of scintigraphic defecography is that it provides quantitative

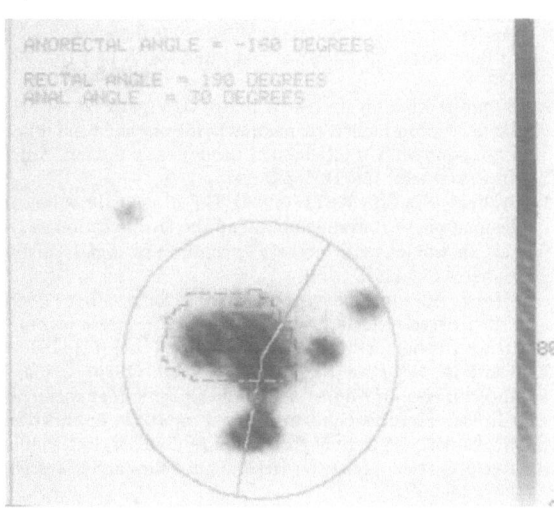

Figure 3.8 An example of a rectocele on scintigraphic defecography.

and dynamic information on rectal evacuation. Functionally significant pelvic floor descent and rectocele can be assessed. The other main advantage is the minimal radiation dose administered to the patient. This technique can be safely and effectively used in the follow up of treatment as well as the primary assessment of patients with disordered defecation.

Conclusion

The lower intestinal tract, like the urinary tract, can be studied by a variety of investigations. The selection of appropriate investigations should depend on the patient's symptoms and signs.

References

1. Blaivas JG, Bhimani G, Labib KB (1979) Vesicourethral dysfunction in multiple sclerosis. J Urol 122: 342–7.
2. Abrams P, Blaivas JG, Stanton SL, Anderson JT (1988) The standardization of terminology of lower urinary tract function. Neurourol Urodyn 7: 403–27.
3. Abrams P, Blaivas JG, Stanton SL, Anderson JT (1988) The International Continence Society Committee on Standardization of Terminology: the standardization of terminology of lower urinary tract function. Scand J Urol Nephrol 114S: 5–19.
4. Blaivas JG, Appell RA, Fantl JA et al. (1997) Definition and classification of urinary incontinence: recommendations of the Urodynamic Society. Neurourol Urodyn 16: 149–51.
5. DeBeau CE, Resnick NM (1991) Evaluation of the causes and severity of geriatric incontinence. Urol Clin N Amer 18: 243–56.
6. Videla FLG, Wall LL (1998) Stress incontinence diagnosed without multichannel urodynamic studies. Obstet Gynecol 91: 965–8.
7. Carey MP, Dwyer PL, Glenning pp. (1997) The sign of stress incontinence- Should we believe what we see? Aust NZ J Obstet Gynaecol 37: 436–9.

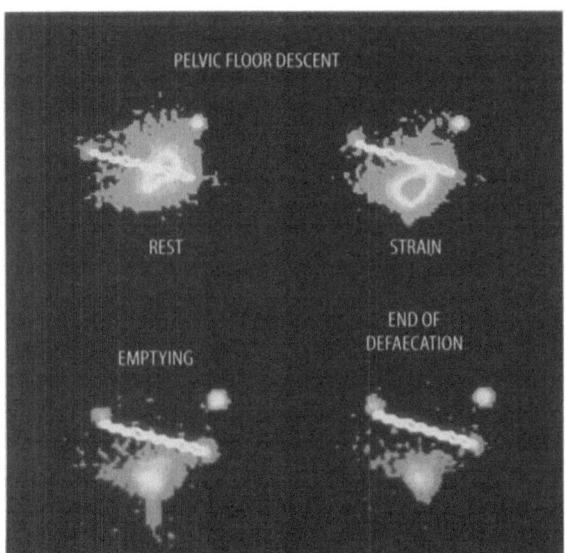

Figure 3.7 A scintigram showing the measurement of pelvic floor descent using the surface markers. The movement of the pelvic floor in relation to the pubococcygeal line joining the pubic and coccygeal markers gives an indication of normal or abnormal pelvic floor movements.

8. Haylen BT, Sutherst JR, Frazer MI (1989) Is the investigation of most stress incontinence really necessary? Br J Urol 64: 147–9.

9. Summitt RL, Stovall TG, Bent AE, Ostergard DR (1992) Urinary incontinence: correlation of history and brief office evaluation with multichannel urodynamic testing. Am J Obstet Gynecol 166: 1835–44.

10. Walters MD, Shields LE (1988) The diagnostic value of history, physical examination, and the Q-tips cotton swab test in women with urinary incontinence. Am J Obstet Gynecol 159: 145–9.

11. Diokno AC, Dimaculangan RR, Lim EU, Steinert BW (1999) Office based criteria for predicting type II stress incontinence without further evaluation studies. J Urol 161: 1263–7.

12. Fantl JA, Newman DK, Colling J et al. (1996) Urinary Incontinence in Adults: Acute and Chronic Management. Clinical Practice Guideline, No. 2. AHCPR Publication No. 96-0682. US Dept of Health and Human Services. Public Health Service, Agency for Health Care Policy and Research, Rockville, MD.

13. Bump RC, Mattiasson MD, Bo K et al. (1996) The standardization of terminology of female pelvic organ prolapse and pelvic floor dysfunction. Am J Obstet Gynecol 175: 10–17.

14. Snyder JA, Westmacott R (1991) Treatment of mild, moderate and severe cystoceles. Probl Urol 5: 85–93.

15. Stamey TA (1980) Endoscopic suspension of the vesical neck for urinary incontinence in females. Ann Surg 192: 465.

16. Versi E, Orrego G, Hardy E et al. (1996) Evaluation of the home pad test in the investigation of female urinary incontinence. Br J Obstet Gynaecol 103: 162–7.

17. Siltberg H, Victor A, Larsson G (1997) Pad weighing tests: the best way to quantify urine loss in patients with incontinence. Acta Obstet Gynecol Scand 76(166S): 28–32.

18. Ryhammer AM, Djurhuus JC, Laurberg S (1999) Pad testing in incontinent women: a review. Int Urogynecol J 10: 111–15.

19. Elser DM, Fantl JA, McClish DK (1995) The Continence Program for Women Research Group. Comparison of subjective and objective measures of severity of urinary incontinence in women. Neurourol Urodyn 14: 311–16.

20. Weber AM, Walters MD, Ballard LA, Booher DL, Piedmonte MR (1998) Posterior vaginal prolapse and bowel function. Am J Obstet Gynecol 179: 1446–50.

21. Wyman JF, Choi SC, Harkins SW, Wilson MS, Fantl JA (1988) The urinary diary in evaluation of incontinence in women: a test-retest analysis. Obstet Gynecol 71: 812–17.

22. Steele AC, Kohli N, Mallipeddi P, Karram M (1999) Pharmacologic causes of female incontinence. Int Urogynecol J 10: 106–10.

23. Barber MD, Cundiff GW, Weidner AC et al. (1999) Accuracy of clinical assessment of paravaginal defects in women with anterior vaginal wall prolapse. Am J Obstet Gynecol 181: 87–90.

24. Sampselle CM, DeLancey JOL (1998) Anatomy of female continence. J Wound Ostomy Continence Nurs 25: 63–74.

25. Hall AF, Theofrastous JP, Cundiff GW et al. (1996) Interobserver and intraobserver reliability of the proposed International Continence Society, Society of Gynecologic Surgeons, and American Urogynecologic Society pelvic organ prolapse classification system. Am J Obstet Gynecol 175: 1467–71.

26. Blaivas JG, Olsson CA (1988) Stress incontinence: classification and surgical approach. J Urol 139: 727–31.

27. Haab F, Zimmern PE, Leach GE (1996) Female stress urinary incontinence due to intrinsic sphincteric deficiency: recognition and management. J Urol 156: 3–17.

28. Bump RC, Coates KW, Cundiff GW, Harris RL, Weidner AC (1997) Diagnosing intrinsic sphincteric deficiency: comparing urethral closure pressure, urethral axis, and Valsalva leak point pressures. Am J Obstet Gynecol 177: 303–10.

29. Ghonheim GM, Walters F, Lewis V (1994) The value of the vaginal pack test in large cystoceles. J Urol 152: 931–4.

30. Blaivas JG, Zayed AAH, Labib KB (1981) The bulbocavernosus reflex in urology: a prospective study of 299 patients. J Urol 126: 197–9.

31. Bergman A, McKenzie C, Ballard C, Richmond J (1988) Role of cystourethrography in the preoperative evaluation of stress incontinence in women. J Reprod Med 33: 372–6.

32. Greenwald SW, Thornburg JR, Dunn LJ (1967) Cystourethrography as a diagnostic aid in stress incontinence: an evaluation. Obstet Gynecol 29: 324–7.

33. Pelsang RE, Bonney WW (1996) Voiding cystourethrography in female stress incontinence. AJR 166: 561–5.

34. Dietz HP, Wilson PD (1998) Anatomical assessment of the bladder outlet and proximal urethra using ultrasound and videocystourethrography. Int Urogynecol J Pelvic Floor Dysfunct 9: 365–9.

35. Schaer GN, Koechli OR, Schuessler B, Haller U (1995) Perineal ultrasound for evaluating the bladder neck in urinary stress incontinence. Obstet Gynecol 85: 220–4.

36. Mostwin JL, Yang A, Sanders R, Genadry R (1995) Radiography, sonography, and magnetic resonance imaging for stress incontinence. Contributions, uses, and limitations. Urol Clin N Amer 22: 539–49.

37. Huddleston HT, Dunnihoo DR, Huddleston PM, Meyers PC (1995) Magnetic resonance imaging of defects in DeLancey's vaginal support levels I, II, III. Am J Obstet Gynecol 172: 1778–82.

38. Aronson MP, Bates SM, Jacoby AF, Chelmow D, Sant GR (1995) Periurethral and paravaginal anatomy: an endovaginal magnetic resonance imaging study. Am J Obstet Gynecol 173: 1702–8.

39. Hock D, Lombard R, Jehaes C et al. (1993) Colpocystodefecography. Dis Colon Rectum 36: 1015–21.

40. Altringer WE, Saclarides TJ, Dominguez JM, Brubaker LT, Smith C (1995) Four-contrast defecography: pelvic. Dis Colon Rectum 38: 695–9.

41. Govier FE, Pritchett TR, Kornman JD (1994) Correlation of the cystoscopic appearance and functional integrity of the female urethral sphincteric mechanism. Urology 44: 250–3.

42. Labasky RF (1997) Endoscopic Evaluation. In: Donnell PD (ed) Urinary Incontinence. Mosby, St. Louis, Mo., pp. 115–22.

43. Cundiff GW, Bent AE (1996) The contribution of urethrocystoscopy to evaluation of lower urinary tract dysfunction in women. Int Urogynecol J 7: 307–11.

44. Aagaard J, Bruskewitz R (1991) Are urodynamic studies useful in the evaluation of female incontinence? Probl Urol 5: 11–22.

45. Labasky RF (1972) Urodynamics. In: Smith JA (ed) High Tech Urology: Technologic Innovations and Their Clinical Applications. WB Saunders, Philadelphia, pp. 140–8.

46. Coates KW, Harris RL, Cundiff GW (1997). Uroflowmetry in women with urinary incontinence and pelvic organ prolapse. Br J Urol 80: 217–21.

47. Coates KW (1998) Physiologic evaluation of the pelvic floor. Obstet Gynecol Clin N Amer 25: 805–25.

48. Dmochowski R (1996) Cystometry. Urol Clin N Amer 23: 243–52.

49. Kulseng-Hanssen S (1997) Reliability and validity of stationary cystometry, stationary cysto-urethrometry and ambulatory cysto-urethro-vaginometry. Acta Obstet Gynecol Scand 76(166S): 3–8.

50. Brown K, Hilton P (1997) Ambulatory monitoring. Int Urogynecol J Pelvic Floor Dysfunction 8: 369–76.

51. Vereecken RL, Nuland T Van (1998) Detrusor pressure in ambulatory versus standard urodynamics. Neurourol Urodyn 17: 129–33.

52. Swithinbank LV, James M, Shepherd A, Abrams P (1999) Role of ambulatory urodynamic monitoring in clinical urological practice. Neurourol Urodyn 18: 215–22.

53. McGuire EJ, Fitzpatrick CC, Wan J et al. (1993) Clinical assessment of urethral sphincter function. J Urol 150: 1452–4.

54. Nitti VW, Combs AJ (1996) Correlation of Valsalva leak point pressure with subjective degree of stress urinary incontinence in women. J Urol 155: 281–5.

55. McGuire EJ (1995) Urodynamic evaluation of stress incontinence. Urol Clin N Amer 22: 551–5.

56. Bump RC, Elser DM, Theofrastous JP, McClish DK (1995) Continence Program for Women Research Group. Valsalva leak point pressures in women with genuine stress incontinence: reproducibility, effect of catheter caliber, and correlation with other measures of urethral resistance. Am J Obstet Gynecol 173: 551–7.

57. Theofrastous JP, Cundiff GW, Harris RL (1996) [14] RC. The effect of vesical volume on Valsalva leak point pressures in women with genuine stress urinary incontinence. Obstet Gynecol 87: 711–14.

58. Petrou S, Kollmorgen TA (1998) Valsalva leak point pressure and bladder volume. Neurourol Urodyn 17: 3–7.

59. Miklos JR, Karram MM (1995) A critical appraisal of the methods of measuring leak-point pressures in women with stress incontinence. Obstet Gynecol 86: 349–52.

60. Cummings JM, Boullier JA, Parra RO, Wozniak-Petrofsky J (1997) Leak point pressures in women with urinary stress incontinence: correlation with patient history. J Urol 157: 818–20.

61. McGuire EJ, Appell RA (1991) Collagen injection for the dysfunctional urethra. Contemp Urol 3(9): 11–19.

62. Appell RA (1994) Collagen injection therapy for urinary incontinence. Urol Clin N Amer 21: 177–82.

63. Wan J, McGuire EJ, Bloom DA, Ritchey ML (1993) Stress leak point pressure: a diagnostic tool for incontinence children. J Urol 150: 700–2.

64. Theofrastous JP, Bump RC, Elser DM, Wyman JF, McClish DK (1995) The Continence Program for Women Research Group. Correlation of urodynamic measures of urethral resistance with clinical measures of incontinence severity in women with pure genuine stress urinary incontinence. Am J Obstet Gynecol 173: 407–14.

65. Hextall A, Boos K, Cardozo L et al. (1998) Video-cystourethrography with a ring pessary in situ. A clinically useful preoperative investigation for continent women with urogenital prolapse? Int Urogynecol J Pelvic Floor Dyfunct 9: 205–9.

66. Choe JM, Gallo ML, Staskin DR (1999) A provocative maneuver to elicit cystometric instability: measuring instability at maximum infusion. J Urol 161: 1541–4.

67. Chancellor MB, Blaivas JG, Kaplan SA, Axelrod S (1991) Bladder outlet obstruction versus impaired detrusor contractility: the role of uroflow. J Urol 145: 810–12.

68. Farrar DJ, Whiteside CG, Osborne JL, Turner-Warwick RT (1975) A urodynamic analysis of micturition symptoms in the female. Surg Gynecol Obstet 141: 875–81.

69. Lose G (1997) Urethral pressure measurement. Acta Obstet Gynecol Scand 76(166S): 39–4.

70. McGuire EJ, Cespedes RD, Cross CA, O'Connell HE (1996) Videourodynamic studies. Urol Clin N Amer 23: 309–21.

71. Ouslander JG, Leach GE, Staskin DR (1989) Simplified tests of lower urinary tract function in evaluation of geriatric urinary incontinence. J Am Geriatr Soc 37: 706–14.

72. Sand PK, Brubaker LT, Novak T (1991) Standing incremental cystometry as a screening method for detrusor instability. Obstet Gynecol 77: 453–7.

73. Fonda D, Brimage PJ, D'Astoli M (1993) Simple screening for urinary incontinence in the elderly: comparison of simple and multichannel cystometry. Urology 42: 536–540.

74. Frenckner B, Van Euler C (1975) Influence of pudendal block on the function of the anal sphincters. Gut 16: 482–489.

75. Read NW, Harford WV, Schmulen AC, Read MG, Santa Ana C, Fordtran JS (1979) A clinical study of patients with faecal incontinence and diarrhoea. Gastroenterology 76: 757–756.

76. Read NW, Haynes WG, Bartolo DCC (1983) Use of anorectal manometry during rectal infusion of saline to investigate sphincter function in incontinent patients. Gastroenterology 85: 105–13.

77. Nivatvongs S, Stern HS, Fryd DS (1981) The length of the anal canal. Dis Colon Rectum 67: 216–20.

78. Roe AM, Bartolo DC, Mortensen N (1986) New method for assessment of anal sensation in various anorectal disorders. Br J Surg 73: 310–312.

79. Kiff E (1983) The clinical use of anorectal physiology studies. Sir Alan Parks Memorial Symposium. Ann R Coll Surg Engl 158: 498–512.

80. Neal ME, Swash M (1980) Increased motor unit fiber density in the external anal sphincter muscle in ano-rectal incontinence: a single fibre EMG study. J Neurol Neurosurg Psychiatry 43: 343–7.

81. Lubowski DZ, Swash M, Nicholls RJ, Henry MM (1988) Increase in pudendal nerve terminal motor latency with defecation straining. Br J Surg 75: 1095–7.

82. Vernava AM III, Longo WE, Daniel GL (1992) Pudendal neuropathy and the importance of EMG evaluation of faecal incontinence. Dis Colon Rectum 35: 11.

83. Deen KI, Kumar D, Williams JG, Oliff J, Keighley MRB (1993) The prevalence of anal sphincter defects in faecal incontinence: a prospective endosonic study. Gut 34: 685–8.

Part III

Sphincter Surgery

4 Congenital Abnormalities

Gynaecological Congenital Abnormalities

Karen D. Bradshaw

Anatomic gynecologic anomalies including congenital absence of the vagina, defects in lateral and vertical fusion of the müllerian ducts, as well as disorders of sexual development, occur with surprising frequency in referral practices of reproductive endocrinology and genitourinary surgery. This section serves to review the embryology and development of the reproductive system and to describe common genital tract anomalies. Details of surgical or nonsurgical correction of these anomalies are

presented. Obstetrical, gynecologic, and urologic consequences of these defects are described.

Embryology and Development

The reproductive organs consist of gonads, a ductal system, and external genitalia. Although the final maturation of the reproductive organs occurs after birth, the critical developmental steps occur during the embryonic and fetal periods of development. Initially, the reproductive system is capable of developing along either male or female lines. Sexual differentiation is dependent upon the genetic sex that is determined at fertilization by the presence or absence of the Y chromosome. In the presence of the Y chromosome, the gonads develop as testes leading to the production of hormones that promote the development of the male or wolffian ductal system and the regression of the female or müllerian ductal system.

Gonadal Differentiation

Under the influence of the sex-determining region of the Y-chromosome (SRY), the embryonic genital ridges form testes. The presence of the SRY gene sets in motion a cascade of events that ultimately results in testicular development.[1] Other genes that are important in mediating sexual differentiation include *SF-1*[2,3] and *DAX-1*.[4] Initially, cells in the medullary region of the primitive sex cord differentiate into the Sertoli cells and these cells organize to form the testicular cords. Testicular cords are identifiable at 6 weeks and consist of tightly packed germ cells. Early in the second trimester the cords develop a lumen and become seminiferous tubules.[5,6]

The developing Sertoli cells begin to secrete müllerian-inhibiting substance (MIS) during the weeks 7–8 of development. MIS secreted by the Sertoli cells cause the ipsilateral paramesonephric (müllerian) duct system to regress (Fig. 4.1). The

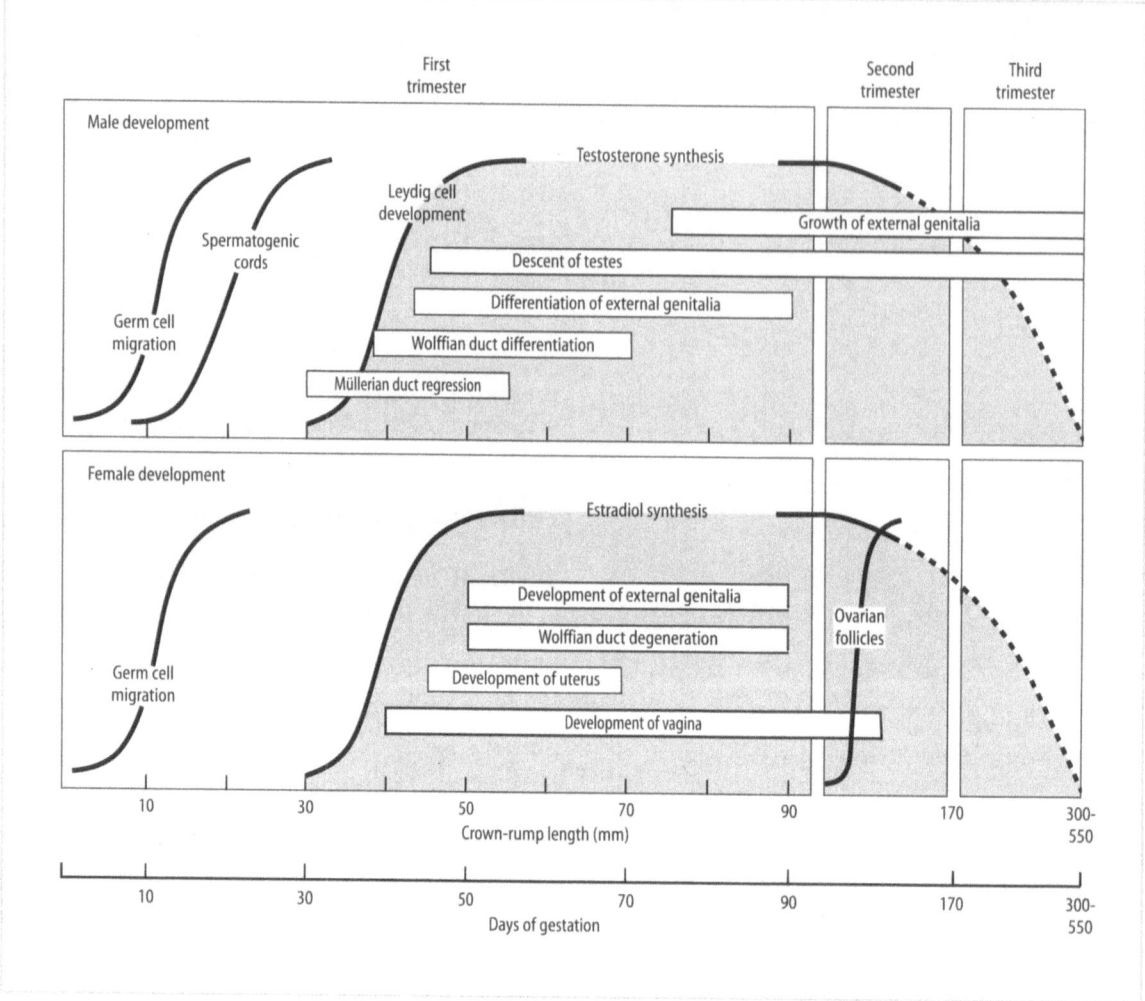

Figure 4.1 Scheme of prenatal development of reproductive system in relation to embryonic/fetal length and age. Reprinted with permission from Wilson JD, George FW, Griffin JE. The hormonal control of sexual development. Science 1981; 211:1279. Copyright 1981 American Association for the Advancement of Science.

disappearance of the müllerian ducts in the male fetus is completed by weeks 9–10 of gestation. MIS may also control the rapid gubernacular growth necessary for the transabdominal descent of the testes.[7] Serum MIS levels remain elevated in boys during childhood and then decline at puberty to the low levels seen in adult men. In contrast, girls have undetectable levels of MIS until the onset of puberty when serum MIS levels become measurable.[8]

Leydig cell differentiation begins 1 week after Sertoli cell development. The Leydig cells begin to secrete testosterone by week 8 of gestation and testosterone production peaks at weeks 15–18 as a result of stimulation of the testes by human chorionic gonadotropin (hCG). Testosterone acts in a paracrine manner on the ipsilateral mesonephric (wolffian) duct to accomplish virilization of the wolffian duct into the epididymis, vas deferens, and seminal vesicle. Dihydrotestosterone, derived from 5-a reduction of testosterone, causes the differ-

entiation of the external genitalia from the urogenital sinus and genital tubercle. Testosterone and dihydrotestosterone are essential for the development of the male phenotype. Androgens produced by the testes control the differentiation and growth of the internal and external genitalia and also prime male differentiation of the brain.[9,10]

In the female embryo, without the influence of the Y chromosome, the bipotential gonad develops into an ovary. This occurs about 2 weeks after testicular development in the male and is characterized by the absence of testicular cords. The primitive sex cords degenerate and the mesothelium of the genital ridge forms secondary sex cords. These secondary sex cords become the follicles that surround the germ cells, while the medullary portion regresses and forms the rete ovarii within the hilum of the ovary. The primordial germ cells proliferate by mitosis and reach a maximum number of 5–7 million by 20 weeks of gestation. At this time, the fetal ovary demonstrates mature organization with the presence of primordial follicles containing oocytes and stroma. The oocytes within the primordial follicles begin meiosis and are arrested at the diplotene phase of meiosis I until that oocyte undergoes ovulation after menarche. Atresia of the oocytes occurs, leading to the reduction of the number of germ cells present at birth.[5,6]

Ductal System Development

Sexual differentiation of the reproductive ducts begins early in the fetal period (35 mm) and is attributed to the influence of gonadal hormones (testosterone and MIS) on the dual mesonephric (wolffian) and paramesonephric (müllerian) ducts.[5,6] In the XX embryo, in the absence of fetal testes, the lack of testosterone and MIS secretion allows for the maturation of the müllerian ducts. In the XY embryo, the male ductal system of the vas deferens, epididymis, and seminal vesicle develops as a result of the local secretion of testosterone by the ipsilateral testes while the müllerian ducts degenerate under the influence of MIS. Although heterologous ducts in each sex mostly regress, remnants can be found and may become clinically apparent by forming cysts.[5,6]

In the female, in the absence of MIS, the paramesophric ducts persist. The paramesonephric ducts grow caudally and along with the mesonephric ducts become enclosed in peritoneal folds that later give rise to the broad ligaments of the uterus to which the ovaries (mesovarium), fallopian tubes (mesosalpinx), and uterus (mesometrium) are attached. The paramesonephric ducts approach each other and begin to fuse even before they reach the urogenital sinus. The fused ducts form a tube with a single lumen called the uterovaginal canal which forms the uterus and upper portion of the vagina while the unfused cranial portions of the paramesonephric ducts become the fallopian tubes.[5,6] Vaginal agenesis is caused by failure of caudal migration of the paramesonephric ducts. In the normal female, the uterine corpus and uterine cervix differentiate and the uterine wall thickens by 12 weeks.

The distal third of the vagina develops from bilateral proliferations known as the sinovaginal bulbs which may arise from the urogenital sinus.[5,6] Meanwhile, the most inferior portion of the uterovaginal canal becomes occluded by a cellular mass termed the vaginal plate. The cells of the vaginal plate desquamate during the second trimester, allowing for canalization of the vaginal lumen. Defects in vertical fusion occur when there is incomplete canalization of the vaginal plate. This may take the form of a transverse septum, which can occur at varying sites and various thicknesses in the vagina.

The hymen is the partition that persists to a varying degree between the dilated, canalized, fused sinovaginal bulbs and the urogenital sinus. The hymen usually becomes perforated shortly before or shortly after birth. An imperforate hymen, which represents persistence of the membrane separating the canalized caudal end of the paramesonephric ducts from the evaginated urogenital sinus, is another example of a lateral fusion defect.

External Genitalia

The early development of the external genitalia is similar in both sexes. By week 6 of gestation, three external protuberances have developed surrounding the cloacal membrane; these are the left and right genital swellings which meet anterior to the cloacal membrane to form the genital tubercle.[5] Ultimately, the genital swellings become the labioscrotal folds. The urogenital sinus extends on to the surface of the enlarging genital tubercle to form the urethral groove which is flanked on either side by the urethral folds and lie within the labioscrotal folds. By week 7 of gestation, the urogenital membrane ruptures exposing the cavity of the urogenital sinus to the amniotic fluid. The genital tubercle elongates to form the phallus. The coronary sulcus that surrounds the phallus represents the primordium of the glans penis and glans clitoris[5] (Fig. 4.2).

It is not until the week 12 of gestation that one is able to visually identify a difference between male and female external genitalia.[5,9,10] In the male fetus, because of the effects of dihydrotestosterone formed locally by the 5-a reduction of testosterone, the anogenital distance lengthens, the labioscrotal folds fuse to form the scrotum, and subsequently the urethral folds fuse to enclose the penile urethra.[5] In the female fetus, in the absence of testosterone, the anogenital distance does not lengthen and the labioscrotal and urethral folds do not fuse. The genital tubercle bends caudally to become the clitoris and the urogenital sinus becomes the vestibule of the vagina. The labioscrotal folds become the labia majora while the urethral folds persist as the labia minora.[5]

Anomalies of the Female Ductal System

Anomalies of the female ductal system are classified into three separate groups on the basis of similar embryonic developmental defects and clinical presentation (Table 4.1).[11]

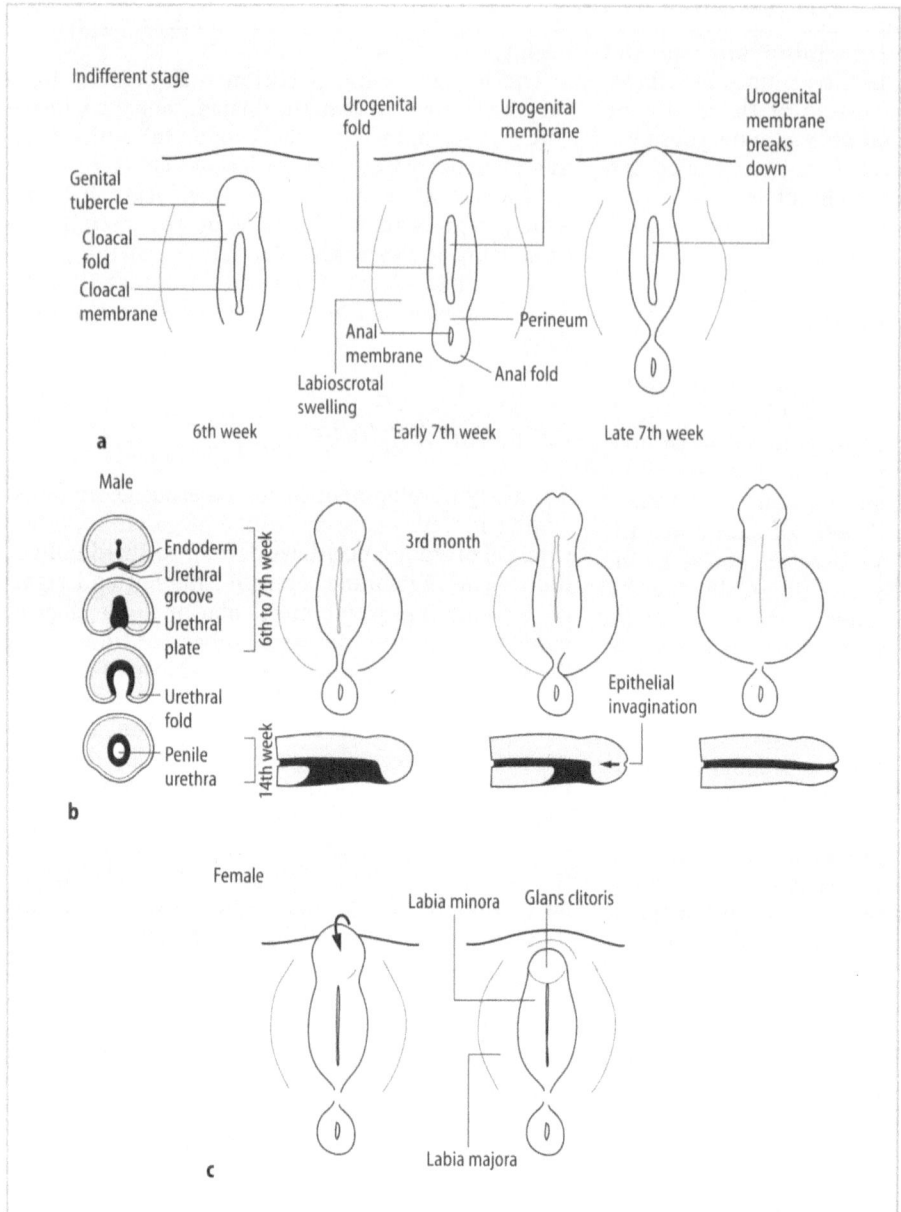

Indifferent stage

Figure 4.2 Development of external genitalia. **a** Indifferent stage. **b** Under influence of testosterone and dihydro-testosterone, virilization of external genitalia occurs. **c** In the absence of androgens, feminization occurs.

Table 4.1. Anomalies of the female ductal system

I	Agenesis of the uterus and vagina (Rokitansky–Kuster–Hauser syndrome)
II	Defects in vertical fusion
A	Obstructive
B	Nonobstructive
III	Defects in lateral fusion
A	Obstructive
B	Nonobstructive

Agenesis of the Uterus and Vagina (Rokitansky–Kuster–Hauser syndrome)

The most serious developmental anomaly of the female reproductive tract is congenital absence of the uterus and vagina. In this disorder, the müllerian derivative of the vagina and the remaining müllerian ducts destined to become the uterus fail to develop. The incidence of this disorder among newborn females is approximately 1 per 2000–5000.[12]

Clinical Presentation

Females with müllerian agenesis have normal external genitalia and the diagnosis of müllerian agenesis is therefore rarely made in infancy. Individuals with this disorder usually present at or after the expected time of puberty with primary amenorrhea. These patients have a normal karyotype (46XX) and normal secondary sex characteristics. Because the ovaries are not müllerian structures, they are present and function normally allowing for normal breast development, a female body habitus, and a normal female escutcheon. However, either complete absence of the vagina is noted or a small dimple representing the urogenital sinus origin of the distal vagina is present. Rectal examination reveals the absence of the uterus. Rarely, in less than 1% of patients, these rudimentary horns contain functioning endometrium causing cyclic abdominal pain due to obstructed hematometra. Surgical excision of functioning rudimentary horns is the only condition requiring intra-abdominal exploration.[11]

Müllerian agenesis is associated with abnormalities of the upper urinary tract as well as with spine and skeletal abnormalities. The incidence of major urinary tract anomalies such as unilateral renal agenesis, unilateral or bilateral pelvic kidney, or horseshoe kidney is approximately 15%.[11,12] If more minor anomalies, such as hydronephrosis, hydroureter, malrotation of the kidney and collecting system duplication are included the incidence rises to approximately 40%.[11-13] Anomalies of the skeletal system occur in approximately 5-10% of women with müllerian agenesis.[11-13] These abnormalities primarily affect the spine and include wedge vertebrae, fusions, rudimentary and supernumerary vertebrae, and scoliosis. Rarely deafness is associated with müllerian agenesis, because of abnormalities of the small bones of the middle ear.

Diagnosis

Since most women with müllerian agenesis have normal external genitalia, this condition does not often become apparent until the time of expected menarche. The patients generally present with normal breast and pubic hair development, but primary amenorrhea. Although the presence or absence of a uterus may often be appreciated on rectal examination, sonography is often necessary to confirm the absence of a uterus. More recently, magnetic resonance imaging (MRI) has been utilized to delineate the extent of genital and urinary tract abnormalities.[14,15] Imaging of the renal system is also essential.

Müllerian agenesis may also be confused with androgen resistance syndrome in which there may also be a shallow vaginal pouch and no uterus. Complete androgen resistance syndrome is more likely in patients with scant or absent pubic and axillary hair. The definitive method for distinguishing between müllerian agenesis and complete androgen resistance syndrome is to determine the karyotype of the patient. Patients with müllerian agenesis have a 46XX karyotype, whereas those with complete androgen resistance have a 46XY karyotype and normal male levels of testosterone.

Etiology

The etiology of müllerian agenesis is not completely understood, but mutations or defects in embryonic gene expression of a series of genes known as homeobox or HOX have been described. These genes share an expressed region which define positional identities along the anterior-posterior body axis. This suggests that normal müllerian development may be dependent upon the specific balance of HOX gene expression.[16,17,18]

Treatment

The goal of treatment for women with müllerian agenesis is to restore normal sexual function through the creation of a neo-vagina. Before the 1930s, treatment of congenital absence of the vagina was notoriously unsuccessful. Use of small or large bowel to provide a mucosal lining after perineal cavitation was abandoned because of unacceptably high morbidity and mortality. Pedunculated skin grafts have been attempted, but these have been abandoned because of marked scaring, the need for multiple operations, and poor functional results.

In the late 1930s, Frank developed a nonsurgical technique for the successful creation of a neo-vagina.[19] Frank demonstrated that systematically applied pressure to the perineal dimple can result in a functional neo-vagina in some women with congenital absence of the vagina. Initially, the patient places a dilator measuring 1.5 cm at its outside diameter and 15 cm in length at the vaginal dimple and applies pressure downward daily for 20 minutes. This is performed for the first week to stretch the mucosa and to prevent distorting the urethral meatus. Subsequently, the direction of the dilator is changed so that it is parallel to the axis of the normal vagina. The dilator is held in place with enough pressure to cause minimal discomfort for 20-30 minutes each day. Within 6-8 weeks, a vaginal length of 7.5 cm can be obtained.[19,20] The vagina will lengthen further with regular coital activity. In the absence of coitus, dilation with the dilators must be done several times weekly to maintain the vaginal depth and caliber. Although it is agreed that when a neo-vagina can be created by the intermittent pressure technique it is equal in function to that achieved by a contemporary surgical procedure, only 10–25% of women[21] can successfully create a neo-vagina using the Frank technique. Reasons cited for the high failure rate include the inability to generate adequate perineal pressure manually for the required periods of time each day, the difficulty and boredom of maintaining the physical position required to manually apply perineal pressure for an adequate time, and the difficulty in devoting the requisite time necessary each day.

In order to overcome these problems, Ingram described a modified approach which utilizes the patient's own body weight in a sitting position to obtain passive dilation.[21] Ingram developed a simple bicycle seat stool on which the patient sits to apply pressure to lucite vaginal dilators. The patient places the appropriate dilator at the vaginal dimple and it is held in place by a light girdle. The patient may then wear any outer clothing and sits on the bicycle stool, leaning slightly forward, for intervals of 15–30 minutes for a total of 2 hours per day. Ingram initially reported a 71% success rate.[21] As with the Frank method, success is dependent on the maturity of the patient and her willingness to commit the necessary time.

The most commonly used method for surgical creation of the neo-vagina is the McIndoe procedure.[22] McIndoe emphasized three important principles governing the success of this procedure:

- the dissection of an adequate space between the rectum and the bladder
- the placement of a split thickness skin graft
- the necessity of continuous and prolonged stenting of the neo-vagina during the healing process.

Although McIndoe was not the first to use skin grafts after perineal cavitation, he was the first to emphasize the importance of prolonged stent dilation during the postoperative period (Fig. 4.3).

The procedure itself consists of obtaining the graft followed by creating a neo-vaginal space. First, the patient is positioned to harvest a skin graft from the buttocks. For cosmetic reasons, the buttocks are the preferred site rather than the thigh or the hip. An electrodermatome is set to obtain a graft 0.5 mm thick and 8–9 cm wide. The total graft length should be 20–25 cm. If an adequate graft length cannot be obtained from one buttock, a graft can be taken from each buttock and the resultant skin grafts can be sutured together. The donor site is dressed with fine mesh gauze and the patient is repositioned in dorsal lithotomy. The skin graft is then sutured around a vaginal form using 4-0 nonreactive suture.

The form for the vaginal cavity is shaped from foam rubber and then covered with sterile condoms.[12,23] Alternatively, a Hayer–Schulte inflatable stent can be used.

The neo-vaginal space is created by incising the vaginal dimple with a transverse incision and then bluntly dissecting the space between the rectum and bladder along each side of the median raphe. The dissection is carried to the peritoneum and the median raphe is excised sharply. The dissection is completed when a button of peritoneum is seen. After obtaining meticulous hemostasis, the vaginal form covered with the skin graft is inserted into the vaginal cavity and sutured to the perineum with interrupted nonreactive 3-0 suture. The mold is further retained by suturing the labia minora across the mold.[12,23] It is essential that the vaginal bed is dry. Bleeding between the graft and the vaginal bed will prevent the graft from adhering to the vaginal bed and increases the chance of failure.

Immediately postoperatively, the patient remains on strict bedrest with a Foley catheter in place. She is also placed on a low-residue diet and stool softeners to minimize her need to strain for a bowel movement. Prophylactic antibiotics are prescribed until the stent is removed. One week after surgery, the patient returns to the operating room, the vaginal form is removed, the neo-vagina is copiously irrigated and the graft is inspected. The patient is then instructed on removing, cleaning, and replacing the form daily.

Early postoperative complications which have been reported include bleeding, failure of the graft to take and injury to adjacent structures.[12] Formation of postoperative rectovaginal, urethrovaginal, and vesicovaginal fistulae have also been described. Granulation tissue may also develop and may be treated by silver nitrate cauterization or excision. Finally, postoperative stricture may occur possibly requiring additional dilation or reoperation to maintain patency of the neo-vagina. Patient satisfaction ranges from 78% to 100%.[11,24] In general, the success of the procedure depends on the maturity of the patient and her motivation to retain and care for the postoperative stent. A recent modification of the McIndoe procedure involves utilizing Interceed absorbable adhesion barrier in place of the skin graft.[25]

Problems of Vertical Fusion

Problems of vertical fusion occur when there is incomplete cavitation of the vaginal plate formed by the down-growing müllerian ducts and the up-growing urogenital sinus. These disorders may be considered in two categories: imperforate hymen

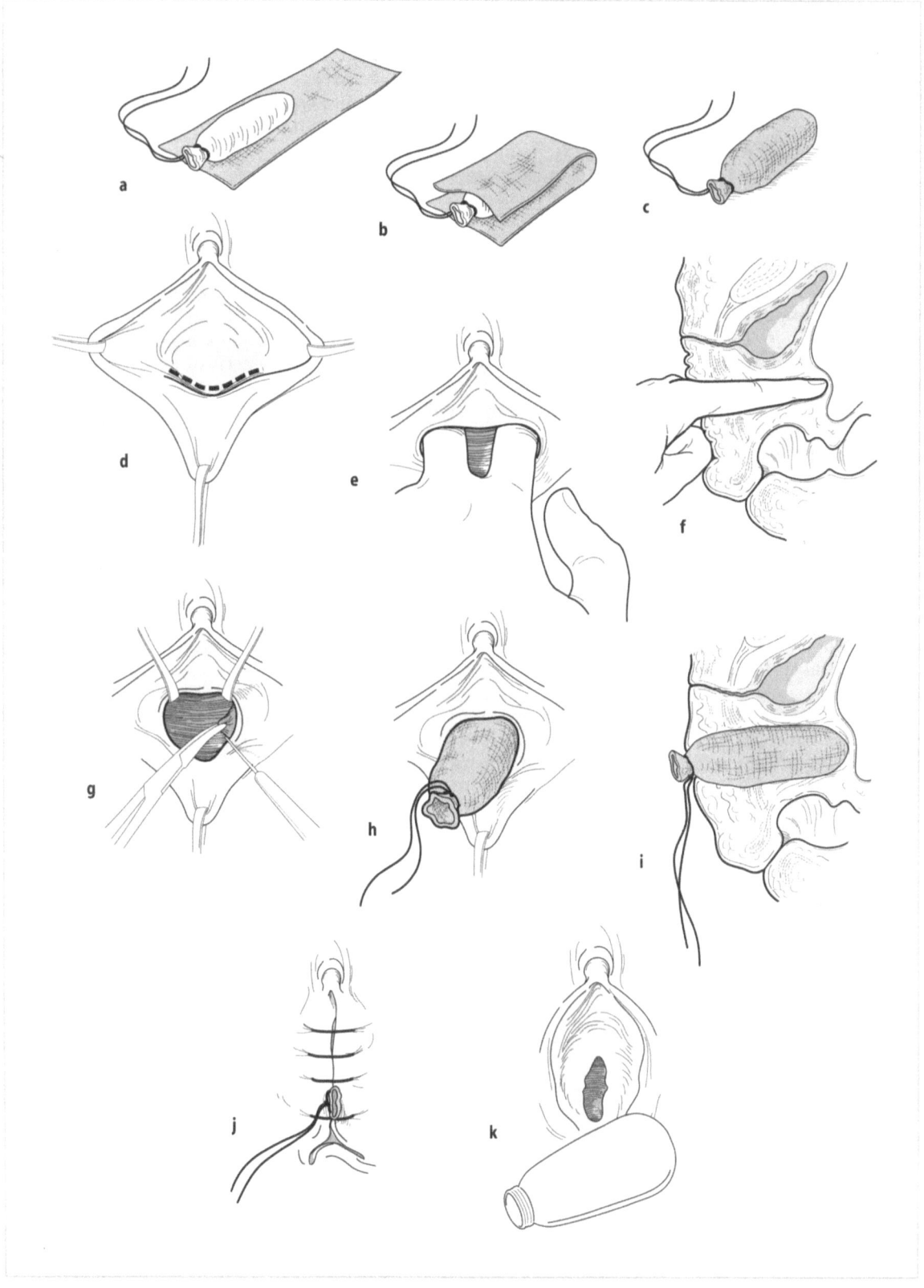

Figure 4.3 Steps involved in McIndoe vaginoplasty. Step 1: Split thickness skin graft is obtained (**a**). Step 2: Skin graft sutured in place over vaginal mold (**b**, **c**). Step 3: McIndoe vaginoplasty incision in perineum (**d**). Sharp and blunt dissection to create opening for neovagina (**e**, **f**). Hemostasis obtained (**g**), skin graft placed (**h**, **i**). Labia sutured (**j**). Postoperative dilation (**k**).

and transverse vaginal septum, each of which can be obstructive or nonobstructive.

Clinical Presentation

Most patients with an obstructive transverse vaginal septum or imperforate hymen are diagnosed as having these conditions at or shortly after menarche. At this time, there is usually development of cyclic pelvic pain due to hematocolpos or hematometra. A hymeneal membrane or a blind-ending pouch of varying depth is found on vaginal exam. Rectal examination reveals a vaginal mass representing hematocolpos. These conditions may also be encountered in infancy when large amounts of mucus collect behind the obstructing membrane.

Patients with imperforate hymen usually present after the initiation of menses when accumulated menstrual blood bulges behind the imperforate hymen. As menstruation recurs, the vagina becomes greatly overdistended and the cervix begins to distend allowing for the formation of a hematometra and hematosalpinx. In the case of a transverse vaginal septum, there is no bulging at the outlet, but the mass can be appreciated by rectal exam or visualized by sonography. The hydromucocolpos or hematocolpos can sometimes become quite large and be mistaken for a lower abdominal or pelvic mass.

The incidence of transverse septum has been reported as 1 in 2100 to 1 in 72 000.[26] Transverse vaginal septum can vary in thickness and the septum can be present at varying sites within the vaginal canal (Fig. 4.4). Occasionally, a transverse vaginal septum is not complete. Women with a partial transverse vaginal septum may present because of dyspareunia or because of a complication pertaining to reproduction.

Diagnosis

It is usually straightforward to distinguish between an obstructive transverse vaginal septum and an imperforate hymen. Rectal examination and ultrasonography can be used to identify the presence or absence of a uterus. If there is no uterus, the diagnosis of müllerian agenesis or androgen resistance should be considered. If a uterus is present, then, by definition, the diagnosis is either imperforate hymen or transverse vaginal septum. The goal at this point is to ascertain the exact location of the obstruction and its thickness. MRI is a useful tool to determine preoperatively the location of the obstruction as well as its extent and the anatomy proximal to the obstruction. Finally, in contrast to müllerian agenesis, transverse vaginal septum are rarely associated with urologic or other congenital anomalies.

Treatment

Imperforate hymen is treated in a sterile, operating room environment. The hymenal membrane is incised with a cruciate incision at the 2, 4, 8 and

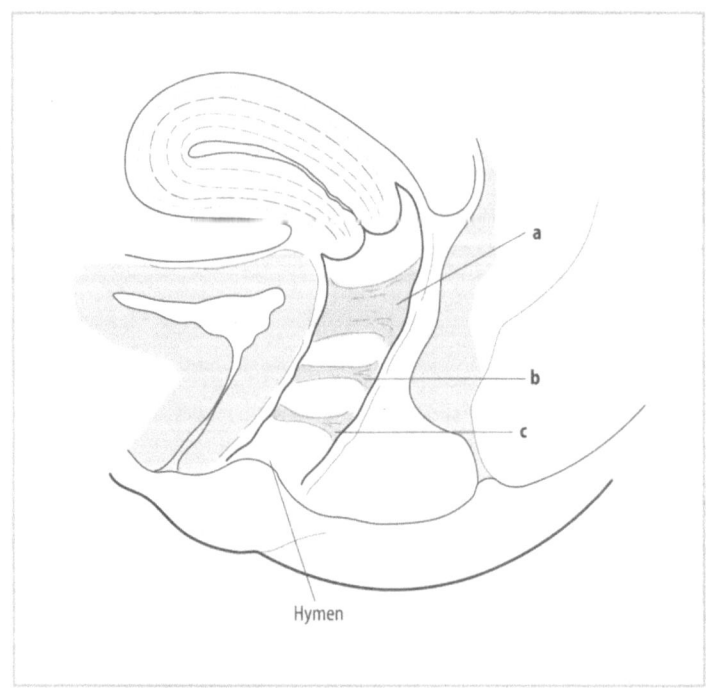

Hymen

Figure 4.4 Positions of septa responsible for complete vaginal obstruction. **a** High transverse vaginal septum is in most instances thicker than septum in middle and lower vagina. **b** Transverse septum in middle third of vagina. **c** Transverse septum in lower third of vagina.

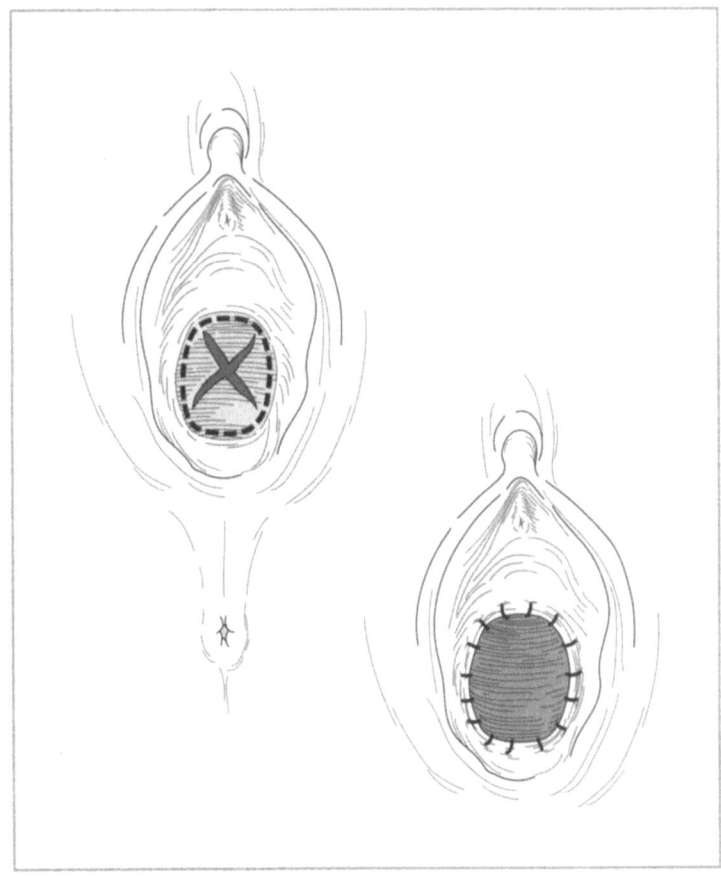

Figure 4.5 Excision of imperforate hymen. Stellate incisions are made through hymenal membrane at 2-, 4-, 8-, and 10-o'clock positions. Individual quadrants are excised along the lateral wall of the vagina, avoiding excision of the vagina. Inset, Margins of vaginal mucosa are approximated with fine delayed-absorbable suture.

10 o'clock positions and the accumulated hemato-colpos is evacuated. The quadrants of the hymen are then excised and the vaginal mucosa is re-approximated using fine delayed-absorbable suture (Fig. 4.5).

In the case of a transverse vaginal septum, a prudent first step is simply to aspirate a small amount of accumulated fluid behind the obstructing membrane or septum with a needle using sterile technique. This provides information on the location of the distended cavity behind the obstruction so that one can avoid the urethra above and the rectum below. Also, manipulation of the needle provides information on the thickness of the obstruction. A transverse incision is made in the vaginal septum followed by blunt and sharp dissection to identify the cervix[11] (Fig. 4.6). It is important to note that the cervix behind a transverse vaginal septum does not have the characteristic appearance of vaginal mucosa. Instead, it appears adenomatous like that of the endocervical canal. The upper vagina that was present behind the obstruction also has this appearance. However, once the obstruction is removed, these cells undergo squamous metaplasia and eventually will resemble the distal vagina. After identification of the cervix, the lateral margins of the septum are excised and the edges of the upper and lower vaginal mucosa are anastomosed.

Occasionally, the thickness of the transverse vaginal septum is such that anastomosis of the upper and lower vagina is not possible. In this circumstance, it is necessary to use an indwelling stent. Jones describes a Lucite form with a bulbous tip at one end.[27] These forms also have an internal channel to allow the egress of menstrual blood. This form is inserted into the upper vagina after the transverse vaginal septum is excised. As the dissected area contracts, the Lucite form will retain its shape. The stent is left in place for 4–6 months, allowing for epithelization of the area between the upper and lower vagina. Following removal of the Lucite stent, vaginal dilation should be performed daily for 2–4 months to prevent contracture of the space.

In very thick transverse septums a modified Pena procedure approach may be indicated. With the patient in the prone position the rectum is mobilized and the obstruction is resected via the posterior approach. The vagina is then mobilized and brought down to the perineum, or a skin graft is placed. A temporary colostomy may be necessary if dissection of the rectum is extensive.[28]

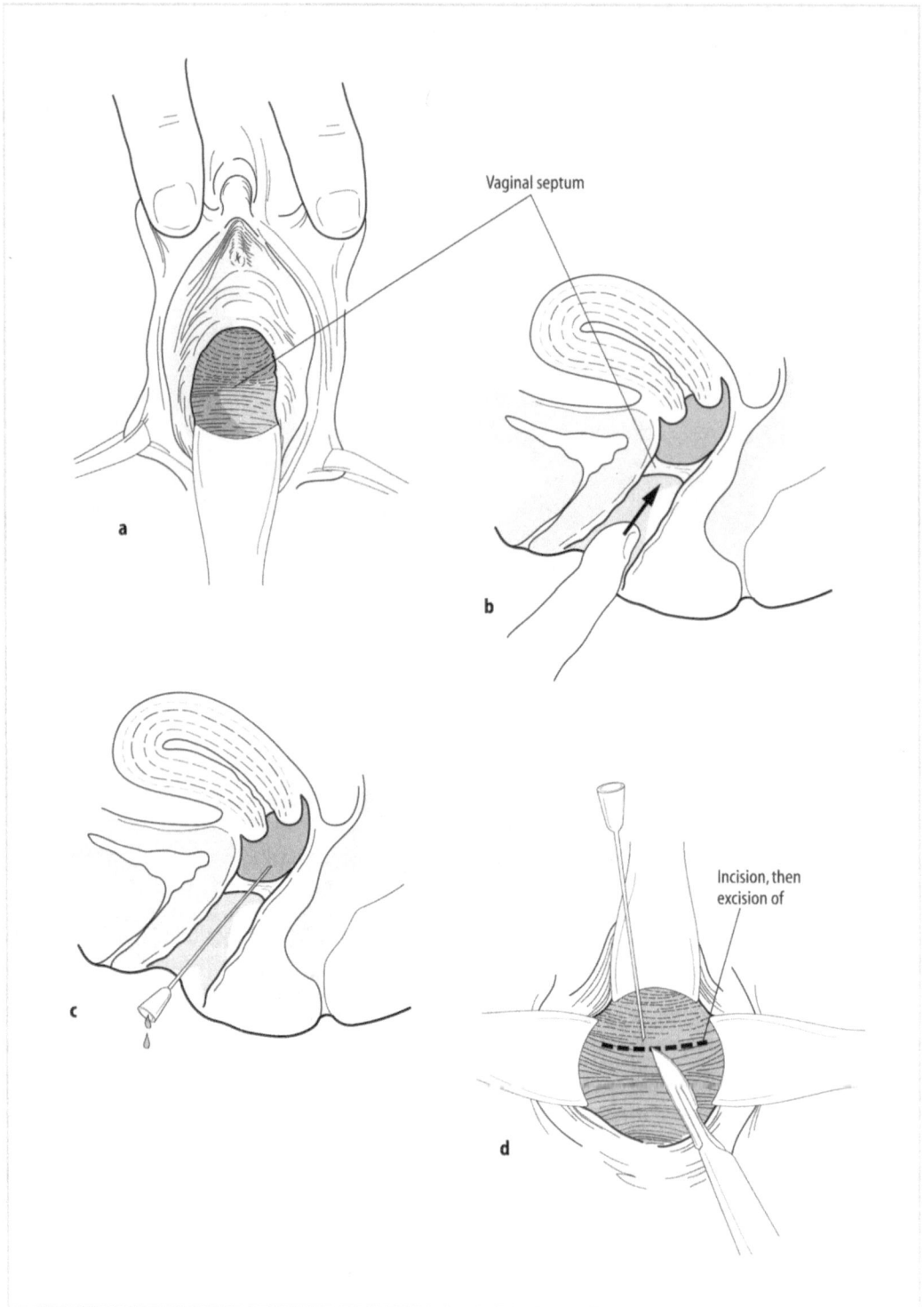

Figure 4.6 High transverse vaginal septum. **a** Neovaginal space is dissected revealing a high obstructing vaginal septum. **b** This may be palpated with the middle finger. **c** A needle is then placed into the mass over which the incision is made with a sharp knife. **d** Excision of septum is performed.

It is recommended that a laparoscopy be performed in patients undergoing surgery for transverse vaginal septum to identify the presence and extent of endometriosis. Endometriosis is common in these patients due to the retrograde flow of menstrual blood. Endometriosis can be treated laparoscopically, and postoperative treatment can consist of GnRH agonist, continuous oral contraceptive, or

Depo-Provera injections. It should be noted, however, that endometriosis associated with vaginal obstruction often resolves spontaneously once the obstruction is removed.

Normal coital function can be achieved in virtually all cases after excision of the obstructing septum. The only failures occur in cases where a thick vaginal septum was excised and there is poor compliance maintaining the postoperative stent.

Pregnancy success following surgical correction of imperforate hymen or a transverse vaginal septum has been reported by Rock and colleagues,[29] who treated 22 patients for imperforate hymen. Of 15 patients attempting pregnancy, 86% conceived and 66% had a living child. In the case of transverse vaginal septum, 19 patients attempted pregnancy, 47% conceived, and 36% had a living child. Pregnancy was more likely when the transverse vaginal septum was in the lower or middle third of the vagina.

Rarely, cervical agenesis or cervical atresia is diagnosed in association with a defect in vaginal development. MRI has been demonstrated to be useful in diagnosing cervical agenesis.[30] The goal of treatment is to relieve cyclic abdominal pain and to prevent the development of endometriosis. Although some authors have reported the surgical creation of a fistulous tract between the uterus and vagina, only one successful pregnancy has been reported. Most of these women require multiple surgical procedures to keep the fistula tract patent and have a high incidence of infectious morbidity. Ultimately, most require hysterectomy. Therefore, the preferred form of treatment for cervical agenesis is hysterectomy.[31]

Problems of Lateral Fusion

Problems of lateral fusion can conveniently be grouped into two categories: obstructive and non-obstructive. These will be discussed in turn.

Problems of Lateral Fusion with Obstruction

Problems of lateral fusion with obstruction develop when there is failure of lateral fusion of two müllerian ducts, and also failure of one duct to communicate with the outside. Thus, there is unilateral obstruction.

Problems of lateral fusion with obstruction can be classified according to the site of obstruction. Typically, these patients have a double uterus, double cervix, and double vagina. They vary in terms of whether there is complete obstruction low in the vagina, communication between the two vaginas or communication laterally between the two uteri (panels a, b, and c respectively in Fig. 4.7). Occasionally, the obstruction is at the level of the uterine fundus and involves an isolated horn of the uterus with minimal connection to the unobstructed side.[24]

Clinical presentation

Patients present with varying degrees of dysmenorrhea, abdominal pain, and vaginal mass depending on the level of the obstruction and the presence of any lateral communication. For instance, patients characterized by panel a in Fig. 4.7 present with a paravaginal mass (hematocolpos), severe dysmenorrhea, and lower abdominal pain. Regular menses

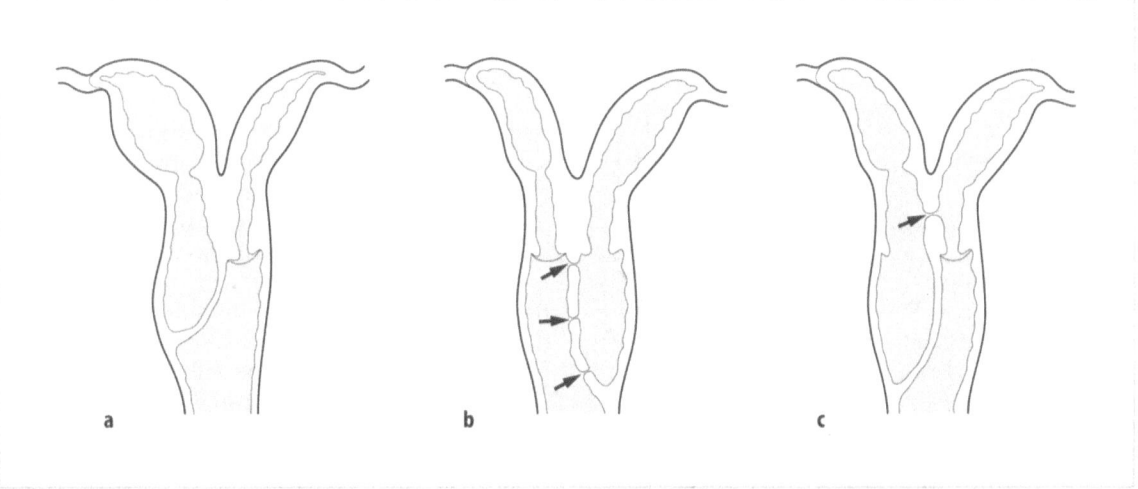

Figure 4.7 Findings in uterus didelphis with obstructed hemivagina. **a** Complete obstruction. **b** Partial vaginal communication. **c** Partial uterine communication.

occur, but are associated with progressively severe dysmenorrhea from the time of menarche. An IVP shows renal agenesis on the obstructive side in virtually all cases. Patients characterized by panel **b** (Fig. 4 7) present with lower abdominal pain, moderate to severe dysmenorrhea, and intermittent, foul, mucopurulent discharge. Commonly, there is also unpredictable staining between menstrual cycles. Finally, patients characterized by panel **c** (Fig. 4.7) report dysmenorrhea and a vaginal mass that disappears after menstruation. In this group, although symptoms begin shortly after menarche, diagnosis is often delayed for 5–10 years. When there is an isolated uterine horn with minimal connection to the unobstructed side, there can often be dysmenorrhea, and the development of endometriosis associated with retrograde menstruation.

Diagnosis

Diagnosis of these conditions is often extremely difficult. If obstruction occurs low in the vagina, as in panel **a** of Fig. 4.7, a large amount of blood may accumulate and the condition may go unrecognized for some time. Evidently, the vagina can distend to accommodate the increments of blood resulting from each successive menstrual period, and in the early stages there is sufficient absorption of blood between menstrual periods to prevent the development of severe pain.[32]

Patients who report intermittent, foul, mucopurulent discharge without evident etiology, or a disappearing vaginal mass associated with intermenstrual bloody vaginal discharge, should be suspected as having a problem of lateral fusion. A careful pelvic examination should be performed to identify a paravaginal mass. Sometimes a tract can be identified in the vagina through which a fine metal probe can be passed. Ultrasound and hysterosalpingography are extremely helpful in pinpointing the nature of the problem.

Treatment

Treatment consists of complete excision of the vaginal septum. So long as retrograde menstruation has not caused severe tubal damage due to hematosalpinx, and there has not been the development of a significant amount of endometriosis, reproductive capacity should not be compromised.[11,32]

In cases where an isolated horn of the uterus has minimal connection to the unobstructed side, treatment consists of excising the obstructed uterine horn. This is advised in order to prevent the development of endometriosis from retrograde men-

struation, and to prevent the development of a pregnancy in the rudimentary horn.

Problems of Lateral Fusion Without Obstruction

Several conditions may be considered in this category (Fig. 4.8): didelphic uterus, unicornuate uterus, bicornuate uterus, and septate uterus.

Didelphic uterus

In this condition, there is nonobstructed failure of lateral fusion involving both the uterus and the vagina. In effect, there is a double uterus, double cervix, and double vagina. Reproductive capacity is essentially normal, although there are anecdotal case reports in which it is suggested that the didelphic uterus is associated with primary infertility, pregnancy wastage, and premature labor. In many cases, intercourse is possible in both vaginal cavities, and there have been reports of simultaneous pregnancies in the two uterine horns. Occasionally, the vagina may be narrowed by the vertical septum and dyspareunia may result. This is the only circumstance in which the vaginal septum should be excised. No other treatment is generally necessary.

Unicornuate uterus

Since the didelphic uterus represent a mirror-image duplication of the unicornuate uterus, reproductive potential is approximately the same (i.e. essentially normal) in both situations. Since no vaginal septum is present, there is no indication for surgical intervention in the unicornuate situation.[12,24]

Bicornuate and septate uterus

As can be seen in Fig. 4.8, the bicornuate uterus has a very different external configuration from the septate uterus. It may also be appreciated that a hysterosalpingogram would not be particularly useful in distinguishing between the two. This distinction, however, is of critical importance because the bicornuate uterus is associated with only minimal reproductive difficulties, whereas the septate uterus is frequently involved with repeated miscarriage.[33]

In the bicornuate uterus, two distinct horns (or at least a midline depression in the uterine contour) can be appreciated. It is important to go to such lengths to make the diagnosis, because a septate uterus is a surgically correctable condition that has a firm association with repeated miscarriage,

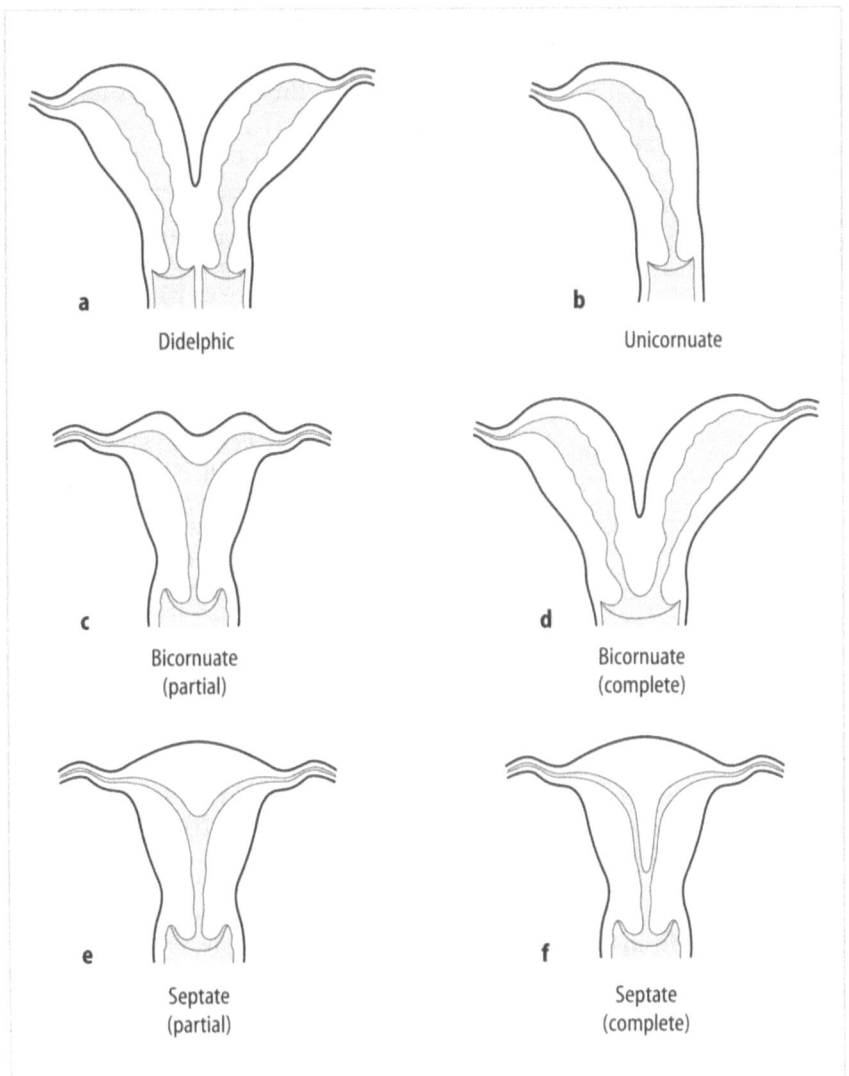

Figure 4.8 Various forms of double uterus. **a** Didelphic. **b** Unicornuate. **c** Bicornuate (partial). **d** bicornuate (complete). **e** Septate (partial). **f** Septate (complete). From: Rock JA, Murphy AA, Jones HW Jr (1992) Female Reproductive Surgery. Williams & Wilkins, Baltimore.

whereas a bicornuate uterus probably represents an incidental finding.[34-37]

After all other causes of habitual abortion have been ruled out, and a septate uterus is documented, treatment consists of excising the septum. Historically, this has been most commonly accomplished with a transabdominal metroplasty following either the Jones or Tompkins technique. Currently, the hysteroscopic approach for resection of an uterine septum either with scissors or electro-cautery has become the procedure of choice. Recent large studies evaluating the pregnancy rate after hysteroscopic metroplasty report 36 month cumulative pregnancy rates ranging from 63% to 89%. In addition, the spontaneous loss rate decreases significantly following hysteroscopic metroplasty.[36,39-41]

Abnormal Sexual Differentiation (Congenital Genital Ambiguity)

One of the most delicate responsibilities of the obstetrician is the assignment of sex to the newborn. A profound dilemma exists in the event of ambiguity of the external genitalia. Ambiguous external genitalia in a newborn is a true medical emergency and represents a diagnostic challenge. The development of ambiguous external genitalia is

Table 4.2. Classification of ambiguous genitalia

Category I	Female pseudohermaphroditism
Category II	Male pseudohermaphroditism
Category III	Disorders of genetic or gonadal development
a	Gonadal dysgenesis
b	True hermaphroditism
c	Embryonic testicular regression

due to abnormal or inappropriate androgen exposure in utero. Table 4.2 and Fig. 4.9 present a classification scheme for the evaluation of the newborn with sexual ambiguity.

Female Pseudohermaphroditism (Category I)

Too much androgen exposure in an embryo or fetus destined to be a female results in the development of female pseudohermaphroditism. The karyotype is 46XX. The ovaries and the female internal genital structures such as the uterus, cervix, and upper vagina are present. The external genitalia are virilized, with the degree of virilization dependent on the amount and the timing in embryonic development of the androgen excess. Virilization may result in an entire spectrum from modest clitoromegaly to posterior labial fusion and development of a phallus. Are all potentially fertile.

The etiology of female pseudohermaphroditism is excessive androgen exposure in utero due to adrenal abnormalities or nonadrenal sources of androgen. Congenital adrenal hyperplasia due to deficiency of 21-hydroxylase is the most common cause of female pseudohermaphroditism. 11-β-hydroxylase and 3-β-hydroxysteroid dehydrogenase deficiency can also result in ambiguous genitalia.[42] Nonadrenal causes include maternal exposure to drugs such as danazol or testosterone. Virilizing ovarian tumors, such as luteoma of pregnancy, Sertoli–Leydig cell tumor or virilizing adrenal tumors, or other undetermined causes may be the source of androgen excess.[43]

Male Pseudohermaphroditism (Category II)

Too little androgen exposure in utero in an embryo or fetus destined to be a male leads to male pseudohermaphroditism. The karyotype is 46XY and testes are present. The uterus is absent because of the normal embryonic production of müllerian inhibitory factor. These patients are most often sterile due to abnormal spermatogenesis and an inadequate phallus for sexual function.

The etiology of male pseudohermaphroditism is due to:

● enzyme defects in the biosynthesis of testosterone, or
● peripheral enzyme defects, or
● abnormalities in the androgen receptor.

There are five enzyme defects associated with impairments in testicular testosterone production. Cholesterol side-chain cleavage or 20–22 desmolase deficiency and 3β-hydroxysteroid dehydrogenase deficiency are also associated with congenital adrenal hyperplasia. 17-α-hydroxylase deficiency, 17,20-desmolase deficiency, and 17-β-hydroxysteroid dehydrogenase deficiency also lead to impaired testosterone production.

A defect in the peripheral enzyme 5-α-reductase leads to impaired conversion of testosterone to dihydrotestosterone. DHT is the active androgen in the peripheral tissue. Androgen resistance or testicular feminization is due to defects in the androgen receptor. There may be a complete resistance with no genital ambiguity, or an incomplete form associated with genital ambiguity. Complete androgen resistance, which is also described as testicular feminization, is caused by either impaired androgen receptor function or decreased number of androgen receptors. The gene for the androgen receptor is found on the long arm of the X chromosome. Mutations in this gene cause the phenotypic abnormalities of male sexual development ranging from complete androgen resistance and a female phenotype to that of undervirilized or infertile men.[44] Mutations may result in the production of a nonfunctional receptor which will not bind androgen or may lead to receptors which bind androgen but are unable to effect transcriptional activation. Patients with complete androgen resistance appear as phenotypically normal girls at birth and often present at puberty secondary to amenorrhea. These girls develop breasts at puberty but are found to have a blind-ending vagina and scant pubic hair. Laboratory evaluation demonstrates elevated LH levels, normal or slightly elevated male testosterone levels, and a 46XY karyotype. Treatment consists of surgical excision of the gonads after puberty, estrogen replacement, and creation of a functional vagina.

Disorders of Genetic or Gonadal Development (Category III)

Gonadal dysgenesis is due to chromosomal abnormalities leading to abnormal gonadal development and streak gonads. True hermaphroditism is due to the presence of male and female elements in the gonads, known as ovotestis. Embryonic testicular regression or agonadism may occur in a 46XY individual. All these conditions may all lead to the development of ambiguous genitalia. Müllerian inhibitory factor may or may not have been produced, therefore the uterus may be present or absent. The karyotype may or may not be abnormal, i.e., 46XY/45X (mixed gonadal dysgenesis), 46XX (true hermaphroditism), 46XY(embryonic testicular regression). There is variable androgen secretion and phenotype presentation in these disorders of genetic or gonadal development.[43]

Principles of Management

When an infant with ambiguous genitalia is delivered, it is essential that proper decisions and consultations are carried out in the delivery room. Fig. 4.9 outlines steps in evaluation of a child born with ambiguous genitalia. Of primary importance is to rule out congenital adrenal hyperplasia (CAH), which is a life-threatening disorder. Gender assignment is usually made in the delivery room. However, if there is uncertainty, the correct sex assignment

should be made within a few days to weeks. The vast majority of the time, sex assignment is female. A male gender assignment is made only if there is adequate phallus (>2 cm) with the presence of erectile tissue, and no more than minimal to moderate hypospadias. The testes should be present in the scrotum or inguinal canal. All other cases are assigned a female gender role. If necessary, under extenuating circumstances, final sex assignment can be reassigned up until 18 months of age. It is important to describe the defect to parents as "incomplete or unfinished". If possible one should avoid the use of terms such as hermaphrodite and, later, of chromosome discrepancies.[42]

The parents should be encouraged to examine and hold the infant, as this may stimulate bonding and allay some of the parent's fears of their infant's abnormalities. A family history of members with similar defects, unexplained death of siblings in newborn period suggestive of CAH, maternal drug exposure (progestins, androgens), antiandrogens (spironolactone, flutamide), or maternal virilization during pregnancy can help in determining diagnosis and etiology of the defect.

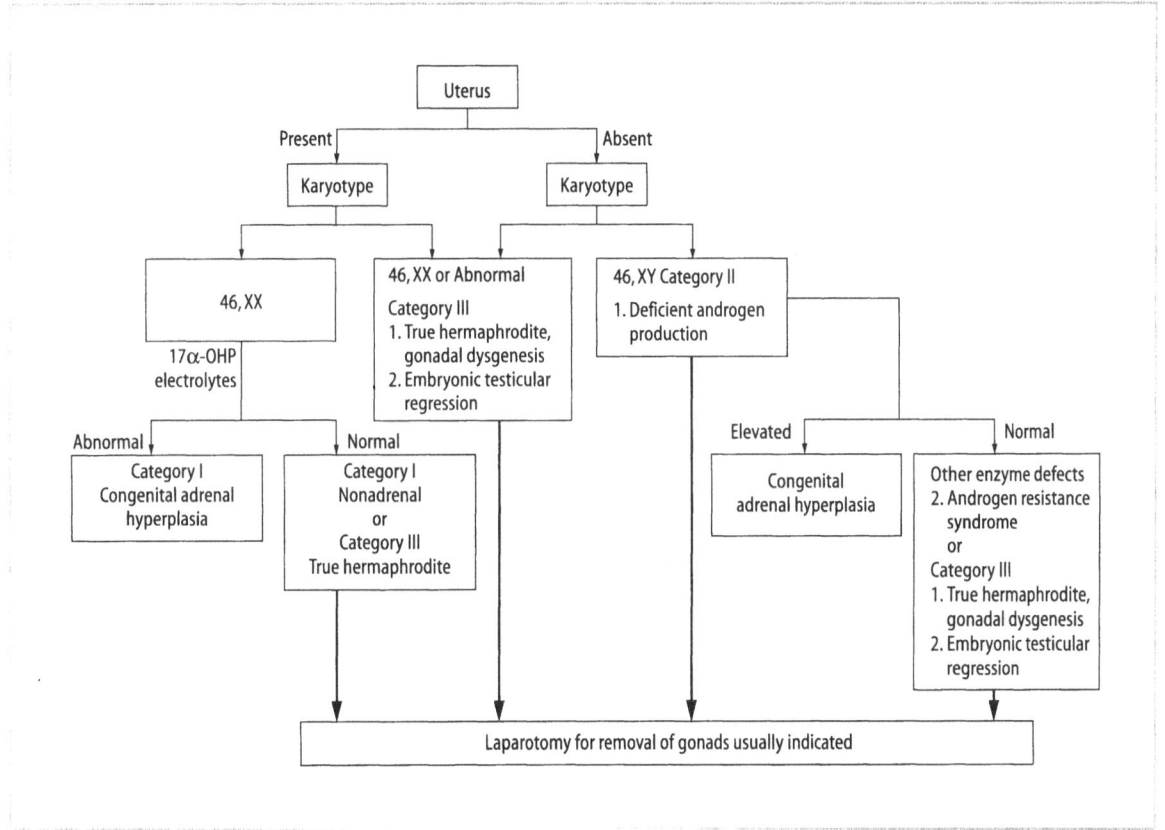

Figure 4.9 Evaluative steps for a child with ambiguous genitalia. 17α-OHP, 17-alpha-hydroxyprogesterone.

Physical Examination of the Newborn with Ambiguous Genitalia

Physical examination of the infant should target the presence of extra-adrenal malformations such as cardiac, renal, or gastrointestinal anomalies. In evaluation of the phallus, it is important to document the degree of hypospadias, the length, width, and degree of erectile tissue. The degree of labial fusion and the presence of a palpable gonad in scrotum or inguinal hernia or canal should be documented. The presence of a uterus is indicative of absence of müllerian inhibiting substance, either due to absent testes (i.e. presence of ovaries) or embryonic testicular regression. A uterus in the newborn can usually be palpable by rectal examination, or by ultrasound, radiographic dye studies, or endoscopy. Laboratory tests should be begun immediately and completed by 1 week. Preliminary results of chromosome analysis should be available in 5 days. The presence of a fluorescent Y-body in buccal smear upon guinacrine staining can speed the diagnosis of genetic sex. Electrolytes should be obtained to look for salt wasting in CAH. 17β-OH progesterone or urinary 17-ketosteroids and pregnanetriol will be elevated in cases of CAH. Other laboratory tests may be required to make the final diagnosis such as a complete steroid hormonal profile associated with a HCG stimulation test, androgen receptor determination from sexual skin fibroblasts, or 5α-reductase determination also from sexual skin fibroblasts.

Surgery may be indicated in these patients, but it is important that only experienced surgeons approach these patients. Phallus reduction should be done early. Vaginal or vulvar reconstruction is performed around puberty. Intraabdominal streaks or gonads should be removed in all individuals with congenital sexual ambiguity with a Y chromosome before puberty, since there is a higher incidence of gonadal tumors in these patients.

Intersex and Androgenization of the Female Vulva

Problems that arise in the external genitalia associated with overvirilization of the female or undervirilization of the male are considered intersex states, and sex of rearing needs to be determined. In this section we consider female intersex induced by congenital adrenal hyperplasia, endogenous and exogenous androgen production, incomplete androgen insensitivity, and 5-α-reductase deficiency.

Congenital Adrenal Hyperplasia

The endocrine problems produced by congenital adrenal hyperplasia (CAH) result in excess production of androgen, which is converted peripherally to dihydrotestosterone in the perineal region, resulting in cloacal virilization. The degree of virilization depends on the dose of the androgen exposure, and results in a wide range of physical changes, with increasing masculinization. There are two aspects of the cloaca that deserve attention: those related to the vulva and that associated with clitoral or phallic growth. The urogenital sinus in its normal development allows the urethra to exit in the midvulvar position between the clitoris and the vaginal opening. As masculinization increases, the urethra may become enclosed and open at the base of the phallus, almost like a hypospadias. More commonly, as the vulva becomes occluded by labial fusion, the urethra opens high on the anterior vaginal wall. The increasing severity of androgenization is associated with increased thickening of the lower vagina, which may open into the urethra in severe cases. A vagina is always present in CAH, and drainage of the uterus at the time of menstruation through the vagina and urogenital sinus is possible.[42]

Prenatal Diagnosis

Prenatal diagnosis of CAH is possible, and women who are known to be at risk may undergo either chorionic villus sampling or amniocentesis to diagnose the condition. A direct DNA probe can be used and intrauterine treatment of the affected fetus is commenced. This is performed by administering steroids (dexamethasone) to the mother, which are then transferred across the placenta to suppress ACTH release, preventing adrenal hyperplasia and excessive androgen production in utero.

Diagnosis

In the child born with an intersex problem, it is extremely important to establish the diagnosis as quickly as possible. A pelvic ultrasound is advised to determine the presence of a normal uterus and vagina, which makes the diagnosis of CAH most likely. Chromosomal studies can be obtained on blood, and samples sent for the measurement of serum 17-α-hydroxyprogesterone (17-α-OH). Thus, within 2 or 3 days of life, a diagnosis of both gender and sex of rearing can be established. The most common abnormality is 21-hydroxylase deficiency, and associated mineralocorticoid therapy and management of water and sodium intake must be considered.[43]

Surgical Management

Once the diagnosis of CAH has been confirmed, the child is reared as a female, regardless of the degree of masculinization of the external genitalia. The ovaries and uterus are normal and function at puberty for the initiation of normal female fertility. Having established that the child is female, enlargement of the clitoris and excessive fusion of the labial folds is addressed. Reduction of the clitoral enlargement with labial fold division is performed, with correction of the masculinization of the external genitalia between 6 and 18 months. Vaginoplasty is commonly delayed until later pubertal years when the young girl is mature enough to use vaginal dilators to maintain adequacy of the vaginal canal. The procedures are outlined in Fig. 4.10.[42]

The outcome of these surgical procedures is generally very good, with menstruation generally delayed slightly beyond the norm. Fertility rates in patients with CAH are also related to compliance with therapy, which influences the onset of menstruation and subsequent normal hypothalamic–pituitary–ovarian function and the degree of virilization.

In the largest review published, fertility was addressed in a group of 80. In those patients with simple virilization, satisfactory surgical correction was achieved in 73%, but 56% of those in the salt-losing group had an inadequate introitus. In 15 of 25 patients with the simple virilizing form, 25 pregnancies resulted in 20 normal children; only 1 of 15 women with the salt-losing form became pregnant.[45] Thus, achieving adequate medical control and using good surgical technique to ensure normal sexual function are imperative.

Endogenous Androgen Production

Androgenization of the vulva has been described in various circumstances. The most common conditions are adrenal adenomas, luteomas, and virilization in pregnancy due to other androgen-producing tumors. In the case of hyperreactio luteinalis, however, maternal virilization may occur in the absence of female fetus virilization due to the potent aromatization of androgens in the normal placenta. These are extremely rare phenomena, and the degree of virilization depends on the dose of androgen. Surgical management is similar to that described for CAH.

Exogenous Androgen Production

This is also a rare situation, with virilization due to administration of virilizing drugs such as danazol or methyltestosterone. Again, surgical management is as described for CAH.

Incomplete Androgen Insensitivity

This condition covers a wide spectrum of disorders ranging from gynecomastia with azoospermia to the presence of a pseudovagina. The most common presentation is a male neonate with perineal–scrotal hypospadias and associated cryptorchidism. The testes are small but contain normal Leydig cells. Endocrinologically these individuals undergo normal postpubertal development, with high levels of testosterone, and are similar to 46XY females. Depending upon the degree of masculinization, the choice is between a male role with a microphallus that may not be reconstructible and a female role with removal of the gonads and subsequent perineal reduction.[46] The latter is most commonly chose, because creation of a vagina is almost always feasible, whereas building and construction of a functional penis is extremely difficult. Vaginoplasty may be performed in a manner similar to that described for the absent vagina. Labial fold creation may be difficult if the perineum is flat.

5-α-Reductase, 17-β-Hydroxysteroid Dehydrogenase Deficiency

In these rare conditions, children are born with a markedly bifid scrotum that appears similar to the labia, but the phallus is enlarged, and a urogenital sinus with a blind ending vaginal pouch is seen. There are no müllerian structures present and the wolffian ducts are normally developed. It is important to establish this diagnosis soon after birth, because at puberty, rising levels of testosterone will cause rapid virilization, with deepening of the voice and phallus growth.[48] Failure to remove the gonads before puberty will result in significant virilization. Surgical management involves reduction clitoroplasty and subsequent development of a vagina as described earlier for vaginoplasty.

When to do a Gonadectomy

Gonadectomy should be performed in any individual with a Y-bearing cell line who is to be raised as a female. The karyotype may range from a mosaic with minimal Y cells, limited to the gonads, to a mosaic gonadal dysgenesis (45X, 46XY) to individuals with a normal 46XY karyotype with complete or incomplete androgen receptor deficiency, or male pseudohermaphrodites with a defect in either

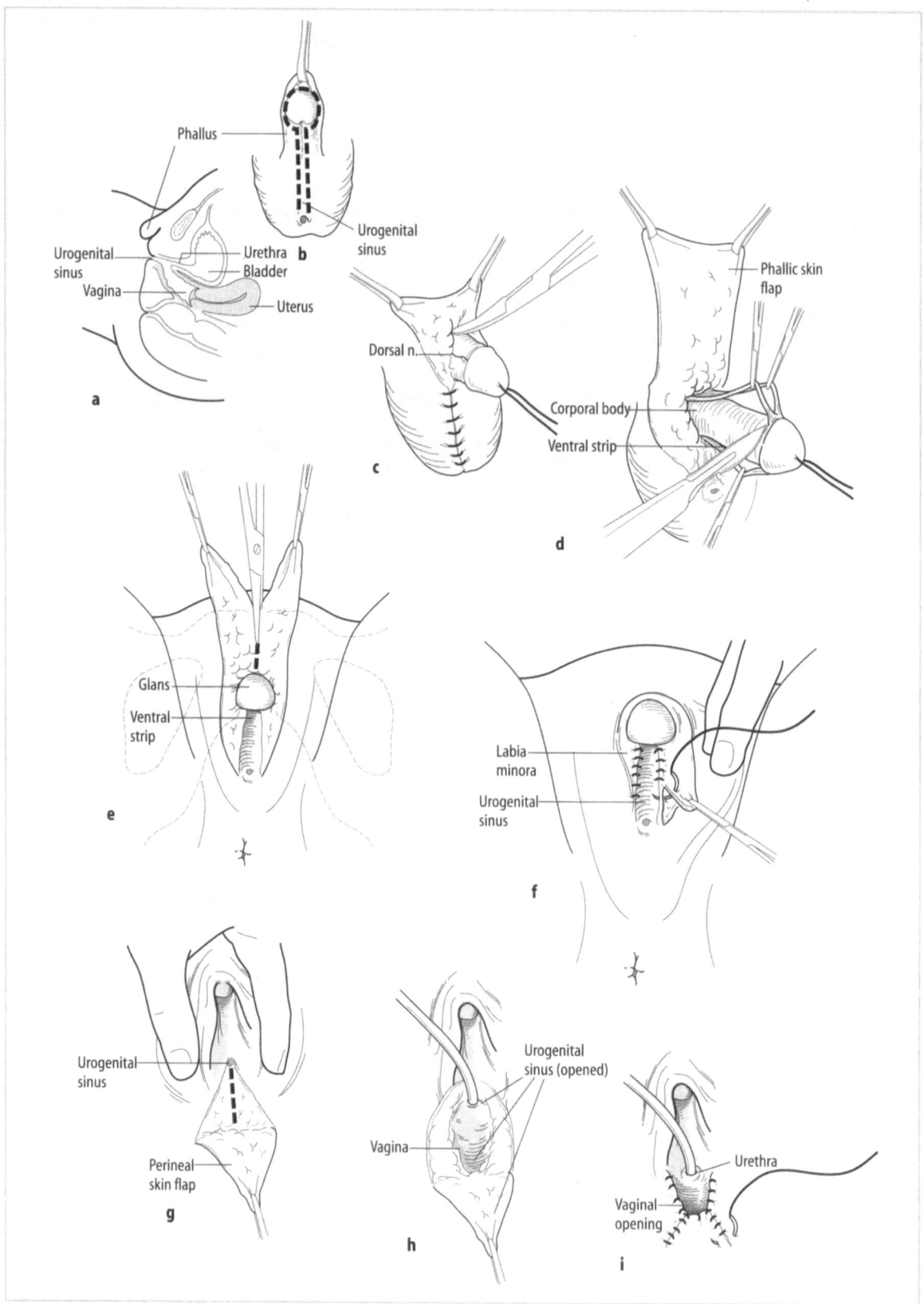

Figure 4.10 Surgical management of ambiguous genitalia in CAH. **a** Typical anatomic findings in virilized female patients with phallic hypertrophy and labioscrotal fusion forming a urogenital sinus. **b** Hatched lines show incision site for phallic reduction. **c** Phallic skin flap dissected. **d** Corporal body dissected and excised preserving dorsal nerve. **e** Clitoral recession, division of phallic skin flap. **f** Formation of labia minora using phallic skin flap. **g** Incision site in perineum for vaginoplasty. **h** Opening of urogenital sinus. **i** Suturing of vaginoplasty. From: Chantilis SJ, Bradshaw KD (1994) Infertility and Reproductive Endocrinology Clinics of North America 5:90.

5-α-reductase or 17-beta-hydroxysteroid dehydrogenase. In all but complete androgen receptor deficient patients, gonadectomy should be performed prior to puberty, to prevent pubertal virilization of the genitalia. Patients with complete androgen insensitivity will benefit from delayed orchiectomy with superior breast development by testicular estrogen production.

Techniques of gonadectomy vary with the position of the gonad and the vascular supply. Most intraabdominal and inguinal testes can easily be removed laparoscopically in much the same manner as oophorectomy. Diagnosis of symptomatic inguinal hernias are important and may be closed at the same procedure. Occasionally the testes will be extremely difficult to locate and imaging studies or selective venous catheterization must be performed.

Conclusions

Successful management of congenital anomalies of the genital tract demands both intense psychological support and a high degree of surgical skill. In-depth consultation should be obtained or patients should be referred to centers where such expertise exists and long-term follow up can be provided. Certain guidelines can be applied to each of the categories of congenital genital tract anomalies, importantly each case has to be dealt with individually depending on the patients anatomy, desires, and age.

Congenital Causes of Urinary Incontinence

Anthony M.K. Rickwood and Ashish Wakhlu

Although but a tiny fraction of the many girls troubled by diurnal urinary incontinence have some congenital lesion as a cause (Table 4.3), it is essential that they be identified since:

- in contrast to almost all those with functional enuresis, their incontinence is not a self-limiting complaint
- even if not curable, most are still eminently treatable
- some lesions, principally those neurological, also pose a potential threat to renal function.

With few exceptions, these various conditions can be diagnosed on the basis of history and examination, supplemented, in selected instances, by ultrasonography of the urinary tracts.

Embryology and Pathology

Ureteric Ectopia (Duplex System, Singleton System)

Complete duplication anomalies of the upper urinary tracts occur when two ureteric buds arise separately from the mesonephric (wolffian) duct. In ureteric ectopia, the more cranially disposed bud, subserving the *upper renal pole*, is involved. The caudally disposed bud comes to lie normally on the trigone while the accessory bud is carried inferiorly to emerge at some point in the lower urinary tract incorporating the mesonephric ducts, in females the bladder neck, the urethra, the vestibule and the distal vagina (ectopia at this last site may derive from Gartner's duct). Only *infrasphincteric* ectopia (Fig. 4.11) (vestibular, vaginal) causes urinary incontinence and in approximately 10% of cases the anomaly exists bilaterally.

In singleton-system ectopia there is a solitary ureteric bud but one arising at a more than usually cranially disposed level so that it too emerges at some point in the lower urinary tract deriving from the mesonephric ducts. In unilateral lesions, the

Table 4.3. Congenital causes of urinary incontinence	
Structural	**Neurological**
Ureteric ectopia	Open lesions
duplex-system	myelomeningocele
singleton-system	Occult lesions
Urovaginal confluence	lumbosacral lipoma
Congenital short urethra	diastematomyelia
Exstrophic anomalies	intraspinal cysts
vesical exstrophy	tethered cord
epispadias	Sacral agenesis
cloacal exstrophy	

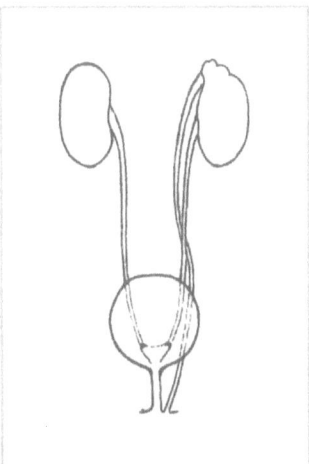

Figure 4.11 Infrasphincteric duplex-system ureteric ectopia. The left upper renal pole is dysplastic and its ureter drains ectopically at the vestibule.

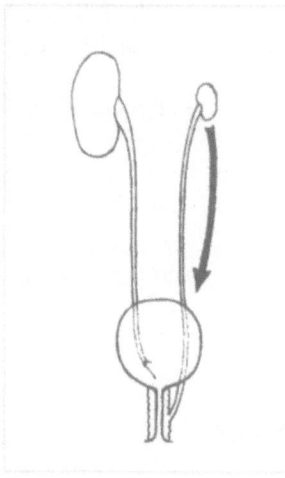

Figure 4.12 Infrasphincteric singleton-system ureteric ectopia. The ureter of the small dysplastic left kidney drains ectopically into the distal vagina. As indicated by the arrow, such kidneys may be located ectopically.

great majority, only those infrasphincteric (Fig. 4.12) cause incontinence and with few exceptions the ectopic orifice lies within the vagina, typically at the junction of its lower and middle thirds. Bilateral singleton-system ectopia is almost always *suprasphincteric* but the child is incontinent because both the bladder neck and external urethral sphincter are deficient while the bladder itself is usually small and ill-formed.

In all varieties of ectopia, the developing aberrant ureteric bud makes abnormal contact with the metanephric blastema to give rise to renal dysplasia, of the upper pole in duplication anomalies and of the entire kidney in singleton-system lesions. As a general rule, the more extreme the ectopia, the more severe the dysplasia.

Common Urogenital Sinus (Urovaginal Confluence)

These anomalies, all characterized by a single, abnormal, vulval orifice (Fig. 4.13), arise when development of the müllerian ducts arrests at some point following their fusion with the urogenital sinus. Persistent urogenital sinus anomalies, the cloacal deformity especially, may be associated with sacral agenesis or some other abnormality of the lower spine so that the child is incontinent as a result of neuropathic bladder. Only urovaginal confluence (Fig. 4.14), occurring with very early arrest (9th week of gestation) of müllerian development, causes incontinence in its own right since the bladder neck, confluent with the anterior wall of the vagina, is wholly incompetent.

Congenital Short Urethra

The embryogenesis of this anomaly is unknown. The urethra seldom exceeds 2 cm in length and its orifice is typically wide and patulous (Fig. 4.15). Although the bladder is normal, the sphincteric mechanism is wholly deficient.

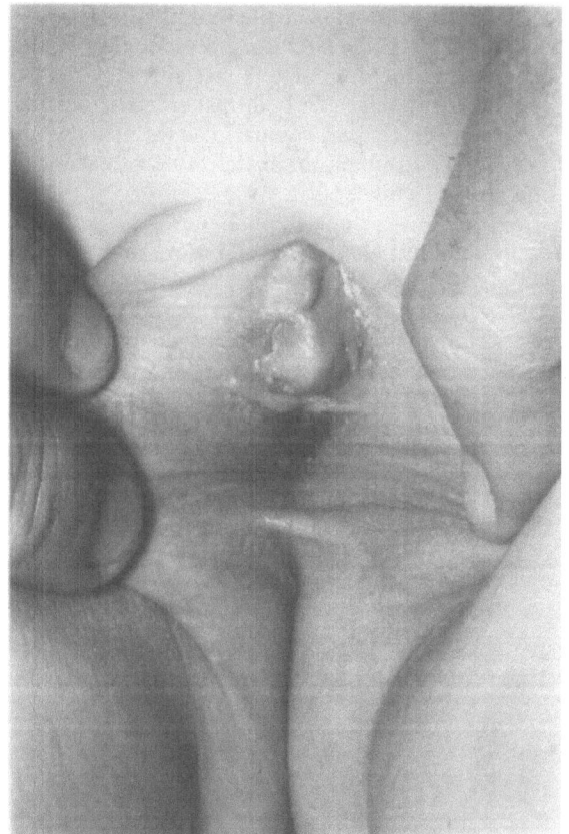

Figure 4.13 Persistent urogenital sinus. There is a single, abnormal, vulval orifice.

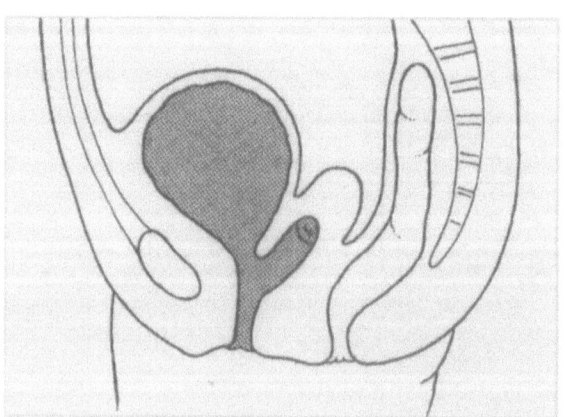

Figure 4.14 Urovaginal confluence.

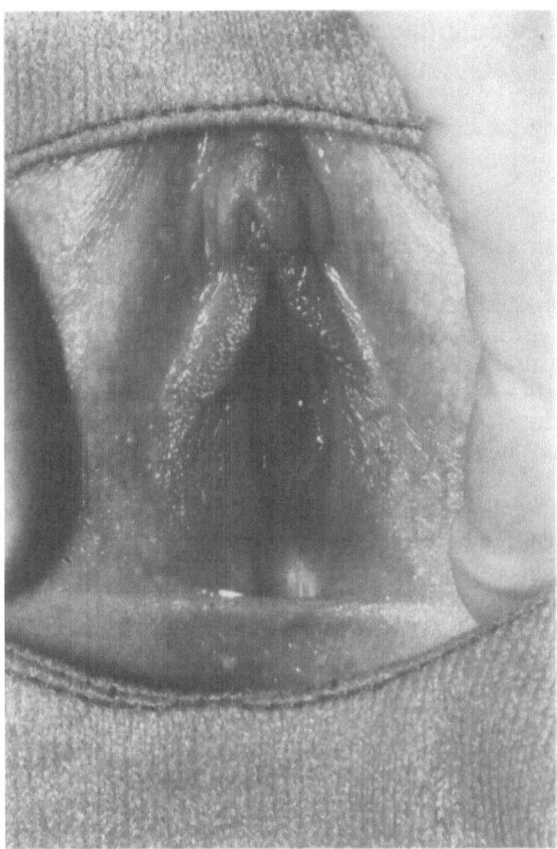

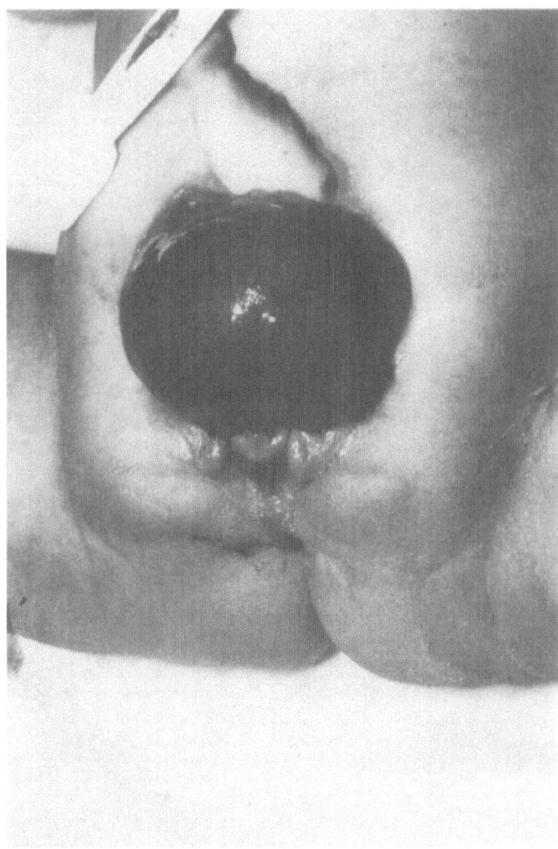

Figure 4.15 Congenital short urethra. The urethral meatus is wide and patulous (in this case there was also vaginal atresia).

Figure 4.16 Vesical exstrophy. The bladder is of almost normal size and the bifid clitorises are situated either side inferiorly.

Exstrophic Anomalies

The developmental abnormality common to this spectrum of anomalies is failure of primitive streak mesoderm to invade the allantoic extension of the cloacal (infraumbilical) membrane so that ectoderm and endoderm remain abnormally in contact in the developing lower abdominal wall, an unstable state leading to disintegration of the membrane and thus to the pelvic viscera being laid open onto the lower abdominal surface. The abnormally extensive cloacal membrane produces a wedge effect holding apart the developing lower abdomen and so results in a wide linea alba (or occasionally an exomphalos) superiorly and, inferiorly, in pubic diastasis, clitoral duplication and, sometimes, duplication of müllerian-derived structures. The nature of the visceral exstrophy depends upon the extent of the allantoic extension of the cloacal membrane and upon the timing of its dehiscence. An extensive membrane breaking down after formation of the urorectal septum leads to the most common lesion, vesical exstrophy with epispadias, while similarly timed

dehiscence of a less extensive membrane, limited to the pubic area, causes epispadias only. The most severe anomaly, cloacal exstrophy, arises when dehiscence of the membrane occurs prior to formation of the urorectal septum.

In classical vesical exstrophy, occurring in approximately 1 in 50 000–80 000 liveborn females, the bladder surface area varies from almost normal dimensions (Fig. 4.16) to a state in which little more than the trigone is represented. The urethra is completely epispadiac. The upper urinary tracts are usually normal but following bladder closure there is almost always vesico-ureteric reflux. At birth the bladder mucosa is thin and smooth but, with exposure, becomes thickened and friable and may later undergo squamous metaplasia. The detrusor, initially pliable, becomes edematous and rigid and may eventually lose innervation or become replaced by fibrous tissue.

In female epispadias (Fig. 4.17), one-tenth as prevalent as exstrophy, it is usual for the entire urethra to be affected up to and including the bladder neck, with the latter incompetent to cause continuous leakage of urine.

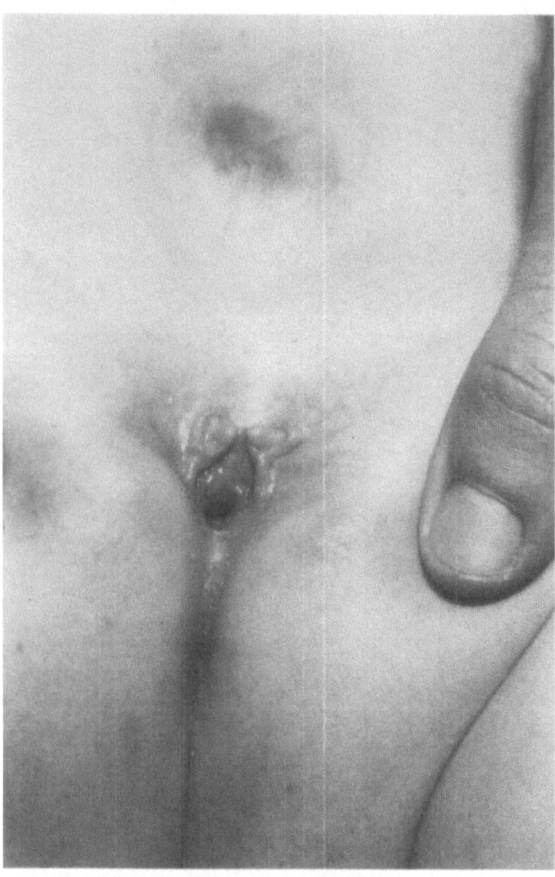

Figure 4.17 Female epispadias. Bifid clitorises lie either side of the epispadiac urethral strip, the latter extending up to a gaping bladder neck (in this case the abdominal wall is imperfectly formed over the bladder).

Myelomeningocele and Other Congenital Spinal Anomalies

Myelomeningocele, much the commonest of these anomalies, results from failure of tubularization of the neural crest and because this process commences at the mid-point, to proceed both cranially and caudally, the conus medullaris is almost invariably involved to cause neuropathic bladder. The untubularized crest lies exposed at the surface as the neural plaque (Fig. 4.18) and within the plaque neural tissue is grossly disorganized, although some reflex arcs may be preserved. Myelomeningocele is almost always associated with hydrocephalus and hence, in many instances, with some degree of intellectual impairment.

Among other congenital spinal anomalies, some (e.g. lumbosacral lipoma) may be associated with an inherent neurological deficit, whereas in others (e.g. intraspinal dermoid cyst) the deficit occurs secondarily as a result of compression of, or traction on, the cord or roots. Sacral agenesis, an example of the caudal regression syndrome, may occur in isolation or in association with anal imperforation.

Classically, the *pathophysiology* of neuropathic bladder dysfunction had been considered in relation to the site of the cord lesion, although in patients with congenital neuropathic bladder an intermediate pattern of activity is the most common finding.[47]

In *suprasacral* cord lesions (*contractile* bladder, anocutaneous reflex positive), the conus medullaris, along with the innervation of detrusor and sphincters, is intact but isolated from higher centers. The sphincteric mechanism is competent and

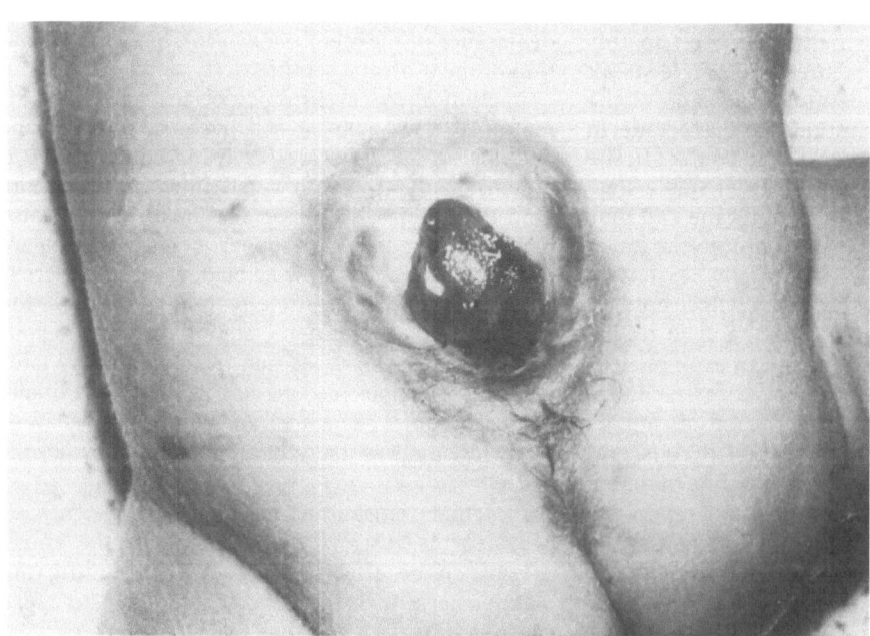

Figure 4.18 Myelomeningocele. The neural plaque lies centrally, surrounded by meningeal tissue.

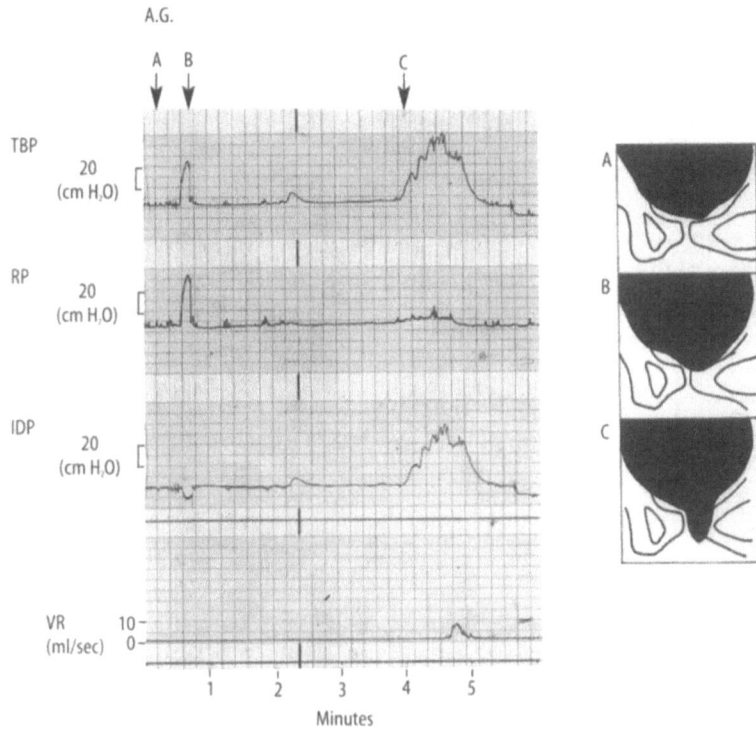

A.G.

Figure 4.19 Video-urodynamics, contractile bladder. The bladder neck is closed at rest (**a**) and remains so during raised intra-abdominal pressure (**b**). A reflex voiding contraction is accompanied by detrusor-sphincter dyssynergia (**c**). IDP, intrinsic detrusor pressure; RP, rectal pressure; TBP, total bladder pressure. Reprinted from Mundy AR et al (1984) Urodynamics, Principles, Practice and Application, 1st edn, 331, by permission of Churchill Livingstone.

voiding occurs only by reflex detrusor contractions (Fig. 4.19). Detrusor-sphincter dyssynergia is the rule, leading to high-pressure detrusor contractions and, often, to significant residual urine. A minority of patients have an incomplete cord lesion, with sacral sensory sparing and sometimes motor sparing also, and, because of bladder sensation, may achieve urinary continence, albeit precariously so and at the expense of marked urgency of micturition. Their upper renal tracts are at no less risk than those with complete cord lesions. In *sacral* cord lesions (*acontractile* bladder, anocutaneous reflex negative), the conus medullaris is destroyed along with the innervation of both detrusor and sphincters. Detrusor activity is absent and voiding occurs by overflow or by raising intra-abdominal pressure (Fig. 4.20). Although there is always a measure of sphincteric incompetence, paradoxically there is often partial fixed outflow obstruction at the level of the external urethral sphincter, possibly resulting from denervation fibrosis. Termed static sphincteric obstruction,[48] this varies widely from one patient to another. When severe it leads to good bladder capacity at the expense of large residual urine (Fig. 4.20a) and vice versa when minimal (Fig. 4.20b). Detrusor

noncompliance exists in some patients, leading to pathologically elevated intravesical pressure in the presence of marked static sphincteric obstruction or further compromising bladder capacity when such obstruction is minimal.

Intermediate bladder dysfunction (anocutaneous reflex negative) is characterized by a combination of reflex detrusor activity and sphincteric incompetence (Fig. 4.21). Static sphincteric obstruction is common and similarly detrusor noncompliance (Fig. 4.22), the latter often in association with the sacculation classical of neuropathic bladder (Fig. 4.23).

Factors impairing capacity of the neuropathic bladder are summarized in Table 4.4. In patients with congenital cord lesions, secondary upper renal tract complications are common and occur when a combination of outflow obstruction (detrusor-sphincter dyssynergia or static sphincteric obstruction) and detrusor hyperreflexia and/or noncompliance leads to persistently raised intravesical pressure. This, in turn, causes secondary ureterovesical obstruction or reflux, the effects of which are often further compounded by urinary infection.

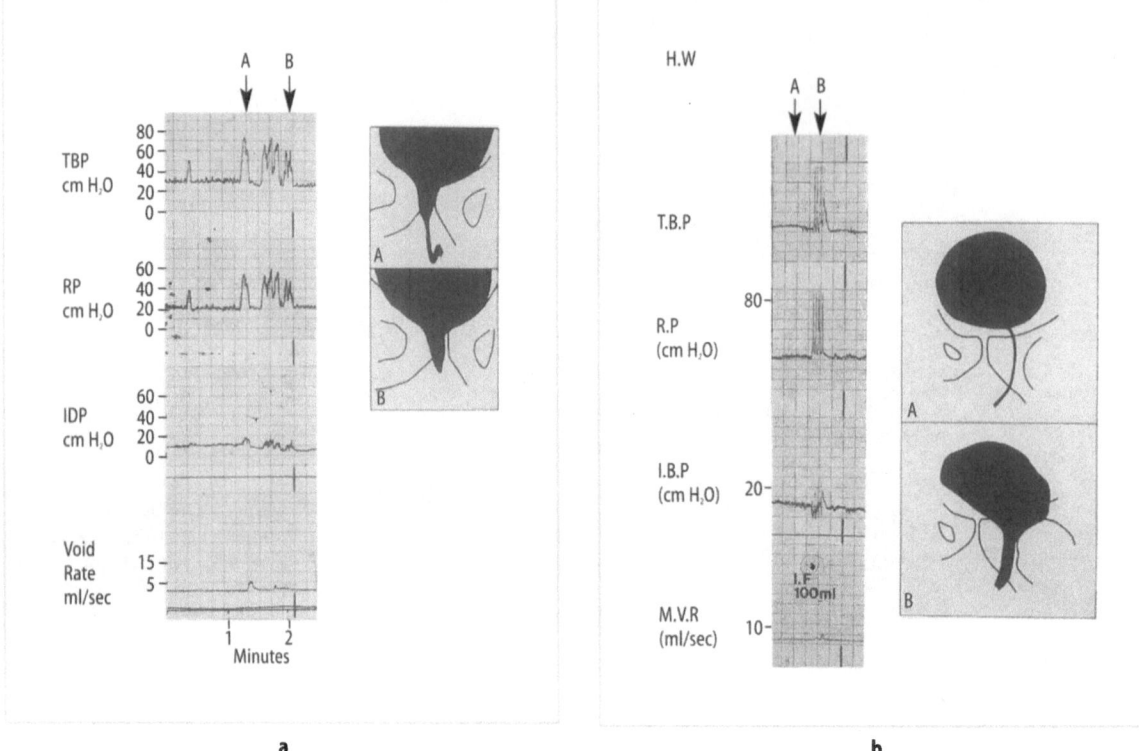

a   b

Figure 4.20 Video-urodynamics, acontractile bladder. **a** During voiding by abdominal straining there is static sphincteric obstruction (**i**) which ultimately becomes complete to leave a large residual urine (**ii**). **b** The bladder neck, although closed at rest (**i**), exhibits gross incompetence on coughing and without static sphincteric obstruction (**ii**). Reprinted from Mundy AR et al (1984) Urodynamics, Principles, Practice and Application, 1st edn, 332/3, by permission of Churchill Livingstone.

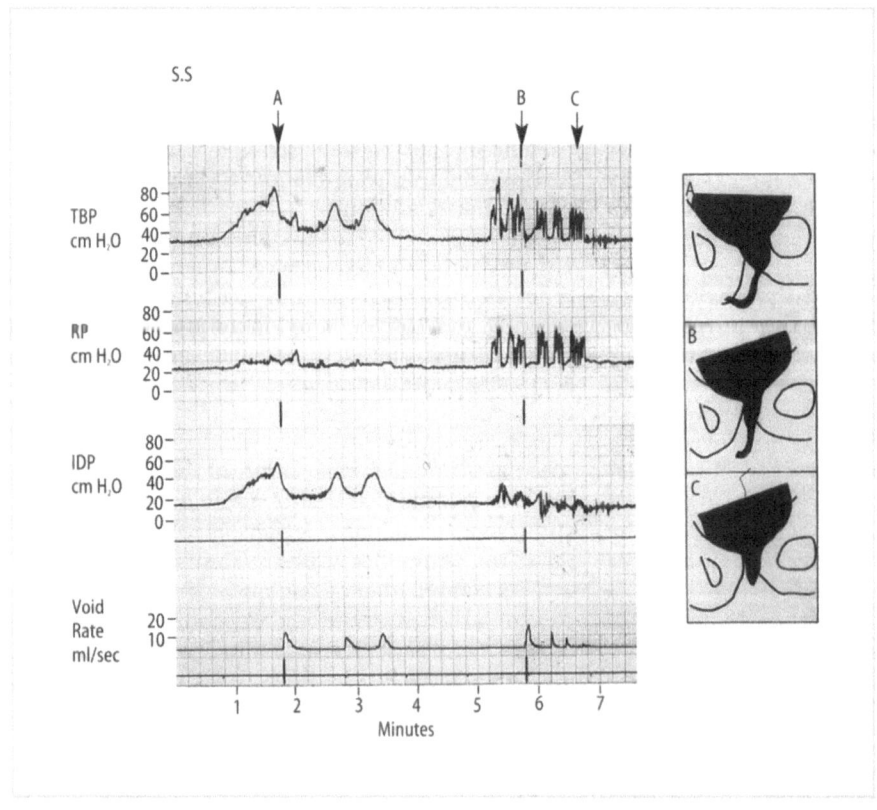

Figure 4.21 Video-urodynamics, Intermediate bladder. Voiding occurs both by reflex detrusor contractions (**a**) and by abdominal straining (**b**). There is static sphincteric obstruction (**c**). Reprinted from Mundy AR et al (1984) Urodynamics, Principles, Practice and Application, 1st edn, 331, by permission of Churchill Livingstone.

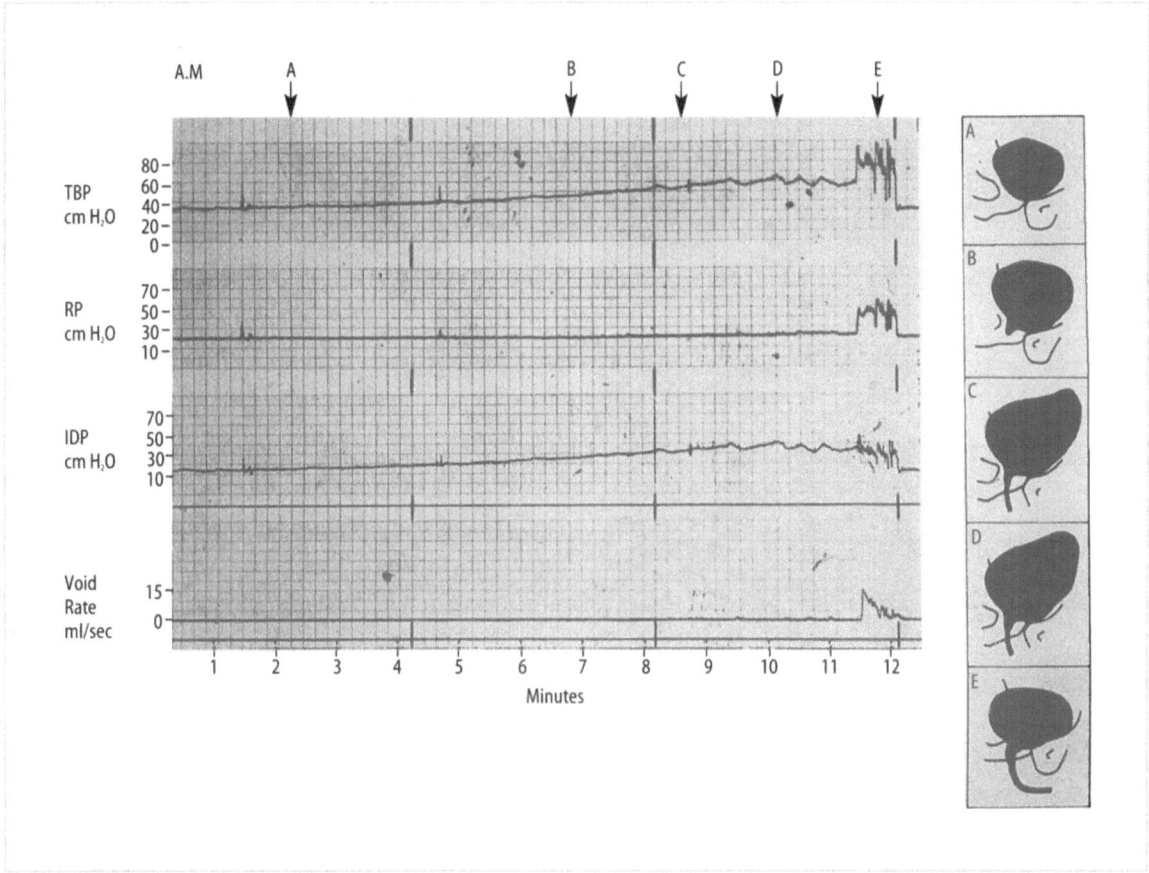

Figure 4.22 Video-urodynamics, intermediate bladder. Detrusor non-compliance during filling. Low-pressure detrusor contractions occur approaching capacity (**d**) and voiding is principally by abdominal straining (**e**). Reprinted from Mundy AR et al (1984) Urodynamics, Principles, Practice and Application, 1st edn, 335, by permission of Churchill Livingstone.

Clinical Presentation

The *exstrophic anomalies, urovaginal confluence* and *congenital short urethra* are all characterized by continuous urinary leakage, without any micturition otherwise, and except for congenital short urethra the diagnosis is obvious on physical examination.

Duplex-system ureteric ectopia and *unilateral singleton-system ectopia* classically present with the unique and pathognomonic features of continuous (and usually slight) urinary leakage superimposed upon an otherwise normal pattern of micturition. Not all cases are so straightforward. Some girls are dry overnight, and a few are able to remain dry for brief periods during the day. Secondary changes may occur in the normal micturition, typically gross frequency occasioned by the parents' desperate efforts to have their daughter dry. Lastly, in cases with severe dysplasia and vaginal ectopia the small quantity of urine produced pools within the vagina, becomes infected, and presents as vaginal discharge.

Bilateral singleton-system ureteric ectopia is characterized by continuous urinary leakage without micturition otherwise, and in cases where both kidneys are markedly dysplastic there may also be symptoms of renal insufficiency.

In most cases of *congenital neuropathic bladder* there is an evident spinal anomaly (myelomeningocele, lipoma, hairy patch, haemangioma, dermal sinus), although the existence of such lesions does not necessarily imply bladder involvement, a matter better determined by the history. Sacral agenesis is more readily overlooked, but palpable absence of the lower-most sacral segments and flattening of the upper buttocks (Fig. 4.24) are diagnostic of this condition. In some cases without an apparent spinal anomaly there are peripheral neurological signs (e.g. calf-wasting, claw toes) but in a few there are neither. Some patients leak urine continuously; others void only intermittently, but usually unknowingly. A few achieve precarious urinary continence although always with gross urgency of micturition. Urinary infections are common. Simultaneous disturbance of bowel habit, especially if with frank fecal incontinence, points to a diagnosis of neuropathic bladder.

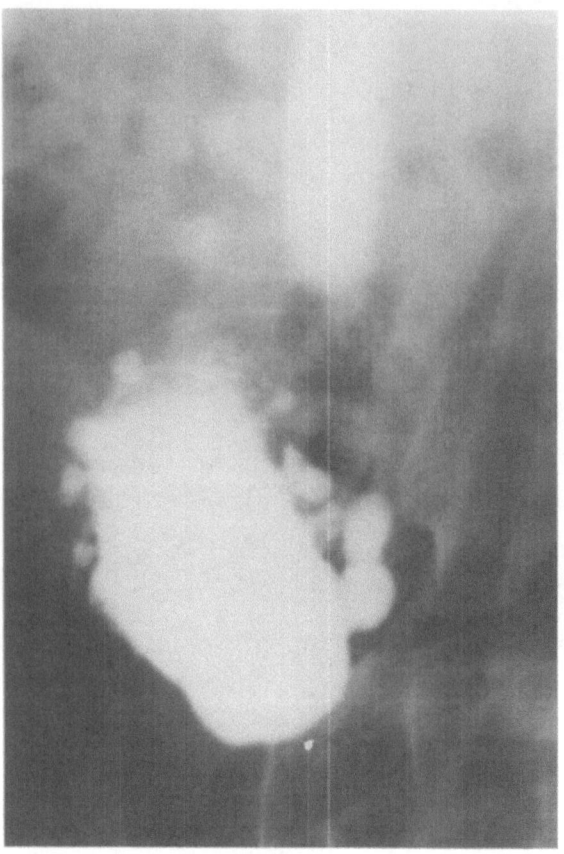

Figure 4.23 Cystography, intermediate bladder, and showing typical neuropathic sacculation (also unilateral vesico-ureteric reflux).

Table 4.4 Factors limiting the capacity of the neuropathic bladder

Contractile bladder	Acontractile bladder	Intermediate bladder
Detrusor hyperreflexia	Sphincteric incompetence	Detrusor hyperreflexia
	Detrusor noncompliance	Detrusor noncompliance
	Combinations	Sphincteric incompetence
		Combinations

Investigation

Exstrophic Anomalies, Urovaginal Confluence, Congenital Short Urethra

Ultrasonography is advisable to exclude any abnormality of the upper renal tracts. *Endoscopy* is undertaken in cases of urovaginal confluence and congenital short urethra both for diagnostic purposes and as pre-therapeutic assessment.

Ureteric Ectopia (Duplex System, Unilateral Singleton System)

Although usually suspectable from the history, confirmatory diagnostic imaging can present major difficulties since, because of dysplasia, the affected renal tissue and its drainage system are rarely directly demonstrable by intravenous urography. *Ultrasonography* is the investigation of first choice

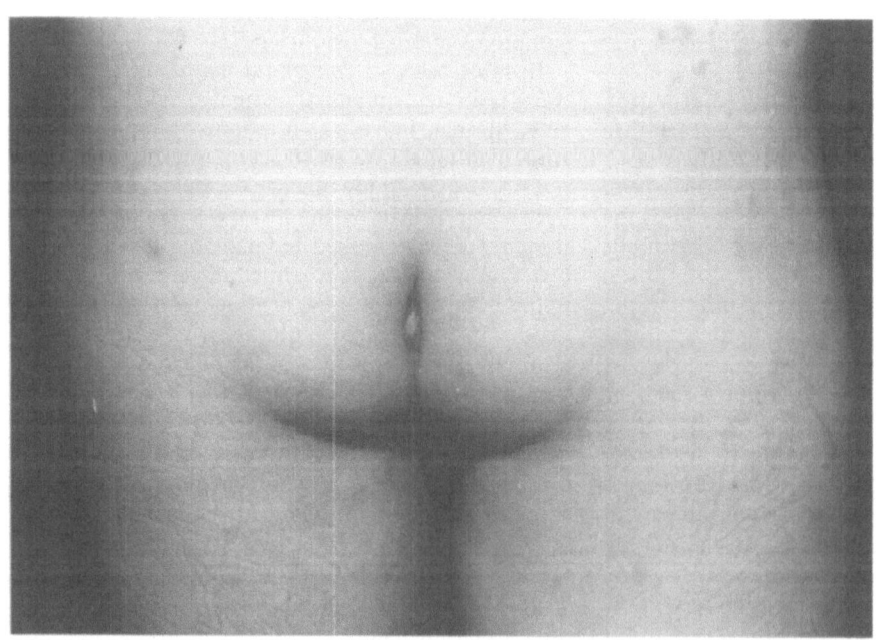

Figure 4.24 Sacral agenesis with typical wasting of the buttocks superiorly.

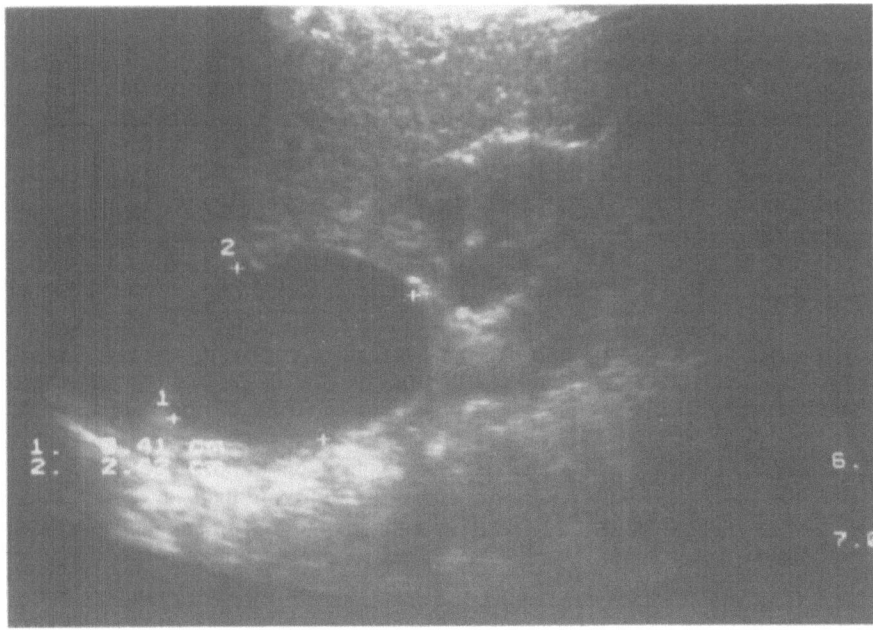

Figure 4.25 Ultrasonography (longitudinal section of kidney), infrasphincteric duplex-system ureteric ectopia. The upper renal pole is grossly hydronephrotic with no visible renal substance. The lower pole is normal.

and upper polar hydronephrosis in a duplication anomaly (Fig. 4.25) or a small singleton kidney is found, the diagnosis is confirmed. Often, however, an affected upper pole is small, nonhydronephrotic and hence difficult to detect by ultrasonography. The same is true of singleton kidneys which are minute or ectopic. *DMSA scintigraphy* may be diagnostic, especially in demonstrating singleton kidneys (Fig. 4.26), and is in any case routinely advisable to assess function (Fig. 4.27). In duplication anomalies, *intravenous urography* is occasionally helpful in demonstrating a "missing" (i.e. nonfunctioning) upper polar calyx. *Examination under anesthetic* may locate an ectopic orifice, although failure to do so by no means excludes the diagnosis. In the last resort, a *methylene blue* test is undertaken. The dye

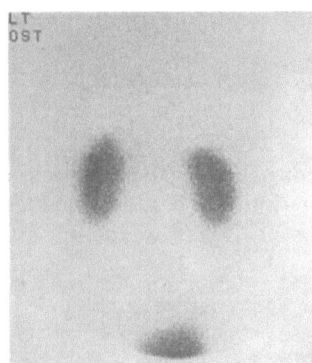

Figure 4.27 DMSA scintigraphy, infrasphincteric duplex-system ureteric ectopia. The small defect at the left upper pole represents the small, nonfunctioning, upper moiety.

is introduced into the bladder via a catheter which is then removed, and a pad is placed on the vulva. If subsequent urinary leakage is blue the problem is one of bladder malfunction, but if it is colorless the diagnosis of ectopia is confirmed.

Bilateral Singleton System Ureteric Ectopia

Ultrasonography typically finds small kidneys, often associated with a degree of hydroureteronephrosis. The diagnosis is confirmed by *endoscopy*.

Congenital Neuropathic Bladder

Diagnostically, ultrasonography may find some combination of a thick-walled bladder, significant

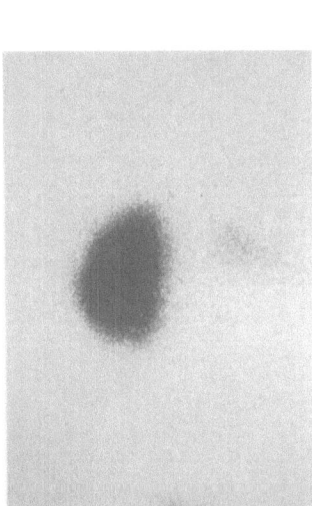

Figure 4.26 DMSA scintigraphy, singleton-system infrasphincteric ureteric ectopia. The examination demonstrates a small minimally-functioning right kidney which, in this case, is situated orthotopically

residual urine or hydroureteronephrosis, unilaterally or bilaterally. The examination also finds use in routine monitoring of the state of the upper renal tracts. *DMSA* scintigraphy is undertaken in those troubled by febrile urinary infections while *micturating cystourethrography*, to confirm or exclude vesico-ureteric reflux, is best combined with a simultaneous *urodynamic examination*. This latter is routinely advisable in the event of secondary upper renal tract complications or when planning treatment for incontinence.

Treatment

Duplex System and Unilateral Singleton System Ureteric Ectopia

Upper polar heminephrectomy or nephrectomy, as appropriate, is curative. Ureteric reimplantation is employed only in the rare event of the ectopic ureter draining usefully functioning renal tissue.

Bilateral Singleton System Ureteric Ectopia

This calls for major reconstruction involving reimplantation of the ureters into the bladder, bladder neck repair and, in most instances, augmentation cystoplasty.

Urovaginal Confluence

If, as is usual, the bladder has adequate capacity, a continent sphincteric zone may be constructed from an anterior detrusor tube.[49] An alternative approach[50] is to detach the bladder neck from the vagina and to construct a urethra distally by means of a tubed strip of anterior vaginal wall, closing the resulting defect in the latter by a transposed flap of perineal skin.

Congenital Short Urethra

Standard bladder neck repair[51–53] is usually curative.

Vesical Exstrophy

Whenever possible, the bladder, urethra, pelvic ring, and lower abdominal wall are repaired neonatally, before secondary changes occur in the mucosa and detrusor, and if the procedure is undertaken within 48 hours of birth it is usually possible to approximate the pubic bones anteriorly without need of osteotomies (Fig. 4.28). Vesico-ureteric reflux ensues, but this is inconsequential since the bladder neck remains incompetent and urine dribbles from an empty bladder. Surgery for continence is delayed until the child is older, usually 5–7 years of age, and always includes bladder neck repair, a procedure which, in involving tubularization of the trigone, requires reimplantation of the ureters at a higher level in the bladder and thereby correcting the vesico-ureteric reflux. Although some centers report good results from bladder neck repair alone,[54] these have not been widely replicated, usually because the bladder lacks capacity. Augmentation cystoplasty rectifies this problem but often at the expense of poor emptying, a complication calling for intermittent self-catheterization, either per-urethrally or via a Mitrofanoff stoma. In the event of persistent sphincteric incompetence, the bladder neck may be obliterated in conjunction with a Mitrofanoff[55] procedure for the necessary intermittent catheterization.

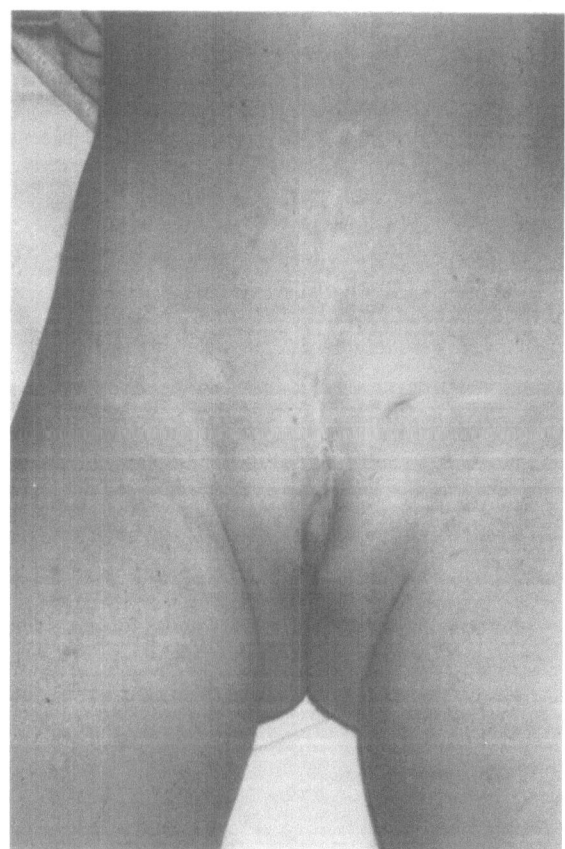

Figure 4.28 Long-term appearances following neonatal closure of vesical exstrophy (same case as in Figure 4.16).

Epispadias

Because the bladder has normal capacity and innervation, bladder neck repair and urethral reconstruction afford consistently better results than in the case of exstrophy.

Congenital Neuropathic Bladder

Treatment has two fundamental objectives:

- preservation of the integrity of the upper renal tracts
- appliance-free urinary continence.

These are achieved by replicating, so far as is possible, the two basic functions of a normal bladder:

- adequate, low-pressure, functional capacity, definition of "adequate" being determined by the patient's mobility
- complete voluntary voiding.

The latter is nowadays almost always effected by intermittent self-catheterization and in the 10–20% of cases naturally having adequate low-pressure capacity no more is required. Treatment otherwise is directed to correcting the factors responsible for inadequate or high-pressure capacity (Table 4.4) and although, in an individual patient, two or more factors may apply, so calling for combined treatment (e.g. augmentation cystoplasty plus a sphincter enhancing procedure), for present purposes their management is described individually.

Detrusor hyperreflexia

As a rule this responds adequately to detrusor antispasmodics, notably oxybutynin and tolterodine. The former may be delivered intravesically, during catheterisation, in the event of unacceptable side-effects with oral intake. Augmentation cystoplasty is needed only for the minority of patients unresponsive to medication.

Detrusor noncompliance

Unresponsive to medication, this calls for augmentation cystoplasty, either employing a detubularized bowel segment or, if there is a grossly dilated ureter, by means of ureterocystoplasty.

Sphincteric Incompetence

This is the most difficult problem to manage, as evidenced by the many means that continue to be employed. α-adrenergic agonists (e.g. ephedrine) are effective in only marginal degrees of sphincteric incompetence and much the same is true of periurethral bulking agents. The artificial urinary sphincter is seldom employed in girls since there exist cheaper and equally effective alternatives. These include bladder neck slings,[56] bladder neck suspension,[56] and an anterior detrusor flap valve.[58] In most instances it is necessary to combine these procedures with augmentation cystoplasty.

Management of the Severely Disabled

Extra or alternative measures may be required for these patients. For those unable to practice urethral self-catheterization, a Mitrofanoff procedure represents an alternative means of access to the bladder, if necessary in conjunction with bladder neck obliteration. Self-catheterization in any form requires good sitting balance to leave both hands free. Where this is lacking more elementary management is called for, either long-term indwelling urethral catheterization, if properly handled,[59] or an old-fashioned conduit urinary diversion.

Congenital Anorectal Anomalies

Keith Holmes, Madan Samuel and Liam McCarthy

Embryology

Anorectal anomalies in the female arise from disturbances in the development of the terminal hindgut or cloaca (presumptive bladder and rectum) and paramesonephric ducts, (presumptive vagina, uterus, and oviducts).

The concept is simpler in the male (Fig. 4.29) where defective separation of the cloaca results in a persisting connection between urogenital sinus (presumptive bladder and urethra) and rectum, which gives rise to the *recto-urinary fistula*. The other consequence is failure of the hind gut to reach the perineum, which results in the anorectal anomaly or *imperforate anus*.

These developments occur between 4 and 6 weeks and are coincident with the evolution of the paramesonephric ducts in the female (Fig. 4.30). Defective development of the Rathke and Tourneau folds which separate the cloaca result in a connection between the rectum and inferior uterovaginal canal (presumptive vagina) or definitive urogenital sinus (presumptive vaginal vestibule). This leads to the anorectal anomaly and the *rectovaginal or rectovestibular fistula*.

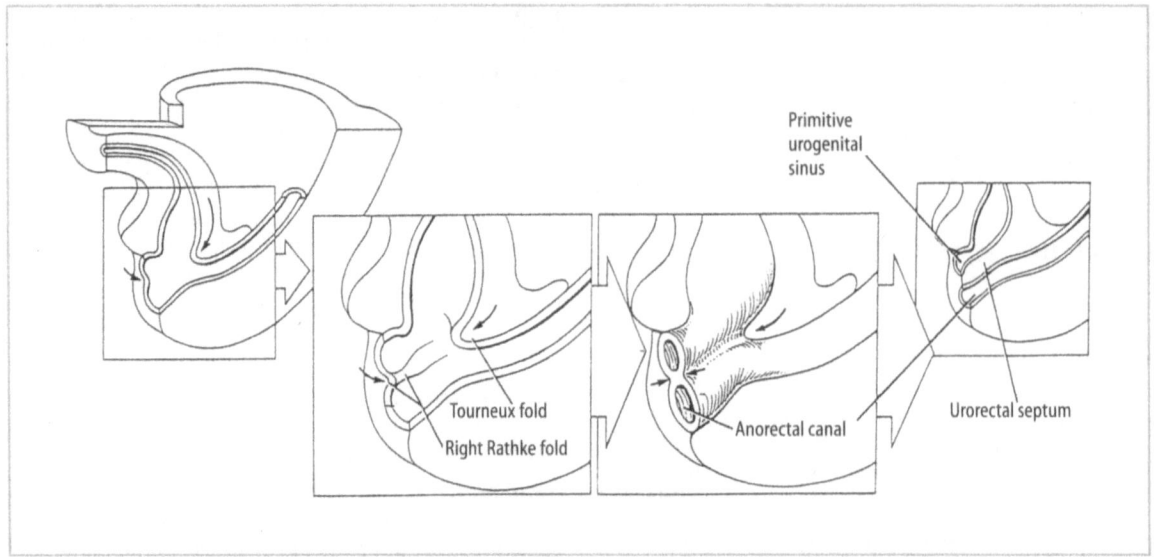

Figure 4.29 Cloacal partition (male). From: Larsen WJ (1998) *Essentials of Human Embryology*, Churchill Livingstone, New York, p. 244.

In both sexes, variation in the extent of cranio-caudal partition of the cloaca accounts for the spectrum of anorectal anomalies. A long gap between the terminal hindgut and perineum results in a *high* anomaly, for example rectovaginal fistula, whereas more distal, but incomplete, progression of the partition results in a *low* anomaly, for example *anovestibular fistula*. The end result is a rectum which terminates anterior to and sometimes higher than the normal level and is not therefore surrounded by the levator funnel.

The perineum is also deficient because of a failure of expansion of the mesodermal folds inferiorly. These folds, which partition the cloaca, normally result in further separation of vagina from anus when they reach the perineum.

Classification

It is perhaps not surprising that the complicated embryological events in the hind gut and pelvic floor may become disordered at different stages, resulting in a spectrum of anomalies. These anomalies have been the subject of detailed examination by expert groups on a number of occasions over the past 30 years, and the classification in Table 4.5 has gained wide international acceptance.[60] The complexity of treatment and the prognosis for anorectal function vary with the severity of the abnormality. Examples of the female anomaly are shown in Fig. 4.31.

Incidence and Associated Anomalies

Anorectal anomalies occur approximately once in every 5000 live births. The teratogenic event, as yet unknown, affects a number of other organ systems, which leads to an extra-ordinarily high co-incidence of equally rare anomalies. These are described by the acronym *VACTERL*, and the incidence in association with the primary abnomality is shown in brackets:

<u>V</u>ertebral (30–50%)
<u>A</u>norectal (100%)
<u>C</u>ardiac (10%)
<u>T</u>racheo-<u>E</u>sophageal (10%)
<u>R</u>enal tract (40–50%)
<u>L</u>imb (5%).

The fetus is rarely so compromised that the predicted quality of life would justify termination of the pregnancy.

Management

In the Newborn Child

All of these babies must be carefully examined by a neonatologist and pediatric surgeon, to check for associated abnormalities and determine the precise anatomy of the anorectal anomaly. In the majority of patients, careful clinical inspection will reveal the presence of a low lesion and thus the strategy for treatment.

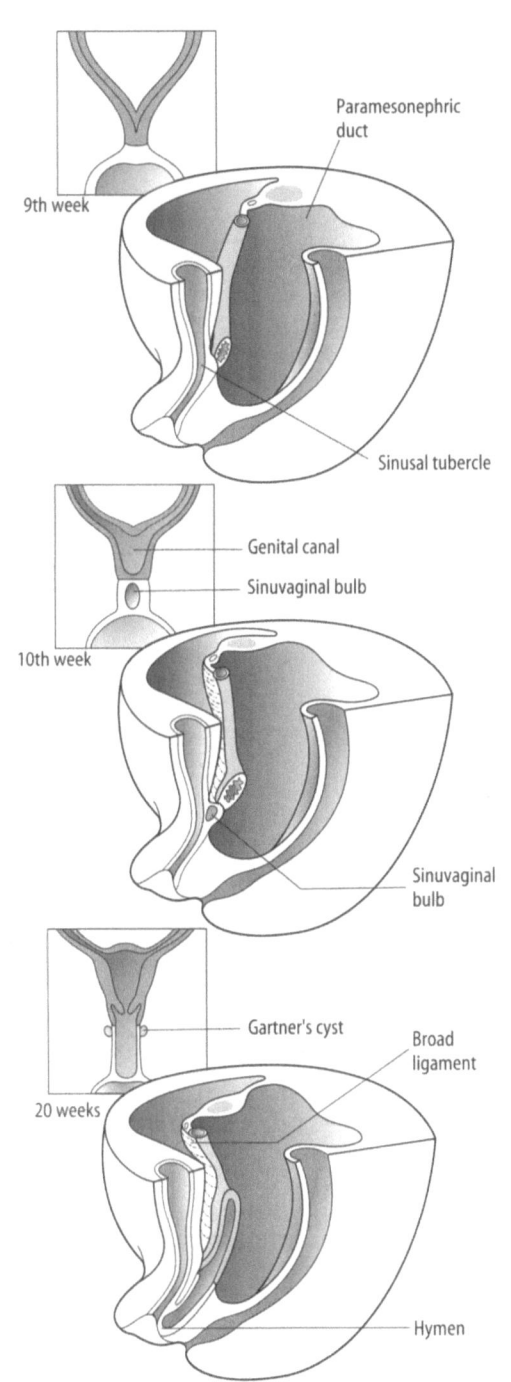

9th week

Paramesonephric duct

Sinusal tubercle

10th week

Genital canal

Sinuvaginal bulb

Sinuvaginal bulb

20 weeks

Gartner's cyst

Broad ligament

Hymen

Figure 4.30 Cloacal partition (female). From: Larsen WJ (1998) *Essentials of Human Embryology*, Churchill Livingstone, New York, p. 281.

Investigations should include a plain radiograph of chest and abdomen to exclude vertebral anomalies, an abdominal ultrasound scan to examine the renal tract and an echocardiogram.

Table 4.5. The 1984 Wingspread classification of anorectal anomalies

Female	Male
High	*High*
Anorectal agenesis with/without rectovaginal fistula	Anorectal agenesis with/without rectoprostatic fistula
Rectal atresia	Rectal atresia
Intermediate	*Intermediate*
Rectovestibular fistula	Rectobulbar urethral fistula
Rectovaginal fistula	
Anal agenesis without fistula	Anal agenesis without fistula
Low	*Low*
Anovestibular fistula	Anocutaneous fistula
Anocutaneous fistula	
Anal stenosis	Anal stenosis
Other	
Cloacal malformations	
Rare malformations	Rare malformations

A lateral radiograph of the pelvis at 24 hours of age, originally with the child inverted but more recently lying prone with the buttocks raised, gives an indication of the gap between the distal bowel and the perineum.

In practice, if clinical inspection does not reveal the anal opening, examination under anesthesia will allow sufficiently precise diagnosis to decide between primary reconstruction or colostomy.

Anal opening on perineum (low lesion)

If the anus is visible on the perineum and the baby is passing meconium without evidence of intestinal obstruction, there is no need for immediate intervention; indeed, the patient may never need surgical treatment.

There is an hierarchy of problems, not mutually exclusive, which vary with age.

- *In infancy* the main problem is constipation, which has been attributed to anterior angulation of the anal canal. This may arise with the introduction of solid food in a child who was previously coping with soft stool and may necessitate some form of reconstruction.
- *In adult life* when the woman becomes sexually active the aesthetic appearance of the perineum becomes relevant. Problems of this nature are difficult to anticipate in early childhood but should be raised with the parents. Provided there is a reasonable space between anus and vestibule there is no indication for reconstruction as the, albeit small, risk of fecal incontinence outweighs the aesthetic benefit.
- *During childbirth* the risk of sphincter damage may be increased as a consequence of the anorectal anomaly. As effective obstetric measures

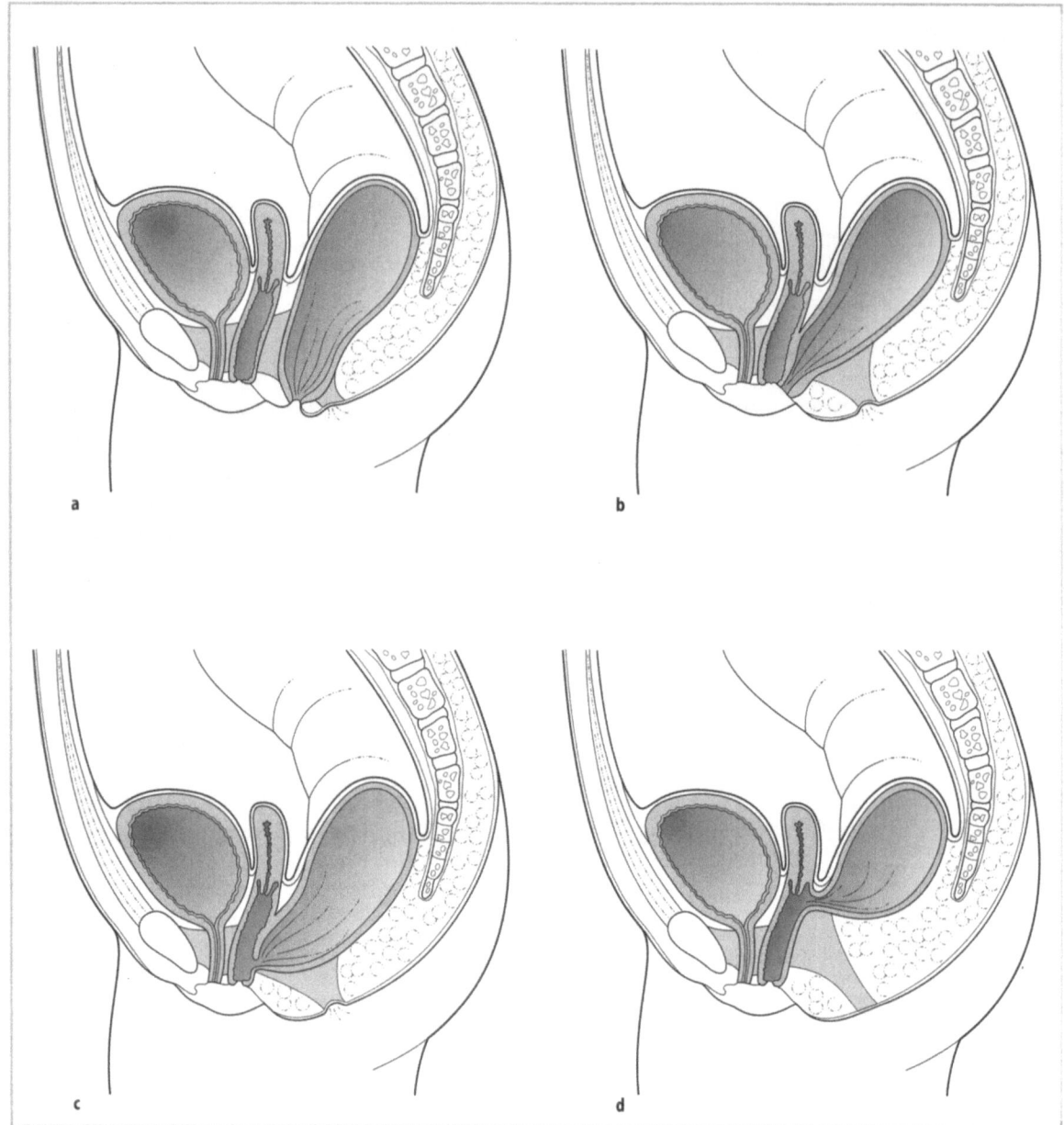

Figure 4.31 Anorectal anomalies in the female. **a** Perineal (cutaneous) fistula. **b** Vestibular fistula. **c** Low rectovaginal fistula **d** High rectovaginal fistula. From: Pena A (1990) Surgical Management of Anorectal Malformations, Springer-Verlag New York, 55.

may be employed to avoid such damage, this last does not equate to an indication for reconstruction. It is axiomatic that the patient be aware of this potential problem and inform her obstetrician.

Decision-making in patients with low lesions calls for fine judgment. It should be emphasized that these girls have the best prognosis for normal anorectal function and that a misguided attempt at perineal reconstruction may irrevocably damage the pelvic floor and anorectum, creating lifelong problems.

The work of Pena and deVreis would indicate that the anus is not completely surrounded by the external sphincter complex in anything other than a minor variation from normal, when the anocutaneous fistula is just anterior to the normal anal position. Effective reconstruction must therefore involve more than a simple "cutback" procedure in which the perineal skin covering the fistula is divided.

The exact position of the external sphincter in relation to the anal opening must be determined by electrical stimulation. If the external sphincter does surround the anus then the posterior "shelf" of perineal skin may be divided safely to open up the relatively normally sited anus. A posteriorly based VY-plasty gives a better result than a simple sagittal "cutback" incision.

If the anus is not surrounded by the external sphincter then a limited posterior sagittal anoplasty (see above) is the best way to reconstruct the perineum and reposition the anus in a correct relationship to the external sphincter.

If there is any doubt about the feasibility of primary reconstruction then the only safe strategy is to form a sigmoid colostomy and defer definitive correction until the anatomy has been defined more accurately.

No anal opening on perineum (high lesion)

Although definitive reconstruction is feasible in the neonatal period without a covering colostomy, most pediatric surgeons would elect to manage patients with an high or intermediate anomaly by formation of a sigmoid colostomy in the left iliac fossa. Division of the colon making two stomata has strong advocates, but many find a loop colostomy a satisfactory means of diverting fecal flow. Definitive reconstruction may be undertaken a few weeks later, after decompression and cleansing of the often dilated distal rectum and appropriate investigation.

Definitive Reconstruction

The pioneering work of Stephens in the early 1950s,[61] and others since, emphasized the importance of the relationship of the reconstructed anorectum to the muscular pelvic floor, in particular the puborectalis muscle and external anal sphincter. In 1982 deVries and Pena[62] described a novel posterior approach which allowed direct access to the primary abnormality and the pelvic floor. This technique has gained wide acceptance and will be described.

Posterior Sagittal Anorectoplasty

The principle is a sagittal approach in the posterior midline which divides the levatores ani in the same plane and gives access to the posterior wall of anorectum and vagina (Fig. 4.32, 4.33). Dissection is by knife and fine pointed diathermy and the extent dependent on the severity of the anomaly. The site of the external anal sphincter is identified by electrical stimulation and a posterior midline incision made from mid sacrum to its center. A narrow band of *parasagittal* muscle fibers should be bisected as they indicate that the incision is continuing in the true midline. Extension of the incision towards the exter-

nal *sphincter complex* and division of its posterior part will also open the inferior portion of the levator muscle *funnel*. The levator funnel is then opened completely in the posterior midline from coccyx to sphincter.

In the case of a rectovaginal fistula, the terminal rectum is opened vertically at its termination to expose the fistula orifice. A number of *parachute* sutures are placed around the orifice and the rectum is dissected from the posterior vaginal wall. The plane between rectum and vagina is thin inferiorly and the vagina tends to envelop the rectum on each side. As dissection proceeds superiorly both vaginal and rectal walls become independent. Mobilization should continue to the level of the cervix uteri.

Reconstruction involves closure of the vaginal fistula and approximating pelvic connective tissue between rectum and vagina. This should result in a triangular profile between vagina in front, anterior wall of rectum behind, and perineum at the base. Finally, the posterior element of the levator funnel is recreated around the rectum and sphincter complex around the anus. The skin is closed overlying the reconstructed perineum and in the posterior midline. A near normal appearance of the anus can be achieved by using the Nixon anoplasty to create a skin-lined anal canal.[63]

When the anal opening is low, in the vaginal vestibule for example, dissection may be less extensive but it is important to separate the rectum from the vagina for a sufficient length to create an adequate perineal body and place the mobilized rectum completely within the levator funnel.

Results of Treatment

Operative and early postoperative complications are rare after the posterior sagittal approach; indeed patients are usually feeding a few hours after surgery and most are discharged from hospital within a few days.[64]

The major long-term problems faced by these patients are fecal incontinence or constipation. Precise comparison of published data is difficult because of a lack of uniformity in the parameters used to describe outcome, but all workers acknowledge the above difficulties

Continence

The largest series reported to date is that of Pena[64] who studied anorectal function in 387 of 792 patients treated by the posterior sagittal approach. Voluntary bowel movement was used as an indicator of good anorectal function and was present in 74% of the group, varying with the severity of the lesion

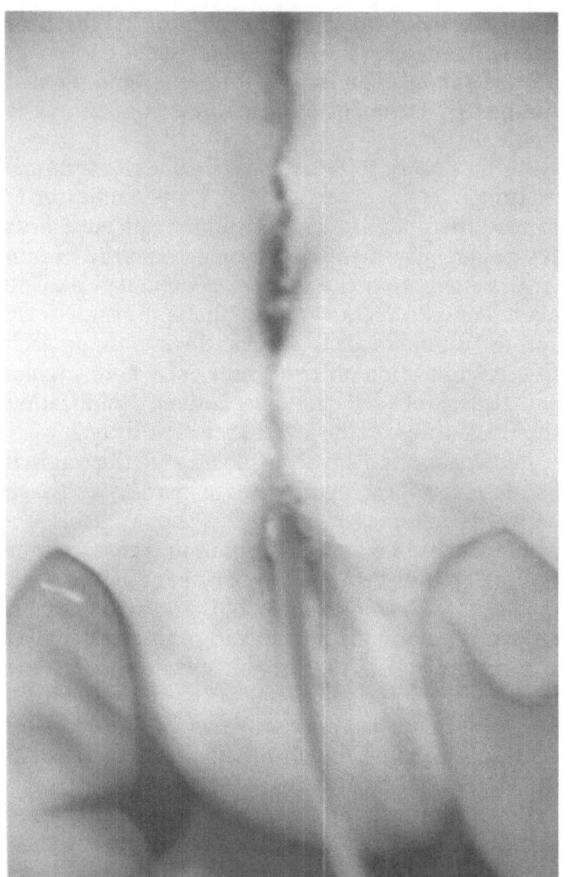

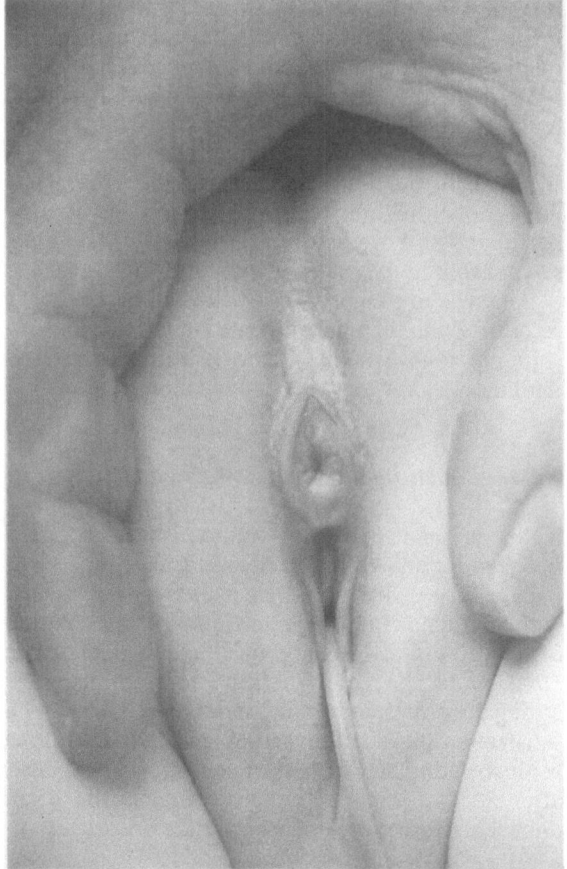

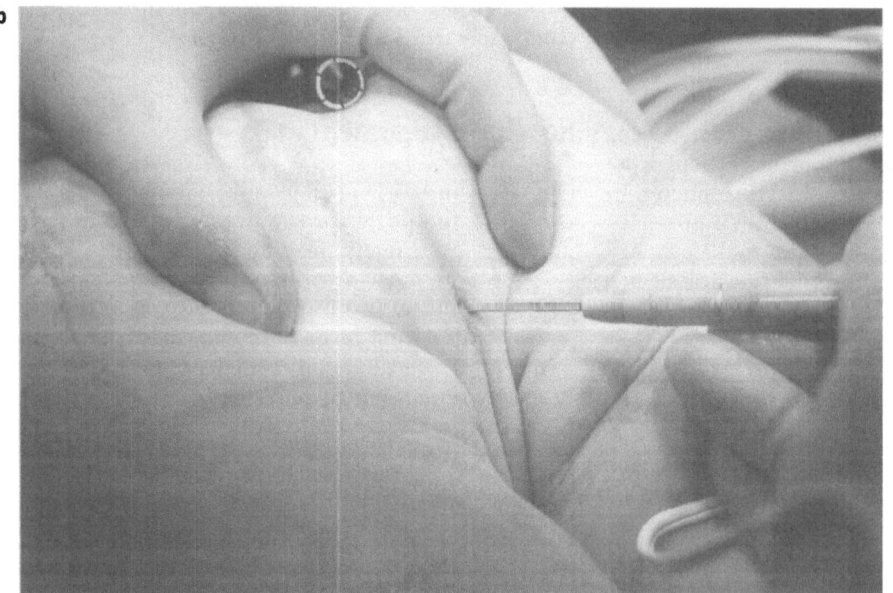

Figure 4.32. Posterior sagittal anorectoplasty. **a** Rectovestibular fistula. **b** Muscle stimulation. **c** Completed reconstruction.

from near 100% in patients with a cutaneous or vestibular fistula to 71% in those with a cloacal anomaly. Patients with voluntary bowel movement who did not soil were considered continent and comprised 41% of the group. Continence, thus defined, varied from 100% in patients with an

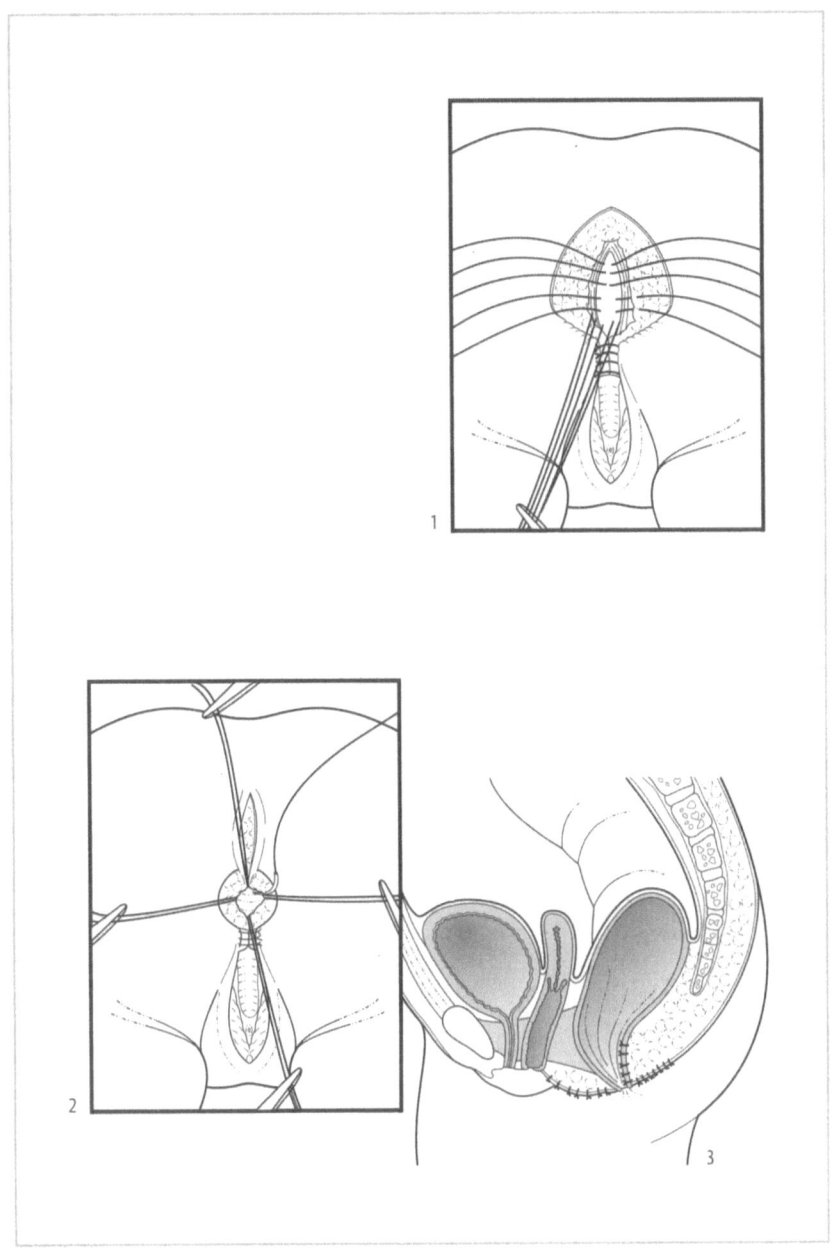

Figure 4.33 Posterior sagittal anorectoplasty. 1. Muscle complex suture, anchoring the rectum. 2. Anoplasty. 3. Operation completed. From: Pena A (1990) Surgical Management of Anorectal Malformations, Springer-Verlag New York, 55.

anocutaneous fistula to 66% in patients with a vestibular fistula.

Other published reports of results from posterior sagittal anorectoplasty vary widely in outcome and in the parameters used for assessment.[65-68] A study from Helsinki reported 35% "normal" plus 35% "good" outcome for continence after correction of high and intermediate anomalies, whereas another from Rotterdam[68] found that all of 50 patients with an high anomaly were incontinent following correction.[66]

Long-term reviews of adult patients treated before the advent of the posterior sagittal approach reveal that very few have normal control.[69-72]

Curiously, in spite of this, most reports indicate that the patients are satisfied with their cleanliness and have "acceptable social continence".[73]

Although considerable improvements in bowel control occur around puberty and most adults seem to cope with their disability, we no longer accept incontinence through early childhood. By using a bowel training program it is usually possible to get these children clean and out of diapers by the time they start school. The principle of this technique is to stimulate defecation at a predictable time by means of oral laxatives or enemas.

In our institution all children are carefully monitored both clinically and by anorectal physiology tests. Of children treated by us, 82% are clean or soil once per month or less and have a stool frequency in the normal range. None of this group has any social embarrassment. Anal sensation was the physiology test which correlated most closely with continence. Constipation was found in 36%.

If conservative measures do not achieve acceptable continence, then the Malone Antegrade Colonic Enema procedure[74] or similar may be employed. This allows thorough irrigation and emptying of the colon, using the appendix as a continent stoma, and has transformed the lives of many incontinent children.

Constipation

Patients with impaired sphincter function find cleanliness easier to achieve with hard rather than soft stools, but hard stools may be associated with problematic constipation and ultimately work against acceptable bowel function.

The origins of constipation are many, but include dilation of the left colon and rectum which may be present at birth. Although adequate rectal capacity is necessary as a "reservoir" especially if sphincter function is diminished, there is a tendency for these patients to develop pathological rectal and colonic distension.

In addition, many of these patients have disordered colonic motility[75] as a primary or secondary phenomenon, with the result that at least half of the patients will suffer from constipation requiring treatment, sometimes surgical resection.[74–76] The condition is more common in those with low anomalies and those with a high anomaly with a good external sphincter.

Summary

The aim of therapy in patients with this rare congenital anomaly is to allow a near normal quality of life. In most cases the anorectum can be reconstructed in a normal relationship to the pelvic floor structures. Continence is possible in many of these patients, but even if it is not achieved there are very effective measures to achieve cleanliness and avoid social embarrassment.

References

1. Haqq CM, King C-Y, Ukiyama E et al. (1994) Molecular basis of mammalian sexual determination: activation of mullerian inhibiting substance gene expression by SRY. Science 266: 1494.

2. Parker KL, Schimmer BP (1996) The roles of the nuclear receptor steroidogenic factor 1 in endocrine differentiation and development. Trends Endocrinol Metab 7: 203.

3. Sadovsky Y, Crawford PA (1998) Developmental and physiologic roles of the nuclear receptor steroidogenic factor-1 in the reproductive system. J Soc Gynecol Invest 5: 6.

4. Swain A, Narvaez V, Burgoyne P, Camerino G, Lovell-Badge R (1998) Dax1 antagonizes Sry action in mammalian sex determination. Nature 39: 761.

5. Larsen WJ (1993) Human Embryology. Churchill Livingstone, New York.

6. Langman J (1975) Medical Embryology. Williams & Wilkins, Baltimore, MD.

7. Lee MM, Donahoe PK (1993) Mullerian inhibiting substance: a gonadal hormone with multiple functions. Endo Rev 14: 152.

8. Gustafson ML, Lee MM, Asmundson L, MacLaughlin DT, Donahoe PK (1993) Mullerian inhibiting substance in the diagnosis and management of intersex and gonadal abnormalities. J Ped Surg 28: 439.

9. Edman CD, Winters AJ, Porter JC, Wilson J, MacDonald PC (1977) Embryonic testicular regression: A clinical spectrum of XY agonadal individuals. Obstet Gynecol 49: 208.

10. Wilson JD, George FW, Griffin JE (1981) The hormonal control of sexual development. Science 211: 1278.

11. Rock JA (1986) Anomalous development of the vagina. Semin Reprod Endocrinol 4: 13.

12. Thompson JD, Rock JA (1992) Te Linde's Operative Gynecology, 7th edn. Lippincott, Philadelphia.

13. Lindenman E, Shepard MK, Pescovitz OH (1997) Mullerian agenesis: an update. Obstet Gynecol 90: 307.

14. Reinhold C, Hricak H, Forstner R et al. (1997) Primary amenorrhea: evaluation with MR imaging. Radiology 203: 383.

15. Togashi K, Nishimura K, Itoh K et al. (1987) Vaginal agenesis: classification by MR imaging. Radiology 162: 675.

16. Taylor HS, Vanden Heuvel GB, Igarashi P (1997) A conserved Hox axis in the mouse and human female reproductive system; late establishment and persistent adult expression of the Hoxa cluster genes. Biol Reprod 57: 1338.

17. Warot X, Fromental-Ramain C, Fraulob V, Chambon P, Dolle P (1997) Gene dosage-dependent effects of the hoxa-13 and hoxd-13 mutations on morphogenesis of the terminal parts of the digestive and urogenital tracts. Development 124: 4781.

18. Stelling JR, Bhagavath B, Gray MR, Reindollar RH (1997) Hoxa13 homeodomain mutation analysis in patients with mullerian system anomalies. Abstract. Society for Gynecologic Investigation, 1997, Atlanta GA, p. 140A.

19. Frank RT (1938) The formation of an artificial vagina without operation. Am J Obstet Gynecol 35: 1053.

20. Wabrek AJ, Millard R, Wilson WB, Pion RJ (1971) Creation of a neovagina by the Frank nonoperative method. Obstet Gynecol 37: 408.

21. Ingram JM (1981) The bicycle seat stool in the treatment of vaginal agenesis and stenosis: a preliminary report. Am J Obstet Gynecol 140: 867.

22. McIndoe A (1950) The treatment of congenital absence and obliterative conditions of the vagina. Br J Plast Surg 2:254.

23. Wheeless CR, Parker J (1997) Atlas of Pelvic Surgery. Williams & Wilkins, Baltimore, MD.

24. Rock JA, Murphy AA, Jones HW Jr (1992) Female Reproductive Surgery. Williams & Wilkins, Baltimore, Md.

25. Jackson ND, Rosenblatt PL (1994) Use of interceed absorbable adhesion barrier for vaginoplasty. Obstet Gynecol 84: 1048.

26. Wenof M, Reynick JV, Novendstern J, Castadot MJ (1979) Transverse vaginal septum. Obstet Gynecol 54: 61.

27. Rock JA, Jones HW Jr (1984) Vaginal forms for dilatation and/or to maintain vaginal patency. Fertil Steril 42: 187.

28. Pena A (1997) Total urogenital mobilization–an easier way to repair cloacas. J Pediatr Surg 32: 263–7.

29. Rock JA, Zacur HA, Dlugi AM, Jones HW Jr (1982) Pregnancy success following surgical correction of imperforate hymen and complete transverse vaginal septum. Obstet Gynecol 59: 448.

30. Markham SM, Parley TH, Murphy AA, Huggins GR, Rock JA (1987) Cervical agenesis combined with vaginal agenesis diagnosed by magnetic resonance imaging. Fertil Steril 48: 143.

31. Rock JA, Schlaff WD, Zacur HA, Jones HW Jr (1984) The clinical management of congenital absence of the uterine cervix. Int J Gynaecol Obstet 22: 231.

32. Rock JA, Jones HW Jr (1980) The double uterus asociated with an obstructed hemivagina and ipsilateral renal agenesis. Am J Obstet Gynecol 138: 339.

33. Gant NF, Cunningham FG (1993) Basic Gynecology and Obstetrics. Appleton and Lange, Norwalk, CT.

34. Daly DC, Walters CA, Soto-Albors CE, Riddick DH (1983) Hysteroscopic metroplasty: surgical technique and obstetrical outcome. Fertil Steril 39: 623.

35. Israel R, March GM (1984) Hysteroscopic incision of the septate uterus. Am J Obstet Gyencol 149: 66.

36. Fedele L, Arcaini L, Parazzini F, Vercellini P, Di Nola G (1993) Reproductive prognosis after hysteroscopic metroplasty in 102 women: life-table analysis. Fertil Steril 59: 768.

37. McShane PM, Reilly FJ, Schiff I (1983) Pregnancy outcomes following Tompkins metroplasty. Fertil Steril 40: 190.

38. Muasher JJ, Acosta AA, Garcia JE, Rosenwaks Z, Jones HW (1984) Wedge metroplasty for the septate uterus: an update. Fertil Steril 42: 515.

39. Goldenberg M, Sivan E, Sharabi Z, Mashiach S, Lipitz S (1995) Seidman DS. following hysteroscopic management of intrauterine septum and adhesions. Hum Reprod 10: 2663.

40. Cararach M, Penella J, Ubeda A, Labastida R (1994) Hysteroscopic incision of the septate uterus: scissors versus resectoscope. Hum Reprod 9: 97.

41. Baggish MS, Barbot J, Valle RF (1993) Diagnostic and Operative Hysteroscopy: A Text and Atlas. Year Book Medical Publishers, Chicago, IL

42. Chantilis SJ, Bradshaw KD (1994) Clinical and molecular aspects of steroidogenic enzyme deficiencies. Infertil Clin North Am 5: 81.

43. Sanfilippo JS, Muram D, Lee PA, Dewhurst J (eds) (1994) Pediatric and Adolescent Gynecology. WB Saunders, Philadelphia, PA.

44. McPhaul MJ, Marcelli M, Zoppi S, Griffin JE, Wilson JD (1993) The spectrum of mutations in the androgen receptor gene that causes androgen resistance. J Clin Endocrinol Metab 76: 17.

45. Mulkaikal RM, Migeon CJ, Rock JA (1987) Fertility rates in female patients with congenital adrenal hyperplasia due to 21-hydroxylase deficiency. N Engl J Med 316: 178.

46. Money J, Norman BF (1987) Gender identity and gender transposition: Longitudinal outcome study of 24 male hermaphrodites assigned as boys. J Sex Marital Ther 13: 75.

47. Rickwood AMK, Thomas DG, Spicer RD (1982) Assessment of congenital neuropathic bladder by combined urodynamic and radiological studies. Br J Urol 54: 512–18.

48. Mundy AR, Shah PJR, Borzyskowski M, Saxton HM (1985) Sphincter behaviour in myelomeningocele. Br J Urol 57: 647–51.

49. Williams DI, Snyder H (1976) Anterior detrusor tube repair for urinary incontinence in children. Br J Urol 48: 671–7.

50. Hendren WH (1980) Construction of the female urethra from the vaginal wall and perineal flap. J Urol 123: 657–64.

51. Young HH (1919) An operation for the cure of incontinence of urine. Surg Gynaecol Obstet 28: 24–90.

52. Dees JE (1949) Congenital epispadias and incontinence. J Urol 62: 513–20.

53. Leadbetter GW (1964) Surgical correction of total urinary incontinence. J Urol 91: 738–45.

54. Lepor H, Jeffs RD (1983) Primary bladder closure and bladder neck reconstruction in males with bladder exstrophy. J Urol 130: 1142–5.

55. Mitrofanoff P (1980) Cystostomic continente transappendiculair dans le traitement des vesies neurologiques. Chir Paediatr 21: 297–305.

56. McGuire EJ, Wang C, Usitaki H (1986) Modified pubovaginal sling in girls with myelodysplasia. J Urol 135: 94–6.

57. Freedman ER, Singh G, Donnell SC, Rickwood AMK, Thomas DG (1994) Combined bladder neck suspension and augmentation cystoplasty for neuropathic incontinence in female patients. Br J Urol 73: 621–4.

58. Pippi Salle JL, Fraga JCS de Aramante A et al. (1994) Urethral lengthening with anterior bladder wall flap for urinary incontinence: a new approach. J Urol 152: 803–6.

59. Rickwood AMK, Thomas DG, Philip NH (1983) Long-term catheterisation for congenital neuropathic bladder. Arch Dis Child 58: 111–16.

60. Stephens FD, Smith ED (1986) Classification. Ped Surg Int 1: 200–5.

61. Stephens FD (1953) Imperforate rectum: A new surgical technique. Med J Aus 1: 202–6.

62. Vries PA De, Pena A (1982) Posterior sagittal anorectoplasty. J Ped Surg 17: 638–43.

63. Nixon HH (1971) Nixon's operation for ectopic anus. In: Ano-rectal malformation in children. Eds Stephen FD and Smith ED. Year Book Medical Publishers, Inc. Chicago. p 269.

64. Pena A (1995) Anorectal malformations. Semin Pediatr Surg 4: 35–47.

65. Bliss DP Jr, Tapper D, Anderson JM et al. (1996) Does posterior sagittal anorectoplasty in patients with high imperforate anus provide superior fecal continence? J Ped Surg 31: 26–30.

66. Langemeijer RA, Molenaar JC (1991) Continence after posterior sagittal anorectoplasty. J Ped Surg 26: 587–90.

67. Rintala RJ, Lindahl HG, Rasenen M (1997) Do children with repaired low anorectal malformations have normal bowel function? J Ped Surg 32: 823–6.

68. Rintala RJ, Lindahl HG (1995) Is normal bowel function possible after repair of intermediate and high anorectal malformations? J Ped Surg 30: 491–4.

69. Rintala R, Mildh L, Lindahl H (1992) Feacal continence and quality of life in adult patients with an operated low anorectal malformation. J Ped Surg 27: 902–5.

70. Hassink EA, Rieu PN, Severijnen RS et al. (1993) Are adults content or continent after repair for high anal atresia? A long term follow-up study in patients 18 years old or older. Ann Surg 218: 196–200.

71. Rintala R, Mildh L, Lindahl H (1994) Fecal continence and quality of life for adult patients with an operated high or intermediate anorectal malformation. J Ped Surg 29: 777–80.

72. Hassink EA, Rieu PN, Brugnan AT et al. (1994) Quality of life after operatively corrected high anorectal malformation: a long term follow-up study in patients aged 18 years and older. J Ped Surg 29: 773–6.

73. Rintala R, Lindahl H, Louhimo I (1991) Anorectal malformations–Results of treatment and long term follow-up in 208 patients. Ped Surg Int 6: 36–41.

74. Rintala R, Lindahl H, Marttinen E et al. (1993) Constipation is a major functional complication after internal sphincter saving posterior anorectoplasty for high and intermediate anorectal malformations. J Ped Surg 28: 1054–8.

75. Rintala R, Marttinen E, Virkola K et al. (1997) Segmental colonic motility in patients with anorectal malformations. J Ped Surg 32: 453–6.

76. Rintala R, Lindahl H, Rasanen M (1997) Do children with low anorectal malformations have normal bowel function? J Ped Surg 32: 823–6.

5 Injectables for the Treatment of Female Stress Urinary Incontinence

Sender Herschorn

Since the first report of injection of sodium morrhuate around the urethra by Murless in 1938,[1] various materials have been injected into and around the urethra for urinary incontinence, as an alternative to surgery. Quackels[2] reported paraffin wax in 1955 and Sachse[3] used sclerosing agents in 1963. The initial results were poor, and significant complications such as pulmonary emboli and urethral sloughing were seen. Polytetrafluoroethylene (Teflon) paste was first introduced by Berg[4] and then popularized by Politano[5] in the 1970s. Shortliffe et al.[6] published the first report on glutaraldehyde cross-linked collagen, and more recently autologous fat injection[7] has been described. Newer agents, such as silicone microparticles[8] and injectable microballoons, have also been reported.[9]

Recently there has been growing interest in injectable agents, because of their minimally invasive nature. This chapter summarizes the properties, results, and complications of the various agents as well as examining some of the controversies and the yet unanswered questions.

Mechanism of Action of Injectables

It is generally thought that injectable agents improve intrinsic sphincter function. Collagen injections have been reported[10,11] to augment urethral mucosa, improve coaptation and intrinsic sphincter function, as evidenced by an increase in post-treatment abdominal leak pressure[12-14]. Initial investigators with collagen[15,16] postulated obstruction as a mechanism of action, but Monga et al.[11] showed that successfully treated patients have an increased area and pressure transmission ratio in the first quarter of the urethra. They suggested that placement of the injectable at the bladder neck or proximal urethra prevents bladder neck opening under stress. Proper placement of the injectable, possibly just below the bladder neck, rather than actual quantity[17] of the agent, improves intrinsic sphincter deficiency (ISD).

The ideal injectable agent[18] should be easily injectable and conserve its volume over time. If unsuccessful, it should not interfere with subsequent surgical intervention. It should also be biocompatible, nonantigenic, noncarcinogenic and nonmigratory. To date, no substance has met all of these requirements.

Patient Selection

Patients with ISD and normal detrusor function are candidates for treatment with injectable agents.[19]

The identification of these patients has been described by McGuire et al.[20] with the use of abdominal leak pressures to measure the strength of the intrinsic sphincter. Low leak pressures (<65 cm water) correlate well with type 3 videourodynamic findings, i.e., a poorly functioning bladder neck and proximal urethra (ISD), and higher leak pressures correlated with types 1 or 2 hypermobility.

Normal continence in women, according to Raz et al.[21], results from the musculofascial components maintaining normal anatomic support and position of the bladder along with an intrinsically intact urethra with its coapting mucosal surface. Failure of one of the components will not invariably produce stress incontinence because of the compensatory effect of the other component. This may explain why many patients with bladder and urethral prolapse do not have stress incontinence. The intrinsic urethral mechanism or "sphincter" maintains a "washer effect" for continence by directing submucosal expansile forces toward the mucosa. This creates a seal that is a major contributor to continence.

When women with hypermobility do not leak with increases in intra-abdominal pressure, continence may be attributed to a compensating intrinsic sphincter mechanism.[21] If women with hypermobility have stress incontinence, even with high abdominal leak pressures, the intrinsic sphincter mechanism may not be compensating.

The presence of a poor or nonfunctioning proximal urethra (ISD) is the primary indication for the use of collagen in patients with stress incontinence.[10] Since ISD can co-exist with hypermobility, injectables have also been administered to patients with hypermobility, to improve the ISD component of their incontinence. The results of these trials are presented below. Furthermore, elderly women with stress incontinence who may be poor operative risks have also been injected.[22]

Injection Techniques

The materials can usually be administered under local anesthesia with cystoscopic control as an outpatient procedure. The two commonly used routes are *periurethral* or *transurethral*, but both methods are done to implant the agent within the urethral wall, preferably in the submucosa or lamina propria. It is thought that the implant should be positioned at the bladder neck or proximal urethra. Different sites can be chosen, such as 3 and 9 o'clock or 4 and 8 o'clock positions. The needle size depends on the viscosity of the injectable. Collagen can be injected through a 20 or 22-gauge whereas Teflon, fat, and silicone microparticles require 16–18-gauge needles.

Pre- and postoperative antibiotics are usually administered.

With the periurethral approach, subcutaneous blebs are raised with 1% or 2% lignocaine (lidocaine) at the 3 o'clock and 9 o'clock or 4 o'clock and 8 o'clock positions approximately 3–4 mm lateral to the urethral meatus. A 20F urethroscope with a 30° telescope is inserted into the urethra after instillation of topical urethral lignocaine (lidocaine). The periurethral needle is introduced and advanced parallel to the endoscope sheath until its position can be seen cystoscopically just below the bladder neck within the mucosa. Care must be taken to prevent the needle from getting too close to or entering the urethral lumen, as rupture of the mucosa and extravasation will occur is this happens. Rocking the needle will allow confirmation of the tip position. If penetration of the mucosa occurs, the needle should be removed and repositioned. Once in place, a small amount of lignocaine (lidocaine) can be injected into the needle for confirmation of the position and for additional pain control. The substance is injected either unilaterally or bilaterally to create the appearance of prostatic lobes. Care should be taken to prevent the cystoscope from compressing the freshly injected substance. The patient is asked to cough or strain in the supine and then upright position. If leakage still occurs, more agent may be given. If no leakage is seen, the procedure may be terminated. The patient then voids and can be discharged. Acute retention can be treated by insertion of a fine 8F catheter.

The implant can also be injected through the cystoscope directly into the mucosa with specially designed transurethral needles. Collagen can be injected manually but Teflon, silicone microparticles, and fat, because of their high viscosity, may require the use of injection guns. Various sites at or just below the bladder neck can be injected to achieve a similar appearance of an obstructing prostate.

Collagen

Glutaraldehyde cross-linked collagen or Gax-collagen is a highly purified suspension of bovine collagen in normal saline containing at least 95% type I collagen and 1% to 5% type III collagen[23]. It is prepared by selective hydrolysis of the N-terminal and C-terminal segments (telopeptides) of the collagen molecules to reduce its antigenicity. Cross-linking reduces the hypersensitivity to below 1% to the bovine collagen.[23] Gax-collagen is cross-linked with 0.0075% glutaraldehyde. This cross-linking makes the Gax-collagen resistant to the fibroblast-secreted collagenase. As a result of this, the Gax-collagen is only very slightly resorbed. The implant causes no inflammatory reaction or granuloma formation and is colonized by host fibroblasts and blood vessels. It is not known to migrate, but it does degrade over time and is replaced by host collagen, which explains its persistence[23].

Since 2–5% of patients[24] are previously sensitized to collagen through dietary exposure, all patients must undergo a skin test into the volar aspect of the forearm 30 days prior to treatment. Positive responders should be excluded.

Results

Since the first description of collagen injections for urinary incontinence there have been numerous reports of its clinical efficacy, safety, ease of administration, and relative lack of morbidity. Our original report, with short-term follow-up of 6 months,[12] showed a cured and improved rate of 90.3%. As expected, with longer follow-up the success rate has deteriorated, but there still are long-term cures. Table 5.1 lists results from a number of reported clinical series.

Long-term durability of the collagen procedure is an important factor in assessing its value and cost.

Persistence of the implant itself has been demonstrated with magnetic resonance imaging of the urethra at intervals of up to 22 months after injection although the measured volume was less than that injected.[25] Early results are generally good with success rates of 72–100% (Table 5.1). Maintenance of good results in the long term may be from durability of the initial procedure itself or from reinjections with additional collagen. It is important for authors to differentiate the durability of the original procedure(s) from reinjections or top-ups by reporting the follow-up period starting from after the last injection.

Longer-term results of more than 1–2 years, vary from 57%, cure and improved,[17] to 94%.[33] Most patients need 1–2 treatment sessions with means of 5.6–15 ml of collagen. Since patients are treated at different times and durations of follow-up vary, the Kaplan–Meier curve can be useful to display the persistence of a good result. In our series,[30] the probability of remaining dry was 72% at 1 year, 57% at 2 years, and 45% at 3 years (Fig. 5.1). Winters and Appell[13] also reported a similar 50% rate of complete continence in the multicenter trial after 2 years. Additional administration of collagen usually resulted in restoration of continence and this has to be factored into the reporting.

Table 5.1. Comparison of collagen parameters and results

Study	No. of patients	Type of incontinence	Follow-up (mo)	No. dry (%)	No. improved (%)	No. failed (%)
Stricker and Haylen[26]	50	ISD	Mean: 11 Range: 1–21	21 (42)	20 (40)	7 (14)
Kieswetter et al.[27]	16	Not specified	9	7 (44)	7 (44)	2 (12)
Eckford and Abrams[15]	25	Not specified	3	16 (64)	4 (16)	5 (20)
O'Connell et al.[28]	44	42 with ISD 2 hypermobile	1–2 (longest 7)	20 (45)	8 (18)	16 (37)
Moore et al.[29]	11	Types 1 and 3	2	1 (9)	7 (63)	2 (18)
Winters and Appell[13]	50	ISD	>12	48 (96) dry or socially continent		2 (4)
McGuire and Appell[10]	17 137	Mobile ISD	>12 >12	8 (47) 63 (46)	3 (17) 47 (34)	6 (35) 29 (19)
Faerber[22]	12	Type 1	10.3 (Range 3–24)	10 (83)	2 (17)	0
Monga et al.[11]	60	Some hypermobile	3 (N=59) 12 (N=54) 24 (N=29)	27 (46) 24 (40) 14 (48)	22 (40) 20 (37) 6 (20)	
Richardson et al.[14]	42	ISD	46 (10–66 after 1st injection)	17 (40)	18 (43)	7 (17)
Herschorn et al.[30]	181	Type 1: 54 Type 2: 67 Type 3: 60	Mean: 22 (Range 4–69) >=24 (N=62) >=36 (N=25)	42 (23) 27 (43.5) 13 (52)	94 (52) 29 (46.8) 8 (32)	45 (25) 6 (9.7) 4 (16)
Smith et al.[31]	94	Type 3	Median: 14	36 (38.3)	27 (28.7)	31 (33)
Khullar et al.[17]	21	Not specified	24 (minimum)	10 (48)	2 (9)	9 (43)
Swami et al.[32]	107	Some hypermobile	24 (minimum)	27 (25)	43 (40)	37 (35)
Cross et al.[33]	103	Type 3	Median: 18 (Range 6–36)	Substantially improved 103 (74)	29 (20)	7 (6)

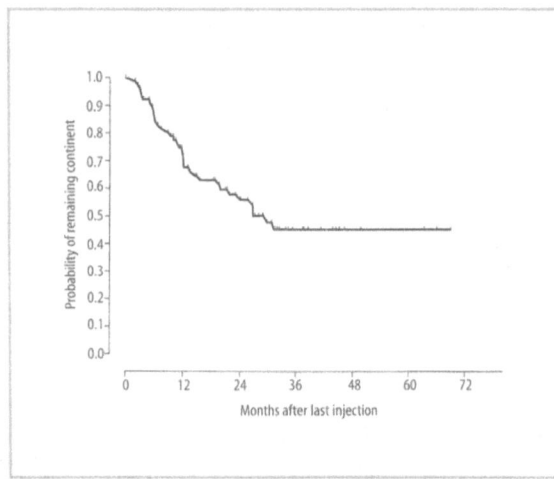

Figure 5.1 Durability: Kaplan–Meier curve showing durability of cure of incontinence after the last collagen injection in 78 patients.[30] Reprinted with permission from Herschorn S, Radomski SB (1997). Collagen injections for genuine stress urinary incontinence: Patient selection and durability. *Int Urogynecol J* 8:21.

Berman and Kreder[34] analysed the cost effectiveness of collagen versus sling cystourethropexy for type 3 incontinence. They concluded that surgery may be more cost effective than collagen.

Injections in Patients with Hypermobility

Although controversial, the use of collagen for patients with hypermobility has also been reported. Moore et al.[29] included patients with both type 1 and type 3 abnormalities. Faerber[22] treated elderly patients with type 1 abnormality. In the report by McGuire and Appell,[10] the results at more than one year in women with ISD were similar to those in women with hypermobility, although there were far more women with ISD. However, Appell[19] subsequently reported that these patients with hypermobility all required bladder neck surgery within 2 years. Monga et al.[11] included patients with hypermobility and found that cure rates were not reduced for women with up to 2.5 cm of movement. In our series of 181 patients there was no significant difference in outcome with or without hypermobility.[30]

Complications

Early treatment-related morbidity has been minimal. Urinary retention ranges from 1–21%[12,13,19] and can be managed with intermittent catheterization or short-term Foley. Urinary tract infection occurs in 1–25%.[12,13,19] Extravasation resolves quickly with flushing away of the dilute collagen suspension and sealing over of the small needle site. Hematuria can occur in 2% of patients.[19] Other rare complications include periurethral abscess formation.[35]

Changes in bladder function have also been reported. De novo instability was seen in 11 of 28 elderly women (39%) treated by Khullar et al.[17] and Stothers et al. reported de novo urgency with urgency incontinence in 43 of 337 patients (12.9%), 21% of whom (9) did not respond to anticholinergic agents.

Delayed hypersensitivity reaction in the previously negative skin test site following a urethral collagen injection has also been reported.[24] This occurred in 3 patients (1.9%) and was associated with arthralgias in 2. These investigators pretested the patients 2 weeks rather than the usual 4 weeks prior to the planned treatment. This reaction has been reported before in the dermatologic literature[37] and two negative pretreatment skin test have been suggested to prevent it. Since antibody production is stimulated by collagen injection,[38] the potential for hypersensitivity reactions is present.

Polytetrafluoroetylene Paste (PTFE, Teflon, Urethrin)

Polytetrafluoroetylene paste (Teflon) is composed of equal parts Teflon paste and glycerine with polysorbate 20.[39] The paste consists of many small particles, most of which are smaller than 40 μm in diameter. Teflon is a resin polymer with a very high molecular weight and high viscosity. It does not dissolve in any common solvent. It is inert, stable, and does not induce an allergic response. However, it does cause a local inflammatory response with histiocytes phagocytizing the particles and coalescing to form foreign body giant cells and a granuloma. There is also fibrous tissue ingrowth which adds to the bulk formed by the Teflon. Due to the small particle size, Malizia et al.[40] in experimental animals also showed distant migration of Teflon particles to pelvic nodes, lung, brain, and kidneys.

Teflon paste has been used to treat urinary incontinence since 1964, but was not reported in the literature until 1975 by Berg.[4] Since that time, numerous reports on clinical findings relating to its use in treating incontinence have appeared in the literature documenting treatment methods, success rates, complications and complication rates. Although it is not approved in the USA, Teflon has been approved in Canada and Europe (including the UK). Table 5.2 lists results published in peer-reviewed journals.

Because of its high viscosity, Teflon usually requires an injection gun. It is injected into four quadrants below the bladder neck via the periurethral route. Volumes of 10–20 ml are injected. The procedure is under local or spinal anesthesia and repeat injections may be done after 6 months.

Table 5.2. Results of using Teflon for female stress incontinence

Study	No. of patients	Follow-up (mo)	No. dry (%)	No. improved (%)	No. failed (%)
Politano et al.[42]	51	6	26 (51)	10 (20)	15 (29)
Lim et al.[43]	28	–	6 (21)	9 (33)	13 (46)
Schulman et al.[44]	56	3	39 (70)	9 (16)	8 (14)
Deane et al.[29]	28	3–24	9 (32)	8 (28)	11 (40)
Beckingham et al.[46]	26	36	2 (7)	7 (27)	17 (66)
Harrison et al.[47]	36	61	4 (11)	8 (22)	24 (67)
Lotenfoe et al.[48]	21	11	8 (38)	4 (19)	9 (43)
Lopez et al.[49]	74	31	41 (56)	15 (20)	18 (24)
Vesey et al.[50]	36	9 (3–36)	20 (56)	4 (11)	12 (33)
Herschorn and Glazer[41]	46	12	14 (31)	19 (41)	13 (28)

We have recently modified the procedure by injecting small amounts (2.5 ml) via the periurethral approach under local anesthetic, similar to the collagen technique.[41] Heating the Teflon reduces its viscosity and allows injection without a gun.

Results

Table 5.2 lists the various series. There is a wide range of results with long-term series showing poorer results (33–76% cure and improved) than those of short-term series (57–86%).

Complications

Since relatively large volumes of Teflon have been injected with the patient under general anesthetic, the incidence of urinary retention at 25%[42] is higher than that of collagen. Irritative voiding symptoms may also be seen transiently in 20%.[44] Urinary infection is rare at 2%.[43] Perineal discomfort may occur in 5%[42] and transient fever in 10–15% of patients. Perforation and extravasation can occur and, if recognized at the time of injection, the Teflon should be removed.

Although Teflon particles can migrate,[40] only one case of clinical significance has been reported in the literature in humans. Claes et al.[51] described a woman previously treated with large volumes of periurethral Teflon for urinary incontinence who later presented with lymphocytic alveolitis and fever. Light microscopy showed Teflon particles in the lungs. She was treated successfully with steroids. Mittleman and Marraccini[52] reported an incidental finding of postmortem interstitial pulmonary granulomas in a previously asymptomatic man who had received 20–30 ml of Teflon. Kiilhoma et al.[53] reported 3 complications out of 22 women: a sterile periurethral abscess, a urethral diverticulum, and a

urethral granuloma that all required surgical intervention. In another case, the material migrated into the bulbar corpus spongiosum causing perineal pain for 3 months necessitating medication for pain relief.[54]

Although Malizia hypothesized about neoplastic transformation,[40] there has never been a clinical occurrence reported since its initial use in the urethra or in the vocal cords. Furthermore, in a long-term rat study, Dewan et al.[55] demonstrated no increase in tumor risk and no tumor found at the injection site.

Despite the potential for complications with Teflon the actual rate of reported problems is low.

Autologous Fat

Autologous fat has been used for aesthetic and defect reconstruction since the 1980s. Free fat grafts are used for facial and body contouring, vocal cord augmentation, and in many other areas.[56] Although fat is biocompatible and readily available, 50–90% of the transferred adipose tissue graft may not survive.[57] Graft survival depends on minimal handling, low suction pressure during liposuction, and the use of large bore needles. Smaller grafts survive better than larger ones.[58]

The procedure involves harvesting abdominal wall fat by liposuction either under local[59] or general anesthesia.[60] The injection is usually carried out via the periurethral route with a 16 or 18 gauge needle. Postprocedure care may involve intermittent catheterization or even a suprapubic tube.[60]

Results

A number of reports of intraurethral fat injections have been published (Table 5.3). Most of the series report short-term results with success apparently

Table 5.3. Results of autologous fat injection

Study	No. of patients	Follow-up (mo)	No. dry (%)	No. improved (%)	No. failed (%)
Cervigni and Panei[7]	14	9.7	8 (57)	4 (29)	2 (14)
Santarosa and Blaivas[61]	12	11	7 (58)		5 (42)
Trockman and Leach[59]	32	6	4 (12)	14 (44)	14 (44)
Haab et al.[62]	45	7	6 (13)	13 (29)	26 (58)
Su et al.[60]	26	Mean; 17.4 (range 12–30)	13 (50)	4 (15)	9 (35)
Palma et al.[63]	30	12	1 injection: 4/13 (34) 2 injections: 11/17 (67)		

lower than that of other injectables, apart from the study of Su et al.[60] with a follow-up of more than 12 months. Palma et al.[63] showed that repeat injections improved the cure rate from 31% to 64%. Haab et al.[62] reported a comparative study with collagen. After a mean of 7 months 13% of the women with fat injection were cured versus 24% of the women with collagen injections. The subjective improvement rate was also higher with the collagen.

Complications

Reported complications are similar to those for other injectables: urinary infection, retention, hematuria, and extravasation. Additional problems with donor site, the abdominal wall, such as pain, hematomas, and infection may also be seen. Other noteworthy complications are urethral pseudolipoma[64] and fat embolism.[35,65]

Silicone Microimplants

Silicone microimplants[8] are sterile solid polydimethylsiloxane (silicone rubber) particles suspended in a nonsilicone carrier gel that is absorbed by the reticuloendothelial system and excreted unchanged in the urine. Since 99% of the particles are between 100 μm and 450 μm in diameter, the likelihood of migration is low. Henly et al.[66] demonstrated distant migration of small particles, less than 70 μm, but no migration of particles greater than 100 μm in diameter. Furthermore, although there was a typical histiocytic and giant cell reaction within the injection site, there was no granuloma formation in response to the larger particles. These factors theoretically make silicone advantageous over Teflon.

The technique is similar to that used for Teflon. Because the substance is viscous an injection gun is used, through a specially designed transurethral needle with 16 gauge tip.

Results

Hariss et al.[8] reported on 40 patients followed for a minimum of 3 years at which time 16 (40%) were dry, 7 (18%) were improved, and 17 (42%) failed. Twelve of the 16 required only one injection and 4 needed 2 injections to become dry. Sheriff et al.[67] reported an overall success of 48% in 34 patients after unsuccessful stress incontinence surgery and Koelbl et al.[68] reported a 60% success rate in 32 women after 12 months but noted a time-dependent decrease in success.

Complications

Self-limited side-effects of hematuria, dysuria, frequency, and retention have been reported in a minority of patients. The lack of a granulomatous reaction and migration of the large silicone particles may provide some benefit over Teflon, although long-term data are not yet available. Despite the laboratory and clinical evidence of safety with the large particles, concerns still exist about the migration of small silicone particles and long-term tissue response to the injection[57].

Implantable Microballoons

In order to obviate the degradation and movement of injectable materials, Atala and co-workers[69] developed a self-detachable implantable balloon system. The balloon is a silicone elastomer with a check valve that prevents escape of the solution that is injected at the time of implant. The filling solution is a biocompatible cross-linked hydrogel that maintains its volume within the silicone shell. The balloons are inserted into the submucosal area, usually periurethrally, with cystoscopic control.

Pycha et al.[9] reported that 8 (42%) of 19 women were dry and 7 (36.8%) were improved after a mean of 14.4 months. The patients with hypermobility had a poor outcome. Rare complications included bladder instability and balloon extrusion.

Conclusions

Considerable progress has been made in the last decade since the introduction of collagen injections. The injectable agents are used for buttressing the ISD component of the incontinence, but patients with concomitant hypermobility may benefit as well. There are still a number of areas in which further study is needed. Durability of the injectable is a concern. Although long-term successes have been reported with collagen and Teflon, the results of both deteriorate over time. Similarly, autologous fat and silicone microimplants also yield poorer long-term than short-term results. Comparisons of different injectables, and of injectables to surgery, have been done only to a limited degree and prospective studies have yet to be reported. Despite the ease of the technique and the attractiveness to patients of an outpatient procedure that can be repeated if necessary, the cost-effectiveness of injectable agents relative to other treatments still has to be addressed.

Safety of the material is another concern. All of the injectables have excellent safety profiles, although with Teflon the risk of migration and granuloma formation has prevented its widespread use. Rare but serious complications have also been reported with collagen and autologous fat. The long-term risks of silicone microparticles and balloons are unknown.

Newer agents are being tested, and regulatory and approval requirements dictate that comparative studies be carried out. These studies will answer some of the questions, but, as with surgical outcomes, reporting of 5-year and longer data may be necessary to answer the rest.

References

1. Murless BC (1938) The injection treatment of stress incontinence. J Obstet Gynaecol Br Emp 45: 67–73.
2. Quackels R (1955) Deux incontinences après adénectomie guéries par injection de paraffine dans la périnée. Acta Urol Belg 23: 259–262.
3. Sachse H (1963) Treatment of urinary incontinence with sclerosing solutions. Indications, results, complications. Urol Int 15: 225–244.
4. Berg S (1973) Polytef augmentation urethroplasty. Correction of surgically incurable urinary incontinence by injection technique. Arch Surg 107: 379–381.
5. Politano VA, Small MP, Harper JM, Lynne CM (1974) Periurethral Teflon injection for urinary incontinence. J Urol 111: 180–183.
6. Shortliffe LMD, Freiha FS, Kessler R, Stamey TA, Constantinou CE (1989) Treatment of urinary incontinence by the periurethral implantation of glutaraldehyde cross-linked collagen. J Urol 141: 538–541.
7. Cervigni M, Panei M (1993) Periurethral autologous fat injection for type III stress urinary incontinence. J Urol 149: 403A.
8. Harriss DR, Iacovou JW, Lemberger RJ (1996) Peri-urethral silicone microimplants (Macroplastique) for the treatment of genuine stress incontinence. Brit J Urol 78: 722–8.
9. Pycha A, Klingler CH, Haitel A, Heinz-Peer G, Marberger M (1998) Implantable microballoons: An attractive alternative in the management of intrinsic sphincter deficiency. Eur Urol 33: 469–75.
10. McGuire EJ, Appell R (1994) Transurethral collagen injection for urinary incontinence. Urology 43: 413–15.
11. Monga AK, Robinson D, Stanton SL (1995) Periurethral collagen injections for genuine stress incontinence. Brit J Urol 76: 156–60.
12. Herschorn S, Radomski SB, Steele DJ (1992) Early experience with intraurethral collagen injections for urinary incontinence. J Urol 148: 1797–800.
13. Winters JC, Appell R (1995) Periurethral injection of collagen in the treatment of intrinsic sphincter deficiency in the female patient. Urol Clin N Amer 22: 673–8.
14. Richardson TD, Kennelly MJ, Faerber GJ (1995) Endoscopic injection of glutaraldehyde cross-linked collagen for the treatment of intrinsic deficiency in women. Urology 46: 378–81.
15. Eckford SD, Abrams P (1991) Para-urethral collagen implantation for female stress incontinence. Br J Urol 68: 586–9.
16. Appell RA (1990c) New developments: Injectables for urethral incompetence in women. Int Urogynecol J 1: 117–19.
17. Khullar V, Cardozo LD, Abbott D, Anders K (1997) GAX collagen in the treatment of urinary incontinence in elderly women: a two year follow up. Br J Obstet Gynaecol 104: 96–9.
18. Kershen RT, Atala A (1999) New advances in injectable therapies for the treatment of incontinence and vesicoureteral reflux. Urol Clin North Am 26: 81–94.
19. Appell RA (1998) Periurethral injection therapy. In: Walsh PC, Retik AB, Vaughan ED Jr, Wein AJ (eds) Campbell's Urology, 7th edn. WB Saunders, Philadelphia, pp. 1109–20.
20. McGuire EJ, Fitzpatrick CC, Wan J et al. (1993) Clinical assessment of urethral sphincter function. J Urol 150: 1452–4.
21. Raz S, Little N (1992) Juma S. Female Urology. In: Walsh PC, Retik AB, Stamey TA, Vaughan ED (eds) Campbell's Urology, 6th edn. WB Saunders, Philadelphia, pp. 2782–828.
22.. Faerber GJ (1996) Endoscopic collagen injection therapy in elderly women with type I stress urinary incontinence. J Urol 155: 512–514.
23. Remacle M, Bertrand B, Eloy P, Marbaix E (1990) The use of injectable collagen to correct velopharyngeal insufficiency. Laryngoscope 100: 269.
24. Stothers L, Goldenberg SL (1998) Delayed hypersensitivity and systemic arthralgia following transurethral collagen injection for stress urinary incontinence. J Urol 159: 1507–9.
25. Carr LK, Herschorn S, Leonhardt C (1996) Magnetic resonance imaging of intraurethral collagen injected for stress urinary incontinence. J Urol 155: 1253–5.
26. Stricker P, Haylen B (1993) Injectable collagen for type III female stress incontinence: the first 50 Australian patients. Med J Aust 158: 89–91.
27. Kieswetter H, Fischer M, Wöber L, Flamm J (1992) Endoscopic implantation of collagen (GAX) for the treatment of urinary incontinence. Br J Urol 69: 22–5.
28. O'Connell HE, McGuire EJ, Aboseif S, Usui A (1995) Transurethral collagen therapy in women. J Urol 154: 1463–5.
29. Moore KN, Chetner MP, Metcalfe JB, Griffiths DJ (1995) Periurethral implantation of glutaraldehyde cross-linked collagen (contigen) in women with type I or type III stress

incontinence: quantitative outcome measures. Br J Urol 75: 359–63.

30. Herschorn S, Radomski SB (1997) Collagen injections for genuine stress urinary incontinence: Patient selection and durability. Int Urogynecol J 8: 18–24.

31. Smith DN, Appell RA, Winters JC, Rackley RR (1997) Collagen injection therapy for female intrinsic sphincteric deficiency. J Urol 157: 1275–8.

32. Swami S, Batista JE, Abrams P (1997) Collagen for female genuine stress incontinence after a minimum 2-year follow-up. Br J Urol 80: 757–61.

33. Cross CA, English SF, Cespedes RD, McGuire EJ (1998) A followup on transurethral collagen injection therapy for urinary incontinence. J Urol 159: 106–8.

34. Berman CJ, Kreder KJ (1997) Comparative cost analysis of collagen injection and fascia lata sling cystourethropexy for the treatment of type III incontinence in women. J Urol 157: 122–4.

35. Sweat SW, Lightner DJ (1999) Complications of sterile abscess formation and pulmonary embolism following periurethral bulking agents. J Urol 161: 93–6.

36. Stothers L, Goldenberg SL, Leone EF (1998) Complications of periurethral collagen injection for stress urinary incontinence. J Urol 159: 806–7.

37. Elson ML (1986) The role of skin testing in the use of collagen injectable materials. J Derml Surg Oncol 15: 301.

38. McClelland M, DeLustro F (1996) Evaluation of antibody class in response to bovine collagen treatment in patients with urinary incontinence. J Urol 155: 2068–73.

39. Diagnostic and Therapeutic Technology Assessment (DATTA) (1993) Use of Teflon preparations for urinary incontinence and vesicoureteral reflux. JAMA 269: 2975–80.

40. Malizia AA, Reiman HM, Myers RP et al. (1983) Migration and granulomatous reaction after periurethral injection of Polytef (Teflon). JAMA 251: 3277–281.

41. Herschorn S, Glazer AA (2000) Early experience with small volume periurethral teflon for female stress urinary incontinence. J Urol 163: 1838–1842.

42. Politano VA (1982) Periurethral polytetrafluoroethylene injection for urinary incontinence. J Urol 127: 439–42.

43. Lim KB, Ball AJ, Feneley RCL (1983) Periurethral teflon injection: A simple treatment for urinary incontinence. Br J Urol 55: 208–10.

44. Schulman CC, Simon J, Wespes E et al. (1984) Endoscopic injections of teflon to treat urinary incontinence in women. Br Med J 288: 192.

45. Deane AM, English P, Hehir M, Williams JP, Worth PHL (1985) Teflon injection in stress incontinence. Br J Urol 57: 78–80.

46. Beckingham IJ, Wemyss-Holden G, Lawrence WT (1992) Long-term follow-up of women treated with periurethral Teflon injections for stress incontinence. Br J Urol 69: 580–3.

47. Harrison SC, Brown C, O'Boyle PJ (1993) Periurethral Teflon for stress urinary incontinence: medium-term results. Br J Urol 71: 25–7.

48. Lotenfoe R, O'Kelly JK, Helal M, Lockhart JL (1993) Periurethral polytetrafluoroethylene paste injection in incontinent female subjects: surgical indications and improved surgical technique. J Urol 149: 279–82.

49. Lopez AE, Padron OF, Patsias G, Politano VA (1993) Transurethral polytetrafluoroethylene injection in female patients with urinary incontinence. J Urol 150: 856–8.

50. Vesey SG, Rivett AO, Boyle PJ (1988) Teflon injection in female stress incontinence. Effect on urethral pressue profile and flow rate. Br J Urol 62: 39–41.

51. Claes H, Stroobants D, Meerbeek J van et al. (1989) Pulmonary migration following periurethral polytetra-fluoroethylene injection for urinary incontinence. J Urol 142: 821–2.

52. Mittleman RE, Marraccini JV (1983) Pulmonary teflon granulomas following periurethral teflon injection for urinary incontinence. Arch Pathol Lab Med 107: 611–12.

53. Kiilhoma PJ, Chancellor MB, Makinen J, Hirsch IH, Klemi PJ (1993) Complications of teflon injection for stress urinary incontinence. Neurourol Urodyn 12: 131–7.

54. Stanisic TH, Jennings CE, Miller JI (1991) Polytetrafluoro-ethylene injection for post-prostatectomy incontinence: experience with 20 patients during 3 years. J Urol 146: 1575–7.

55. Dewan PA, Owen AJ, Byard RW (1995) Long-term histologic response to subcutaneously injected Polytef and Bio-plastique in a rat model. Br J Urol 76: 161–4.

56. Billings E, May JW (1989) Historical review and present status of free fat graft autotransplantation in plastic and reconstructive surgery. Plast Reconst Surg 83: 368–81.

57. Horl HW, Feller AM, Bieuner E (1991) Technique for lipo-suction fat re-implantation and long-term evaluation by magnetic resonance imaging. Ann Plast Surg 26: 248–58.

58. Bircoll M, Novack BH (1987) Autologous fat transplantation employing liposuction techniques. Ann Plast Surg 18: 327–9.

59. Trockman BA, Leach GE (1995) Surgical treatment of intrinsic urethral dysfunction: injectables (fat). Urol Clin North Am 22: 665–71.

60. Su T-H, Wang K-G, Hsu C-Y et al. (1998) Periurethral fat injection in the treatment of recurrent genuine stress incontinence. J Urol 159: 411–14.

61. Santarosa RP, Blaivas JG (1994) Periurethral injection of autologous fat for the treatment of sphincteric incontinence. J Urol 151: 607–11.

62. Haab F, Zimmern PE, Leach GE (1997) Urinary stress incontinence due to intrinsic sphincteric deficiency: experience with fat and collagen periurethral injections. J Urol 157: 1283–6.

63. Palma PC, Riccetto CL, Herrmann V, Netto NR Jr (1997) Repeat lipoinjections for stress urinary incontinence. J Endourol 11: 67–70.

64. Palma PC, Riccetto CL, Netto NR Jr (1996) Urethral pseudo-lipoma: a complication of periurethral lipo-injection for stress urinary incontinence in a woman. J Urol 155: 646.

65. Currie I, Drutz HP, Deck J, Oxorn D (1997) Adipose tissue and lipid droplet embolism following periurethral injection of autologous fat: case report and review of the literature. Int Urogynecol J 8: 377–80.

66. Henly DR, Barrett DM, Weiland TL et al. (1995) Particulate silicone for use in periurethral injections: local tissue effects and search for migration. J Urol 153: 2039–43.

67. Sherriff MKM, Foley S, McFarlane J, Nauth-Misir R, Shah PJR (1997) Endoscopic correction of intractable stress incontinence with silicone micro-implants. Eur Urol 32: 284–8.

68. Koelbl H, Saz V, Doerfler D et al. (1998) Transurethral injec-tion of silicone microimplants for intrinsic sphincter deficiency. Obst Gynecol 92: 332–6.

69. Yoo JJ, Magliochetti M, Atala A (1997) Detachable self-sealing membrane system for the endoscopic treatment of incontinence. J Urol 158: 1045.

6 Retropubic Suspensions

Open Retropubic Suspensions

Menachem Alcalay and Stuart L. Stanton

Procedures

Retropubic procedures for treatment of stress urinary incontinence due to urethral sphincter incompetence (USI), which were introduced in the middle of the twentieth century, opened a new era in the treatment of this devastating condition. Marshall, Marchetti and Krantz[1] reported their first series in 1949, describing the operation as "a simple elevation and mobilization of the bladder neck and urethra by suturing them to the pubis and rectus muscles." The procedure was first performed on incontinent males following prostatectomy, with good results. However, the rationale of applying retropubic procedures to females with urinary stress incontinence is credited to Bailey,[2] Green,[3] and Hodgkinson.[4] Burch described a modification to the retropubic procedure and found that he could correct incontinence and cystocele by suturing the paravaginal tissue to the ileopectineal (Cooper's) ligament.[5] He recognized that the support to the urethra could be achieved by elevation of the vaginal fascia lateral to the urethra, and, to avoid the tech-nical difficulty of retaining sutures in the peri-osteum, inserted the sutures into the ipsilateral ileopectineal ligament, which is better defined. Burch published his initial experience utilizing this modification in 53 patients in 1961. Jarvis[6] reported the results of a meta-analysis of the success rates of the operations, where the diagnosis of urethral sphincter incompetence was made preoperatively. This report summarized 15 666 patients who had been assessed subjectively and 4815 patients with an objective assessment. It seems that both the Burch and the MMK procedures are good options for primary operation, as they have an objective cure rate of 89.8% and 89.5% respectively.

Various modifications to retropubic procedures were reported subsequently,[7] but these did not gain the same popularity among surgeons as the Burch and the MMK procedures. The retropubic procedures became the standard of surgical care of patients with stress urinary incontinence and bladder neck mobility. They were popularized by both gynecologists and urologists[8] as most efficacious procedures with a reliable long-term success rate. In the UK twice as many gynecologists perform the Burch colposuspension as the MMK.[9] A recent review on the Burch procedure found 85 articles in the English literature and approximately 3500 cases,[10] and concluded that this successful procedure has been minimally modified since its first description. The most quoted reference for Burch procedure is the Tanagho modification,[11] and the Mayo Clinic modification[12] for MMK is one of the best known.

Laparoscopic retropubic procedures are discussed in the second part of the chapter.

Indications

Preoperative evaluation is essential to ensure that the patients are properly selected for surgical correction of USI, and also, very importantly, to choose the right operation for the individual patient. The preoperative evaluation should include detailed patient history, preferably with a standardized database questionnaire. The physical examination concentrates on a careful neurological and pelvic examination, including assessment of vaginal wall prolapse and uterine descent, using the POP-Q standardized scoring system[13] or another scoring system, and evaluation of vaginal capacity and mobility. The patient is examined lying and standing with a full bladder for signs of urinary incontinence and prolapse. Elevation of the lateral paravaginal fornices towards the ileopectineal ligaments is performed to evaluate the vaginal capacity and mobility, which are essential components for patients undergoing a Burch colposuspension. The "Q-tip test" may be used to evaluate the support of the urethra. This test was standardized by Karram and Bhatia,[14] who suggested that an angle of less than 30º on exertion demonstrated good anatomical support, while an angle of more than 30º indicates poor support with urethral hypermobility. It is a more popular test in the USA than in Europe.

Further investigations include a urine culture to exclude cystitis, uroflowmetry, measurement of residual urine volume and twin-channel subtracted cystometry. Other dynamic tests to evaluate the lower urinary tract should diagnose USI and detect detrusor instability or voiding dysfunction. Valsalva leak point pressure (VLPP) is usually recorded at 200 ml of fluid in the bladder. Videocysto-urethrography (VCU), or pelvic fluoroscopy, pelvic floor EMG, and cystoscopy may also be relevant in selected patients. Urethral pressure profilometry (UPP) has little role in the diagnosis of USI, as there is an overlap of parameters between continent and incontinent patients.[15]

The major indication for a retropubic urethropexy is the objective diagnosis of USI with good vaginal capacity and mobility. The MMK urethropexy is suitable for patients with USI with only grade I cystocele, whereas the Burch procedure is a good option for a coexistent grade I–III cystourethrocele.[16]

The major contraindication for retropubic urethropexy is the presence of a scarred and immobile anterior vaginal wall, where elevation of the bladder neck and lateral vaginal fornices is unlikely. The bladder neck mobility can be assessed on clinical exam, using a Q-tip test or various imaging techniques such as videourodynamics and perineal ultrasound. This is supported by a small series by Bergman et al.[17] who found 53% failure rate in 9 patients following Burch colposuspension who had an anatomically supported bladder neck preoperatively, determined by a negative Q tip test (<30º change of angle on straining). However, Bowen et al.[18] have found no association between preoperative Q-tip test and operative success.

The patients with the worse type of stress incontinence are those with incompetence of their urethral sphincter, who were previously defined by Green as having a rigid and nonmobile urethra,[19] and are referred to now as "intrinsic sphincter deficiency' (ISD). There is still controversy on the definition of ISD. Sand et al.[20] suggested that maximum urethral closure pressure (MUCP) less than 20 cm of water should be used to prefer a sling procedure rather than a retropubic surgery, while McGuire et al.[21] suggested that VLPP less than 65 cm of water should be used for ISD diagnosis. As both parameters have nonoptimal correlation with incontinence severity,[22,23] a combination of clinical, urodynamic and imaging tools should be used for ISD diagnosis. However, it is naive to believe that patients can be divided into type I, type II, and type III without overlap. We believe that all patients with urethral sphincter incompetence (GSI) have a degree of intrinsic sphincter deficiency, with the worst case having a rigid, nonmobile and totally incompetent urethra. Some patients will have lack of support of the whole urethra and bladder neck, but as the TVT procedure shows, support can also be given to the mid urethra rather than the bladder neck, to ensure continence. More work needs to be done to define the truly critical urodynamic values and techniques that would help in selecting the most appropriate procedure for patients with ISD. In a recent prospective randomized study by Sand et al.[24] it was shown that Burch colposuspension is as effective as sling procedure for patients with low pressure urethra and hypermobile bladder neck. However, this study had a short follow-up of only 3 months, and there is a need for a longer follow-up to recommend this approach. Patients with previous failures of retropubic procedures are difficult to deal with. The dissection in the scarred retropubic space is more challenging, and therefore the best operation for recurrent USI is debatable. Studies from Australia[25] and the UK[26] reported promising results where the Burch colposuspension was chosen. The 53 women who were reoperated in Mahers's et al report had an 80% subjective cure and a 72 % objective cure,[25] while in Cardozo's study 52 patients who had previous bladder neck surgery had an 80% subjective cure and a 78% objective cure at 9 months follow-up.[26]

Concomitant detrusor instability (DI) with stress incontinence is not considered a contraindication to retropubic procedures. Some authors found that preoperative DI reduced the cure rate of the operation,[27] but others found no effect on the results, or even cure of the urge incontinence following surgery.[28]

Depending upon its severity, voiding difficulty is a relative contra-indication to retropubic procedures. The various urodynamic parameters to assess voiding difficulty are urine flow rate, residual urine volume, pressure–flow curves and maximum voiding pressure. It has been shown that preoperative low-pressure voiding with maximum voiding pressure less than 15 cm of water predispose to immediate postoperative voiding difficulty,[29] although other follow up studies did not confirm this.[30]

Operative Technique

Both MMK and Burch procedures may be performed under general or regional anesthesia with no special patient preparation. Administration of first-generation cephalosporin is used perioperatively to reduce infectious morbidity. The use of pneumatic compression boots for antithrombotic prophylaxis is recommended. The patient is placed in Allen Universal Stirrups (Allen Medical Systems, Inc., Cleveland, OH), and the abdomen and vagina are sterilely prepared and draped for surgery. We usually use a transurethral resection drape to cover the perineum, allowing access to the vagina with a sterile condom during the operation. A 14 Foley catheter is placed in the bladder to allow continuous drainage throughout the operation and to facilitate urethral and bladder neck identification. The bladder can later be filled through the same catheter prior to the placement of the suprapubic catheter. If a posterior repair is required, this should be performed first so that maximum access to the rectocele is achieved.

A Pfannenstiel or a Cherney incision is made approximately one finger breadth above the symphysis pubis, and the retropubic space is exposed. If an intraperitoneal procedure is needed, it is performed first. Uterosacral ligament plication is performed in all patients with a deep cul-de-sac, or a grade II cystourethrocele. Attention is now directed to the retropubic space, and a self-retaining retractor (Turner-Warwick) is inserted (Fig. 6.1). The bladder is carefully dissected from the posterior aspect of the symphysis by blunt or sharp dissection until the paravaginal tissues lateral to the urethra, bladder neck and bladder base is identified as a conspicuous white area.

Burch Colposuspension

Once the retropubic space has been exposed, the operator inserts the nondominant forefinger into the vagina, covered with the sterile condom, and elevates the lateral vaginal fornix (Figs 6.2 and 6.3). The bladder neck and bladder base are identified and care is taken to place sutures without breaching them. The obturator foramen and its neurovascular bundle define the lateral margin of the dissection field, and injury to its contents should be avoided. The bladder is dissected medially from the pelvic side-wall, exposing the paravaginal endopelvic fascia. Usually this dissection is accomplished bluntly using a sponge stick (Fig. 6.4). However, in cases with previous bladder neck surgery, a scissors or a Bovey cautery dissection is needed. Large perivesical vessels may be encountered. Tearing of these vessels

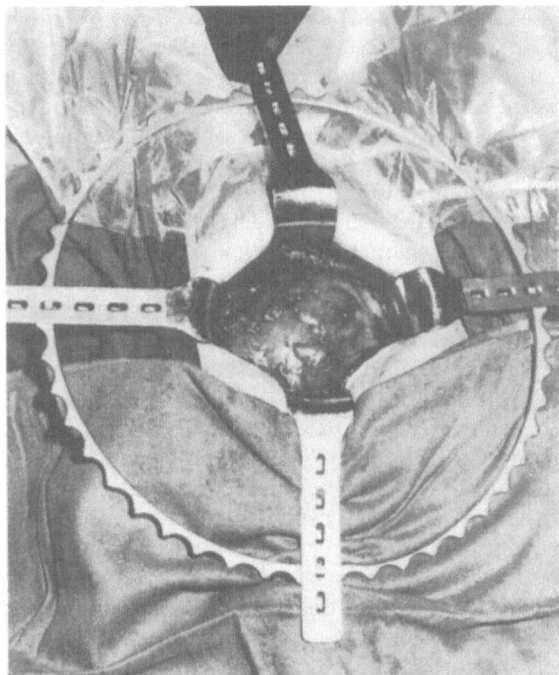

Figure 6.1 Pfannenstiel incision with Turner Warwick four-bladed self-retaining ring retractor in place. From Stanton SL, Tanagho EA (ed.) (1986), *Surgery of Female Incontinence*, Springer-Verlag, Berlin Heidelberg.

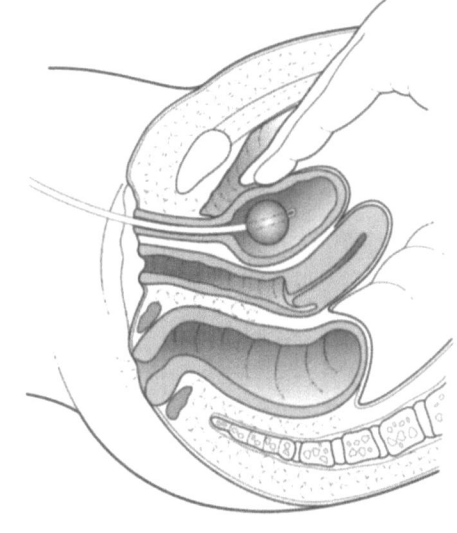

Figure 6.2 Sagittal section showing blunt finger dissection in the retropubic space, between the symphysis pubis and the anterior surface of the bladder and urethra.

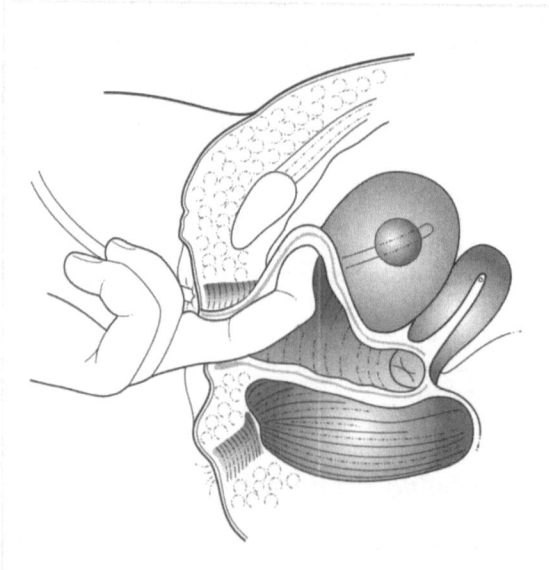

Figure 6.3 Sagittal section showing surgeon's forefinger in a lateral vaginal fornix, to aid the abdominal dissection.

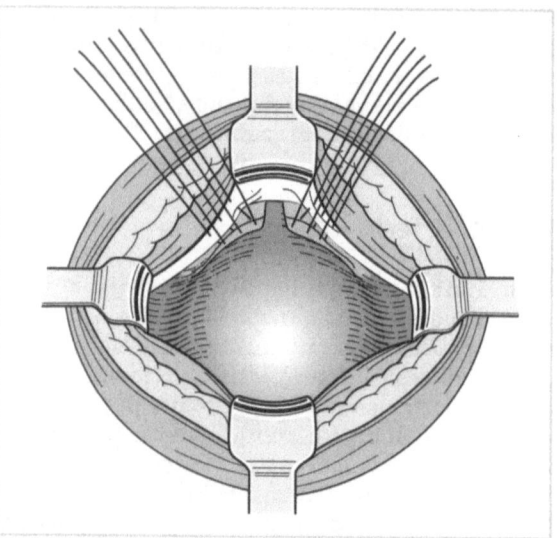

Figure 6.5 Three pairs of suture in place between the paravaginal fascia and ileopectineal ligaments, before being tied. The most distal (caudad) suture is level with the bladder neck, but the most proximal suture (cephalad) is as high as the surgeon's forefinger will reach, to enable as much support to be given as possible to the bladder base.

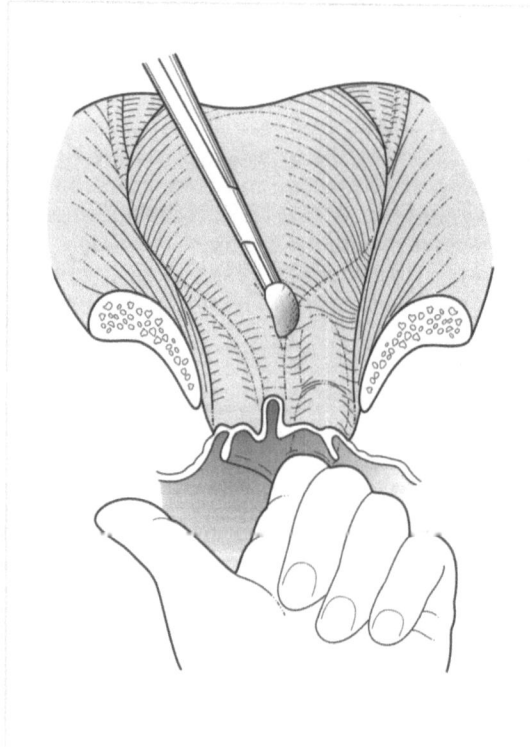

Figure 6.4 Medial dissection of the bladder base on the paravaginal fascia using a peanut swab, aided by the surgeon's forefinger in the vagina.

may result in considerable hemorrhage and should either be clipped, cauterized, or ligated. Exposure of the "glistening" white paravaginal fascia is a key step in this procedure, as it facilitates correct suture placement.

Using the vaginal finger to elevate the paravaginal fascia, 2–4 figure-of-eight pairs of No. 1 non-absorbable polybutylate-coated polyester sutures (Ethibond, Ethicon Ltd., Edinburgh, UK) are placed through the paravaginal fascia. The use of a curved needle holder (Finochette) and a heavy J needle facilitate proper suture placement. The first most proximal (cephalad) suture is placed first through the paravaginal fascia, as proximal as the operator can reach to correct cystocele (Fig. 6.5). This suture is tied on the fascia to provide hemostasis and to prevent sliding through the fascia. The operator's finger is then placed in the vagina once again to elevate the paravaginal tissue toward the ipsilateral ileopectineal ligament, to select the site of placement through the ligament. Following the site determination, the suture is placed through the ligament, obtaining a healthy bite of tissue. The most distal (caudad) suture is placed opposite the bladder neck, 1.5–2 cm lateral to the urethra, as delineated by the Foley bulb with the catheter under gentle traction. This suture is then passed through the ipsilateral ileopectineal ligament in the predetermined site. This suture serves to correct the stress incontinence, while the remaining cephalad sutures support the bladder base and correct any cystocele. The surgeon has to assess at this stage whether more sutures are needed according to the previous suture placement and the relation to the bladder neck and the cystocele degree. If needed, the remaining sutures are placed in the ipsilateral paravaginal fascia, 1–2 cm apart. The same steps are repeated, i.e. securing knots on the fascia, ileopectineal ligament site deter-

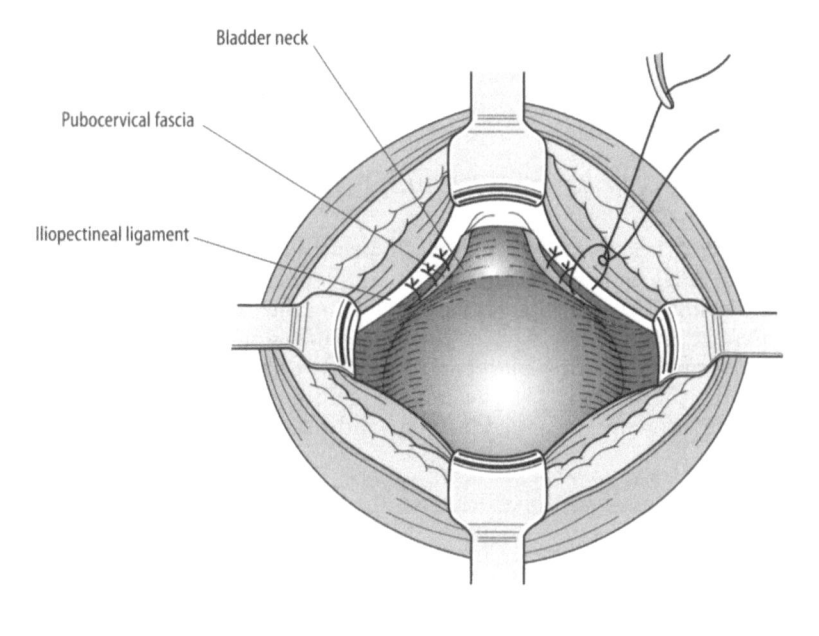

Figure 6.6 The sutures are tied, showing approximation of the paravaginal tissue to the ileopectineal ligaments with some bowstringing on either side. Elevation is produced by holding taut the suture which passes through the ileopectineal ligament and tying the other limb of the suture around this. The operator gauges the amount of tension required, avoiding excess tension which can lead to obstruction. This technique obviates the need for an assistant to elevate the vagina.

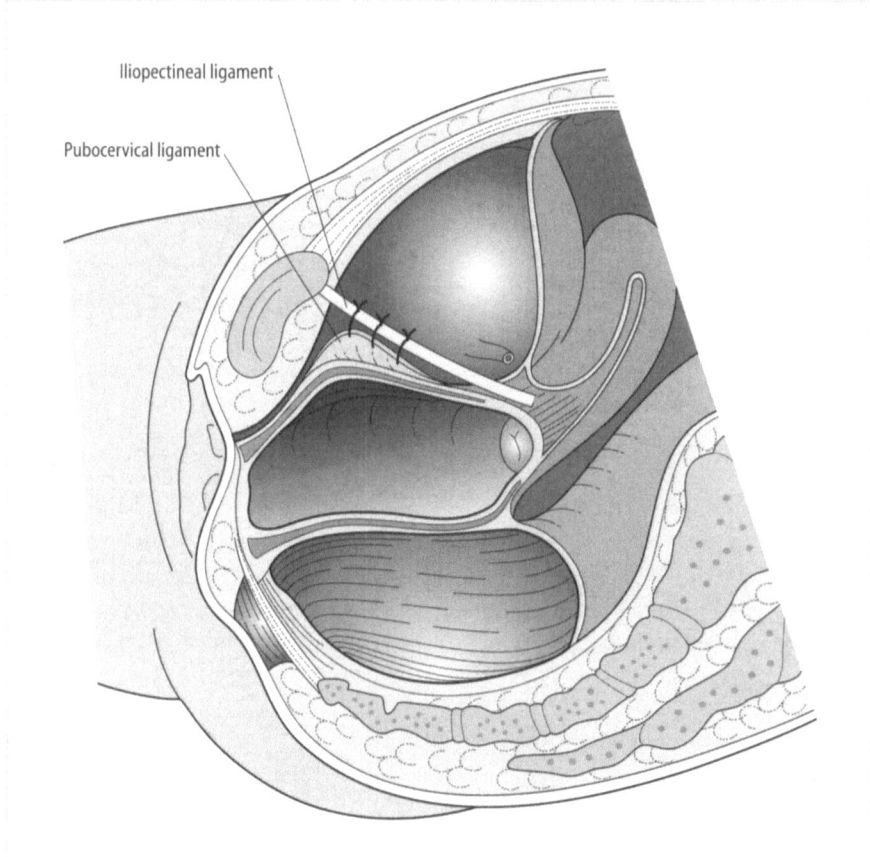

Figure 6.7 Sagittal section showing elevation of the bladder neck and bladder base on the shelf of paravaginal fascia, sutured to an ileopectineal ligament.

mination and passing through the ligament. After the sutures are placed on one side, the bladder is dissected off the paravaginal fascia on the opposite side, and the sutures placed in a similar way.

Only after all the sutures are placed through the ligament bilaterally are they tied. The most caudad sutures are tied first, and then the remaining sutures are tied on alternating sides to ensure balanced support with some elevation to the bladder neck, and approximating paravaginal fascia to the ileopectineal ligament or pelvic side wall (Figs 6.6 and 6.7). It is common to have a suture bridge between the paravaginal fascia and the ileopectineal ligament. Tying the sutures too tightly can result in overcorrection and possible postsurgical voiding difficulties. It is the practice of some surgeons to

inspect the bladder endoscopically or initially to instill dye into the bladder to ensure that no sutures have perforated the bladder wall. A suprapubic catheter is inserted, and a retropubic suction drain through a separate stab wound is inserted.

Marshall–Marchetti–Krantz

In the MMK procedure a 20 or 22 French Foley catheter is recommended to facilitate better urethral palpation. Following the exposure of the retropubic space, the surgeon's nondominant forefinger is placed in the vagina, which is already covered with a sterile condom, and the paravaginal fascia near the bladder neck and the urethra is identified. Using a

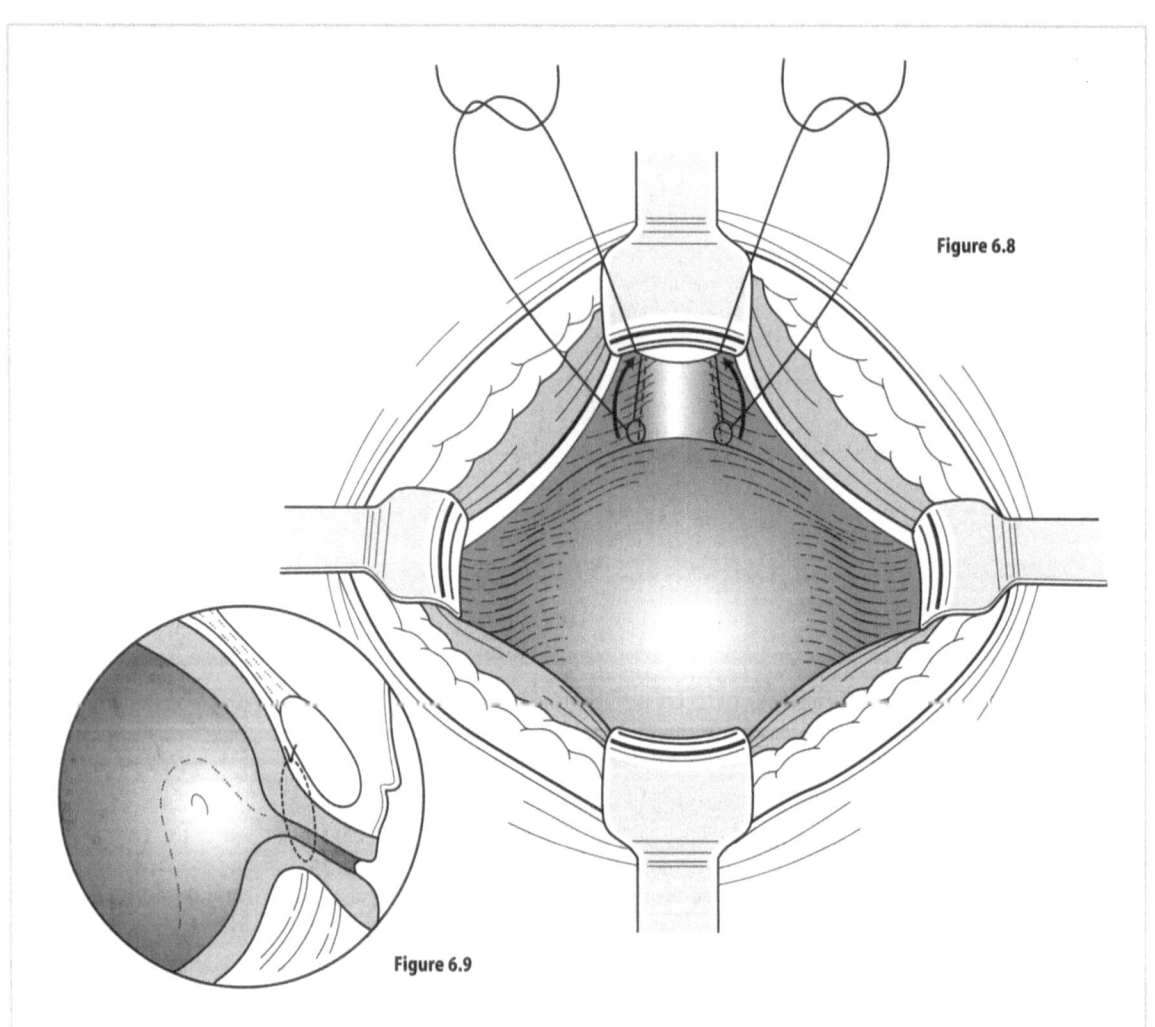

Figure 6.8

Figure 6.9

Figure 6.8 Marshall–Marchetti–Krantz procedure: The sutures are placed at the urethrovesical junction and lateral to the urethra.

Figure 6.9 Marshall–Marchetti–Krantz procedure: To illustrate first suture placement between the vaginal wall and paravaginal fascia and fibrocartilage of the symphysis. Succeeding sutures are placed more distally.

permanent suture, such as 0-Ethibond (Ethicon Ltd., Edinburgh, UK), a double bite of suture is placed incorporating the full thickness of the vaginal wall, but avoiding the vaginal epithelium. The most cephalad suture is placed at the level of the bladder neck, 2–3 mm lateral to the urethra (Fig. 6.8). Additional sutures in each side are dependent on urethral length, and usually 2–3 sutures in total are needed. After all the periurethral sutures have been placed, they are secured into the fibro-cartilage of the symphysis, at their corresponding location (Fig. 6.9) and are tied, starting from the most caudal one. At this stage some surgeons will perform cystoscopy with intravenous indigo carmine (American Reagent, Shirley, NY) to assess ureteric patency and urethral integrity. A suprapubic catheter is placed, and a retropubic suction drain is used as needed.

The Mayo modification of MMK procedure, which was popularized by Lee[31] and Symmonds,[12] advocates cystotomy during the procedure for direct inspection and palpation of bladder neck and proximal urethra. After assessment, the first suture is placed at the level of the bladder neck. A Russian forceps is used to press against the catheter to define the urethral margins to confirm that the tip of the needle is 2–3 mm lateral to the urethra. The insertion of the paraurethral suture should include almost the entire thickness of the anterior vaginal wall. Usually two sutures are placed in each side, the second set being placed approximately 0.5 cm distal to the bladder neck. The cystotomy incision is used for placement of the suprapubic catheter.

Complications

The most common intraoperative complications include damage to the lower urinary tract, pelvic blood vessels and nerves.[32]

Hemorrhage and Hematoma

During retropubic dissection, rupture of a thin-walled venous plexus in the bladder or vagina causes considerable blood loss. The retropubic space has no dependent drainage, so the surgeon must dissect carefully and secure hemostasis at the time of surgery, and, if necessary, place suction drains in the retropubic space to prevent formation of hematomas.

If a hematoma is suspected it may be diagnosed by ultrasound. If it is increasing in size and causing cardiovascular deterioration, bleeding may be arrested either using interventional radiology to identify and thrombose either the artery or vein, or a laparotomy to evacuate the clot and secure the bleeding vessel.

Nerve Injury

Nerve injuries associated with retropubic surgery most often result either from placing patients in a "frog leg" or lithotomy position, or by compression of a nerve by a surgical retractor. The peroneal, femoral, or sciatic nerves are the most likely to be injured by these maneuvers. Dissection and placement of sutures are more likely to injure the obturator or entrap the ilioinguinal nerves.

Lower Urinary Tract Injury

Damage to the ureter is rare, and has been described following the Burch procedure[33] or MMK, where two cases of bilateral ureterovesical obstruction were reported.[34] The bladder is more likely to be transfixed by suture, crushed by an instrument, or surgically incised. Inadvertent cystotomy is associated infrequently with both procedures, mainly in cases with difficult exposure and dissection,[34,35] and the incidence is less than 1% of cases. Urethral obstruction were reported mainly in the MMK procedure. One series reported 13 cases of female urethral obstruction that were treated with transvaginal urethrolysis and needle bladder neck suspension from 1 to 6 years after MMK.[35] In a survey of reported 2712 MMK cases, Mainprize found 9 cases (0.3%) of various lower urinary tract fistulae.[36] Burch himself[5] reported a single vesicovaginal fistula in a case with concomitant total abdominal hysterectomy.

Urinary Infection

Urinary tract infections may follow lower urinary tract surgery. Bacteriuria and cystitis are the most common postoperative infection, with a rate of 8.0%.[6] The incidence of such infections is reduced if the urine is sterile preoperatively and if the bladder is drained postoperatively by a suprapubic catheter rather than a transurethral catheter. Antibiotic prophylaxis is not prescribed just for the presence of an indwelling catheter, but symptomatic bladder infections are treated when an indwelling catheter is in place.

Voiding Difficulty

Voiding dysfunction following retropubic procedures is a well-documented complication, with a highly variable incidence reported from 1.7% to 25%.[30,32,37–40] The Burch colposuspension produces significant changes in postoperative voiding function even 3 months after surgery.[40] Usually the resumption to a normal voiding pattern often takes 10–14 days, and persistent voiding dysfunction is quite low. Various preoperative urodynamic factors were suggested to predict which patients are prone to have voiding difficulties, such as detrusor pressure <15 cm of water,[29] or voiding with Valsalva maneuver and without a detrusor contraction.[39] Other reports were not able to confirm this.[40] However, it is suggested that careful preoperative evaluation should identify these patients so that they may be appropriately counseled regarding their surgical risks and offered alternative forms of therapy. In cases of postoperative delayed voiding, the patients should be managed with prolonged catheter drainage, preferably self-catheterization or suprapubic catheter.

Detrusor Instability (Bladder Overactivity)

Occurrence of detrusor instability in a previously stable bladder is another well-recognized complication of colposuspension, and is often cited as a cause of failure.[41] Vierhout et al.[42] reviewed six studies with a total of 396 patients, and found a prevalence of 5–27%, with cure rate between 64% and 98%. Early onset of postoperative detrusor instability may be due to inflammation of the surgical site, a lower urinary tract infection, a foreign body such as a suture within the bladder, or bladder outlet obstruction. If a likely cause is found, it should be treated. Heslington and Hilton,[43] using ambulatory monitoring, found that 68% of asymptomatic patients might demonstrate some spontaneous uninhibited detrusor contractions on ambulatory urodynamics. It is likely that routine preoperative urodynamic assessment failed to detect these, which then presented postoperatively.

Enterocele

Postoperative enterocele formation following Burch procedure is a known long-term complication, with an incidence between 2% and 27%[5,32,44]. However, the rate of enterocele repair following Burch is lower, and in a follow-up of 109 patients for 10–20 years, only 5 patients (4.6%) needed surgical repair.[30] Wiskind et al.[44] tried to identify preoperative risk factors to predict postoperative prolapse, and the only factor found was the presence of a grade II or III cystocele. Although prophylactic obliteration of the cul-de-sac was suggested by some surgeons during retropubic urethropexy, there is no clear evidence in the literature whether enteroceles occur predominantly when a Burch procedure is performed with hysterectomy, or whether McCall or Halban's culdoplasties are effective in preventing enterocele formation.

Osteitis Pubis

Osteitis pubis is a rare inflammatory process of the symphysis, which appears to result from periosteal trauma. This complication was reported up to 5% of the patients who underwent MMK procedure. The condition may be incapacitating for several weeks or months. The recommended treatment includes rest, analgesics, and systemic corticosteroid injections. A survey from the Mayo clinic revealed 15 cases of osteitis pubis among 2030 cases of MMK, which is a prevalence of 0.74%.[45] Half of their cases were relieved conservatively, and half needed surgical treatment. Interestingly, 71% had positive bone cultures. They did not find any correlation to postoperative complication or clinical sign that could predict osteitis pubis.

Thrombosis

The incidence of postoperative thrombosis or thromboembolism is reported as low for both Burch and MMK procedures. Various preventive measures are used during the procedures and in the postoperative period such as intra- and postoperative compression stockings, "mini-dose" heparin, and early ambulation.

Results

Of the various surgical options to treat stress urinary incontinence, the retropubic procedures are the most investigated procedures in the literature, with more than 150 articles documenting subjective or objective short- and long-term follow-up. The long-term results are an important factor in tailoring the right procedure for the patient, as the cure rate is time dependent, with a tendency to decrease significantly after 5 or 10 years.[6,10,30] Another important factor in evaluating the efficacy of the procedure is whether the results are reported with objective or subjective assessment, as it has been shown that subjective evaluation gives better results than objective testing.[25,30]

The range of cure rate for Burch colposuspension is 75–98%,[6,10,26,27,30,46] and several factors were suggested to affect cure rate, such as patient selection (clinical and urodynamic parameters), patient's weight, prior bladder neck surgery, age over 65, and excessive blood loss. Short-term results of the colposuspension for patients who had previous failed surgery have been reported by Cardozo et al.[26] and Maher et al.[25] The former achieved an objective success rate at 9 months of 78% cure of stress incontinence with a 13% incidence of voiding difficulty. Maher and colleagues achieved a 72% cure rate with a 6% incidence of postoperative detrusor instability and a 4% incidence of voiding difficulty. Alcalay et al.[30] reviewed 109 patients who between them had had 48 previous operations, the majority of which (83%) were anterior colporrhaphy. The objective cure rate at 1 year for recurrent surgery was 78%, which decreased to 61% at 15 years, indicating the relevance of long-term follow-up.

The success rate of the MMK procedure reveals similar results to the Burch. The review by Mainprize found success rate ranging from 29% to 100%.[36] This review summarizes 2712 reported cases with 86.1% deemed to be successful, 2.7% improved, and 11.2% failed. The reasons for failure were similar to the reported causes of failure in Burch, such as poor patient selection, severe scarring of the retropubic space, and previous bladder neck surgery. Vesico-vaginal fistula was also reported as a cause for failure in MMK procedure.[36]

The comparable success rate in both retropubic procedures was also reflected in a prospective randomized study that compared Burch and MMK operations. Colombo et al.[47] compared 80 women who underwent the two types of operation and followed them for up to 7 years. The outcome measures included subjective and objective assessment and revealed non significant changes (Burch vs. MMK subjective cure: 92% vs. 85%; objective rate: 80% vs 65%). The MMK group showed a longer hospital stay (7.4 vs 6.3 days, p = 0.001), a later resumption of spontaneous voiding (13.8 vs 8.5 days, $p = 0.002$), and was associated with considerable complications.

Conclusion

Retropubic urethropexies have high subjective and objective cure rates and are suitable for patients with urethral sphincter incompetence and bladder neck mobility. As these procedures were reported to have more than 80% cure rate for at least 5 years of follow-up from numerous medical centers in the world, with reasonable rate of complications, they have become the "gold standard" of surgical choice for patients with stress incontinence. New minimally invasive procedures for stress urinary incontinence should be compared to these standards.

Laparoscopic Bladder Neck Suspension

Howard N. Winfield

Numerous surgical procedures for the management of females with anatomical stress urinary incontinence (SUI) have been advocated, including transabdominal, transvaginal, or a combination of approaches. The fact that no one procedure prevails is indicative of the fact that the long-term efficacy and morbidity of each operation is not optimal. The literature does, however, contain prospective randomized clinical trials as reported by Bergman and associates showing that the 1 year cure rate is over 85% following Burch colposuspension compared to a cure rate of 72% with the vaginal Pereyra urethropexy.[48] A long-term randomized prospective study comparing the Burch to Marshall–Marchetti–Krantz procedure indicates superior results with the former, with persistent cure rates of 92% and 80% at 2–7 years follow-up.[47]

However, it is generally believed, although not definitively proven, that the postoperative pain and hospitalization are greater after retropubic suspension. In an extensive review Jarvis noted that the surgical and postoperative morbidity of the vaginal approach appears to be no less than for the open retropubic operation.[49]

In order to potentially diminish postoperative pain, hospitalization, and morbidity as well as maintain efficacy, the laparoscopic Burch-type bladder neck suspension gained increasing attention and favor since Vancaillie and Schuessler first described this minimally invasive approach in 1991.[50]

Indications

After assuring that the patient does have type I or II SUI on the basis of clinical history, physical examination, voiding lateral cystourethrogram, urodynamics, and cystourethroscopy, she is informed of the possibility of laparoscopic correction. Women with suggestion of intrinsic sphincter deficiency (type III) stress urinary incontinence or neurogenic bladder are not good candidates for laparoscopic Burch urethropexy. Furthermore, women who have failed previous open or vaginal colposuspension are also not considered optimal candidates and most likely would benefit from a sling procedure.

Preoperative Preparation

All women must be carefully educated about the treatment options available, as well as advantages and disadvantages of each. Should a laparoscopic approach be considered, potential risks and complications of this form of intervention should be described in detail including injury to pelvic or abdominal viscera possibly necessitating conversion to formal laparotomy. The patients should also be counseled on the possibility of postoperative urinary retention requiring intermittent self-catheterization. A mechanical bowel preparation without oral antibiotics is suggested prior to laparo-scopic bladder neck suspension (L-BNS).

Technique

Extraperitoneal Laparoscopic Bladder Neck Suspension

A transperitoneal approach to L-BNS was initially utilized, but it has become apparent that the extraperitoneal route is simpler and more expeditious. After general anesthesia is obtained the patient is positioned in low lithotomy and pneumatic boots are placed on the lower extremities. The abdomen and genitalia are prepared and an 18 French Foley is placed into the bladder.

A midline incision is made approximately 4 cm below the umbilicus. The extraperitoneal space is created with a balloon inflation device. Commercially available or "home-made" balloon-type inflation devices are available which are effective in creating such a working space. A 10/11 mm Hassan cannula is secured and the laparoscope is inserted for the subsequent insertion of three working ports directly into the extraperitoneal space. These ports may vary in size from 5 to 10 mm and are placed in a diamond configuration (Fig. 6.10). Much of the dissection is often already accomplished after extra-peritoneal balloon inflation. Care is exercised to

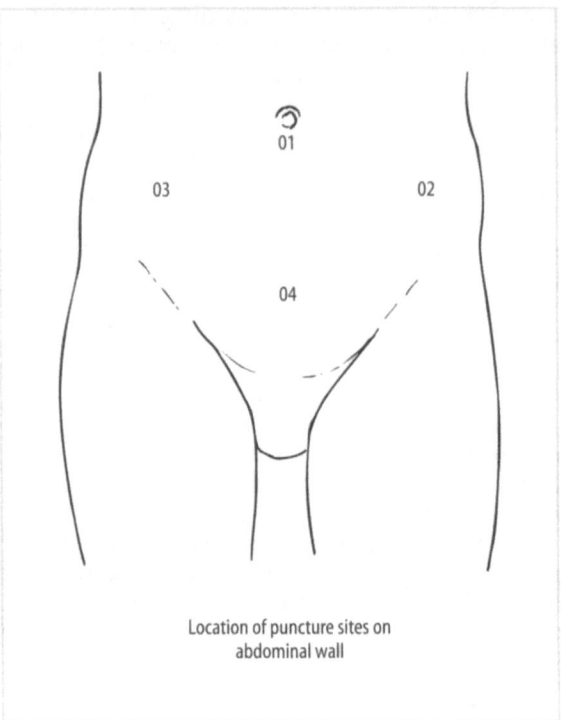

Location of puncture sites on abdominal wall

Figure 6.10 Placement of laparoscopic ports in a diamond-shaped configuration for bladder neck suspension.

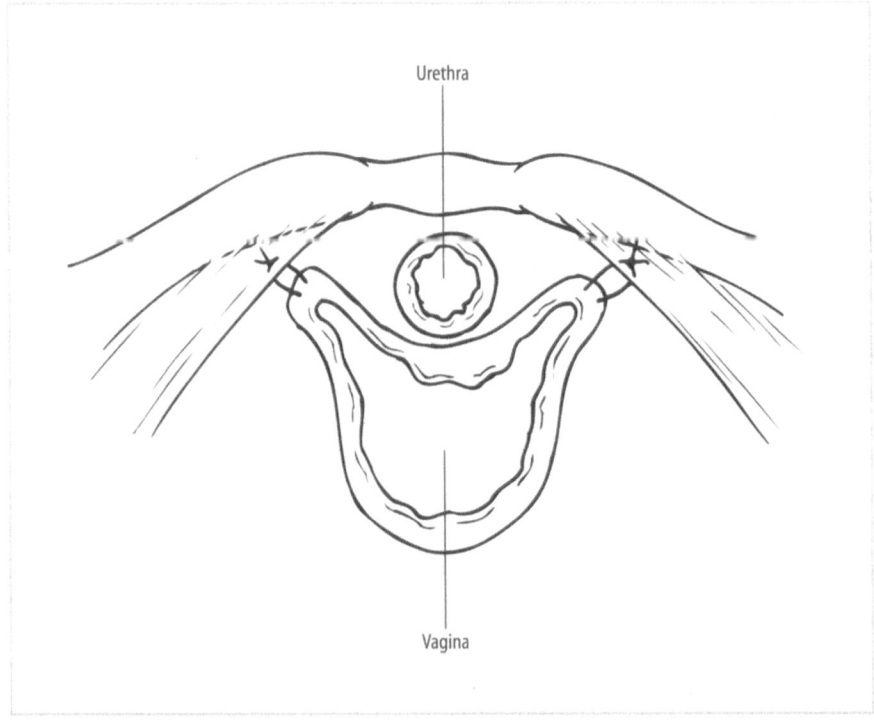

Urethra

Vagina

Figure 6.11 Placement of two stitches in a "hammock" position on either side of the bladder neck in order to complete the laparoscopic bladder suspension.

clear fibrofatty tissue away from the periurethral-bladder neck region, to improve exposure to the endopelvic fascia covering the anterior vaginal wall.

For a right-handed surgeon the left lateral port and the SP port are best for laparoscopic suture placement. A long strand (120 cm, 48 in) of 2-0 Goretex on a CV-2 tapered style needle is inserted into the working space and then solid bites into the endopelvic fascia at the level of the bladder neck are obtained using the index finger of the operator's left hand or the assistant's hand in the vagina as a guide to correct placement. The suture is then transferred through the ileopectineal ligament and the two ends are brought out through a 5 or 10 mm port. Extra-corporeal knots are secured while the assistant lifts the bladder neck anteriorly by digital transvaginal upward pressure. Ideally, two stitches are placed on each side of the bladder neck (Fig. 6.11). With this approach, the goal is to elevate the bladder neck sufficiently in a type of "hammock" position but not to overcorrect. Attempting to bring the vaginal endopelvic fascia directly in contact with ileopectineal ligament will cause excessive tension and certain postoperative urinary retention.

Indigo carmine is administered intravenously and then cystoscopy is normally performed, prior to carbon dioxide desufflation of the abdomen and laparoscopic port removal, so as to examine the bladder wall and to visualize efflux of colored urine from the ureteric orifices. The Foley catheter is left in place overnight and, if necessary, intermittent catheterization is used if temporary urinary retention occurs.

Numerous other variations of the L-BNS approach as well as techniques to place and secure the sutures have been advocated. Absorbable or non-absorbable mesh,[51] bone anchors,[52] and a laparoscopic clip applier[53] have been found useful in order to avoid the technical difficulties of laparoscopic suturing. Each laparoscopic surgeon seems to develop his or her own method.

Intraperitoneal Laparoscopic Bladder Neck Suspension

This approach was utilized initially and is occasionally necessary in cases where previous lower abdominal surgery has been performed and creation of a suitable extraperitoneal space is not feasible. After establishment of pneumoperitoneum, four laparoscopic ports are placed in the diamond configuration. A vertical incision is made just medial to the left obliterated umbilical ligament aiming towards the pubic bone (Fig. 6.12). The surgeon must be cognizant of the possibility of injury to the inferior

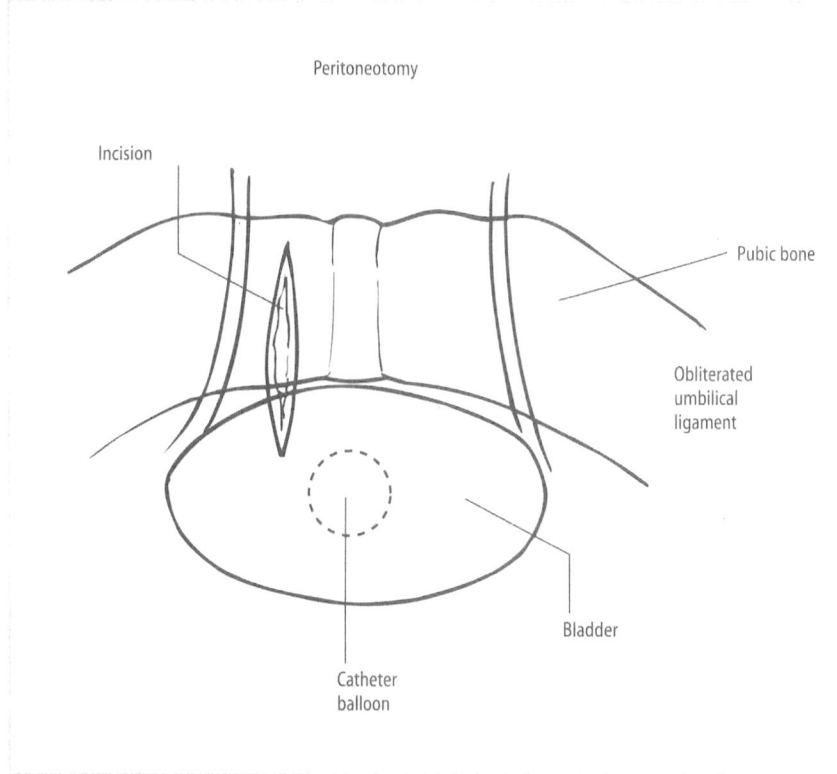

Peritoneotomy

Incision

Pubic bone

Obliterated umbilical ligament

Bladder

Catheter balloon

Figure 6.12 Vertical peritoneotomy made just medial to the left obliterated umbilical ligament in order to gain entrance into the retropubic space.

epigastric vessels or perforation of the bladder, especially in women who have undergone previous bladder or uterine surgery.

Once the pubic bone has been located and the left ileopectineal ligament exposed, the dissection is carried medially in order to expose the symphysis pubis and region of the right ileopectineal ligament. Manipulating the Foley catheter allows identification of the urethra and bladder. Fibrofatty tissue is gently cleared in the region of the vesicourethral junction so as to expose the endopelvic fascia covering the anterior vaginal wall. There are often some unnamed blood vessels traversing through this area which require careful electrocoagulation. Placement of sutures through the endopelvic fascia at the level of the bladder neck proceeds as described for the extraperitoneal approach.

Complications

To date in our hands, this procedure has been shown to be safe and relatively effective on the basis of short-term results. Complications of any type of laparoscopic procedure have been well described previously.[54] In relation to L-BNS, risk of bladder perforation during exposure of the bladder neck region is higher in patients who have undergone previous pelvic or bladder surgery as a result of surgical adhesions. Placement of laparoscopic sutures at the bladder neck region runs the risk of bladder, urethral, or ureteral injury, especially in patients who have undergone previous pelvic surgery, where the expected anatomy may be distorted.[33,55] Without a clear understanding of the laparoscopic pelvic anatomy, injury to vessels with significant hemorrhaging is feasible during dissection or suture placement. No significant difference in infection rate, blood loss, or de novo detrusor instability have been reported.[56] Femoral or lower extremity neuropathy although rare, may be due to prolonged thigh abduction during L-BNS.[6]

Enterocele and rectocele formation following the Burch procedure is not uncommon when performed either in an open or laparoscopic fashion.[44] Ross found a threefold decrease in symptomatic enteroceles and rectoceles when he began performing apical vaginal vault repair in conjunction with the laparoscopic Burch procedure. However, this required a transperitoneal approach to perform the apical vault repair.[56]

Results

In comparative studies between L-BNS, transvaginal, or open Burch colposuspension, the estimated blood loss is similar. Operative time seems consistently longer with the laparoscopic approach, but does show an improvement as the learning curve is overcome. The immediate postoperative course is significantly improved with the laparoscopic approach compared to open or transvaginal bladder suspension surgery. Patients require significantly less parenteral and oral analgesia and have shortened hospitalization, often reduced to a 23-hour stay in many centers (Table 6.1). Interestingly, the return to normal voiding pattern appears to be consistently faster in the laparoscopic group. Taken together, these laparoscopic postoperative characteristics help to correct for any financial differences caused by the longer operative times and intraoperative expenses compared to the open or transvaginal approaches. In fact, in the hands of laparoscopic surgeons with extensive experience in BNS, the operative time and expenses may be less than for the alternate surgical approaches.[57]

A brief review of published contemporary series, as outlined in Table 6.2, shows that the short-term results up to 18 months after laparoscopic bladder neck suspension for cure of stress urinary incontinence are good, and comparable to those of the open and transvaginal approaches. Despite the fact that these authors use different laparoscopic techniques

Table 6.1. Perioperative comparison of laparoscopic to open or transvaginal bladder neck suspension

Author	N	Procedure	Av. OR time (min)	Av. analgesia parenteral (mg)	Hospitalization (days)	Length of catheterization (days)
Das[52]	10	Abdominal colposuspension	55	75[a]	2.3	1.7
	10	L-BNS	155	52.5[a]	1.5	1
	10	Vaginal suspension	53	187[a]	2.6	n/a
McDougall[53]	19	L-BNS	124	6.3[b]	1.4	0.6
	23	Raz vaginal BNS	44	15.6[b]	2	13
Polascik[66]	12	L-BNS	190	14.2[b]	1.9	n/a
	10	Abdominal Burch colposuspension	109	131.4[b]	4.9	n/a

[a] meperidine HCl, [b] morphine.

Table 6.2. Comparative follow-up of laparoscopic bladder neck suspension

Author	N	Procedure	Follow-up: % cured of stress urinary incontinence				
			1 year	2 years	3 years	4 years	5 years
Das[59]	10	Abdominal colposuspension	100	70	50		
	10	L-BNS	90	70	40		
	10	Vaginal needle BNS	100	60	20		
McDougall[53]	19	L-BNS	78				
	23	Raz vaginal BNS	82				
McDougall[60]	58	L-BNS				30	
	42	Raz vaginal BNS					35
Polascik[66]	12	L-BNS	83				
	10	Burch colposuspension			70		
Burton[58]	30	Burch colposuspension	96		93		
	30	L-BNS	73		60		
Ross[56]	47	L-BNS					85–89
Blander[51]	22	Mesh L-BNS	90		70		

such as suturing, mesh, or bone anchor material, and points of fixation into ileopectineal ligament as well as the symphysis pubis, the eradication of significant stress urinary incontinence at 12 months is 78–90%. As has been historically shown with the multitude of other approaches to treating genuine stress urinary incontinence, the success rate with L-BNS begins to drop after 18 months. Table 6.2 also shows rather dismal results beyond 3 years. In one of the few prospective randomized reports, Burton reports a success rate of only 60% at 36 months compared with 93% with the open approach.[58] One might question whether there was a learning curve associated with Burton's poor results using L-BNS. Perhaps it was the needle used, the absorbable suture material or some other reason? However, other authors, in retrospective long-term studies beyond 24 months, seem to support these disappointing results. Das et al.[59] and McDougall et al.[60] in separate studies report complete continence with the laparoscopic approach at 36 months follow-up of only 40 and 35%, respectively. The comparative alternate open or transvaginal treatment approaches did not fare much better. Only select series seem to indicate durable objective success of 85–89% out to 5 years with the L-BNS.[56]

Discussion

On the basis of limited available prospective long-term follow-up data of 5 years or more, the open Burch colposuspension appears to be the gold standard for treatment of urinary incontinence not associated with intrinsic sphincter deficiency.[61] As with other open surgical procedures, considerable associated pain, hospitalization, and convalescence are associated with such a procedure. For this reason

less invasive alternative approaches such as vaginal and laparoscopic surgery have been encouraged.

Early results show L-BNS to have reduced morbidity compared to the abdominal or vaginal approaches and with excellent 1 year cure rates of stress urinary incontinence. Cost evaluation of the L-BNS compared to alternate treatment options is difficult to determine, because of the learning curve associated with this procedure, as well as different healthcare and medical insurance systems prevailing in different locations. However, it appears that once the learning curve is overcome, making operating room time efficient, the L-BNS procedure is cost-effective.[57]

However, longer follow-up of patients undergoing the laparoscopic procedure demonstrates a disappointing decline in women who remain subjectively and objectively dry after 2 years. Very few authors have reported long-term durable results of cure of stress urinary incontinence.[56] What might be the reasons that the L-BNS fails? What can be distilled from the literature might be that, in fact, a true "Burch colposuspension" is not really being done. There may be variations in the suture or mesh material used, as well as the degree of tension on these suspending elements. As described for the Burch procedure with Tanagho modification, it is important to place at least two sutures on each side, one at the level of the bladder neck and one close to the proximal or mid urethra at a reasonable distance from these structures. The sutures through ileopectineal ligament which give the greatest strength should be perpendicular to the ileopectineal fibers and not parallel. How mesh, bone anchors, or other materials apply these principles is unclear. Finally, in many reported studies it may not be clear if in fact the patients had associated pathologies or pelvic floor anomalies that required repair at the same time but were not done.

In order to truly appreciate the value and application of L-BNS it is important to have long-term prospective randomized studies comparing this procedure to the open or transvaginal approaches. As described by Smith and Stanton[62] such a study should clearly describe the indications for surgery, as well as extensive preoperative assessment including urodynamics, leak point pressures, and radiologic imaging when required. The intraoperative morbidity as well as immediate and long-term morbidity including symptoms of bladder dysfunction, voiding difficulty, vaginal prolapse, and dyspareunia must be carefully documented. Follow-up data must be at least 2 years. Remaining dry for 5 years should be considered the gold standard of cure.

In summary, L-BNS has not been proven to be superior or demonstrated durable with long-term cure results for the management of genuine stress urinary incontinence (types I and II). In fact, no bladder suspension surgical approach seems to consistently yield acceptable results, other than perhaps the original Burch colposuspension. As currently advocated by many leading authorities on female urology, the use of the sling urethroplasty may be the preferred treatment for all types of stress urinary incontinence.[63] Attention is also now being directed towards development of a laparoscopic sling procedure.[64-66]

References

1. Marshall VA, Marchetti AA, Krantz KE (1949) The correction of stress urinary incontinence by simple vesicourethral suspension. Surg Gynecol Obstet 88: 509-18.
2. Bailey KV (1954) A clinical investigation into uterine prolapse with stress incontinence. Treatment by modified Manchester colporrhaphy. J Obstet Gynaecol Br Empire 61: 291-8.
3. Green T (1962) The problem of stress incontinence in female: appraisal of its current status. Obstet Gynecol Surv 23: 603-34.
4. Hodgkinson CP (1963) Urinary stress incontinence in the female: a program for preoperative investigation. Clin Obstet Gynecol 6: 154-61.
5. Burch JC (1961) Urethrovesical fixation to Cooper's ligament for correction of stress incontinence, cystocele, and prolapse. Am J Obstet Gynecol 81: 281-290.
6. Jarvis GJ (1994) Surgery for genuine stress incontinence. Br J Obstet Gynecol 101: 371-4.
7. Jarvis GJ (2000) Surgery for urinary incontinence. Baillières Best Pr Res Clin Obstet Gynaecol 14: 315-34.
8. Leach GE, Dmochowski RR, Appell RA et al. (1997) Female Stress Urinary Incontinence. Clinical Guidelines Panel summary report on surgical management of female stress urinary incontinence. The American Urological Association. J Urol 158: 875-80.
9. Hilton P (1988) Bladder drainage: a survey of practices among gynaecologists in Britain (with unpublished observations regarding surgical practices). Br J Obstet Gynaecol 95: 1178-89.
10. Dainer M, Hall CD, Choe J, Bhatia NN (1999) The Burch procedure: a comprehensive review. Obstet Gynecol Surv 54: 49-60.
11. Tanagho EA (1976) Colpocystourethropexy: The way we do it. J Urol 116: 751-3.
12. Symmonds RE (1972) The suprapubic approach to anterior vaginal relaxation and urinary stress incontinence. Clin Obstet Gynecol 15: 1107-21.
13. Bump RC, Mattiasson A, Bo K et al. (1996) The standardization of terminology of female pelvic organ prolapse and pelvic floor dysfunction. Am J Obstet Gynecol 175: 10-17.
14. Karram MM, Bhatia NN (1988) The Q-tip test: Standardization of the technique and its interpretation in women with urinary incontinence. Obstet Gynecol 71: 807-11.
15. Versi E (1990) Discriminant analysis of urethral pressure profilometry data for the diagnosis of genuine stress incontinence. Br J Obstet Gynaecol 97: 251-9.
16. Stanton SL, Cardozo LD (1979) Results of the colposuspension operation for incontinence and prolapse. Br J Obstet Gynecol 86: 693-7.
17. Bergman A, Koonings PP, Ballard CA (1989) Negative Q tip test—a risk factor for failed incontinence surgery in women. J Reprod Med 34: 193-7.
18. Bowen LW, Sand PK, Ostergard DR et al. (1989) Unsuccessful Burch retropubic urethropexy: a case controlled urodynamic study. Am J Obstet Gynecol 160: 452-8.
19. Green TH Jr (1962) Development of a plan for diagnosis and treatment of urinary stress incontinence. Am J Obstet Gynecol 83: 632-6.
20. Sand PK, Bowen LW, Panganiban R et al. (1987) The low pressure urethra as a factor in failed retropubic urethropexy. Obstet Gynecol 69: 399-402.
21. McGuire EJ, Cespedes RD, Cross CA, O'Connell HE (1996) Videourodynamic studies. Urol Clin N Amer 23: 309-21.
22. Hilton P, Stanton SL (1983) Urethral pressure measurement by microtransducer: the results in symptom free women and in those with genuine stress incontinence. Br J Obstet Gynaecol 90: 919-33.
23. Cummings JM (1997) Leakpoint pressures in female stress urinary incontinence. Int Urogynecol J Pelvic Floor Dysfunct 8: 153-5.
24. Sand PK, Winkler H, Blackhurst DW, Culligan PJ (2000) A prospective randomized study comparing modified Burch retropubic urethropexy and suburethral sling for treatment of genuine stress incontinence with low-pressure urethra. Am J Obstet Gynecol 182: 30-4.
25. Maher C, Dwyer P, Carey M, Gilmour D (1999) The Burch colposuspension for recurrent urinary stress incontinence following retropubic continence surgery. Br J Obstet Gynaecol 106: 719-24.
26. Cardozo L, Hextall A, Bailey J, Boos K (1999) Colposuspension after previous failed incontinence surgery: a prospective observational study. Br J Obstet Gynaecol 106: 340-4.
27. Stanton SL, Cardozo L, Williams JE, Ritchie D, Allan V (1978) Clinical and urodynamic features of failed incontinence surgery in the female. Obstet Gynecol 51: 515-20.
28. Langer R, Ron-el R, Newman M, Herman A, Caspi E (1988) Detrusor instability following colposuspension for stress incontinence. Br J Obstet Gynaecol 95: 607-10.
29. Lose G, Jorgensen L, Mortensen SO et al. (1987) Voiding difficulties after colposuspension. Obstet Gynecol 69: 33-8.
30. Alcalay M, Monga A, Stanton SL (1995) Burch colposuspension: A 10-20 year follow up. Br J Obstet Gynecol 102: 740-45.
31. Lee RA (1984) Abdominal operations for urinary stress incontinence. In: Sciarra JJ (ed) Gynecology and Obstetrics. Harper & Row, Philadelphia, pp. 1-10.
32. Chaliha C, Stanton SL (1999) Complications of surgery for genuine stress incontinence. Br J Obstet Gynaecol 106: 1238-45.

33. Rosen DM, Korda AR, Waugh RC (1996) Ureteric injury at Burch colposuspension. 4 case reports and literature review. Aust N Z J Obstet Gynaecol 36: 354–8.

34. Persky L, Guerriere K (1976) Complications of Marshall-Marchetti-Krantz urethropexy. Urology 8: 469–72.

35. Gillon G, Engelstein D, Servadio C (1992) Risk factors and their effect on the results of Burch colposuspension for urinary stress incontinence. Isr J Med Sci 28: 354–6.

36. Mainprize TC, Drutz HP (1998) The Marshall–Marchetti–Krantz procedure: a critical review. Obstet Gynecol Surv 43: 724–9.

37. Zimmern PE, Hadley HR, Leach GE, Raz S (1987) Female urethral obstruction after Marshall-Marchetti-Krantz operation. J Urol 138: 517–20.

38. Stanton SL, Cardozo L, Chandhury N (1978) Spontaneous voiding after surgery for urinary incontinence. Br J Obstet Gynaecol 85: 149–52.

39. Wall LL, Hewitt JK (1996) Voiding function after Burch colposuspension for stress incontinence. J Reprod Med 41: 161–5.

40. Sze EH, Miklos JR, Karram MM (1996) Voiding after Burch colposuspension and effects of concomitant pelvic surgery: correlation with preoperative voiding mechanism. Obstet Gynecol 88: 564–7.

41. Heit M, Vogt V, Brubaker L (1997) An alternative statistical approach for predicting prolonged catheterization after Burch colposuspension during reconstructive pelvic surgery. Int Urogynecol J Pelvic Floor Dysfunct 8: 203–8.

42. Vierhout ME, Mulder AF (1992) De novo detrusor instability after Burch colposuspension. Acta Obstet Gynecol Scand 71: 414–16.

43. Heslington K, Hilton P (1996) Ambulatory monitoring and conventional cystometry in asymptomatic female volunteers. Brit J Obstet Gynaecol 103: 434–41.

44. Wiskind AK, Creighton SM, Stanton SL (1992) The incidence of genital prolapse after the Burch colposuspension. Am J Obstet Gynecol 167: 399–404.

45. Kammerer-Doak DN, Cornella JL, Magrina JF, Stanhope CR, Smilack J (1998) Osteitis pubis after Marshall-Marchetti-Krantz urethropexy: a pubic osteomyelitis. Am J Obstet Gynecol 179: 586–90.

46. Kjolhede P, Ryden G (1997) Clinical and urodynamic characteristics of women with recurrent urinary incontinence after Burch colposuspension. Acta Obstet Gynecol Scand 76: 461–7.

47. Colombo M, Scalambrino S, Maggioni A, Milani R (1994) Burch colposuspension versus modified Marshall-Marchetti-Krantz urethropexy for primary genuine stress urinary incontinence: a prospective, randomized clinical trial. Am J Obstet Gynecol 171: 1573–9.

48. Bergman A, Ballard CA, Koonings pp. (1989) Comparison of three different surgical procedures for genuine stress incontinence: prospective randomized study. Am J Obstet Gynecol 160: 1102–1106.

49. Jarvis GL (1994) Surgery for genuine stress incontinence. Br J Obstet Gynaecol 101: 371–4.

50. Vancaillie TG, Schuessler WW (1991) Laparoscopic bladder neck suspension. J Laparoendosc Surg 1: 169–71.

51. Blander DS, Carpiniello VL, Harryhill JF, Malloy TR, Rovner ES (1999) Extraperitoneal laparoscopic urethropexy with marlex mesh. Urology 53: 985–9.

52. Das S, Palmer JK (1995) Laparoscopic colpo-suspension. J Urol 154: 1119–21.

53. McDougall EM, Klutke CG, Cornell T (1994) Comparison of transvaginal versus laparoscopic bladder neck suspension for stress urinary incontinence. Urology 45: 641–6.

54. Capelouto CG, Kavoussi LR (1993) Complications of laparoscopic surgery. Urology 42: 2–12.

55. Grossman T, Darai E (1996) Role of endoscopy in surgery for urinary incontinence. Ann Chir 50: 896–905.

56. Ross J (1998) Laparoscopy or open Burch colposuspension. Curr Opin Obstet Gynecol 10: 405–9.

57. Loveridge K, Malouf A, Kennedy C, Edgington A, Lam A (1997) Laparoscopic colposuspension. Is it cost-effective? Surg Endosc 11: 762–5.

58. Burton G (1997) A three year prospective randomized urodynamic study comparing open and laparoscopic colposuspension. Neurourol Urodynam 16(1997): 353–4.

59. Das S (1998) Comparative outcome analysis of laparoscopic colposuspension, abdominal colposuspension and vaginal needle suspension for female urinary incontinence. J Urol 160: 368–71.

60. McDougall EM, Heidorn C, Portis A et al. (1999) Laparoscopic bladder neck suspension fails the test of time. J Urol 162: 2078–81.

61. Bergman A, Giovanni E (1995) Three surgical procedures for genuine stress incontinence: five year follow-up of a prospective randomized study. Am J Obstet Gynecol 173: 66–71.

62. Smith AR, Stanton SL (1998) Laparoscopic colposuspension. Br J Obstet Gynecol 105: 383–4.

63. Chaikin DC, Rosenthal J, Blaivas JG (1998) Pubovaginal fascial sling for all types of stress urinary incontinence: long-term analysis. J Urol 160: 1312–16.

64. Narepalem N, Kreder KJ, Winfield HN (1995) Laparoscopic urethral sling for the treatment of intrinsic urethral weakness (Type III stress urinary incontinence). Tech Urol 2: 1.

65. Gilling PJ, Fraundorfer MR, Sealey C, Watts HG (1994) Laparoscopic extraperitoneal approaches to female urinary incontinence: the colposuspension and pubovaginal sling. J Urol 151: 344A.

66. Polascik TJ, Moore RG, Rosenberg MT, Kavoussi LR (1995) Comparison of laparoscopic and open retropubic urethropexy for treatment of stress urinary incontinence. Urology 45: 647–52.

7 Fascial Slings

Kathleen C. Kobashi and Gary E. Leach

Table 7.1. Evolving technique of sling surgery

Author	Technique
VonGiordano (1907)[1]	First sling; gracilis muscle
Stoeckel (1917)[2]	Plication of 'muscular structures'[a] around bladder neck
Price (1933)[3]	Passage of fascial strip beneath urethra from AP incision with fixation to rectus muscle
Aldridge (1942)[4]	Suture two strips of fascia together beneath urethra
Lytton and McGuire (1978)[5]	Fix to rectus fascia
Leach (1988)[6], Appell (1997)[7]	Bone anchors (Suprapubic or transvaginal placement)

[a] Muscles used included gracilis, pyramidalis, levator ani, rectus, and bulbocavernosus.

Since the first pubovaginal sling (PVS) was described by VonGiordano in 1907 (Table 7.1),[1] the PVS has evolved into the gold standard for the surgical treatment of female stress urinary incontinence (SUI) due to intrinsic sphincter deficiency (ISD) and is utilized as first line surgical therapy for SUI associated with urethral hypermobility. PVSs are placed beneath the proximal urethra and bladder neck to provide a hammock effect as well as direct urethral compression. The sling serves as a "backstop" to prevent urethral descensus and opening when increased intraabdominal pressure occurs.

Indications and Patient Selection

Indications

Slings are the most widely accepted treatment for ISD and the authors prefer to use slings for all female patients with any type of SUI should they opt for surgical therapy. However, slings are performed only after confirming the presence of SUI and the absence of detrusor instability or instability that is controlled on medications. Exceptions include urodynamically demonstrated detrusor instability only at high bladder volumes or if the instability does not correlate with the patient's symptoms. Pelvic prolapse, if present, must be repaired at the time of sling placement (see below). Conversely, the bladder neck and proximal urethra must be supported at the time of cystocele repair even if preoperative SUI is not demonstrated in order to prevent the development of SUI postoperatively.

Evaluation and Work-up Specific to Slings

A thorough discussion of the preoperative evaluation of incontinent patients is covered elsewhere in this textbook, so this section covers only the evaluation relevant to the sling.

History

A detailed history is essential, and assessment of the impact of the incontinence on the patient's

Table 7.2. SEAPI Incontinence Score[a] Reproduced with permission from Pat O'Donnell (Ed.), Urinary Incontinence, Mosby, 1997, 450–1

	Subjective	Objective
Stress-related leakage	0 = No urine loss 1 = Loss w/strenuous activity 2 = Loss w/moderate activity 3 = Loss with minimal activity	0 = No leak 1 = Leak @ >80 cm H₂0 2 = Leak @ 30–80 cm H₂0 3 = Leak @ <30 cm H₂0
Emptying ability	0 = No obstructive sxs 1 = Minimal sxs 2 = Significant sxs 3 = Only dribbles or retention	0 = 0–60 ml 1 = 61–100 ml 2 = 101–200 ml 3 = >200 ml or unable to void
Anatomy	0 = No descent w/strain 1 = Descent, not to introitus 2 = Through introitus w/strain 3 = Through introitus at rest	0 = Above symphysis[a] w/strain 1 = <2 cm below symphysis w/strain 2 = >2 cm below symphysis w/strain 3 = >2 cm below symphysis at rest
Protection	0 = Never used 1 = Certain occasions 2 = Daily, occasional accidents 3 = Continually, frequent accidents or constant leakage	0 = Never used 1 = Certain occasions 2 = Daily, occasional accidents 3 = Continually, frequent accidents or constant leakage
Inhibition	0 = No urge incontinence (UI) 1 = Rare UI 2 = UI once/week 3 = UI at least once/day	0 = No pressure rise 1 = Rise late filling (>500 ml) 2 = Medium fill rise (150–500 ml) 3 = Early rise (<150 ml)

[a] Position of bladder neck (BN).

quality of life is important. The SEAPI instrument (Table 7.2) can be useful for objective evaluation of patient symptoms. Patients should be questioned regarding the presence or absence of SUI and urgency or urge incontinence. History pertaining to the possibility of neurogenic bladder dysfunction or sacral arc denervation is essential as this condition puts the patient at higher risk for permanent postoperative urinary retention. Evaluation for neuropathology includes questions concerning the patient's sensation of bladder filling, sensation of complete bladder emptying, and her ability to void spontaneously. Routine questions such as frequency of urination, degree of leakage, number of pregnancies, and history of infections are relevant. Past medical history may reveal neurologic injury, for example secondary to cerebrovascular accident or trauma, or neurologic disease, such as multiple sclerosis or Parkinson's disease, or diabetes mellitus which can affect bladder function. Past surgical history is also important as previous pelvic or abdominal surgery can affect the difficulty of sling surgery or make urethrolysis necessary if abundant scar tissue is present.

Voiding diaries and pad tests are techniques which may help the clinician objectively quantify a patient's voiding pattern and degree of incontinence.

Physical Examination

Pelvic examination is important in the assessment of urethral position, degree of periurethral fibrosis, and urethral mobility as well as the presence of concomitant prolapse. The current trend is toward placing slings for treatment of all types of SUI, regardless of the Valsalva leak point pressure or presence of hypermobility.[9,10] In cases in which there is no pelvic prolapse present, cadaveric transvaginal sling (CaTS) is performed with a 2 × 7 cm strip of cadaveric fascia (see Surgical Technique). However, collagen injection therapy may also be considered in patients with SUI and a well-supported urethra ("classic" ISD). Conversely, if the urethra is hyperelevated and/or severely fixed secondary to scarring following previous anti-incontinence procedures, urethrolysis should be performed in conjunction with sling placement to allow adequate urethral compression from the sling.

The degree and location of concomitant pelvic prolapse, if present, must be assessed for surgical planning. Currently, the authors are utilizing a new technique of simultaneous cystocele repair and pubovaginal sling with a single piece of cadaveric fascia, a procedure entitled cadaveric prolapse repair and sling (CaPS).

Work-up

Urodynamics is performed to demonstrate SUI and evaluate for bladder "overactivity" (detrusor instability or hyperreflexia). In cases in which the patient complains of urgency but cystometry reveals a stable bladder, the urologist must still take into account the possibility of instability that was not demonstrated in the laboratory testing situation.

Correlation of the urodynamic findings with the patient's history is imperative, because approximately 20–40% of patients will have persistent urgency and 10–12% of patients may develop de-novo postoperative urgency.

Preoperative post-void residual should be determined via bladder scan or catheterization to evaluate bladder emptying. Patients with incomplete emptying prior to sling placement are clearly at risk for postoperative urinary retention requiring intermittent catheterization. Nonetheless, the clinician must be aware that post-void residuals are often falsely elevated in the laboratory. In order to confirm preoperative incomplete emptying, patients are asked to keep a log of their post-void catheterized volumes obtained at home prior to surgery.

Finally, cystourethroscopy is performed to evaluate urethral position and mobility and to exclude bladder pathology such as an intravesical suture, stone, or tumor.

Tissue Sources

Numerous materials, including autologous and allogenic tissues as well as synthetic materials, have been used to create slings with varying results (Table 7.3). Although the short-term results have been comparable between autologous, homologous, and synthetic slings, the literature suggests an overall increased complication rate with synthetic materials. Higher infection and erosion rates have been demonstrated with the synthetic materials, although no statistically significant difference in the erosion rates has been demonstrated (Table 7.4).[11]

Table 7.3. Materials used to create slings

Type	Examples
Autologous	Muscle, rectus fascia, fascia lata, dura mater, tendons, vaginal wall, dermis
Allogenic	Cadaveric fascia lata
Xenografts	Porcine dermis
Synthetic materials	Gore-Tex, polyester, nylon, silastic, polytetrafluoroethylene (PTFE), etc.

Table 7.4. Comparison of complications with synthetic versus autologous materials. Figures in brackets are percentages. Reproduced with permission from the American Urological Association.[11]

Complications	#Autologous materials (n = 1715)	#Synthetic materials (n = 1515)
Vaginal erosion	1 (0.0001)	10 (0.007)
Urethral erosion	5 (0.003)	27 (0.02)
Fistula	6 (0.003)	4 (0.002)

This chapter focuses on fascial slings such as the rectus fascia and fascia lata. Although harvesting of rectus fascia may cause less pain than that of fascia lata,[12] fascia lata is reported to be three to four times stronger than rectus fascia.[13] Additionally, harvesting of fascia lata does not require the extensive abdominal dissection which increases the risk of nerve entrapment and postoperative pain associated with rectus fascia harvesting. Moreover, the rectus fascia in patients with a history of multiple abdominal surgeries or radiation therapy may be poor in quality. Cadaveric fascia has recently grown in popularity since no harvesting of fascia is necessary, thereby shortening operative time, hospital stay, and the recuperation period, as well as appreciably decreasing postoperative pain without significantly compromising the results.[14]

In the USA cadaveric tissues are processed by tissue banks licensed by the Food and Drug Administration (FDA). Both freezing and freeze-drying the soft-tissue accomplish elimination of antigenicity,[15,16] although these processes may compromise the integrity of the fascia. Protection against infection transmission is achieved by careful donor selection, antibody testing, and various sterilization techniques.[17] A multistep process is performed to inactivate viral particles.[16] The most common sterilizing treatment is gamma-radiation,[18] which was shown to have no effect on the tensile strength of the fascia up to 4.0 Mrad.[19] There is a wide variability in the processing techniques employed to sterilize the fascia, and no standardized method is required of all tissue banks. One company has developed a patented procedure for tissue processing. Tissue treated using this sterilization technique has been utilized in over 500 000, surgical transplant patients with no reported cases of disease transmission.[20]

Surgical Technique

Preoperative Preparation

A sterile urine culture is essential prior to placement of the PVS. Ideally, the patients are taught how to perform self-catheterization before surgery in case of postoperative urinary retention. In patients who are unable to perform self-catheterization preoperatively, a suprapubic tube (SPT) may be placed at the time of surgery. Vaginal preparation with a betadine douche is performed by the patient the night before and the morning of surgery. Sterile urine must be confirmed before surgery, and all patients receive perioperative intravenous antibiotics. The authors prefer ampicillin or cefazolin together with gentamicin for approximately 24 hours, with the first dose administered on call to the operating room. If the patient is allergic to penicillin, vancomycin is administered for gram-positive coverage.

Patients are placed on intravaginal hormonal cream to improve the quality of the vaginal tissue and urethral mucosa prior to surgery. Timing and dosage of estrogen replacement therapy is controversial. Maximal tissue response to vaginal estrogens takes 3–24 months to achieve.[21] The authors recommend starting patients on local estrogen therapy at least 6 weeks before surgery if the tissue is atrophic.

Placement of the Fascial Sling

Transabdominal Approach

An abdominal incision is made and the proximal urethra is isolated. The fascial strip is passed behind the urethra and secured to the rectus fascia or pubic bone (see below). This technique may be difficult and risks injury to the urethra and bladder, especially in cases of significant pelvic scarring resulting from previous pelvic procedures. For this reason, the authors prefer a transvaginal technique.

Combined Abdominal and Transvaginal Approach

The patient is placed in the dorsal lithotomy position and an inverted U-shaped anterior vaginal incision is made extending from the mid-urethra to the

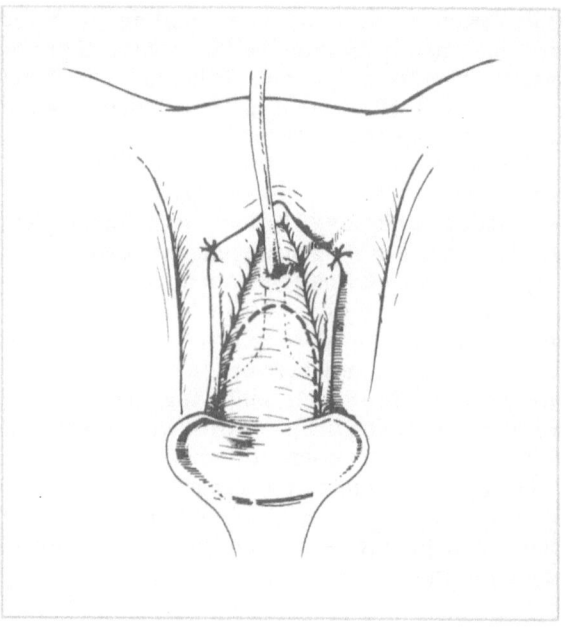

Figure 7.1 An inverted U-incision is made in the anterior vaginal wall. From: Atlas of Urologic Clinics of North America (1994) Courtesy of WB Saunders, 2(1), 67.

bladder neck (Fig. 7.1). Dissection is carried laterally to the ischium, and the endopelvic fascia is perforated. Blunt or sharp dissection is performed to create a tunnel through the retropubic space toward the rectus muscle for the sling (Fig. 7.2). A short suprapubic incision is made and carried down to the rectus fascia, and a 1.5 × 4–8 cm strip of the rectus fascia is obtained. Harvesting of fascia lata involves two or three small incisions in the lateral thigh. A

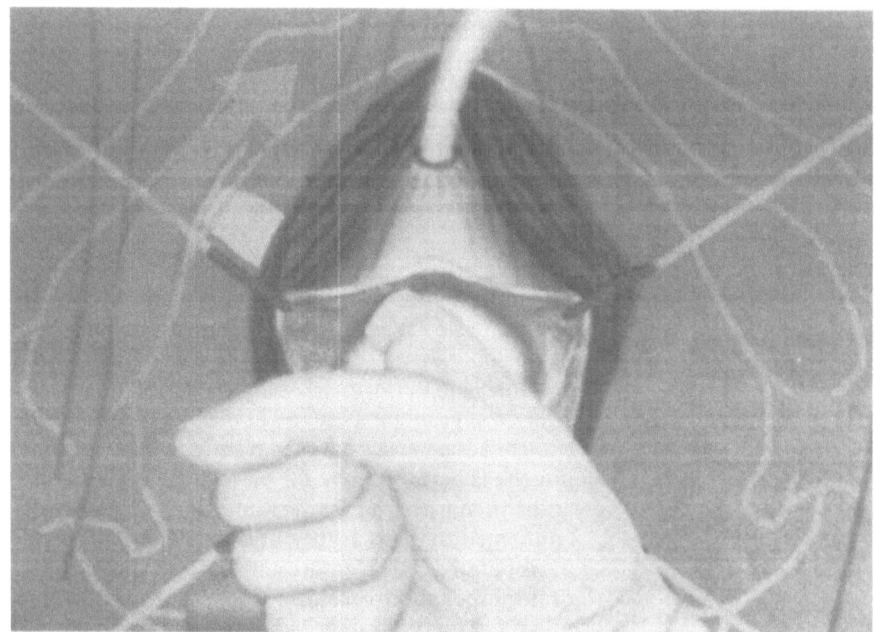

Figure 7.2 Dissection into the retropubic space is made by a combination of sharp and blunt dissection. From: Atlas of Urologic Clinics of North America (1994) Courtesy of WB Saunders, 2(1), 15.

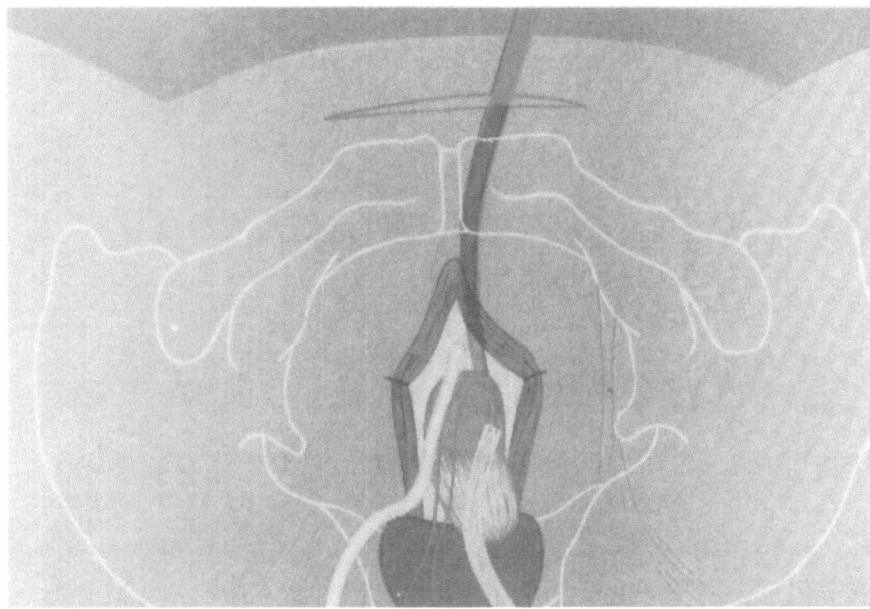

Figure 7.3 The vaginal sutures are transferred to the suprapubic incision. From: Atlas of Urologic Clinics of North America (1994) Courtesy of WB Saunders, 2(1), 68.

1.5–2 cm wide fascial segment is harvested. During dissection, extensive distal dissection should be avoided to prevent injury to the common peroneal nerve. Typically the fascial defect is left open, a drain is placed, and the skin incisions are closed.

A Pereyra needle is used to transfer the Prolene sutures placed at the ends of the fascia from the vagina to the suprapubic incision (Fig. 7.3). Cystoscopy ensures that no bladder perforation has occurred and that no suture material has passed through the bladder or urethra. In cases of concomitant pelvic prolapse repair, cystoscopy also allows visualization of efflux of urine from the ureteral orifices to confirm ureteral patency following the repair. Sutures are used to fix the sling to the periosteum with a #5 Mayo needle[6] or to the rectus fascia. The sling is visualized cystoscopically as the sutures are being secured without excessive tension suprapubically to avoid excessive sling elevation. The free end of the sling is elevated until a minimal indentation of the urethral floor is seen through the 20-French female cystoscope with a 0° lens. The sling is then secured to the pubic tubercle, with care taken to avoid excessive tension.

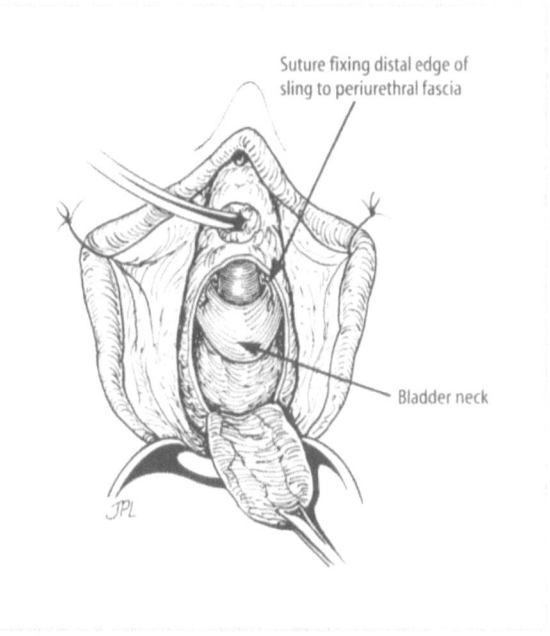

Suture fixing distal edge of sling to periurethral fascia

Bladder neck

Figure 7.4 A vaginal flap is created extending from the distal urethra to the proximal bladder neck. From: Atlas of Urologic Clinics of North America (1994) Courtesy of WB Saunders, 2(1), 69.

Transvaginal (CaTS)

The transvaginal approach for the pubovaginal sling is preferred by the authors since it avoids the pain caused by the passing of the sutures through the abdominal wall. An inverted U-shaped incision is made in the anterior vaginal wall extending from the distal urethra to the bladder neck. The flap is dissected on the white shiny layer on the inside of the vaginal wall. When the correct plane is identified, there is minimal blood loss. The flap is mobilized proximally to the bladder neck which is identified by palpation of the Foley catheter balloon (Fig. 7.4). The pubic bone is exposed lateral to the urethra, and the underside of the bone is cleared of adjacent tissue on the undersurface of the bone. In patients

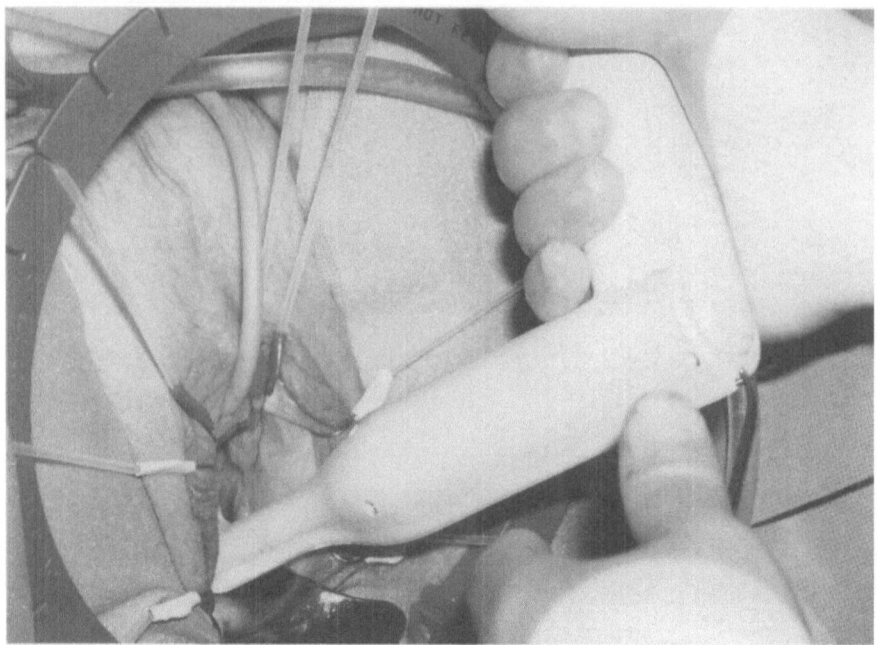

Figure 7.5 A transvaginal drilling device is used to place bone anchors into the pubic bone. Reprinted from Kobashi KC, Leach GE (2001) Better prospects for stress urinary incontinence. Contemp Urol 12(12), 21–25.

who have undergone previous anti-incontinence surgery, this dissection should be performed sharply to avoid inadvertent perforation of the bladder or urethra. The endopelvic fascia is not routinely perforated unless periurethral scarring is present or in cases in which there is inadequate space for placement of the transvaginal anchor.

Bone anchors are placed transvaginally using a transvaginal anchoring system into the underside of the pubic bone (Fig. 7.5). The corners of the 2 × 7 cm cadaveric fascia strip are folded over to prevent tearing-through of the sutures (Fig. 7.6). The 0-prolene sutures attached to the anchors are passed through the fascia using a straight 18-gauge needle to minimize trauma to the fascia. One side of the sling is tied firmly to the bone. The tension of the sling is determined by placing a small right-angle clamp between the urethra and sling while securing the second side of the fascia in place (Fig. 7.7). The sling should lie flat and snug against the right angle such that the right angle can be removed and replaced without problem. The distal edge of the fascia is tacked to the periurethral tissue using a 2–0 absorbable suture to prevent rolling of the fascial patch toward the bladder neck. The vaginal flap is closed with 2–0 vicryl running stitch. An antibiotic-soaked vaginal packing and a 16-French Foley catheter are left in place overnight.

Postoperative Care

The vaginal packing and Foley catheter are removed on the first postoperative day, and the post-void residual volumes are determined by in-and-out catheterization. If the residuals are >100 ml, the technique of CIC is reviewed with the patient before her discharge, and she is instructed to continue CIC at home until the PVR is consistently <100 ml. In the rare case in which a patient has an SPT, the PVRs are measured via the SPT and, if necessary, the patient is discharged home with the tube plugged and instructed on how to check the residuals at home.

Routine precautions are taken to prevent infection. Patients receive approximately 24 hours of perioperative intravenous antibiotics followed by 1 week of oral antibiotics (cephalexin or ciprofloxacin). Most patients need only acetaminophen for adequate analgesia.

Outcomes and Complications

Following an extensive literature review covering surgical techniques for treatment of female SUI, the AUA Clinical Guidelines Panel compiled a set of guidelines for the surgical treatment of female SUI.[11] Slings and retropubic suspensions had the best long-term results with an 83–84% cure/dry rate at 48 months as compared to an only 67% cure/dry rate amongst patients who had undergone needle suspensions (Fig. 7.8). The sling appears to be most efficacious over time for all types of recurrent SUI. One must consider that, in the past, slings were used only for the more severe cases of SUI. Yet slings still maintain excellent long-term results comparable to those of retropubic suspensions which were employed for the less complex cases of SUI.

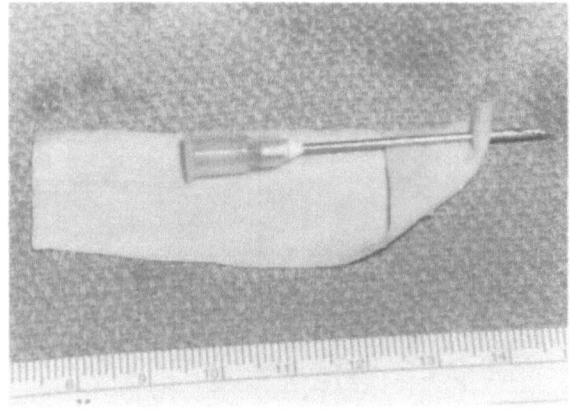

a

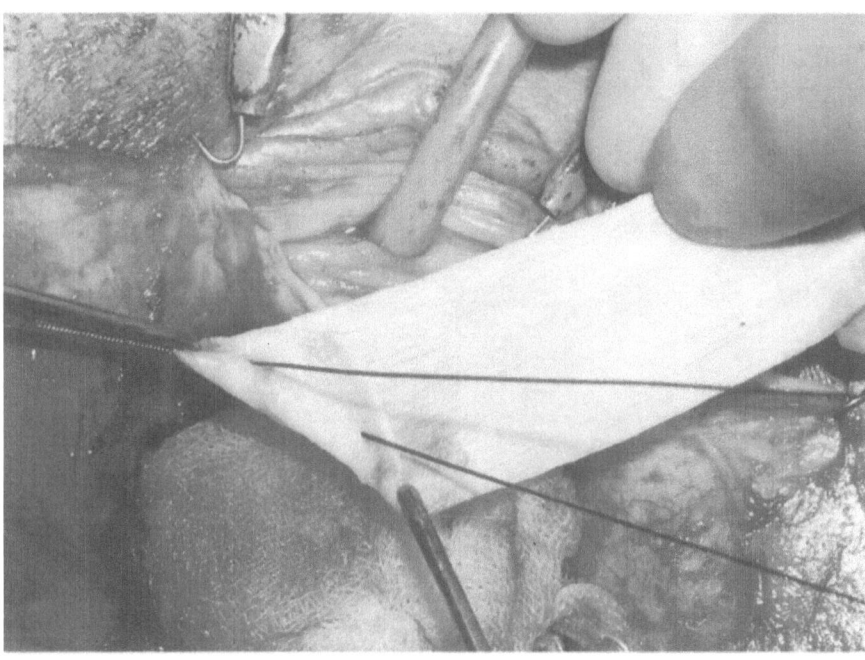

b

Figure 7.6 a The corners of the fascial strip are folded as illustrated to minimize the risk of the sutures pulling through the fascial fibers. **b** The nonabsorbable suture is passed atraumatically through the fascia using an 18-gauge needle. Reprinted from Kobashi KC, Leach GE (2001) Better prospects for stress urinary incontinence. Contemp Urol 12(12), 21–25.

On the Basis of Material Used

Autologous Fascia

Use of fascia lata provides several advantages over other autologous fascia and allogenic tissue. Autologous fascia lata reportedly has a greater tensile strength than rectus fascia,[13] and there is no theoretical risk of infection transmission as there may be with cadaveric fascia. The biggest disadvantage of fascia lata is pain at the harvest site: 67% of patients experience pain with walking, although Wheatcroft et al. showed that pain persists for an average of only 1 week postoperatively.[22] In the authors' experience,

the pain has persisted for approximately 6 weeks. Cosmetic results are also a consideration. 38% of patients in Wheatcroft's series were unhappy with the appearance of the scar, and Naugle reported the complication of herniation of the muscle belly at the fascial harvest site.[23]

Haab et al. studied 40 patients who underwent pubovaginal sling (PVS) placement using autologous fascia for treatment of ISD.[24] Questionnaire analysis was used with a mean follow-up of 48.2 months (range 24–60 months). In this series 13 patients had a rectus fascia sling, and 27 patients underwent fascia lata PVSs. Patients who had preoperative SUI alone were more likely to be dry as compared to patients with mixed incontinence (67% versus 36%).

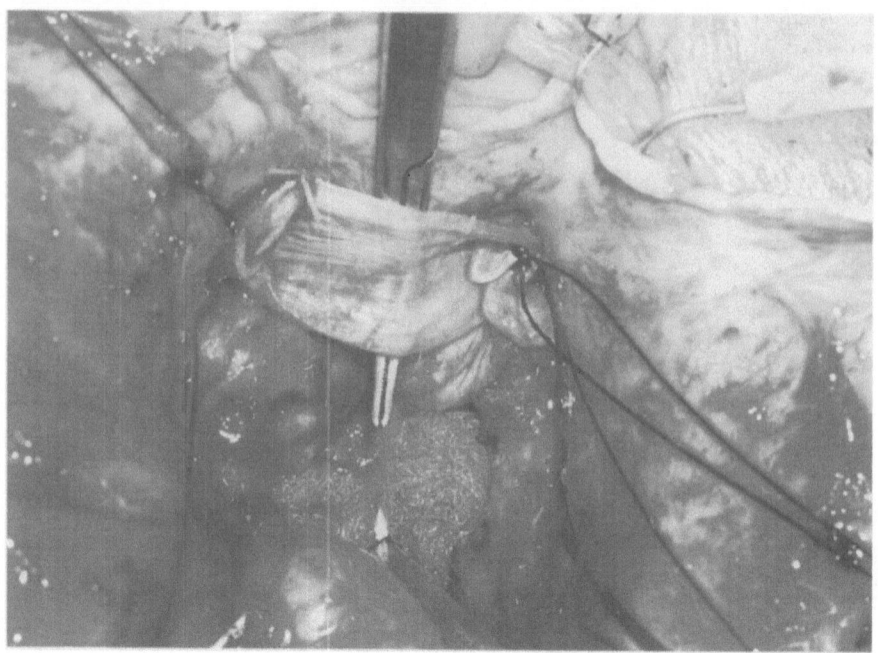

Figure 7.7 A small right angle clamp is placed between the urethra and fascia as the second side of the fascia is secured in place. The suture is secured until the sling lies flat and snug on the clamp without excessive tension. Reprinted from Kobashi KC, Leach GE (2001) Better prospects for stress urinary incontinence. Contemp Urol 12(12), 21–25.

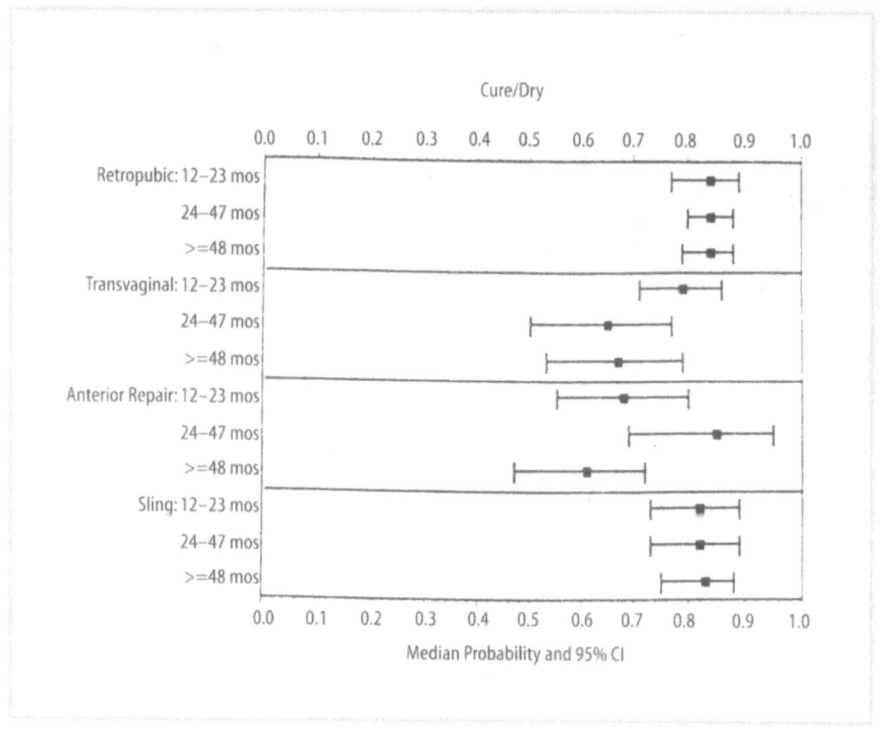

Figure 7.8 The AUA Clinical Guidelines panel for treatment of female stress urinary incontinence concluded that, on the basis of the literature, slings and retropubic suspensions have the best long-term results.

27% (n = 10) had recurrent SUI, 62.2% (n = 23) had postoperative urgency, including 10% (n = 4) who experienced the urgency de-novo, and 8% (n = 3) who had permanent retention, two of whom had sacral arc denervation and were expected pre-operatively to go into retention.

Rectus fascia provides the same excellent long-term results as fascia lata. Disadvantages of rectus fascia include development of abdominal hernia and a "pulling" sensation or pain radiating to the groin, presumably caused by the tension of the suspension sutures on the rectus fascia or suprapubic nerve "entrapment".[6]

Carr et al. studied their results with rectus fascia slings in the geriatric patient population by comparing their outcomes in 19 patients >70 years of age versus 77 patients <70 years old, all with SUI.[25] Mean follow-up was 22 months (range 3–43 months). The symptoms of SUI resolved in 100% of the geriatric patients and 97% of the patients <70 years of age. Urgency symptoms improved postoperatively in 50% of the geriatric patients and 61% of the control group patients who had preoperative detrusor instability. De-novo urgency occurred in 10% of patients in both groups, but was controlled adequately in all patients with anticholinergic medications.

Chaikin et al. studied 251 patients who underwent PVSs using autologous rectus fascia with a mean follow-up of 3.1 years (range 1–15 years).[26] In this series 92% (231) were cured or improved after surgery, 3% (7) had de-novo urge incontinence, 23% (58) had persistent urge incontinence, and 2% (4) experienced unexpected permanent urinary retention.

Cadaveric Fascia Lata

Early results with the transvaginal approach to placement of cadaveric slings (CaTS) have been excellent. Thus far, the authors have performed 106 CaTS using a transvaginal bone anchoring system (Fig. 7.3a, b) with mean follow-up of 10.5 months (range 6–18.5 months). Patients have been evaluated preoperatively and postoperatively using the SEAPI score with early results revealing a significant decrease in the mean SEAPI scores postoperatively (5.67 versus 1.64, p < 0.001). Less than 50% of patients require temporary intermittent catheterization, and only one patient has experienced unexpected permanent postoperative urinary retention (one patient had expected urinary retention). None of the remaining patients has required intermittent catheterization for longer than 1 week. Of the 92 patients available for follow-up, 63 (68.5%) are totally dry, 12 (13.0%) have persistent mild SUI, 4 (4.3%) have persistent urge incontinence, 9 (9.8%) have had de-novo urge incontinence, and 2 (2.2%) have mixed incontinence. Patients who have undergone CaTS alone (no concomitant procedures) have been admitted for 23-hour observation to receive intravenous antibiotics. No abdominal or lower extremity incision for graft harvesting or sling fixation is necessary. Therefore, there is little to no postoperative pain and, in the experience of the authors, the majority of patients require no more than acetaminophen for analgesia.

There is a minimal risk of infection transmission from the transplanted cadaveric fascia. The risk of acquiring HIV-infected tissue from a properly screened donor is reported to be 1/1,667,600[27] and the risk of transmission of HIV from banked cadaveric fascia is 1/8,000,000.[28] There is one reported case of HIV transmission from a seronegative donor. Seroconversion occurred only in the recipients of solid organs (4/4) and unprocessed fresh-frozen bone (3/3). None of the 34 patients who received other tissues, including 3 who received lyophilized soft tissue, became infected with HIV.

Vaginal wound infection or "rejection" has not been seen in the authors' experience to date. Handa reported 2/16 (12%) patients developed abdominal wound infections following placement of cadaveric slings,[14] comparable to the incidence reported by Beck with autologous fascial slings.[28]

Wright et al. evaluated their results in 92 patients with a mean age of 60 years and mean follow-up of 11.5 months.[11] They compared autograft (n = 33) versus allograft (n = 59) fascial PVSs. Preoperative SEAPI scores, number of previous anti-incontinence procedures, and leak point pressure were similar between the two groups. The procedures were equally well tolerated with marked improvement in both groups and without infection or sling erosion. Mean operative time and hospital stay were significantly lower in the allograft patients.

How to Avoid and Treat Complications

The etiology of urinary incontinence after PVS placement can be divided into three main categories:

- persistent stress urinary incontinence
- detrusor instability (persistent or de novo)
- overflow incontinence.

Accurate determination of the cause of incontinence is imperative in order to restore continence. Evaluation includes postoperative physical examination to assess urethral position, determination of post-void residuals to evaluate bladder emptying, urodynamic studies, and cystourethroscopy. Multichannel urodynamic studies may demonstrate detrusor instability or persistent SUI. Cystourethroscopy is performed to exclude urethral erosion of the sling or suture material in the bladder.

Persistent SUI

Persistent SUI after sling placement is usually due to inadequate tension being placed on the sling or urethral fixation not released by urethrolysis. Physical examination is performed to examine for urethral hypermobility. In cases in which SUI persists but urethral hypermobility is absent, collagen injection is a minimally invasive option. Although some sources suggest that injection therapy may be helpful even in cases of SUI involving urethral hypermobility,[29] the authors use collagen only in patients with no urethral hypermobility.

Persistent or De-novo Detrusor Instability

De-novo detrusor instability occurs in 10–12% of patients following placement of a sling.[9] Patients with preoperative instability or symptoms of urgency must be counseled on the 20–40% incidence of persistent symptoms.[9–11] Postoperative anticholinergic medications may successfully relieve urgency and urge incontinence, although if urgency present preoperatively persists following sling placement, it is often difficult to treat. Combination anticholinergic therapy (two medications) or intravesical anticholinergic instillation should be tried. Biofeedback or neuromodulation may also be helpful. In extreme cases, a patient may eventually require an augmentation cystoplasty.

Overflow Incontinence

Postoperative urinary retention following sling placement may be caused by excessive sling tension and outlet obstruction. A 1–2% incidence of permanent urinary retention[9] and up to 60% incidence of temporary retention[10] is reported in the literature. Postoperative overdistension of the bladder must be avoided to prevent myogenic detrusor dysfunction which could contribute to prolonged retention. Additionally, the urologist must be cognizant of the possibility of preoperative poor detrusor function that is evidenced by high preoperative post-void residual volumes. As mentioned previously in this chapter, a preoperative voiding diary and post-void residual log kept by those patients suspected of having poor emptying is essential to confirm elevated post-void residual volumes. Finally, in cases of urethral hyper-elevation or severe periurethral scarring, urethrolysis with Martius fat pad graft placed around the freed urethra may be required in those patients who have urodynamically demonstrated outlet obstruction (Fig. 7.9).

Conclusions

A myriad of techniques for the treatment of female SUI have been described. The current trend in surgical therapy is toward slings for all female patients with SUI. Before sling placement, the surgeon must document the SUI and be aware of potential problems related to detrusor instability or incomplete emptying.

The use of cadaveric fascia avoids complications associated with synthetic slings, is safe, and avoids the pain and complications from harvesting autologous fascia. Technically, the transvaginal approach is simple and, used together with the cadaveric fascia, decreases postoperative pain, operative time, hospital stay, and recuperation period.

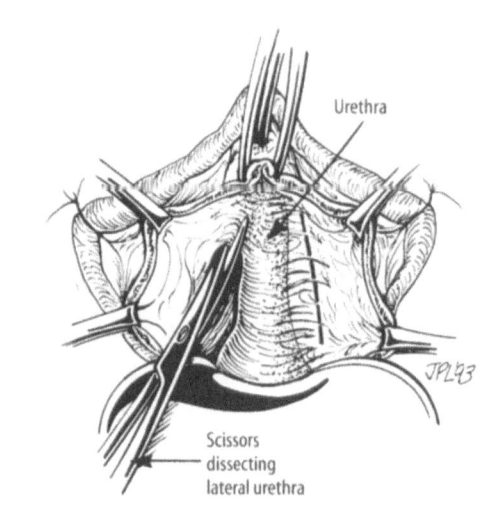

Figure 7.9 Urethrolysis is performed by sharply freeing the urethra from surrounding scar tissue with two lateral incisions. Care is taken to place the incisions very laterally to avoid injury to the urethra. Reprinted from Kobashi KC, Leach GE (2001) Better prospects for stress urinary incontinence. Contemp Urol 12(12), 25.

References

1. Ridley JH (1985) The Goebel–Stoeckel sling operation. In: Mattingly RF, Thompson JD (ed) TeLinde's operative gynecology. Lippincott, Philadelphia.
2. Stoeckel W (1917) Uber die Verwendung der Musculi pyramidales bei der operativen Behandlung der Incontinentia urinae. Zent Gynakol 41: 11.
3. Price PB (1933) Plastic operations for incontinence of urine and feces. Arch Surg 26: 1043.
4. Aldridge AA (1942) Transplantation of fascia for relief of urinary stress incontinence. Am J Obstet Gynecol 44: 398.
5. Lytton B, McGuire EJ (1978) Pubovaginal sling procedure for stress incontinence. J Urol 119: 82–4.
6. Leach GE (1988) Bone fixation technique for transvaginal needle suspension. Urology 31(5): 388–90.
7. Appell RA (1997) The use of bone anchoring in the surgical management of female stress urinary incontinence. World J Urol 15(5): 300–5.
8. Raz S, Stothers L, Chopra A (1997) Anterior vaginal wall sling. In: O'Donnell PD (ed) Urinary Incontinence. Mosby, St. Louis, Mo., pp. 450–1.
9. Blaivas JG, Jacobs BZ (1991) Pubovaginal fascial sling for the treatment of complicated stress urinary incontinence. J Urol 145(6): 1214-18.

10. Zarazoga MR (1996) Expanded indications for the pubovaginal sling: treatment of type 2 or 3 stress incontinence. J Urol 156(5): 1620–2.

11. Leach GE, Dmochowski RR, Appell RA et al. (1997) Female SUI clinical guidelines panel summary report on surgical management of female stress urinary incontinence. The American Urological Association. J Urol 158: 875–80.

12. Sirls LT, Leach GE (1996) Use of fascia lata for pubovaginal sling, Chapter 32. In: Raz S (ed) Female Urology. W. B. Saunders, Philadelphia.

13. Crawford JS (1969) Nature of fascia lata and its fate after implantation. Am J Ophthmol 67: 900.

14. Wright EJ, Iselin CE, Carr LK, Webster GD (1998) Pubovaginal sling using cadaveric allograft fascia for the treatment of ISD. J Urol 160: 759–62.

15. Cooper JL, Beck CL (1993) History of soft-tissue allografts in orthopedics. Sports Med Arthroscopy Rev 1: 2–16.

16. Handa VL, Jensen JK, Germain MM, Ostergard DR (1996) Banked human fascia lata for the suburethral sling procedure: A preliminary report. Obstet Gynecol 88: 1045–9.

17. Bedrossian EH Jr (1989) HIV and banked fascia lata. Trans Pa Acad Ophthalmol Otolaryngol 41: 831–3.

18 Vangesness CT Jr, Triffon MJ, Joyce MJ, Moore TM (1996) Soft tissue for allograft reconstruction of the human knee: a survey of the American Association of Tissue Banks. Am J Sports Med 24(2): 230–4.

19. Cutz A, Reid DB, Basu PK (1977) Tensile strength of fascia lata sutures following gamma radiation. Can J Ophthalmol 12(3): 211–15.

20. Tutoplast® Processed Fascia Lata package insert. Biodynamics International, Inc.

21. Semmens JP, Tsai CC, Semmens EC, Loadholt CB (1985) Effects of estrogen therapy on vaginal physiology during menopause. Obstet Gynecol 66(1): 16–18.

22. Wheatocroft SM, Vardy SJ, Tyers AG (1997) Complications of fascia lata harvesting for ptosis surgery. Br J Ophthalmol 82(3): 333–4.

23. Naugle TC Jr, Fry CL, Sabtier RE, Elliott LF (1997) High leg incision fascia lata harvesting. Ophthalmology 104(9): 1480–8.

24. Haab F, Trockman BA, Zimmern PE, Leach GE (1997) Results of pubovaginal sling for the treatment of intrinsic sphincteric deficiency determined by questionnaire analysis. J Urol 158: 1738–41.

25. Carr LK, Walsh PJ, Abraham VE, Webster GD (1997) Favorable outcome of pubovaginal slings for geriatric women with stress incontinence. J Urol 157(1): 125–8.

26. Chaikin DC, Rosenthal J, Blaivas J (1998) Pubovaginal fascial sling for all types of stress urinary incontinence: long-term analysis. J Urol 160(4): 1312–16.

27. Simonds RJ, Homberg SD, Hurwitz RL et al. (1992) Transmission of human immunodeficiency virus type 1 from a seronegative organ tissue donor. N Engl J Med 326(11): 726–32.

28. Beck RP, McCormick S, Nordstrom L (1988) The fascia lata sling procedure for treating recurrent genuine stress incontinence of urine. Obstet Gynecol 72: 699–703.

29. Herschorn S, Steele DJ, Radomski SB (1996) Followup of intraurethral collagen for female stress urinary incontinence. J Urol 156(4): 1305–9.

8 Tension-free Vaginal Tape

Ulf Ulmsten

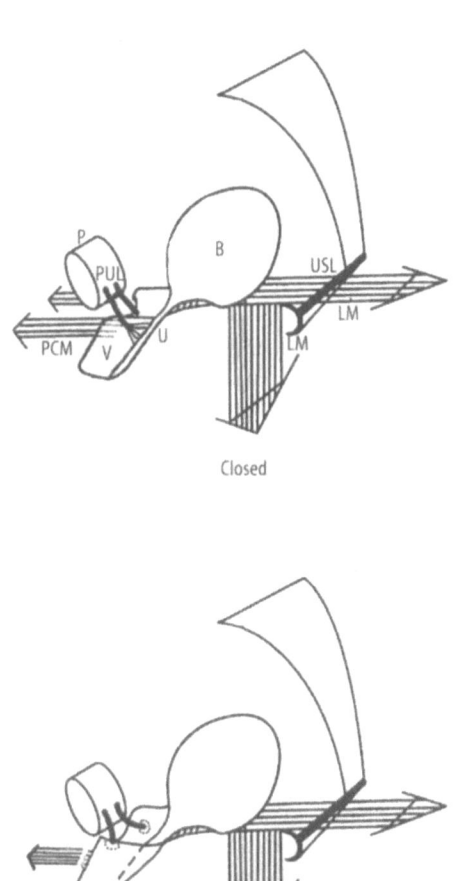

Closed

Open

Figure 8.1 Important anatomical structures involved in urethral closure in women. When the structures are functioning accurately the urethra will be kept closed by forward pressure from the pubourethral ligaments, suburethral anterior vaginal wall and pubococcygeus muscles (upper panel). If there are structural defects the urethra may stay open and allow escape of urine in stress situations (lower panel). B, bladder; LM, levator muscles; P, pubic bone; PCM, pubococcygeus muscles; PUL, pubourethral ligaments; U, urethra; V, vaginal wall.

The tension-free vaginal tape (TVT) technique was introduced into clinical practice in 1994–95, and since then approximately 200 000 operations have been performed worldwide. The operation, which differs significantly from traditional anti-incontinence surgical procedures, is based on the results of a series of experimental investigations of the urethral closure mechanisms in women.[1-3] According to these results, formulated in the integral theory,[1,2] the urethra is not properly closed in stress incontinent women as a result of dysfunctions or defects in pubourethral ligaments (PUL), suburethral vaginal wall (SUW), pubococcygeus muscles (PCM) and paraurethral connection tissue (PCT)[1,2] (Fig. 8.1). The TVT operation aims to correct or reconstruct these dysfunctions or defects. TVT can thus be characterized as a reconstructive surgical procedure of the female lower urinary tract.[1-4]

The operation should preferably be carried out under local anesthesic as an ambulatory procedure, allowing the patient to return home on the same day or the day after surgery, without need for post-operative catheterization.

Indications

TVT is mainly used as the primary operation in patients with genuine stress incontinence (GSI), due to hypermobile urethra or intrinsic sphincter deficiency (ISD, i.e. a resting urethral pressure = 20 cm H$_2$O). TVT can also be carried out as the secondary operation in case of relapses after previous anti-incontinence operations such as the Burch procedure. The procedure is also used in combination with prolapse repair in patients with symptoms and signs of prolapse and stress urinary incontinence.

In patients with mixed incontinence, i.e. symptoms of both stress and urge incontinence, TVT has been found to reduce both stress and urge symptoms, in particular in patients suffering from mainly "sensory" urge.

Surgical Technique

Instruments

The operation is carried out using a specific two-component instrument that comprises a nondisposable metal handle to which two metal or plastic disposable needles are attached (Ethicon) (Fig. 8.2). The needles have an outer diameter of 5 mm. A specific prolene tape (Ethicon) 40 cm long and 10 mm wide covered by a plastic sheath is fixed to the needles. To insert the tape the proximal ends of

the needles are attached to the handle by a coupling, allowing rapid and easy uncoupling once the needle tip has reached the abdominal skin, as described below.

Procedure

Immediately before the operation the patient is premedicated with 1 ml intramuscular ketobemidone 5 mg/ml. In the theatre she is initially sedated with 1 mg intravenous midazolam, which is repeated as necessary to a maximum of 5 mg during surgery. At start of the operation fentanyl 0.05 mg is given intravenously, and this dose is repeated at implantation of the tape.

Initially the bladder is emptied via a transurethral Foley catheter. Local anesthetic (50–60 ml Prilocain with Adrenalin 0.25%) is injected in the abdominal skin just above the pubis symphysis and downwards along the back of the pubic bone to the retropubic space. The injection should be performed "exactly" where the needles are intended to be brought up from below the vagina as described later on. Hence, injections of the local anesthetic should "mimic" the needle passage to be performed later. This also implies a hydrodissection of the tentative tissue

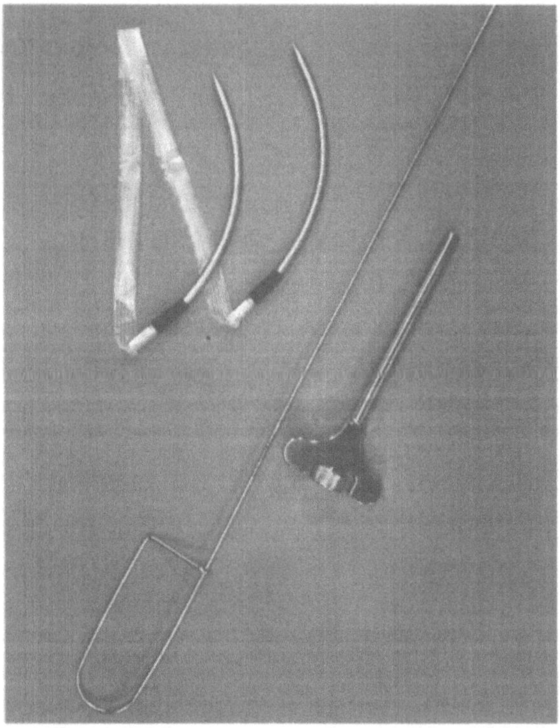

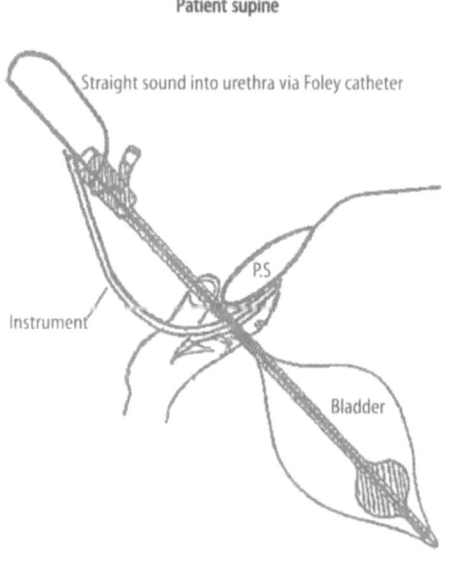

Figure 8.2 The two-component instrument (Ethicon) used for implantation of the tape. The prolene tape (Ethicon) covered by a plastic sheath is connected to two needles which can be coupled to a metal handle (see also text). A rigid (steel) catheter guide introduced into a Foley catheter controls the urethra and the bladder at needle insertion.

Figure 8.3 Schematic outline of the initial part of the surgical procedure. The tip of the needle has perforated the urogenital diaphragm and entered into the retropubic space. The catheter guide in the Foley catheter controls the urethra and bladder neck, whereas the fingertip controls the needle tip at perforation. It is important that immediately after perforation into the retropubic space a direct contact is established between the needle tip and the back of the pubic bone (P.S).

canals. Then two 1cm transverse skin incisions 4–5 cm apart (the width of three fingers) are made on the superior rim of the pubic bone. Vaginally 30–40 ml of 0.25% Prilocain-Adrenalin is injected into the vaginal wall sub- and paraurethrally. A 1.5 cm sagittal incision is made in the midline of the suburethral vaginal wall, starting approximately 0.5 cm from the *outer urethral meatus*. The incision is not allowed to encroach on the bladder neck, to avoid the tethered vagina syndrome and postoperative disturbances of micturition.[2] Laterally from this incision, a minimal blunt dissection (0.5–1.0 cm long) is made with scissors to each side of the urethra. This makes it possible to introduce the tip of the needle in the correct starting position (Fig. 8.3). With a straight steel inserter, i.e. catheter guide, introduced into the Foley catheter, the urethra and the bladder neck are identified. Using the instrument, i.e. the handle with the needle attached, the tape is placed around the *midurethra* as follows: the tip of the needle is inserted into the prepared paraurethral incision on one side of the urethra. The urogenital diaphragm is perforated and when inside the retropubic space the tip of the needle is brought up

to the abdominal incision in *close contact* with the back of the pubic bone (Fig. 8.4). Alternatively the urogenital diaphragm can be perforated with closed scissors to facilitate the introduction of the needles. As soon as the needle tip has reached the abdominal skin incision, the proximal end of the needle is disconnected from the handle. The procedure is then repeated on the other side. At this step of the operation the patient undergoes cystoscopy to confirm an intact bladder. The tape, still covered by the plastic sheath, is then brought into position by gently pulling the needles upward with the tape attached.

With 300 ml of saline in the bladder the patient is then asked to cough vigorously to make sure that continence has been obtained. During coughing the tape is adjusted so that only a few drops of urine escape the urethra. During the adjustment of the tape it is necessary, in particular if there is a heavy leakage and the suburethral vaginal wall is loose, to close the vaginal wall incision beneath the tape temporarily at the cough test. This is easily done by bringing the vaginal flaps together with one or two small forceps. Here the operator mimics the situation when the incision of the vaginal wall is sutured. When the tape has been placed in an ideal U-shape around the *midurethra*, the plastic sheath is withdrawn (Fig. 8.5) with a closed scissors placed between the urethra and tape to prevent undue tension on the tape. The plastic sheath has two aims: it prevents contamination of the tape before insertion, and it enables the ends of the tape to be pulled up to the abdominal incision without trauma. Using the specially designed instrument the tape is thus placed around the *midurethra*, where the pubourethral ligaments and the fascial aspects of the pubococcygeus muscles are assumed to have their functional insertions and not at the bladder neck (Figs 8.1, 8.6).[2,3] Importantly, the tape is only loosely

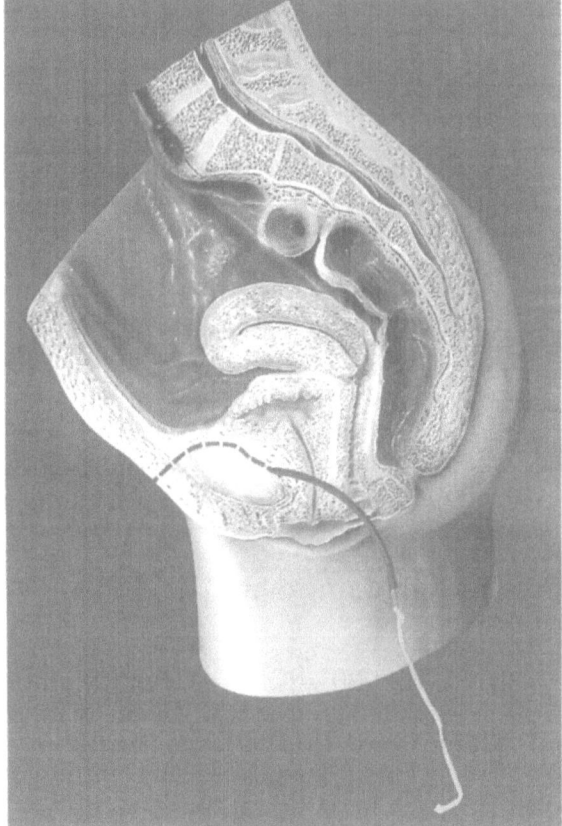

Figure 8.4 Initial step of the TVT procedure. The needle has perforated the urogenital diaphragm and entered the retropubic space. Observe that the needle tip is in close contact with the pubic bone when starting its passage up to the abdominal skin.

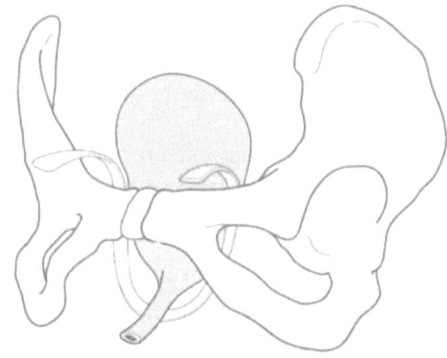

Figure 8.5 The procedure is now completed. The tape has been placed loosely in a U-shape around the mid urethra.

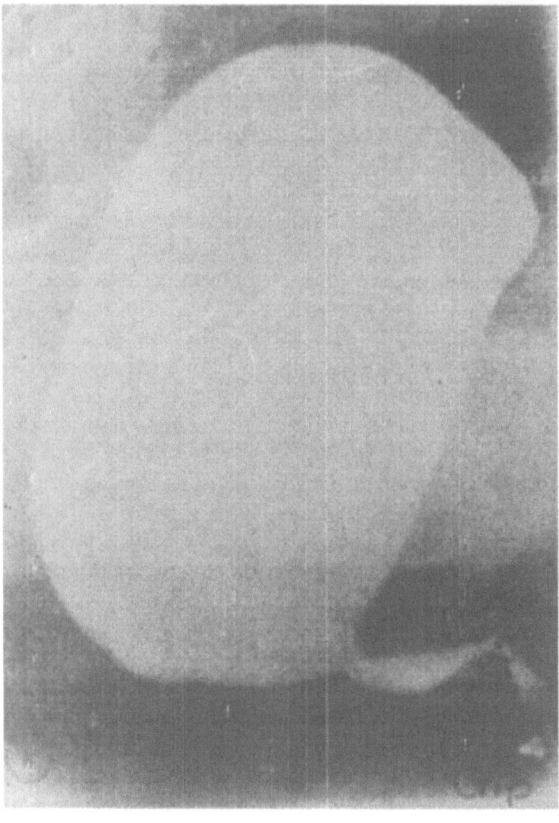

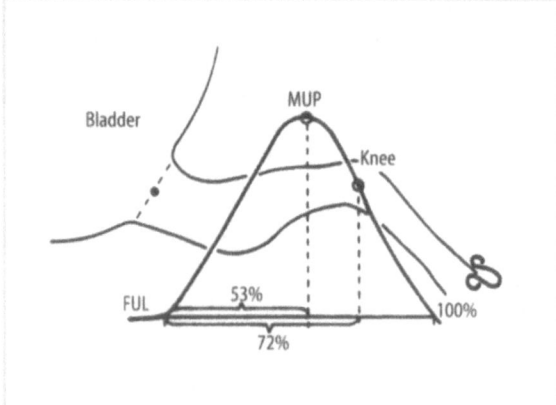

Figure 8.6. Urethral profile measurement and lateral urethrocystography in a continent woman. The 'urethral knee' indicates the main position and fixation of the pubourethral ligaments.[3] As indicated the insertion is located close to the high pressure zone of the urethra. It is important that the tape is positioned at this site. FUL, functional urethral length; MUP, maximum urethral pressure. From: Westby M, Asmussen M, Ulmsten U (1982) Location of maximum intraurethral pressure related to urogenital diaphragm in the female studied by simultaneous urethrocystometry and voiding urethrocystography. In: Am J Obs & Gynae 144: 408–12.

placed around the urethra, without any elevation, and the abdominal ends are not fixed but cut with scissors below the skin surface. Because of the strong adhesive force on the tissue (friction) around the tape, fixation is unnecessary, and should not be done. Finally, the vaginal and skin incisions are sutured.

If there is excessive suburethral vaginal tissue this is cautiously excised, taking special care not to create too much tension in the suburethral vaginal wall. To check that the proximal urethra and bladder neck have an acceptable lumen and mobility, a Hegar no. 7 sound can be passed from the outer meatus into the bladder. Finally, the bladder is emptied and the patient leaves the theatre without an indwelling catheter.

Intraoperatively all patients receive 4 g intravenous penicillin at the start of the operation. Postoperatively antibiotics are given according to local practice.

No immediate postoperative restrictions are given, but the patient is encouraged to move about within the ward as soon as she wishes. Depending on her wishes and general condition she is usually discharged from hospital the same evening or the following morning. In particular, if the patient is old or lives a long distance away, she is given the opportunity to stay overnight in the hospital.

As described above, TVT is a highly standardized procedure. Nevertheless it is also a highly individualized operation, since adjustment of the tape to obtain continence is performed with the patient awake and the adjustments are made according to the prevailing conditions of the particular patient. The tape is not fixed by sutures, but by the patient's own fibroblasts that invade the prolene mesh of the tape and secure its position. Hereby a flexible "natural" reconstruction is obtained which minimizes the risks of overcorrection and postoperative urinary retention.

Results and Comments

As mentioned earlier, over 200 000 TVT operations have been performed so far. On the basis of our own experiences from more than 1000 operations, where the patients have been followed prospectively according to a strict protocol, the following results can be stated:

● When TVT is used as the primary operation for stress urinary incontinence, mean operation time is 20–25 minutes and ~90% of all patients can be discharged from hospital the same day or the next morning. The mean time of absence from work is ~10 days. In some patients who do heavy work an extra week of sick leave is recommended. At subsequent check-ups 80% of patients are dry, with no leakage as confirmed objectively and subjectively. Another 10% are significantly improved according to the protocol. This means that urine leakage may occur occasionally during severe cold, etc.

- Immediate postoperative voiding problems necessitating an indwelling catheter over the first two postoperative nights occur in ~10% of patients. Otherwise no postoperative urinary retention has been recognized, and no long-term catheter treatment is necessary. No defective healing or tape rejection has been observed.[4–10]

- Comparison of the TVT results to those reported using other surgical techniques for SI shows that TVT has a cure rate equal to that of generally accepted standard procedures, or even better. The TVT technique is, however, easier to learn and to carry out than, for example, laparoscopic and traditional Burch colposuspensions. The short operation time and the fact that the procedure can be carried out under local anesthesic makes it also highly cost-effective.

- In patients with a hypermobile urethra, a cure rate of 90% has been obtained. In patients with ISD, i.e. a low resting urethral pressure, the cure rate is 10% lower, also at long-term follow-up, i.e. ≥ 5 years.

- In patients with relapses after previous surgery, TVT in our hands has been able to cure 85% of the patients in the 5 year follow-up period.

- In patients with symptoms and signs of both prolapse and GSI, we have combined TVT with prolapse repairs and obtained cure of stress urinary incontinence of close to 90%. In patients where posterior repairs were necessary, the operations were performed mainly under spinal anesthesia. These results are also consonant with other reports.[6–10]

- In patients with mixed incontinence, i.e. symptoms of both stress and urge incontinence, we have found that TVT can cure or improve both symptoms, in particular if the urge component is mainly "sensory" urge.

- Most encouraging is the finding that so far there have been no rejections of the tape and no defective healing. Most likely this is due to the properties of the tape material, Prolene, which is accepted by the tissues in which it is implanted (unlike, for example, Mersilene and Gore-Tex).[1,2,4] Another important positive effect is the strong adhesive forces created around the tape which prevents sliding, unlike previously used sling materials. In fact, because of the high degree of friction, it is difficult to move the prolene tape as

soon as the surrounding plastic sheath has been removed. This in turn emphasizes the need for the plastic sheath, facilitating placement of the tape in a correct position around the midurethra. The sheath also prevents the tape being contaminated at implantation. Hence the design of the instrument and the surgical technique enables the tape not only to be located in a correct anatomical position, but also to be firmly secured immediately. An interesting observation in this context is that most patients report that directly after the operation they have a far greater sense of "security" than before surgery.

- The small incisions and canals involved with the TVT technique minimize the surgical trauma and enable the operation to be performed under local anesthesia. The technique also makes fairly small demands on postoperative care.

- It must be emphasized that TVT cannot be compared to conventional slingplasties, in which the surgical procedures are more extensive and the sling is located at the bladder neck, which is aimed to be elevated. If the TVT tape was placed too close to the bladder neck there would be a risk of postoperative impairment of urine flow, as is the case in many other surgical procedures for treatment of SI. This is avoided with the present technique in accordance with the theoretical and experimental background to the operation as presented earlier.[1,2]

Complications

As mentioned above, approximately 200 000 TVT operations have been performed since 1994 and remarkably few complications have been reported. A rigorous search yielded the following complications, which were reported at a TVT consensus meeting in Florence in May 1999.

- Bladder perforations seem to occur in 3–5%. All reported to be uneventful. In case of bladder perforation an indwelling catheter is recommended for 1–2 days. To avoid bladder perforation, which is a particular risk in relapse operations, the needle should be kept in close contact with the back of the pubic bone during insertion.

- Haemorrhage has been reported in less than 1%. It is important to avoid TVT surgery in patients on anticoagulants. If excessive bleeding is observed during surgery, the operator should use his or her fingers to compress the retropubic space from the vagina on to the back of the pubic bone for 3–5 minutes. Then a tamponade should be used for 2–4 hours postoperatively. Laparotomy should be performed only in case of circulatory instability.

- In 14 patients out of 50 000 (<1/1000), major vessel injuries have occurred requiring laparotomy. In these cases the needle has been inserted too far laterally. Such a complication will not occur if the operator stays in the midline in close contact with the back of the pubic bone when passing the needle from the vagina to the abdomen.

- Postoperative urinary retention has been reported in 5–10%. This is mainly due to elevation of the urethra. Remember always to place the tape loosely around midurethra, and allow a few drops of urine to escape at final adjustment of the tape. Also remember to close the vaginal wall incision temporarily by two forceps during final adjustment, for fine tuning of the tape.

- Postoperatively, check urine residual using a urethral catheterization (in–out catheter) after first micturition after surgery. This is to make sure of an empty bladder. In case of long-term urinary retention, i.e. 4 weeks, the tape can be cut in the midline via the previous vaginal incision.

Concluding Remarks

Ambulatory surgical procedures have been introduced in gynecologic surgery for several reasons. There is at present great enthusiasm for endoscopic Burch colposuspension, but we are still awaiting long-term follow-up studies. TVT has an operation time which is less than half that of the Burch procedure. It is also carried out under local anesthesia, and the incidence of urinary retention is significantly lower than when the Burch procedure is performed. Another important consideration is that the cost of TVT is about half that of Burch colposuspension, according to the Scandinavian health economic system.

On the basis of the initial results[4] and the results from longer follow-up studies[5–7,9,11] the TVT technique has now been adopted as the primary technique for surgical treatment of genuine stress incontinence in several Scandinavian clinics.

References

1. Petros P, Ulmsten U (1990) An integral theory on female urinary incontinence. Experimental and clinical considerations. Acta Obstet Gynecol Scand 69(suppl): 153.
2. Petros P, Ulmsten U (1993) An integral theory and its method for the diagnosis and management of female urinary incontinence. Scand J Urol Nephrol 153: 1–93.
3. Westby M, Asmussen M, Ulmsten U (1982) Location of maximum intraurethral pressure related to urogenital diaphragm in the female studied by simultaneous urethrocystometry and voiding urethrocystography. Am J Obstet Gynecol 144: 408–12.
4. Ulmsten U, Henriksson L, Johnson P, Varhos G (1996) An ambulatory surgical procedure under local anesthesia for treatment of female urinary incontinence. Int Urogynecol J 7: 81–6.
5. Ulmsten U, Johnson P, Rezapour M (1999) A three-year follow up of tension free vaginal tape for surgical treatment of female stress urinary incontinence. Br J Obstet Gynaecol 106: 345–50.
6. Olsson I, Kroon UB (1999) A three-year postoperative evaluation of TVT (tension free vaginal tape). Gynecol Obstet Invest 48: 267–9.
7. Wang AC, Lo TS (1998) Tension-free vaginal tape. A minimally invasive solution to stress urinary incontinence in women. J Reprod Med 43: 429–34.
8. Ulmsten U, Falconer C, Johnson P et al. (1998) A multicentre study of tension free vaginal tape (TVT) for surgical treatment of stress urinary incontinence. Int Urogynecol J 9: 210–13.
9. Kuuva N, Nilsson C-G (2000) A nationwide analysis on complications associated with the tension-free vaginal tape (TVT) procedure. Neurol Urodynamics 19(4): 394–395.
10. Ward KL, Hilton P, Browning J (2000) A randomised trial of colposuspension and tension-free vaginal tape (TVT) for primary genuine stress incontinence. Neurol Urodynamics 19(4): 386–8.
11. Nilsson JC, Kuuva N, Falconer C, Rezapour M, Ulmsten U (2001) Long term results of the tension free vaginal tape (TVT) procedure for surgical treatment of female stress urinary incontinence. Int Urogynecol J 12 (supple 2) 55–58.

9 Stamey, Raz, and Modified Pereya

Scott Littwiller and Philippe E. Zimmern

For over 40 years, transvaginal needle suspensions have been utilized to treat anatomic or genuine stress incontinence.[1] These procedures have the obvious advantage of avoiding the morbidity from an abdominal incision that was necessary for previous suspension techniques.[2] Since that time, the needle suspension has undergone a number of technical modifications and revisions, all designed to improve cure rates, while simplifying surgical technique. The goals of these procedures have been to correct urethral and bladder neck hypermobility, secure the vaginal wall, and provide support for the proximal urethra during times of increased abdominal pressure. This chapter outlines the various techniques of transvaginal needle suspension for the treatment of stress incontinence, beginning with preoperative assessment through operative technique and postoperative management.

Indications

The ideal patient for transvaginal bladder suspension is one with anatomic stress incontinence who has failed conservative measures such as biofeedback, pelvic muscle exercises, or pharmacologic therapy. Alternately, in a patient with severe anatomic incontinence who wishes to proceed directly to surgery these conservative measures may be omitted. Various authors have speculated on the use of suspension procedures in patients with mixed incontinence (stress and urge incontinence) but, overall, most agree that surgery is not contraindicated in this scenario, provided the patient has a demonstrable anatomic defect and has failed pharmacologic therapy for urge incontinence. Patients should be advised that though some series report an acceptable resolution of urge incontinence with needle suspension,[3,4] the possibility exists for the persistence of urge incontinence or the onset of new urge incontinence. Additionally, patients with a history of intrinsic sphincteric deficiency (ISD, see below) may have a higher rate of failure after conventional needle suspension and are not optimal candidates for this type of surgery. The use of the Valsalva or abdominal leak point pressure is widely accepted and may help in identifying patients with intrinsic sphincteric deficiency who may be at higher risk for failure following conventional needle suspension.[5]

Operative Technique

Patient Preparation

Patient preparation should begin with a detailed description of the chosen procedure as well as the expected risks and benefits. Patients should be given an idea of the customary hospital stay as well as the recuperation time necessary after surgery. Most patients will be advised against lifting heavy objects or straining for up to 2–3 months. Patients will also need to refrain from sexual intercourse for at least 2–3 months. Return to work time is quite variable and dependent on the individual job requirements.

Patients should be counseled as to the published cure rates with their respective procedure, recurrence rates, risk for continued postoperative urgency, de-novo urgency, or urge incontinence. Patients should be made aware of the risk for bladder, urethral or ureteral injury, or fistula, though this is uncommon.

Patients should all have documentation of sterile preoperative urine culture and receive preoperative antibiotics (usually first-generation cephalosporin or ampicillin plus aminoglycoside). Patients may be asked to douche and use an enema on the night before surgery.

Anesthesia and Patient Positioning

In general, needle bladder neck suspension can be performed without difficulty under general or regional (spinal or epidural) anesthesia. Some have advocated performing these procedures under local anesthesia,[6,7] but this is definitely the exception rather than the rule. By their nature these procedures are performed in the lithotomy position with vaginal exposure enhanced by a weighted vaginal speculum and self-retaining vaginal retractor (for example a Lone Star/Scott ring retractor).

Pereyra Suspension

For over 40 years the Pereyra bladder neck suspension (Fig. 9.1) has been used to correct anatomic stress incontinence. As originally described, the procedure involved the blind passage of a special blunt needle introduced through a suprapubic wound and passed out of the vagina. The ends of a stainless steel wire were placed through the eyes of this trocar and withdrawn back to the suprapubic wound leaving a loop of silver wire to encircle the vaginal wall. This wire was tied over the rectus fascia and removed at a later date. All needle suspensions are based on this concept of needle passage. The original procedure was modified in 1967 to include a midline incision in the vaginal wall, substitute chromic cat gut for steel wire, and add a Kelly plication to the procedure. In 1978 the procedure underwent further modifications to prevent suture pull-through; this is the "modified Pereyra" currently known today.[8–10]

In the revised procedure normal saline is injected beneath the vaginal epithelium and a transverse, semicircular incision is made at the distal urethra. A vertical vaginal incision is then made proximally which intersects with the transverse incision. The epithelium is dissected laterally to the edges of the pubic rami. An index finger is then used to perforate the endopelvic fascia at a point 3 cm lateral to the meatus. The freed endopelvic fascia is then grasped

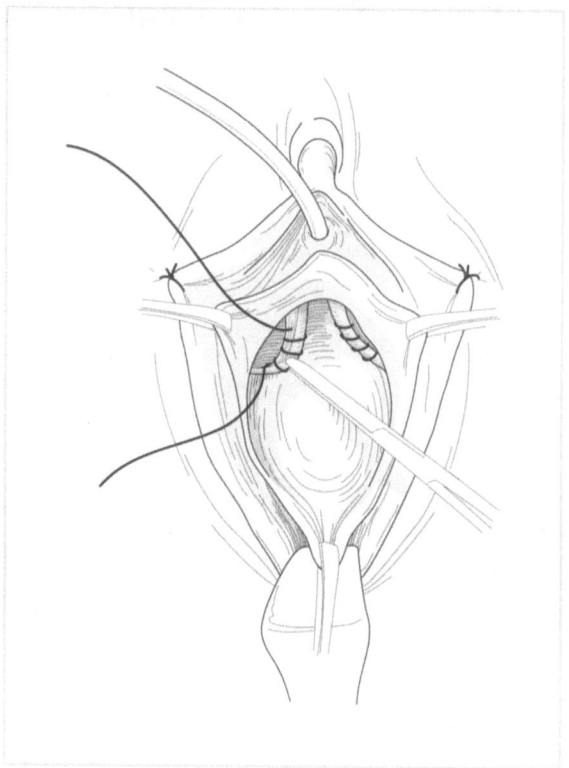

Figure 9.1 Pereyra suspension. Helical passes of non-absorbable suture secure the pubourethral ligament and freed edge of the endopelvic fascia, before retropubic elevation.

with an Allis clamp exposing the freed edge of the pubourethral ligaments. Helical passes of heavy nonabsorbable monofilament suture are used to secure the pubourethral ligament and freed edge of the endopelvic fascia. It is this support complex that forms the basis for the repair. A suprapubic incision is then made and the Pereyra ligature carrier (El Rey Industries Inc., Upland, CA) is passed under finger guidance out through the ipsilateral vaginal incision. The sutures are passed through the eye of the carrier and transferred to the anterior abdominal wall. Cystoscopy is performed to exclude bladder injury or intravesical suture placement. Vaginal incisions are closed with absorbable sutures. Right and left sutures are then tied together while an assistant supports the anterior vaginal wall. The suprapubic incision is closed and a Foley catheter is left to gravity.[9]

Results (see Table 9.1, page 130)

Outcomes with the Pereyra suspension were initially optimistic. In his original article, Pereyra reported success in 28/31 patients at 14 months.[1] In 1967 Pereyra and Lebherz reported on 210 patients undergoing the initial modification of the procedure (chromic suture/Kelly plication). At a follow-up of

12–24 months, 94% cure rate was achieved.[8] Other authors using this technique were not able to reproduce these results, however. Carl and co-workers and Kursh et al. reported cure rates of 54% and 44% respectively.[11,12]

In 1978, Pereyra and Lebherz reported their success with the modified Pereyra procedure as described above. Of 162 patients with at least 1 year of follow-up, 151 had favorable results (143 markedly improved or 8 improved).[13] In 1982, Pereyra again published 4–6 year follow-up in 82 patients undergoing the modified Pereyra procedure. Results were again favorable, with a cure rate of 85.4% and an "improved" rate of 7.3%. Failure was noted in 7.3% of patients.

Methods of outcomes analysis in these and other studies have been questioned. In 1994 Sirls and co-workers evaluated 151 patients with 2 year follow-up following the still further modified Pereyra bladder neck suspension. Patients were evaluated by both chart review and mailed questionnaire. According to outcomes analysis 47% were cured and 64% improved, compared to 72% cured and 89% improved by retrospective review. In this study, questionnaire-based outcomes consistently reported worse results than chart review.[14,15]

Raz Needle Suspension and Raz Vaginal Wall Sling

The Raz bladder neck suspension was reported in 1981 as a modification of the Pereyra procedure.[16] It differs from the original Pereyra procedure in that the retropubic space is entered to facilitate needle passage and prevent bladder injury. Additionally, the procedure incorporates the entire vaginal wall, excluding epithelium (Figs 9.2, 9.3).

An inverted U-shaped flap is raised in the anterior vaginal wall. Dissection is carried laterally toward the pubic bone and the endopelvic fascia is perforated with a scissors. A number 1 polypropylene suture (prolene) is passed in a helical fashion to anchor the anterior vaginal wall (excluding the mucosa) to the endopelvic fascia. A short transverse suprapubic incision is made similar to the one used in the Pereyra procedure and the helical sutures are transferred to the anterior abdominal wall by use of a single- or double-pronged needle carrier.[17] Endoscopy confirms the position of the suspension, the absence of bladder injury, or transvesical suture

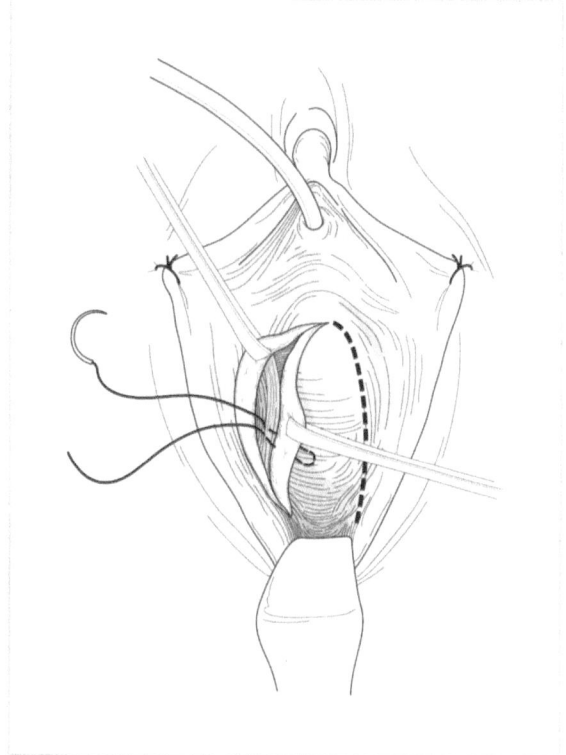

Figure 9.2 Raz needle suspension. Prolene sutures are placed in the vaginal wall and deep into the urethropelvic ligament to provide a secure anchor, before suprapubic transfer with a ligature carrier.

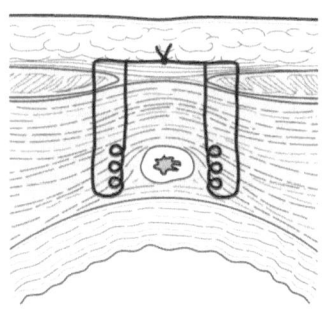 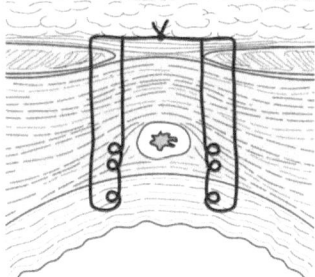 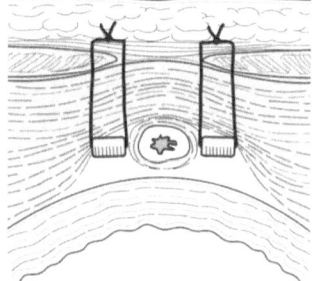

Figure 9.3 Conceptual evolution in the placement of suspension sutures (from left to right: modified Pereyra, Raz, Stamey) These diagrams depict the location and tissue structures incorporated in the suspension "bites" – Stamey recommended Dacron bolsters to reinforce the anchor and add some scarring.

passage. Intravenous indigo carmine may be given to exclude ureteral injury or obstruction. Vaginal incisions are closed with an absorbable suture and the polypropylene sutures are tied over the rectus fascia or over Teflon pledgets to prevent suture pull-through. The abdominal incision is closed with a subcuticular running suture and a catheter is left in the bladder for 1 day.

Results (see Table 9.1)

Initial success was reported in 96 of 100 patients by chart review with an unspecified length of follow-up.[18] In 1992 Raz again presented results in 206 patients (chart review) with a mean follow-up of 15 months. Again results were favorable with success (no protection worn) reported in 90% of patients. In patients with severe stress incontinence (suspected sphincteric deficiency) success fell to 65%. Resolution of urge incontinence occurred in 66% of patients and de-novo urge incontinence occurred in

7.5% of patients. Complications included secondary prolapse in 6% and retention in 2.5%.[19] In 1994, Golomb and colleagues reported the results of the Raz bladder suspension, stratifying patients by age (less than or greater than 65 years). Results were similar in both groups with 85% of younger women and 90.4% of older women completely cured of stress incontinence.[20] Many authors have reported long-term prospective results with failure rates of 50–60%.[21-22] As a result, Raz has modified the original operation as outlined below.

Raz Vaginal Wall Sling (Buried Epithelium)

In 1989, Raz and colleagues reported a new approach to needle suspension, referred to as the vaginal wall sling (Fig. 9.4).[18] This sling is different from the conventional fascial sling in that it is an in-situ patch made of vaginal epithelium which is suspended by monofilament suture and buried by an advancement flap of vaginal epithelium.

Table 9.1. Comparison of needle suspensions

Procedure	N	Follow-up (months)	Follow-up method[a]	% Cure	% Improved	Postoperative urgency	Comment
Pereyra							
Pereyra (1978)[16]	162	12	C	88%	5%	No comment	
Pereyra (1982)[9]	82	48–60	C	85%	7.3%	No comment	
Sirls (1994)[15]	151	25	Q	47%	17%	Correlated with poor outcome	
Raz							
Raz (1981)[16]	100	?	C	96%	–	No Comment	Retention 2.4%
Raz (1992)[19]	206	15	C	83%	7.3%	7.5%	
Gilja (1998)[63]	46	36	Q	80%		13%	
Raz VWS (buried)							
Raz (1989)[18]	32	10–28	C	77%	12%	15%	Retention: 0
Juma (1992)[24]	65	24	C	91%	3.7%	14.8%	Retention: 3.7%
Litwiller (1997)[4]	51	31	Q	71%		9%	Retention: 0.5%
Raz VWS (nonburied)							
Raz (1996)[26]	95	17	Q	93%	–	9%	Retention: 0
Stamey							
Stamey (1980)[31]	206	6–48	C	90%	–	34%	–
Gofrit (1998)[64]	72	90	Q	70%	–	22%	Infected graft/suture: 7%
Kuczyk, MA (1998)[65]	85	61	Q	34%	18%	–	Infected graft/suture: 11%
Conrad (1997)[66]	172	66	Q	36%	27%	–	Infected graft/suture: 15%
Christiansen (1997)[67]	83	84	Q	32%	39%	5%	Infected graft/suture: 6%
Gittes							
Gittes (1987)[39]	38	2–29	C	84%	–	–	–
Foster (1989)[42]	20	2–8	C	60%	10%	–	
Elkabir (1998)	87	46	Q	23%	35%	–	Wound infection: 2%
Kursh (1992)[68]	108	12	C	82%	–	–	
PBNS (Vesica™)							
Schultheiss (1998)[49]	37	6–18	Q	43%	24%	5%	Pelvic pain: 27%
Appell (1997)[47]	71	36	C	82%	–	–	Osteomyelitis: 3%

a C, chart review; Q, questionnaire.

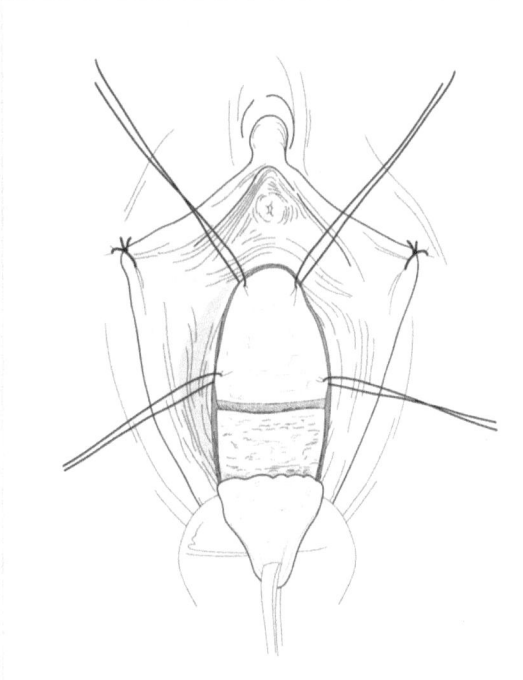

Figure 9.4 Raz vaginal wall sling (buried epithelium). An in-situ patch of vaginal epithelium beneath the urethra is suspended by four monofilament sutures. After suprapubic transfer of theses sutures, a proximal vaginal wall flap is advanced over this in-situ island to cover the sling.

An inverted U-shaped incision is made in the anterior vaginal wall and a distal patch of epithelium is isolated. Lateral dissection is carried out and the endopelvic fascia is perforated as previously described for the Raz bladder neck suspension. Helical sutures of no. 1 polypropylene are placed in the four corners of the patch and transferred to the anterior abdominal wall as for the Raz needle suspension. An anterior vaginal wall flap is advanced and closed over the patch and the suspension sutures are tied under no tension. Despite initial concerns, animal studies in rabbits have revealed no dysplastic or malignant changes in buried vaginal epithelium.[23]

Results *(see Table 9.1)*

Short-term results were reported in 32 patients with sphincteric deficiency by Raz in 1989 with subsequent follow-up in 1992 (54 patients). In the initial report 29/32 (91%) patients were cured of their stress incontinence and no neurogenically intact patient suffered urinary retention.[18] In the follow-up study, results were again favorable with a 94% cure rate of stress incontinence. Urgency and urge incontinence have, however, been a problem for some patients and were seen in 23% of Raz's patients (8% persistent, 15% de novo).[24]

In a similar study by Litwiller and colleagues, questionnaire-based outcome analysis and patient satisfaction were assessed in 51 patients undergoing the vaginal wall sling procedure. At a mean of 31 months, patients enjoyed a 92% cure of anatomical stress incontinence and a 75% cure of incontinence from ISD. Despite these favorable results, postoperative urgency was reported by 59% of patients (51% with preoperative urgency, 8% with de-novo urgency). Persistent postoperative urge incontinence was seen in 33% of patients and was the primary cause for patient dissatisfaction (p < 0.01).[4]

Raz Vaginal Wall Sling (Nonburied Epithelium)

The vaginal wall sling underwent yet another modification which was reported in 1995 by Raz and colleagues (Fig. 9.5). In this new variation, four sets of no. 1 polypropylene sutures are placed to create a hammock of support for the bladder neck and urethra. The first pair of sutures is applied at the level of the bladder neck. Each suture incorporates the vesicopelvic fascia, urethropelvic ligament, and

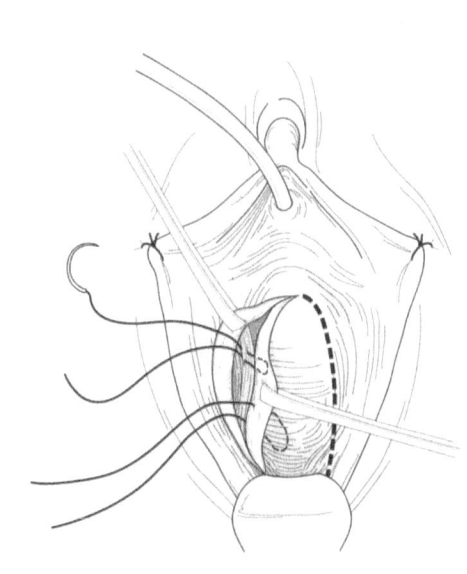

Figure 9.5 Raz vaginal wall sling (nonburied epithelium). Four monofilament sutures are placed to support the bladder neck and urethra. Each suture incorporates the vesicopelvic fascia, the urethropelvic ligament, and the anterior vaginal wall without epithelium. The distal pair of sutures is placed at the midurethral level and the proximal pair is positioned at the level of the bladder neck.

anterior vaginal wall without epithelium. The second pair of no.1 sutures incorporates the levator ani as it inserts near the mid-urethral segment, medial edge of the urethropelvic ligament, and anterior vaginal wall as described above.[25,26] In doing so, a rectangular patch of vaginal epithelium is used for support, without the necessity of a buried vaginal patch. Lateral dissection is carried out as previously described and sutures are transferred to the anterior abdominal wall and tied as described before (under no tension).

Modifications of this technique have been reported and include the "four-corner" anterior vaginal wall suspension which not only supports the entire vaginal wall but may be used to correct minimal to moderate cystocele.[27]

Results

The results of this modification in 160 patients (95 with ISD and 65 with anatomic incontinence) were presented in 1996 by Raz and colleagues.[26] At a median follow-up of 17 months (range 6–32 months), 149 (93%) patients were reported as cured (90.5% with ISD / 96.9% with AI). Eleven patients (7%) developed recurrent stress incontinence as defined by wearing more than 1 pad per day (9 with ISD, 2 with AI). De-novo urge incontinence developed in 12 patients (7.5%). Urodynamic evaluation in these patients revealed detrusor instability with no evidence of obstruction. Prolonged urinary retention was noted in 8 patients (5%) and no patients suffered from permanent retention.[26]

Stamey Endoscopic Needle Suspension

The Stamey bladder neck suspension was originally described in 1973 as a "less morbid", more comfortable, and technically simple alternative to the Pereyra operation (Fig. 9.6). Its cardinal features are the use of knitted Dacron bolsters to support periurethral tissues, blind passage of a blunt needle (straight, 15°, or 30°) through the retropubic space, and intraoperative cystourethroscopy to assure suture placement at the bladder neck.[28]

The operation begins with two 2.5 cm transverse incisions which are made above the symphysis pubis. Blunt dissection is carried down to the rectus fascia. A moist gauze is left in place and attention is focused on the vaginal exposure. The urethral length is measured by inflating a Foley catheter balloon in the bladder and placing it on slight tension. A hemostat is then applied at the urethral meatus. The Foley catheter is then removed and the distance between the clamp and the balloon is measured. The Foley catheter is then replaced and a T-shaped incision is made below the urethral meatus. The vaginal flaps are raised laterally and are carried posteriorly to the level of the bladder neck (beneath the Foley balloon).

The Stamey needle (straight or angled, depending on surgeon preference) is introduced through one of the abdominal incisions, behind the symphysis and out of the vaginal incision at the level of the bladder neck (at the level of the Foley balloon) using finger guidance (see Fig. 9.6) With the needle in place, cystoscopy is performed. By movement of the needle, its position at the level of the bladder neck is confirmed as well as absence of bladder or urethral injury. A no. 2 monofilament nylon suture is then threaded through the eye of the needle and withdrawn suprapubically. The needle is again passed through the same incision 1–2 cm lateral to the original needle entry in the rectus fascia. The needle is brought out through the vaginal incision 1 cm distal to the site of the original needle passage. Again cystourethroscopy confirms the position of the needle and rules out bladder injury. The nylon suture is then passed through a 1 cm length of 5 mm knitted Dacron arterial graft material to buttress the vaginal loop. The vaginal end of the nylon suture is threaded through the eye of the needle which is withdrawn out through the suprapubic incision, leaving a large band of vaginal tissue within the loop of the suture. (see Fig. 9.6) This procedure is then repeated on the other side. Cystourethroscopy is again performed as tension is placed on the sutures. With this maneuver, the bladder neck should coapt leaving the mid and distal urethra intact. If desired, a suprapubic catheter is placed at this time and the vaginal incisions are closed with absorbable suture. As originally described, the nylon sutures are then tied "with considerable tension" and the suprapubic incisions are closed with absorbable suture. Subsequent authors have modified this technique and advocate minimal or no tension on the nylon suture in an effort to avoid over correction.[29,30]

Subsequent technical points have been outlined by Stamey in 1992 in an effort to decrease infectious complications:

- The Dacron graft should be positioned below the suture line to prevent graft erosion through the incision.
- Copious irrigation with aminoglycoside should be used in the vaginal incision before closure to prevent graft infection.

Results (see Table 9.1)

As originally presented, Stamey reported 11/16 patients cured at 3 years following the procedure.[28] In 1979, Stamey again reported results of 203 pa-

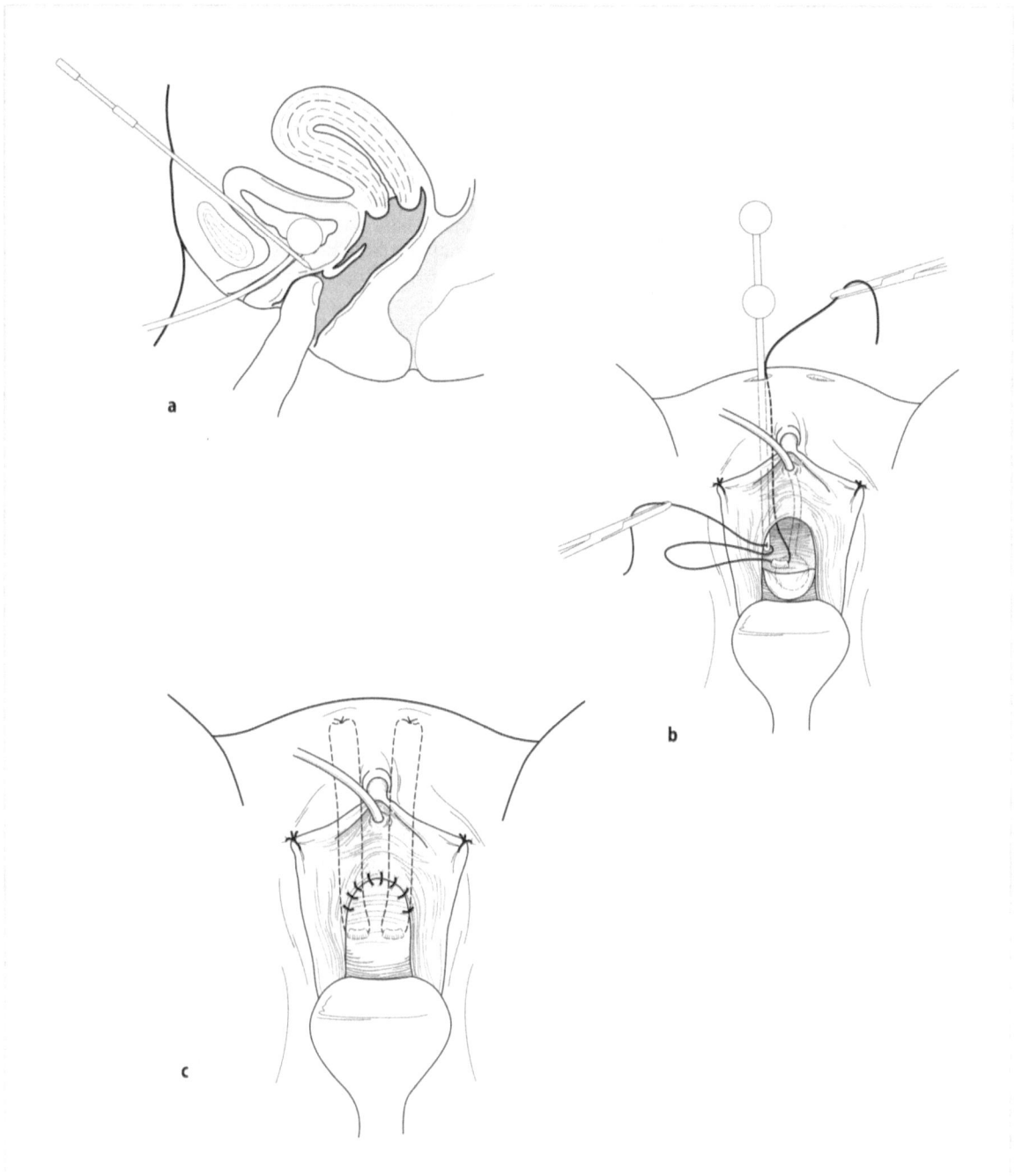

Figure 9.6 a Stamey endoscopic needle suspension. The straight Stamey needle is introduced through one of the short suprapubic incision and then guided behind the symphysis to exit the vagina lateral to and at the level of the bladder neck using finger guidance (**i**). **b** After confirming by endoscopy the lack of bladder injury and the proper placement of the needle at the level of the bladder neck, a nonabsorbable suture is threaded through the eye of the needle and the needle is withdrawn suprapubically **c** At completion of the procedure, the sutures have been tied suprapubically with some tension. Note the Dacron bolster which serves to buttress the vaginal loop to minimize the risk of suture pull-through.

tients followed for 6 months to 4 years. In this chart review, 20% suffered from total incontinence and the remainder from simple stress incontinence. Results were again favorable in 91% of patients.[31] In general, cure rates vary from 53–80% in the English literature.[32,33] The degree to which patients are not cured but "improved" also varies accordingly.

However, the long-term durability of the Stamey procedure has been questioned. Mills found that in 30 patients, an initial cure rate of 67% deteriorated to 33% over a 10 year period.[34] Similar results were reported by O'Sullivan and co-workers who reported results in 65 patients. Initially, 70% were cured and 15% improved. At 6 months, this number decreased to 56% and 21% respectively. At 1 year, 31% of patients were dry and 28% improved. Factors portending a poorer outcome were obesity (p < 0.005) and number of pads used per day (p < 0.05) as well as previous surgery.[35]

Postoperative complications have been extensively reported with the Stamey suspension. The most common complication reported by Clemens and co-workers was postoperative urgency, seen in 70% of patients.[36] In studies by Wang, these patients with postoperative urgency were found to have a significant incidence of bladder outlet obstruction as demonstrated by elevated voiding pressures and decreased flow rates.[37] Other less commonly reported complications included suture abscess (12%), urinary retention (7%), and chronic suprapubic pain (10%).[38]

Gittes Bladder Neck Suspension

The technique of no-incision urethropexy (Fig. 9.7) was first described by Gittes and Loughlin in 1987.[39] This procedure developed out of a desire to perform a less invasive bladder neck suspension which would utilize a natural vaginal bolster to support the vaginal wall, without the infectious risks involved with knitted bolsters as described by Stamey.[38] This procedure is based on the concept that monofilament suture will pull through the vaginal wall and abdominal subcutaneous tissues when placed under tension, creating an autologous pledget of tissue, thus tethering the anterior vaginal wall to the anterior abdominal fascia.[39]

The anterior vaginal wall, just lateral to the balloon (bladder neck) is uplifted toward the abdomen and the most mobile portion is grasped with an Allis clamp. This position will be the location of the first helical suspension suture. In the modified procedure of Morales and VanCott,[69] three or four helical bites are taken with a no.2 Prolene suture along a course parallel to the proximal urethra. Needles are cut off and the procedure is repeated on the other side of the bladder neck (see Fig. 9.7) Subsequently, two suprapubic stab wound incisions are made with an #11 knife blade. Their location should be 2 cm lateral to the midline and just superior to the symphysis pubis. Some surgeons modify this technique and prefer a single transverse incision 4 cm in length (to allow dissection down to the anterior fascia). A Stamey needle is then passed through the anterior abdominal fascia. The tip is levered anteriorly to contact the pubic bone and the needle is "walked" down the pubis toward the operator's non-dominant index finger, which is elevating the vaginal wall near the ipsilateral helical suture. As the bladder may be injured during the course of this maneuver, the Foley catheter is left to drainage and the needle is passed by making sequential medial to lateral sweeps along the symphysis as it is advanced. The vaginal wall is perforated with the needle at the proximal end of the helical suture and one end of the monofilament suture is passed through the eye of the Stamey needle. The needle is withdrawn and brought out through the suprapubic incision. The needle is repassed on the same side and repeated in the same manner (see Fig. 9.7) The procedure is repeated on the other side with the second suture and cystoscopy is performed to exclude the possibility of bladder injury. If a percutaneous suprapubic tube is desired, it may be placed at this time under direct vision. If suture is noted in the bladder wall or lumen, the offending suture is removed and the needle is repassed under direct cystoscopic guidance.

With a Foley catheter in place and the bladder drained, the sutures are tied in the subcutaneous tissues using just enough tension to elevate the anterior vaginal wall. The suprapubic incisions are closed with absorbable suture and a vaginal pack is not usually necessary.

Results

Much of the outcome data regarding the Gittes procedure involves small series, or short follow-up. In their original paper, Gittes and Loughlin reported a 87% continence rate with a follow-up of 2–29 months.[39] More recently, Loughlin and co-workers reported their extended success with this same group over an 8 year period. In this chart review, success was defined as complete absence of incontinence or no requirement of protective pads. Using this criteria, success was reported as 84%.[40]

Other authors have, however, been unable to reproduce these results. Benson and co-workers reported the concomitant use of the Gittes with other pelvic floor surgery. They found an improvement rate of 97% but an objective cure rate of only 58.8% at a 9.5 month mean follow-up.[41]

Similarly, Foster and O'Reilly reported a cure rate of 60% at 5 months,[42] and Kil et al. reported a 44% cure at 14 months.[43] In one of the few long-term outcome studies of the Gittes suspension, Elkabir and Mee reported their series of 87 patients during an 8 year period. With a median follow-up of 46 months, 55 patients responded to a postal questionnaire. In this series, 23% reported no leakage, 26.9.% reported improvement. There was a statistically significant increase in failure among patients with preoperative urgency and urge incontinence and most failures occurred within 2 years.[44]

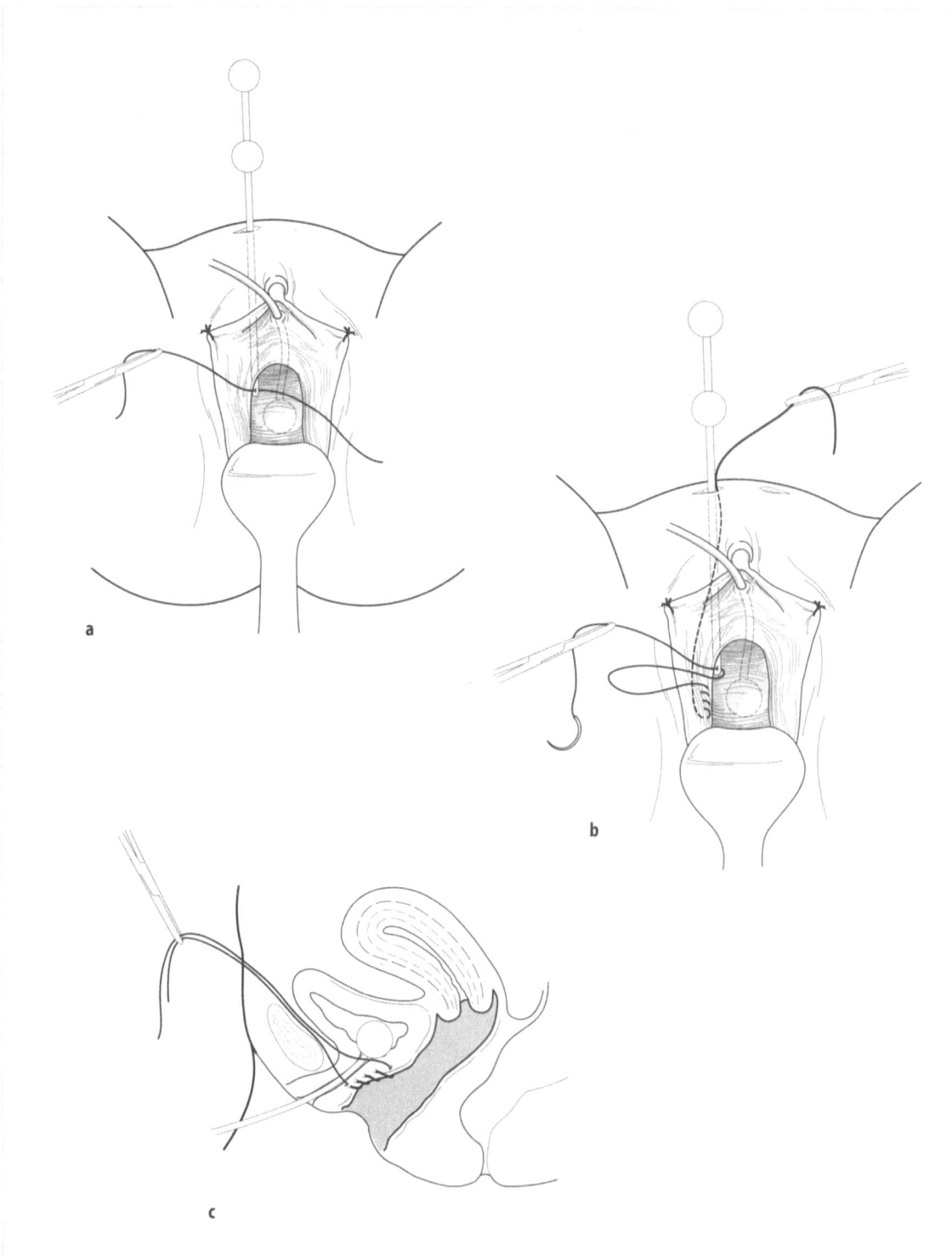

Figure 9.7 Gittes no-incision urethropexy. **a** The ligature carrier is "walked" down the back of the pubis toward the operator's non-dominant index finger which is elevating the vaginal wall. **b** A helical suspension suture is passed through and through the anterior vaginal wall, lateral to the bladder neck. **c** Two passes of the needle are needed on both sides to complete the suspension.

Bone-Anchored Percutaneous Bladder Neck Suspension (PBNS)

The concept of a bone anchored vaginal suspension is not a new concept but has generally combined a conventional vaginal suspension (Pereyra, Gittes, or vaginal wall sling) with pubic bone fixation in lieu of suprafascial fixation (Fig. 9.8).[45,46] The rationale for bone anchor fixation is that stabilization of the suspension sutures in the symphysis pubis prevents movement with Valsalva maneuvers thereby preventing pull-through from the perivaginal tissues.[47] Bone anchor fixation is reported to be less painful than conventional fascial fixation[45] and has been done effectively under local anesthesia.[6] One of the most popular applications of the bone anchoring technique has been its combination with a Z- stitch

anterior vaginal wall modification of the Gittes procedure.[46]

A Foley catheter is placed to aid in localization of the bladder neck and to drain the bladder. Several disposable tools are utilized in this procedure and are available in a kit from the manufacturer (Boston Scientific Corp., Boston, MA). These include a self-retaining vaginal retractor, bone locating device, titanium bone anchoring screw, and needle passer (see Fig. 9.8) A small 2 cm incision is made over each pubic tubercle and dissection is carried down to the level of the fascia overlying the pubic tubercle. The special bone locating device is positioned over the tubercle and the Duratak bone anchor (Davis and Geck St. Louis, MO) with its no.1 monofilament suture is pneumatically drilled into the bone. Next, one end of the no.1 suture is captured in the retractable eye of the disposable suture passer and passed

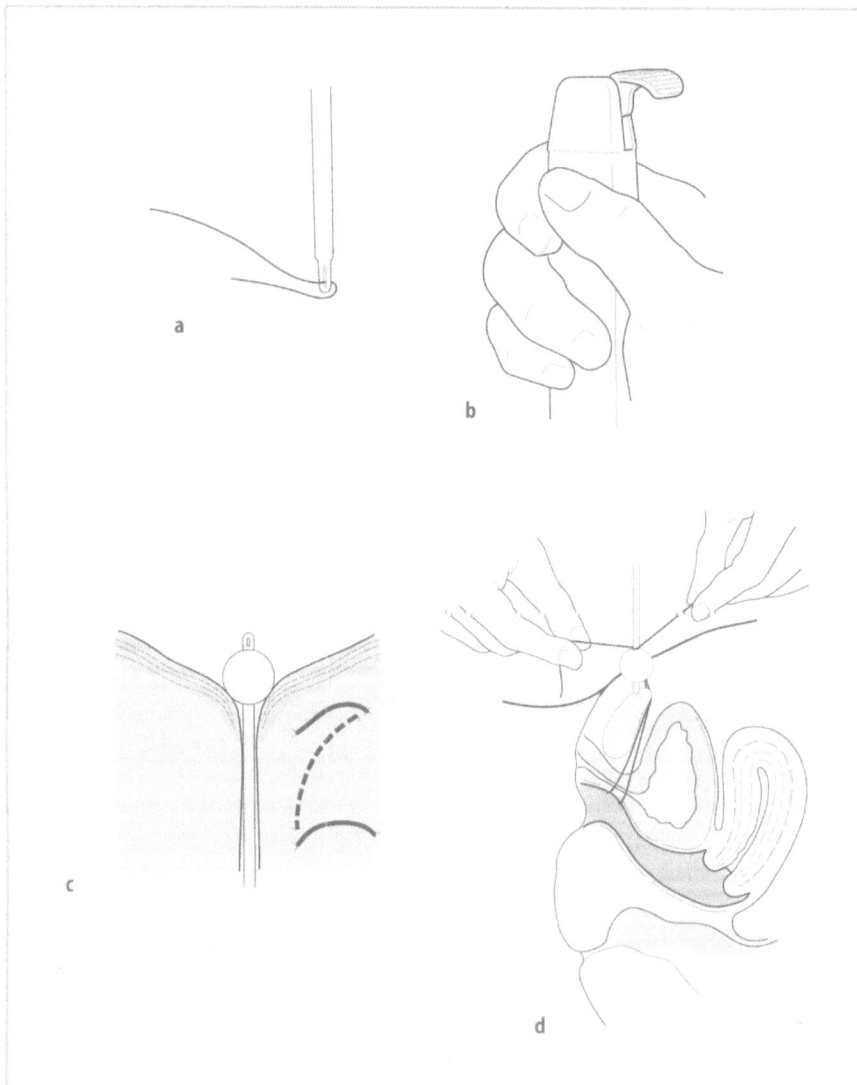

Figure 9.8 Bone-anchored percutaneous bladder neck suspension (Vesica). Disposable tools utilized for this procedure include a needle passer (tip **a**; handle **b**) whose curve facilitates the passage along the posterior aspect of the symphysis pubis. **c** The option of releasing the suture after perforating the vaginal wall lateral to the bladder neck is an advantage of this needle passer. By a series of perforation and retraction of the needle passer in the retropubic space, a "Z" stitch incorporating a broad segment of vaginal wall from the level of the midurethra to the bladder neck is performed with reduced risk of bladder injury. **d** As for the Gittes procedure, nonabsorbable suture is left exposed on the vaginal side. However, the disposable suture spacer allows a more reproducible tension adjustment while tying the suspension sutures suprapubically. The bone anchor fixation additionally stabilizes the suspension suture to avoid pullthrough from the paravaginal tissues.

with the surgeon's dominant hand along the posterior aspect of the symphysis pubis. A finger in the vagina locates the bladder neck and the needle perforates the vaginal wall at a point 1cm distal and lateral to the bladder neck. With the passer still in place, cystoscopy is performed using a 70° lens to exclude bladder injury. When bladder injury occurs, it is usually on the first pass as this is closest to the bladder itself. If bladder injury is noted, the passer and suture are removed and passed under direct cystoscopic guidance. The suture is then released and the passer is withdrawn into the retropubic space. The empty passer is then directed through the vaginal wall on a second pass, 1–2 cm lateral to the first perforation. The suture is grasped with the passer and withdrawn. The passer is then advanced and allowed to perforate the vaginal wall at a point 2 cm distal to the initial pass at the level of the mid-urethra. The suture is released and the passer is again withdrawn. On the final advancement, the passer is brought out at a point 2 cm lateral to the previous point, the suture is grasped and brought out the anterior abdominal wall. The final suture configuration has a Z-shaped configuration, but upon vaginal inspection, only two transverse mono-filament sutures are visible, one at the level of the bladder neck and one at the level of the mid-urethra (see Fig. 9.8) With both sutures at the skin level, they are tied over a special suture spacer to insure no tension and the wound is closed with absorbable suture. Vaginal pack is usually not necessary and voiding trials are commenced on the first post-operative day. If a suprapubic tube is desired, it may be placed at the end of the case under direct vision.

Results

The results of the PBNS were initially presented by Benderev in 1994 in a series of 150 patients. In this series, 49/53 women sampled were "cured" at a follow-up of 15 months.[46] In 1996, Leach and Appell reported 12 month data on 125 women with genuine stress incontinence who achieved a 95% cure of stress incontinence after treatment with the PBNS.[48] At 3 years, this number reportedly fell to 82%.[47] Other authors have reported poorer results utilizing a standardized questionnaire for follow-up. In a study by Schultheiss and co-workers, 37 patients who underwent PBNS were evaluated initially and at a mean of 11 months. Although a 92% continence cure (34/37) was noted at initial questioning, the number fell to 43% completely dry and 24% improved at longer follow-up (6–18 months).[49]

Modifications of the bone anchoring concept have been made and include suspension based on vaginally placed bone anchors as well. In this technique, vaginally placed nitinol bone anchors (Influ-

ence Medical Technologies Ltd., Ramat-Gan, Israel) are placed through the vaginal mucosa and into the medulla of each pubic ramus. Sutures are then passed beneath the vaginal mucosa and tied to the contralateral anchor. In a series by Nativ and co-workers, 50 women underwent this minimally invasive procedure with 12 month chart review. Overall 41 patients (82%) were completely dry and 7 (14%) reported a 50% decrease in pad usage.[50] Recently, this bone anchor technology has been combined with the use of cadaveric fascia lata with good initial results.[51] Clearly, long term (3–5 year) data is needed on these new procedure as nearly all surgical interventions enjoy a good short term (1–2 year) success rate regardless of technique.

Complications

As mentioned already, bladder or urethral injuries arising from needle passage may be dealt with simply by removing the offending suture or needle with little risk for complication. If, however, the bladder is injured bluntly during the dissection of the prevesical space, it should be formally repaired either transvaginally[52] or transabdominally. The decision whether to abort the procedure should be based on the quality of the repair. Ureteral injuries are uncommon but may be easily recognized during cystoscopy using intravenous indigo carmine. Intraoperative bleeding is infrequent and few studies have accurately assessed the blood loss from needle suspension. When significant bleeding occurs, it is usually originating from the rich perivesical, perivaginal and periurethral venous plexus. When simple vaginal packing does not control the hemorrhage and the vessels can not be visually identified, the vagina may be repacked and a Foley balloon inflated within the vagina for tamponade.[53] When clinically significant or life-threatening hemorrhage occurs, consideration should be given to open pelvic exploration. Postoperative pain and nerve injury are infrequently reported and can arise from a variety of causes. In a study by Black and co workers, only 10% of patients felt their postoperative pain control was adequate.[54] Nerve injury is usually due to improper patient positioning (sciatic, obturator, peroneal, femoral) or nerve entrapment from sutures tied laterally over the rectus fascia (ileo-inguinal, genital branch of the genito-femoral nerve).[55] A detailed description of complications and their treatments is beyond the scope of this chapter, but may be found in the bibliography.[54–59]

Conclusion

Despite efficacy that is slightly inferior to that of slings and retropubic suspensions,[60] transvaginal needle suspensions have remained the first line approach for the treatment of anatomic stress incontinence. Though most series report short-term follow-up in an uncontrolled and biased fashion, outcomes have been largely favorable with few complications. The success rates of these procedures should ideally be studied in a prospective randomized fashion with long term follow-up (>5 years). Validated questionnaires should be used to assess quality of life and patient satisfaction.[61,62] As results are fairly similar and randomized trials have not been performed, the choice of which needle suspension to use should be largely be based on surgeon expertise and comfort level. Satisfactory outcomes are, however, achievable with proper patient selection, documenting the presence and degree of anatomical stress incontinence and excluding sphincteric deficiency or severe untreated detrusor instability as underlying causative factors.

References

1. Pereyra A (1959) A simplified surgical procedure for the correction of stress incontinence in women. West J Surg Obstet Gynecol 67: 223-6.
2. Marshall F, Marchetti A, Krantz K (1949) Correction of stress incontinence by simple vesicourethral suspension. Surg Gynecol Obstet 88: 509-18.
3. Dmochowski RR, Zimmern PE, Ganabathi K, Sirls L, Leach GE (1997) Role of the four corner bladder neck suspension to correct stress incontinence with a mild to moderate cystocele. Urology 49: 35-40.
4. Litwiller SE, Nelson RS, Fone PD, Kim KB, Stone AR (1997) Vaginal wall sling:Long term outcome analysis of factors contributing to patient satisfaction and surgical success. J Urol 157: 1279-82.
5. McGuire EJ, Fitzpatrick CC, Wan J, Bloom D, Sanvordenker J, Ritchey M, Gormley EA (1993) Clinical assessment of urethral sphincter function. J Urol 150: 1452-4.
6. Leach G (1996) Local anesthesia for urologic procedures. Urology 48(2): 284-8.
7. Haab F, Leach G (1997) Feasibility of outpatient percutaneous bladder suspension under local anesthesia. Urology 50(4): 585-7.
8. Pereyra A, Lebherz T (1967) Combined urethral vesical suspension vaginal urethroplasty for correction of urinary stress incontinence. Obstet Gynecol 30: 537-46.
9. Pereyra AJ, Lebherz TB, Growdon WA, Powers JA (1982) Periurethral supports in perspective: Modified Pereyra procedure for urinary incontinence. Obstet Gynecol 59(5): 643-8.
10. Pereyra A, Lebherz T (1978) The revised Pereyra procedure. In: Buchsbaum H (ed) Gynecologic and Obstetric Urology. WB Saunders, Philadelphia, pp. 208-22.
11. Christ T, Singleton H, Robertson W (1969) Urethrovesical needle suspension: postoperative loss of vesical neck support demonstrated by chain cystography. Obstet Gynecol 34: 489-93.
12. Kursh E, Wainstein M, Persky L (1972) The Pereyra procedure and urinary incontinence. J Urol 108: 591-4.
13. Pereyra A, Lebherz T (1978) The modified Pereyra procedure. In: Buchsbaum H, Schmidt J (ed) Gynecologic and Obstetric Urology, 2nd edn. WB Saunders, Philadelphia, pp. 259-76.
14. Sirls LT, Keoleian CM, Korman HJ, Kirkemo AK (1995) The effect of study methodology on reported success rates of the modified Pereyra bladder neck suspension. J Urol 154(5): 1732-1735.
15. Korman HJ, Sirls LT, Kirkemo AK (1994) Success rate of modified Pereyra bladder neck suspension determined by outcomes analysis. J Urol 152(5): 1453-1457.
16. Raz S (1981) Modified bladder neck suspension for female stress incontinence. Urology 17(1): 82-5.
17. Golomb J, Klutke C, Raz S (1990) Raz double-prong ligature carrier for transvaginal bladder and bladder neck needle suspension. Urology 36(5): 453-4.
18. Raz S, Siegel AL, Short JL, Snyder JA, Synder JA (1989) Vaginal wall sling. J Urol 141: 43-6.
19. Raz S, Sussman EM, Erickson DB, Bregg KJ, Nitti VW (1992) The Raz bladder neck suspension: results in 206 patients. J Urol 148: 845-50.
20. Golomb J, Goldwasser B, Mashiach S (1994) Raz bladder suspension in women younger than 65 years compared with elderly women: Three years experience. Urology 43(1): 40-3.
21. Fischer R (1998) Transvaginal needle bladder suspension for stress urinary incontinence: practicable methods but not optimal results. Acta Obstet Gynecol Scand 168: 38-43.
22. Kelly MJ, Knielsen K, Bruskewitz R, Roskamp D, Leach GE (1991) Symptom analysis of patients undergoing modified Pereyra bladder neck suspension for stress urinary incontinence: Pre- and postoperative findings. Urology 37(3): 213-19.
23. Phillips T, Zeidman E, Thompson I (1992) The fate of buried vaginal epithelium. J Urol 148: 1941.
24. Juma S, Little N, Raz S (1992) Vaginal wall sling: Four years later. Urology 40(5): 424-8.
25. Stothers L, Chopra A, Raz S (1995) Vaginal wall sling for anatomic incontinence and intrinsic sphincteric damage – Efficacy and outcome analysis. J Urol 153: 525A.
26. Raz S, Stothers L, Young GP, Short J, Marks B, Chopra A, Wahle GR (1996) Vaginal wall sling for anatomical incontinence and intrinsic sphincter dysfunction: Efficacy and outcome analysis. J Urol 156: 166-70.
27. Dmochowski RR, Zimmern PE, Ganabathi K, Sirls L, Leach GE (1997) Role of the four corner bladder neck suspension to correct stress incontinence with a mild to moderate cystocele. Urology 49(1): 35-40.
28. Stamey T (1973) Endoscopic suspension of the vesical neck for urinary incontinence. Surg Gynecol Obstet 136: 547.
29. Ginsberg D, Rovner E, Raz S (1998) Stamey and Gittes bladder neck suspension. In: Graham S Jr (ed) Glenn's Urologic Surgery, 5th ed. Lippincott-Raven, Philadelphia, pp. 313-35.
30. Stothers L, Raz S, Chopra A (1996) Stamey needle suspension for female stress incontinence. In: Raz S (ed) Female Urology, 2nd ed. WB Saunders, Philadelphia, pp. 333-7.
31. Stamey T (1980) Endoscopic suspension of the vesical neck for urinary incontinence in females. Ann Surg 192: 465-71.
32. Ashken M (1990) Follow-up results of the Stamey operation for stress incontinence of urine. Br J Urol 65: 168-9.
33. Hilton P, Mayne C (1991) The Stamey endoscopic bladder neck suspension: A clinical and urodynamic investigation, including actuarial follow-up over four years. Br J Obstet Gynecol 98: 1141-3.
34. Mills R, Persad R, Ashken M (1996) Long-term follow-up results with the Stamey operation for stress incontinence. Br J Urol 77: 86-8.
35. O'Sullivan D, Chilton C, Munson K (1995) Should the Stamey colposuspension be our primary surgery for stress incontinence? Br J Urol 75: 457-60.
36. Clemens JQ, Stern JA, Bushman WA, Schaeffer AJ (1998) Long-term results of the Stamey bladder suspension: Direct

comparison with the Marshall-Marchetti-Krantz procedure. J Urol 160: 372–376.

37. Wang A (1996) Burch colposuspension vs. Stamey bladder neck suspension. J Reprod Med 41(7): 529–33.

38. Spencer J, O'Conor V, Schaeffer A (1987) A comparison of endoscopic suspension of the vesical neck with suprapubic vesicourethrpexy for the treatment of stress urinary incontinence. J Urol 137: 411–15.

39. Gittes R, Loughlin K (1987) No incision pubovaginal suspension for stress incontinence. J Urol 138: 568–60.

40. Loughlin KR, Whitemore WF 3rd, Gittes RF, Richie JP (1990) Review of an 8 year experience with modifications of the endoscopic suspension of the bladder neck for female stress incontinence. J Urol 143: 44–8.

41. Benson J, Agosta A, McClellan E (1990) Evaluation of a minimal-incision pubovaginal suspension as an adjunct to other pelvic floor surgery. Obstet Gynecol 75: 844–7.

42. Foster M, O'Reilly P (1989) Early experience of the Gittes "no incision" pubovaginal suspension for stress urinary incontinence. Br J Urol 64: 590–595.

43. Kil PJ, Hoekstra JW, van der Meijden AP, Smans AJ, Theeuwes AG, Schreinemachers LM (1991) Transvaginal ultrasonography and urodynamic evaluation after suspension operations: Comparison among Gittes, Stamey and Burch suspensions. J Urol 146: 132–7.

44. Elkabir J, Mee D (1998) Long-term evaluation of the Gittes procedure for urinary stress incontinence. J Urol 159(4): 1203–5.

45. Leach G (1988) Bone fixation technique for transvaginal needle suspension. Urology 31: 388–91.

46. Benderev T (1994) A modified percutaneous outpatient bladder neck suspension system. J Urol 152: 2316–20.

47. Appell R (1997) The use of bone anchoring in the surgical management of female stress urinary incontinence. World J Urol 15: 300–5.

48. Leach G, Appell R (1996) Percutaneous bladder neck suspension. Urol Clin N Am 23: 511–16.

49. Schultheiss D et al. (1998) Does bone anchor fixation improve the outcome of percutaneous bladder neck suspension in female stress urinary incontinence? Br J Urol 82: 192–5.

50. Nativ O, Levine S, Madjar S, Issaq E, Moskovitz B, Beyar M (1997) Incisionless per vaginal bone anchor cystourethropexy for the treatment of female stress incontinence: Experience with the first 50 patients. J Urol 158: 1742–4.

51. Leach G (1999) Cadaveric transvaginal sling. J Urol 161(4): 185A.

52. Hernandez R, Himsl K, Zimmern P (1994) Transvaginal repair of bladder injury during vaginal hysterectomy. J Urol 152(6): 2061–2.

53. Katske FA, Raz S (1987) Use of Foley catheter to obtain transvaginal tamponade. Urology 18 (May).

54. Black N, Griffiths J, Pope C, Bowling A, Abel P (1997) Impact of surgery for stress incontinence on morbidity: Cohort study. BMJ 315: 1493–8.

55. Kelly M, Zimmern P, Leach G (1991) Complications of bladder suspension surgeries. Urol Clin N Am 18(2): 339–48.

56. Neale R (1995) Complications of urogynecological surgery. Curr Opin Obstet Gynecol 7: 400–3.

57. Bernier P, Zimmern P (1998) Bone anchor removal after bladder neck suspension. Br J Urol 82: 302–3.

58. Webster G, Kreder K (1990) Voiding dysfunction following cystourethropexy: Its evaluation and management. J Urol 144: 670–3.

59. Cardozo L, Stanton S, Williams J (1979) Detrusor instability following surgery for genuine stress incontinence. Br J Urol 81: 204–7.

60. Leach GE, Dmochowski RR, Appell RA, Blaivas JG, Hadley HR, Luber KM, Mostwin JL, O'Donnell PD, Roehrborn CG (1997) Female stress urinary incontinence clinical guidelines panel summary report on surgical management of female stress incontinence. J Urol 158: 875–80.

61. Blaivas J (1998) Outcome measures for urinary incontinence. Urology 51(2A): 11–19.

62. Uebersax JS, Wyman JF, Shumaker SA, McClish DK, Fantl JA (1995) Short forms to assess life quality and symptom distress for urinary incontinence in women: the incontinence impact questionnaire and the urogenital distress inventory. Neurol Urodynam 14: 131–9.

63. Gilja I, Puskar D, Mazuran B, Radej M (1998) Comparative analysis of bladder neck suspension using Raz, Burch and transvaginal Burch procedures: A 3 year randomized prospective study. Eur Urol 33: 298–302.

64. Gofrit ON, Landau EH, Shapiro A, Pode D (1998) The Stamey procedure for stress incontinence: Long term results. Eur Urol 34: 339–43.

65. Kuczyk MA, Klein S, Grunewald V, Machtens S, Denil J, Hofner K, Wagner T, Jonas (1998) A questionnaire-based outcome analysis of the Stamey bladder neck suspension procedure for the treatment of urinary stress incontinence: The Hanover experience. Br J Urol 82: 174–80.

66. Conrad S, Pieper A, De la Maza SF, Busch R, Huland H (1997) Long-term results of the Stamey bladder suspension procedure: a patient questionnaire based outcome analysis. J Urol 157: 1672–7.

67. Christensen H, Laybourn C, Eickhoff JH, Frimodt-Moller C (1996) Long term results of the Stamey bladder neck suspension procedure and of the Burch colposuspension. Scand J Urol Nephrol 31: 349–353.

68. Kursh E (1992) Factors influencing the outcome of a no incision urethropexy. Surg Gynecol Obstet 175: 254–8.

69. Morales A, VanCott GF (1988) The Gittes procedure as an improved simplification of current techniques for vesical neck suspensions. Surg Gynecol Obstet 167(3): 243–5.

10 The Artificial Urinary Sphincter

Ananias C. Diokno and Thomas M. Rashid

The ultimate goal when treating urinary incontinence is to achieve normal voiding patterns while allowing dry intervals between voiding. In the case of urinary incontinence due to intrinsic sphincter dysfunction (ISD) there are currently three options to offer: behavioral techniques, pharmacotherapy, and surgical intervention. Specifically, for surgical intervention, the options are implantation of an artificial urinary sphincter (AUS), slings, and periurethral injectables. Although all treatment options are appropriate, only the AUS is capable of relieving the artificially created obstruction at the time of voiding, allowing the voiding–continence cycle to be accomplished almost to perfection.[1]

The AUS was one of the first successful applications of a genitourinary prosthetic implant. Foley introduced the first artificial sphincter in 1947.[2] This device had a latex inflatable cuff placed around the corpus spongiosum distal to the penoscrotal junction. This was connected by tubing to a valve and syringe that the patient carried and inflated to prevent incontinence and deflated to empty the bladder. However, pressure necrosis and infections occurred, leading to fistulas and other unmanageable complications.

Modern Devices

The modern AUS was first introduced by Scott and co-workers in 1973.[3] This device, the AMS 721, was made of silicon and consisted of three components: a reservoir, an occlusive cuff, and two pumps. The reservoir was placed in the perivesical space, the cuff around the bladder neck, and one pumps in each labium (Fig. 10.1). This device had an overall success rate of 60–70%.[4] Most complications occurred secondarily to infection and erosion as well as mechanical failure of the four valves that was originally incorporated in the AMS 721. Although this original device offered many patients relief of their incontinence, there were areas for improvement.

Over the next several years American Medical Systems (AMS, Minnetonka, MN) modified the artificial sphincter in an effort to simplify the design, reduce the complications, and reoperation rate, and improve reliability. In 1983, the AMS 800 was introduced. This consists of an inflatable cuff, a pressure-regulating balloon, and a single pump; all components are connected by special kink-resistant and

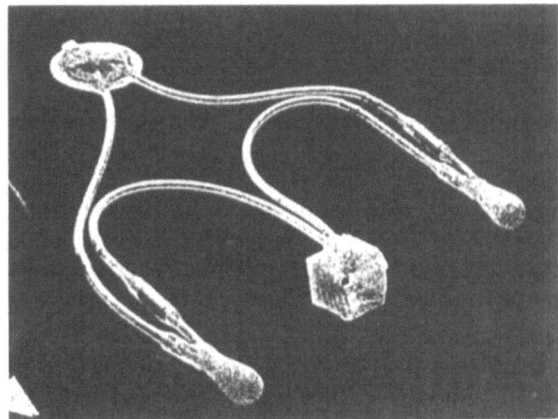

Figure 10.1 AMS sphincter 721™ urinary prosthesis, an artificial urinary sphincter. Courtesy American Medical Systems, Minnetonka, Minnesota; www.visitAMS.com.

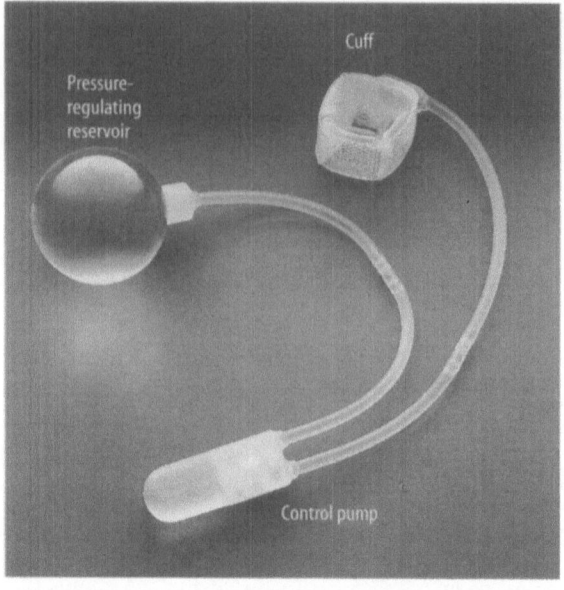

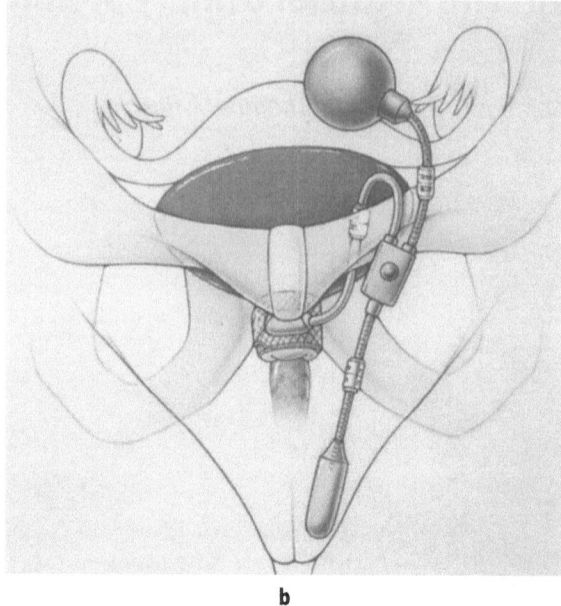

Figure 10.2 AMS Sphincter 800™ Urinary Control System. **a** AMS 800™ with an inflatable cuff, a pressure regulating balloon and a single pump. **b** The pump in place with the cuff around the bladder neck, the pressure regulating balloon in the space of Retzius and the pump in the labium majus. Courtesy of American Medical Systems Inc., Minnetonka, Minnesota; www.visit AMS.com.

color-coded silicone tubing (Fig. 10.2). The inflatable cuff comes in various sizes, is made of silicone and coated with teflon, and is placed around the bladder neck. The cuff fills with fluid from a pressurized balloon, causing the urethra to coapt and provide continence. When the patient wants to urinate, the pump is compressed a few times and fluid is transferred from the cuff into the balloon reservoir, relieving the cuff compression around the urethra thereby allowing micturition or catheterization. The pump is placed in the labia majus. It contains a resistor that provides a 2–3 minute delay before the cuff is automatically refilled to the desired pressure, allowing adequate voiding time. The pump also has a deactivation button located on its cephalad portion that when engaged prevents the cuff to be refilled (Fig. 10.3). When the deactivation button is squeezed the poppet valve moves to a position so no fluid can be transferred. Reactivation is accomplished with a sharp squeeze on the pump that releases the poppet. When deactivating the AUS, it is important to leave some fluid in the pump to offset the poppet valve later. To achieve this, the pump is allowed to refill to the point where a small dimple is palpable before the device is deactivated. The deactivation device is an important addition to the AUS, because deactivation for 6–8 weeks after implantation (to allow tissue healing and decrease periurethral swelling) decreases the incidence of erosion and infection with artificial urinary sphincters.[5] It also allows enough time for the swelling and tenderness in the labium majus to subside before the patient manipulates the pump,

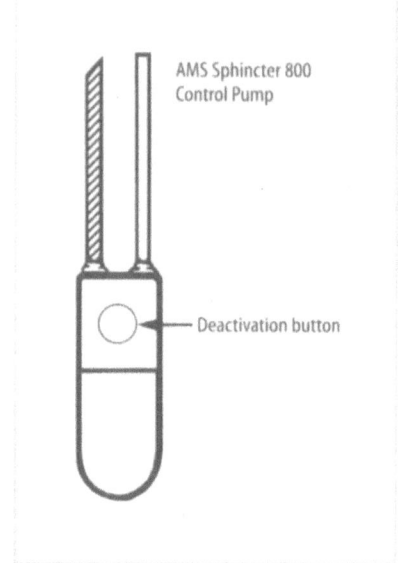

Figure 10.3 AMS Sphincter 800™ Urinary Control System. The control pump of the AMS 800 showing the deactivation button. Courtesy of American Medical Systems, Inc., Minnetonka, Minnesota; www.visitAMS.com.

thereby reducing the discomfort whenever she squeezes the pump to void. When instrumenting or placing a Foley catheter, the AUS should always be deactivated (as described above) to decrease the risk for cuff erosion or infection. If the cuff is not decompressed, the presence of a catheter in the urethral lumen will cause the urethral wall to be sandwiched and compressed by the still inflated compression cuff. This in turn may lead to ischemia and necrosis of the urethral wall.

A seamless pressure regulating balloon is placed in the prevesical retropubic space. The occlusive force of the cuff is determined by the pressure of the regulating balloon, and the balloon is designed so that precalibrated reservoirs are available in different pressure ranges: 51–60, 61–70, 71–80, and 81–90 cm H_2O. The intrabdominal prevesical location of the reservoir also allows transmission of abdominal pressure changes to the cuff, reducing leakage with Valsalva maneuvers.[6]

Indications and Patient Selection for AUS Implantation

When considering patients for artificial urinary sphincter implantation, the physician must realize that AUS is for the treatment of ISD only. A thorough urologic evaluation is necessary to identify these patients. Therefore, careful patient selection by preoperative history, physical examination, and diagnostic testing is imperative.[6,7] The history should entail a general medical history with a detailed genitourinary history. The history should elicit the cause of intrinsic sphincter deficiency. ISD commonly occurs after failed bladder neck suspension procedures, pelvic radiation, denervation, urethral trauma, and urethrotomies. These women classically leak large volumes of urine and soak many pads per day. Among the pediatric age group ISD may be secondary to congenital anomalies such as epispadias or a consequence of neurologic dysfunction such as spina bifida, myelodysplasia, or spinal cord trauma.

The physical examination should include a neurologic examination to identify any disturbances. The patient must have the mental ability to understand and perform the task of cycling the AUS. The physician also needs to be aware of the patient's upper extremity motor skills, because cycling an AUS requires manual dexterity. Finally, a thorough pelvic examination and post-void residual urine are determined. The patient's urine is inspected for signs of infection. If a urinary tract infection is present, it is treated and the cause of such an infection should be elucidated, since recurrent infections in the presence of an AUS can cause prosthesis infection.

Patients suspected of having intrinsic sphincter deficiency should have an adequate evaluation. All patients undergo a cystourethroscopy. The urethra is inspected for any disorders, i.e. strictures, diverticuli, or bladder neck contractures. The integrity of the urethral mucosa should be assessed, particularly at the bladder neck where the cuff is usually implanted. A history of radiation therapy and pale, atrophic-appearing bladder mucosa may call for the lowest balloon pressure or dictate against sphincter placement. Patients with strictures or bladder neck contractures should be treated prior to sphincter placement and patency must be confirmed at least 6 weeks after treatment. A bimanual examination is done at the time of cystoscopy to determine the thickness of the bladder neck and proximal urethra in relation to the vaginal wall thickness, since dissection of this area is critical at the time of implantation.[8] Also, the presence or absence of a hypermobile vesical neck and the presence of an incompetent sphincter at the bladder neck is evaluated cystoscopically.

Appropriate urodynamic testing is also performed to both document the mechanism of incontinence and assess detrusor function. A cystometrogram determines detrusor instability/ hyperflexia, bladder sensation, and capacity. Detrusor hyperreflexia and areflexia are not contraindications for AUS implantation. However, failure to recognize and treat detrusor hyperreflexia before implanting an AUS can cause elevated bladder storage pressures, resulting in upper tract damage and renal deterioration. Therefore, it is imperative to suppress detrusor hyperreflexia with an anticholinergic agent. If this is ineffective, the patient may require a bladder augmentation or placement of a sacral nerve neuromodulator. Detrusor areflexia and elevated post-void residual urine will require patients to perform intermittent self-catheterization after AUS placement.[9,10] If an AUS is to be implanted in these patient, they must be taught clean intermittent catheterization preoperatively. Ideal bladder capacity should be 300–400 ml, but capacities as low as 200 ml are adequate for urinary storage after AUS implantation. During the cystometrogram, the patient is asked to slowly perform a Valsalva maneuver after 200 ml of intravesical fluid is placed, determining the leak point pressure. Leak point pressures less than 60 cm H_2O are consistent with intrinsic sphincter deficiency. However, higher pressures or inability to demonstrate leak point pressure does not exclude ISD. Finally, after bladder capacity is reached during the cystometrogram, lateral static and stress cystograms are obtained to elicit information about the urethral and bladder neck anatomy. Classically, in ISD the bladder neck at rest and at straining view is open or funneled and that bladder neck is fixed behind the symphysis pubis.

After the diagnosis of intrinsic sphincter deficiency the timing for placement of an AUS is planned. Strictures or vesical neck contractures are managed at least 6 weeks before artificial sphincter implantation and patency is confirmed before surgery. For patients performing intermittent catheterization or with a significant history of urinary tract infections, a urine culture is obtained

2 weeks before surgery to ensure sterility. If a urinary tract infection is detected, it should be treated with antibiotics according to the organism sensitivity.

Preoperative Counseling

Preoperative counseling is a necessity prior to implanting an artificial sphincter. The patient needs to be informed of the risk of infection, erosion, or mechanical failure accompanying the device. If any of these events occur there is a risk that the sphincter will have to be removed or replaced. Further, the patient should be informed that complete urinary continence may not be achieved but a marked improvement in leakage is expected.

Operative Approach

In the preoperative care unit the patient is administered broad-spectrum antibiotics, i.e. ampicillin/vancomycin and gentamicin prior to skin incision. A spinal or general anesthetic is administered. The skin is shaved. The patient is prepped and draped in a normal sterile fashion. A 16 French silicone Foley catheter is placed to dependent drainage. A low transverse (Pfannenstiel) incision is made. The retropubic space is entered. Dissection is carried to the level of the bladder neck and proximal urethra. A plane is developed between the urethra and the vagina using right angle clamps. A 2 cm length of proximal urethra is dissected. The cuff size is then measured (usually 6.5 or 7.0 cm cuff).

On the "back table" the pump, cuff and balloon reservoir are placed in an antibiotic solution. Each device is then prepared with an isotonic contrast solution composed of 50 ml of 25% hypaque mixed with 60 ml of sterile water or sterile normal saline solution. All air bubbles are removed from the system. The balloon is instilled with 22 ml of contrast, the cuff is left empty, and the pump is filled with fluid with both the inflow and outflow tubing in the solution. Once full and free of air, the tubes are clamped with rubber shods.

The AUS cuff is then placed around the urethra. The cuff volume is then calibrated by temporarily connecting the balloon with 22 ml of fluid to the empty cuff. The Foley catheter is also removed during this maneuver. The total volume of the device is then calculated as the volume of the cuff added to standard 20 ml volume of the reservoir. The reservoir is then placed underneath the rectus fascia. Next the pump is passed into the left labium majus. The pump is secured in place with a Babcock clamp. The tubing from the three separate components are trimmed appropriately to avoid redundancy and

prevent kinking. Like tubes are connected to each other using straight connectors and a crimping tool. The rubber shods are removed and the device is cycled. The AUS is tested multiple times and then deactivated so the cuff is in the open position. The patient returns to the regular surgical floor with a Foley catheter, receiving two more doses of intravenous antibiotics. On the first postoperative day the Foley catheter is removed, the patient is expected to be incontinent, and discharged home. After 3 weeks the patient is re-examined, and in 6 weeks the sphincter is activated.

Troubleshooting

The complications associated with AUS are infection, erosion, and mechanical malfunction. Typically, complications are identified by changes in the patient's voiding habit or new onset of incontinence. These problems must be diagnosed and treated aggressively.

Patients with infected sphincters present with tenderness, swelling, and erythema over a component or the entire device. The incidence of an infected prosthesis is 1–3%. The most common organism is *Staphylococcus epidermidis*. Infections most commonly occur in the early postoperative period secondary to seeding of the prosthesis during surgery. Infections occurring later usually result from hematogenous spread or from chronic smoldering infections.

All patients with a suspected infected sphincter should undergo urethroscopy to rule out cuff erosion. If there is no erosion, then the patient is started on a prolonged course of intravenous antibiotics to control the infection and salvage the device if possible. If the infection persists, then the device should be removed to its entirety. An omental flap placed around the bladder neck and urethra has been suggested to maintain a plane for a future sphincter implantation.[11] A new sphincter may be placed 3–6 months after removal of the device and resolution of the infection.

Urethral erosion is an uncommon but significant complication. Prior to the development of delayed activation the erosion ratio was as high as 18%; now the incidence is 1.3% with delayed activation techniques.[12] Erosions occurring early in the postoperative period are usually from insertion problems, with violation of the urethra being the most significant factor. Delayed erosion may occur from: decreased vascularity secondary to radiation, infection, high cuff pressures, or small cuff sizes. Placement of the Foley catheter can also cause late erosion when the sphincter is not deactivated. The pressurized cuff squeezes the urethra against the rigid Foley catheter, causing ischemia. This eventually will lead to erosion and infection of the cuff. It is therefore of utmost importance that all health-care providers should be aware of the need to de-activate the sphincter before placing an indwelling Foley catheter. Patients are encouraged to wear an "alert" bracelet or carry a medical card stating that they have an AUS in case of an emergency. The diagnosis of a cuff erosion is made by urethros-copy. Treat-ment involves removal of the cuff or whole device and placement of a Foley catheter for 3 weeks. Reimplantation may be considered at least 3 months after the urethra is healed and a new cuff placed in a different site.[13] Patients with a history of erosion should deactivate their device at night to diminish the time the urethra is compressed and increase vascularity. In cases of erosion involving the pump, removal of the eroding part, and cap-ping the tubing for future implantation is an option if the wound is clean and there is no sign of infection.

The third major category of complications com-prises mechanical dysfunction. When an insufficient amount of fluid is left in the pump, the sphincter cannot be activated. This can be avoided by allowing the pump to refill to a point where a small dimple is palpable prior to deactivating the device. Therefore, enough fluid remains in the pump to release the poppet valve. If this problem is encountered, stabilize the pump, squeeze forcibly over the entire unit to create enough force to open the valve. If this does not work, then squeeze the hardened silicone 90° away from the deactivation button; this will distort the control valve allowing fluid into the pump. However, if this is unsuccessful, operative intervention is required. Another problem infrequently encountered is an

inability to squeeze the pump. This may be caused by an obstruction of the flow in the tubing by debris, blood, crystals, or air. Also, redundant tubing will cause kinking preventing free fluid flow. Prevention is the best way to avoid this complication. Meticulous care should be taken when filling and connecting the components to prevent blood, debris, or crystals from entering the system. Trimming the tubing appro-priately will prevent kinking. The introduction of kink-resistant tubing has also decreased the incidence of kinking. Treatment consists of replacing the affected parts.

After the AUS is activated, urinary incontinence may persist. Leaks along the component are the most common problem, in our experience.[8] This can occur in the tubing, balloon, pump, or most com-monly the cuff. A pelvic radiograph should be obtained (if contrast was used) with the sphincter activated and deactivated to determine if the cuff fills and empties (Fig. 10.4). A partially filled or empty balloon suggests a leak in the system. The source of the leakage should be determined and that com-ponent replaced. In addition to leakage, persistent incontinence after sphincter activation may be due to a low cuff filling pressure, too loose cuff, malfunction of the sphincter, or detrusor instability. If leakage is due to low filling pressure unable to coapt the ure-thra, then the balloon pressure can be increased to 71–80 cm H_2O; however, this may not improve conti-nence and may lead to cuff erosion. In cases when too large a cuff is placed, a smaller cuff may be placed. If detrusor instability is thought to be the source of incontinence, a full urodynamic evaluation needs to be performed. Detrusor instability can usually be treated with anticholinergic medication.

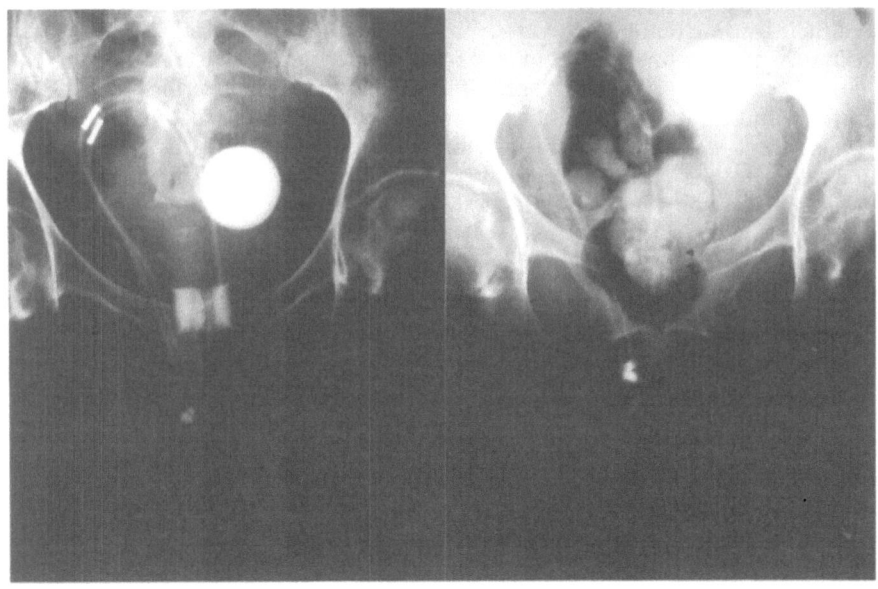

Figure 10.4 a Pelvic radiograph of the AMS urinary sphincter showing it in the activated mode with contrast outlining the cuff. **b** Deactivated mode.

When urinary retention occurs postoperatively the physician needs to cycle the AUS and then deactivate it. Urinary leakage should occur immediately; when leakage does not occur, obtain a pelvic radiograph to assure the cuff is opened. If the cuff remains closed and inflated despite deactivation, then the pump is defective and needs to be replaced. In addition, urinary retention may be secondary to a tight cuff or edema. The urethra should be examined with cystoscopy. The AUS should be deactivated and the patient placed on clean intermittent catheterization to allow time for edema to resolve. Retention occurring late can be caused by: infection, or erosion. The patient needs immediate sphincter deactivation, urethroscopy, and Foley placement.

Results

Women with intrinsic sphincter deficiency have often undergone several unsuccessful earlier incontinence procedures, making placement technically challenging. Noll and Schreiter reported on 106 patients (80 followed for at least 1 year) with 86% cure rate (no pads). However, they had a reoperation rate of 56% of their patients.[14] Webster et al. reported on 24 women undergoing sphincter placement: 92% of patients were dry and 100% socially continent.[15] Moreover, Appell reported 100% dryness in 34 patients using a transvaginal approach with only 3 reoperations.[16]

Between 1984 and 1997, 53 women at our institution underwent AMS 800 AUS placement. 38 patients had complete databases available for evaluation, with a mean follow-up of 8 years. 68% of patients (N = 26) are cured and 92% (N = 35) are socially continent. Moreover, 89% of these women have a much better control of their voiding pattern. Nine patients required revisions of their sphincter (mean of 1.44 procedures).

Children with myelodysplasia and adults with neurogenic bladders have excellent continence results after AUS insertion, despite the added medical, neurologic, and genitourinary considerations. Because of these added considerations, myelodysplastic patients must not only undergo very careful preoperative evaluation of bladder capacity and function but also very close postoperative monitoring of bladder and upper urinary tract function. These patients may require bladder augmentations. Singh et al. reported on 90 patients with neurogenic bladders undergoing sphincter placement. In this group, 92% of patients are dry and 96% are socially continent at a mean of 6 month follow-up; 79% required intestinal cystoplasty and 78% required clean intermittent catheterization.[17] Patients with AUS and augmented bladders must be vigilant about emptying their bladder to prevent

overdistension or rupture of the bladder. Finally, in the management of incontinence in this group of patients, it is important to understand the primary goal is renal preservation, and controlling continence should never overshadow this goal.

Conclusion

The AMS 800 artificial urinary sphincter should be considered in all patients with incontinence secondary to intrinsic sphincter deficiency. In order to have a successful outcome, the patient needs tailored preoperative evaluation. Type III stress urinary incontinence should be documented by endoscopy, urodynamics, and/or video fluorodynamics. The patient and patient's family should be well educated about potential problems, outcome, and life-long vigilance.[18]

During surgery, the urologist must be meticulous about details and surgical technique to prevent peri- and postoperative complications, i.e. mechanical malfunction, infection, and erosion. Postoperatively, the patient needs routine follow-up examinations as long as their device is in place. Any changes in voiding patterns, signs of voiding dysfunction, or infection need prompt evaluation.

With careful preoperative evaluation, intraoperative technique, and postoperative follow-up, the AMS 800 AUS should offer patients a very effective and durable surgical procedure that will greatly improve their quality of life.

Editorial Comment

Placement of an AUS in women can be intraoperatively challenging. Some urethrae are shorter than expected, rendering the placement of the cuff more difficult. In addition, urethral or vaginal injuries can occur during the dissection of the proximal urethra. In a recent series by Costa,[19] the placement of two fingers in the vagina, one to control the balloon at the bladder neck and the other to verify the progression of the dissection between urethral wall and vaginal wall, was recommended. The appropriate plane for dissection is generally found closer to the vagina and is accessed after transection of the periurethral fascia approximately 2 cm away from the bladder neck area on each side. This technical detail is important to prevent local ischemia to the urethral wall.

In case of urethral injury, the bladder may need to be opened and the ureters stented for better identification. Vaginal injury is more difficult to recognize, justifying the recommendation for the placement of two fingers in the vagina at the time of the dissection of the proximal urethra. In case of recognized injury, the closure can be performed transvaginally and the operation continued.

In their large series of 184 non-neurogenic patients operated for type 3 stress incontinence over 10 years, the incidence of explantation rate (5.3%) was higher when an intraoperative injury to the urethra or vagina occurred. There was, however, no correlation between explantation rate and the age of the patient, prior bladder neck suspension procedure, or the patient's neurological status. Clearly, troubleshooting the placement of an AUS in women starts in the operating room.

References

1. Martins FE, Boyd SD (1995) AUS in patients following major pelvic surgery and/or radiotherapy: Are they less favorable candidates. J Urol 153: 1188.
2. Foley FB (1947) An AUS. J Urol 50: 250.
3. Scott FB, Bradley WE, Timm GW (1973) Treatment of urinary incontinence by implantable prosthetic sphincter. Urology 1: 252.
4. Diokno AC, Taub ME (1976) Experience with the artificial urinary sphincter at Michigan. J Urol 116: 496.
5. Furlow WL (1981) Implantation of a new semiautomatic artificial genitourinary sphincter: experience with primary activation and deactivation at 47 patients. J Urol 126: 741.
6. Light JK (1985) The artificial urinary sphincter in children. Urol Clin North Am 12: 103.
7. Mundy AR (1991) Artificial urinary sphincters. Br J Urol 67: 225.
8. Stone KT, Diokno AC (1997) Artificial urinary sphincter. In: O'Donnell PD (ed) Urinary Incontinence. Chap. 36, pp. 258–265.
9. Diokno AC, Sonda LP (1981) compatibility of genitourinary prostheses and intermittent self-catheterization. J Urol 125: 659.
10. Barrett DM, Furlow WL (1984) Incontinence, intermittent self-catheterization and the artificial genitourinary sphincter. J Urol 132: 268.
11. Nurse DE, Mundy AR (1988) One hundred artificial sphincters. Br J Urol 61: 318.
12. Motley RC, Barrett DM (1990) Artificial urinary sphincter cuff erosion: experience with reimplantation in 38 patients. Urology 35: 215.
13. Kowalczyk JJ, Nelson R, Mulcahy JJ (1996) Successful reinsertion of the AUS after removal for erosion or infection. Urology 48: 906.
14. Noll F, Schreiter F (1991) The AS800 artificial sphincter for the treatment of female incontinence. Urology 30(5): 294.
15. Webster GD, Perez LM, Khoury JM, Timmons SL (1992) Management of type III stress urinary incontinence using artificial urinary sphincter. Urology 39: 499.
16. Appell RA (1988) Techniques and results in the implantation of the artificial urinary sphincter in women with Type III stress urinary incontinence by vaginal approach. Neurourol Urodynam 7: 613.
17. Singh G, Thomas DG (1996) Artificial urinary sphincter in patients with neurogenic bladder dysfunction. Br J Urol 77(2): 252.
18. Diokno AC, Lapides J (1970) Urinary Incontinence and Genitourinary Prostheses, Chapter 19. Harper & Row, New York.
19. Costa P, Mottet N, Rabut B, Thuret R, Naoum KB, Wagner L (2000) The use of an artificial urinary sphincter in women with type III incontinence and a negative Marshall test. J Urol 165: 1176.

11 Primary and Secondary Anal Sphincter Repair

Abdul H. Sultan

Definition

Anal sphincter disruption during vaginal delivery remains the commonest reason for performing an anal sphincter repair in women. There is now considerable evidence to suggest that occult mechanical trauma to the anal sphincter sustained during childbirth[1-3] is a major etiological factor in the development of fecal incontinence.[4] Unfortunately, it has not been established whether these injuries are genuinely occult or possibly undiagnosed and therefore missed at delivery. Taken literally, the terms "primary" and "secondary" anal sphincter repair can be somewhat confusing as they may not always refer to a first and second attempt at sphincter repair; a primary repair is usually performed in the immediate postpartum period following a recognized obstetric anal sphincter rupture. When an anterior repair of the anal sphincter is performed to treat fecal incontinence (usually months or years later), it is regarded as a secondary sphincter repair even though a direct primary repair may or may not have been attempted in the postpartum period. As fecal incontinence may only manifest for the first time many years after the initial obstetric injury, it is not always possible to establish whether a primary repair was performed or if the injury was occult or indeed, just missed. Therefore, in this context, a secondary repair refers to a repair performed secondary to the development of symptoms of fecal incontinence. In the UK, primary repair of a fresh tear is conducted by obstetricians whereas secondary repairs are predominantly performed by colorectal surgeons.

Methods of Repair

In 1940, Blaisdell[5] reviewed the results of secondary anal sphincter repair using the end-to-end technique and reported success in 42%. Arnaud et al.[6] published a series of 40 patients undergoing end-to-end repair with a mean follow-up of 17 months; full continence occurred in 62.5%, and partial success in 25%. In 1971, Parks and McPartlin[7] described the overlap technique of repair using stainless steel wire. They noted that anterior sphincter lesions which usually follow obstetric injuries are associated with a better result than posterolateral lesions which frequently involve the puborectalis muscle as well. Browning and Motson[8] reported on the results of Parks' consecutive series of 97 sphincter repairs 4–116 months after surgery. The repair was successful in 78% and partially successful in 13%. The mechanism of success is probably due to the increased surface area of muscle contact with the overlap technique. The external anal sphincter is always in a state of tonic contraction even at rest and therefore with an end-to-end repair there is a risk of ischemia to the muscle ends and a tendency for retraction and disruption of the muscle ends. Attachment by multiple mattress sutures during overlap repair minimizes the risk of sutures tearing out. The overlap technique is now the most widely used technique for secondary repairs, and a fair to good outcome is reported in 74–100% of cases.[9] Engel et al.[4] performed a prospective study of 55 patients with fecal incontinence following obstetric trauma. After a median of 15 months improvement in continence status was noted in 80%. However, at 5 year follow-up only 59% had a successful long-term outcome (defined as no further surgery and infrequent urge fecal incontinence)[10] although a previous retrospective 5 year follow-up study from the same institution reported a 76% improvement.[11]

Primary Anal Sphincter Repair

The incidence of acute obstetric anal sphincter tears vary and is dependent largely on the type of episiotomy performed in that particular institution. It is reported to occur in 0.5–2.5% of deliveries in centers where mediolateral episiotomy is practiced[12–14] and 11% in centers where midline episiotomy is practiced.[15] Midline episiotomies are favored in North American practice and mediolateral episiotomies are favored in Europe.

Classification of Perineal Tears

Earlier classifications in the literature of perineal tears, especially third- and fourth-degree tears,[16] appear to be totally inconsistent. Furthermore, the current classification fails to address internal

sphincter involvement or thickness of external sphincter disruption. Consequently, some obstetricians and midwives are still classifying anal sphincter tears as a second-degree tear.[17–18] This has major implications for clinical management and is therefore a source of increasing litigation. In order to maintain consistency, Sultan[19] proposed a descriptive and standardized classification:

- *First degree*: laceration of the vaginal epithelium or perineal skin only.
- *Second degree*: involvement of the vaginal epithelium, perineal skin, perineal muscles, and fascia but not the anal sphincter.
- *Third degree*: disruption of the vaginal epithelium, perineal skin, perineal body, and anal sphincter muscles. This should be subdivided into:

  3a: partial tear of the external sphincter involving less than 50% thickness.

  3b: complete tear of the external sphincter.

  3c: internal sphincter torn as well.
- *Fourth degree*: a third degree tear with disruption of the anal epithelium.

Isolated tears of the rectal mucosa are rare and should not be included in the above classification.

Outcome of Primary Repair

In the last 12 years, 15 studies[13,20–23] have evaluated outcome following anal sphincter rupture (Table 11.1). These studies show that about 40% of women continue to suffer from anal incontinence

Table 11.1. The incidence of anal incontinence (excluding fecal urgency) following primary repair of acute obstetric anal sphincter rupture

Authors	Year	Country	N	Follow-up (months)	Anal incontinence
Walsh et al.	1996	UK	81	3	20%
Crawford et al.	1993	USA	35	12	23%
Sorensen et al.	1993	Denmark	38	3m	24%
Nielsen et al.	1992	Denmark	24	12	29%
Go and Dusselman	1988	Netherlands	20	6	33%
Uustal Fornell et al.	1996	Sweden	51	6	40%
Poen et al.	1998	Netherlands	117	56	40%
Sultan et al.	1994	UK	34	2	41%
Sorensen et al.	1988	Denmark	25	78	42%
Tetzschner et al.	1996	Denmark	72	24–48	42%
Kammerer-Doak et al.	1999	New Mexico	15	4	43%
Haadem et al.	1988	Sweden	62	3	44%
Bek and Laurberg	1992	Denmark	121	?	50%
Gjessing H et al.	1998	Norway	38	12–60	57%
Goffeng et al.	1998	Sweden	27	12	59%

In all studies except those of Crawford et al. and Kammerer-Doak et al., and in some patients in Go and Dusselman's study, mediolateral episiotomy were practised.

despite primary sphincter repair (Table 11.1). The morbidity is, however, much higher when one considers other symptoms such as fecal urgency,[12] anal discomfort, dyspareunia, and anal incontinence during sexual intercourse.[2,1]

Neurophysiological Investigations

A consistent finding is that anal resting and voluntary squeeze pressures are lower in women who previously sustained anal sphincter rupture[3,14,24] and the anal canal is significantly shorter after repair.[3,14] The development of incontinence does not appear to be directly related to a pelvic neuropathy as demonstrated by EMG[23,25] and pudendal nerve motor latency conduction studies.[3,4,13] Although Tetzschner[24] reported that 3 month pudendal latency measurements are delayed in women with a risk of incontinence, the measurements were still within the normal range and no relationship was demonstrated between abnormal latency and incontinence. Although anal sphincter disruption and repair is invariably associated with some degree of denervation and atrophy, current neurophysiologic tests are not sensitive or specific enough to quantify pudendal neuropathy. There is however, strong evidence that poor outcome following primary[3,13,25] and secondary[4] repair is related to persistent mechanical disruption as demonstrated by anal endosonography rather than "pudendal neuropathy."

Principles of Primary Repair

The unsatisfactory outcome following primary sphincter repair may be attributed either to operator inexperience or to inappropriate technique of repair and subsequent management. Poor training and inexperience of clinicians performing perineal repair have already been highlighted[17,26] and could well contribute to adverse outcome.

Approximation of the external anal sphincter by placing sutures in the outer fascial capsule without traversing the muscle substance was described by Fulsher and Fearl in 1955.[27] However, proper evaluation of outcome with this technique is lacking. The most common type of repair performed by obstetricians is an end-to-end approximation of the anal sphincter by either interrupted or figure-of-eight sutures.[3,28] (Fig. 11.1) There is now overwhelming evidence that this type of repair is associated with an unsatisfactory outcome, as up to 59% have some degree of persistent anal incontinence.[22] By contrast, secondary repair using the overlap repair is associated with a good outcome in 74–100%.[9] Using anal endosonography it has been shown that a poor result is associated with a persistent external sphincter defect and a favorable result when overlapping of the external sphincter was demonstrated. The poor outcome with the end-to-end repair and the good results reported following secondary repair using the overlap technique led Sultan et al. to evaluate the feasibility of this technique for primary repair.[26]

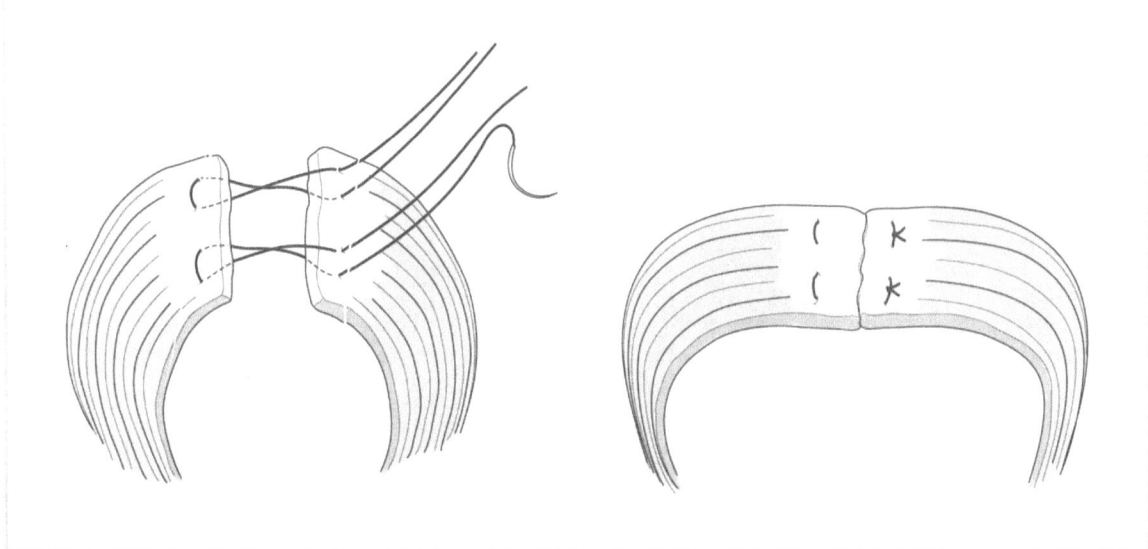

Figure 11.1 Conventional end-to-end approximation following anal sphincter rupture with two figure-of-eight sutures.[26] From Sultan AH, Monga AK, Kumar D, Stanton SL (1999) Primary repair of obstetric anal sphincter rupture using the overlap technique. Br J Obstet Gynaecol 106:318–23.

Technique of Primary Repair

- Repair should be conducted in the operating theatre where there is access to good lighting, appropriate equipment, and aseptic conditions.

- General or regional (spinal, epidural, caudal) anesthesia is an important prerequisite, particularly for overlap repair, as the inherent tone in the sphincter muscle can cause the torn muscle ends to retract within their sheath. Muscle relaxation is necessary to retrieve the ends and overlap without tension.

- The woman is placed in the lithotomy position and the full extent of the injury is evaluated by a careful vaginal and rectal examination.

- In the presence of a fourth-degree tear, the torn anal epithelium is repaired with interrupted Vicryl (polyglactin) 3/0 (Ethicon, Edinburgh, UK) sutures with the knots tied in the anal lumen. A subcuticular repair of the anal epithelium using 3/0 PDS (polydioxanone sulfate, Ethicon) via the transvaginal approach has also been used with equal success.

- The sphincter muscles are repaired with 3/0 PDS clear (Ethicon) sutures. These monofilamentous sutures are less likely than braided sutures to precipitate infection. Nonabsorbable monofilament sutures such as nylon or prolene (polypropylene) Ethicon are preferred by colorectal surgeons and can be equally effective. However they can cause stitch abscesses and the sharp ends of the suture can cause discomfort, necessitating removal.

- The internal anal sphincter should be identified and any tear should be repaired separately from the external sphincter. The internal anal sphincter lies between the external sphincter and the anal epithelium. It is paler than the striated external sphincter and the muscle fibers run in a circular fashion. The ends of the torn muscle are grasped with Allis forceps and an end-to-end repair is performed with interrupted 3/0 PDS sutures (Fig. 11.2). A torn internal sphincter should be approximated with interrupted sutures, as overlapping can be technically difficult. We advocate primary surgical repair of the internal sphincter, as it has been shown to be beneficial when repaired in patients with established anal incontinence.[29]

- The torn ends of the external anal sphincter are then identified and grasped with Allis tissue forceps (Fig. 11.3). In order to perform an overlap, the muscle may need mobilization by dissection with a pair of McIndoe scissors separating it from the ischioanal fat laterally. The external sphincter can now be pulled across to overlap in a "double-breasted" fashion. The torn ends of the external sphincter are then overlapped as shown in Fig. 11.4 using PDS 3/0 (Ethicon) sutures. A conventional end-to-end repair of the external sphincter using figure-of-eight sutures is shown in Fig. 11.1.

- Great care should be exercised in reconstructing the perineal muscles to provide support to the sphincter repair. The anal sphincter would be more likely to be traumatized during a subsequent vaginal delivery in the presence of a short deficient perineum. Muscles of the perineal body are reconstructed with interrupted Vicryl 2/0 sutures (Ethicon) after closing the vaginal epithelium with a continuous Vicryl 3/0 suture. Lastly, the perineal skin is approximated with a Vicryl 3/0 subcuticular suture.

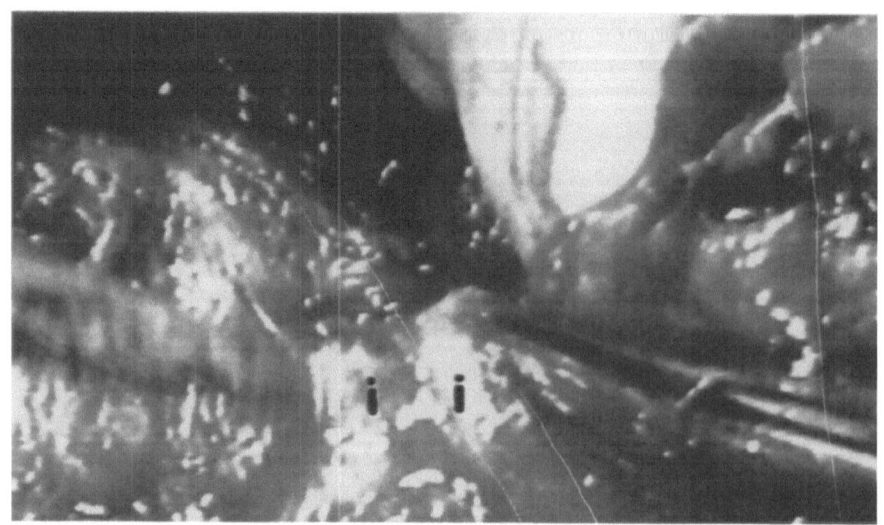

Figure 11.2 End-to-end approximation of the torn ends of the internal anal sphincter (i).[26] Reprinted from Sultan et al (1999) Primary repair. In: Br J Obstet Gynaecol 106: 318–23, with permission from Elsevier Science.

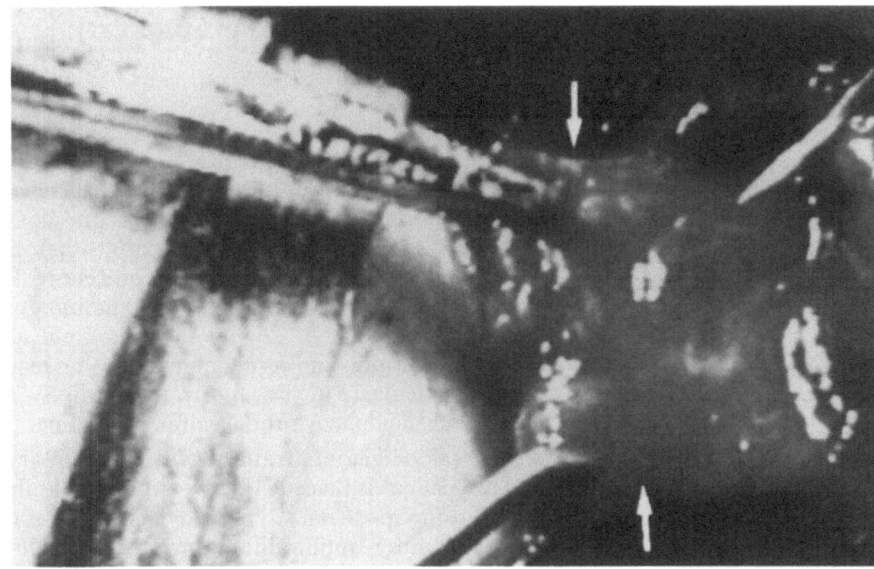

Figure 11.3 Full width of the external sphincter (between arrows) after mobilization.[26] Reprinted from Sultan et al (1999) Primary repair. In: Br J Obstet Gynaecol 106: 318–23, with permission from Elsevier Science.

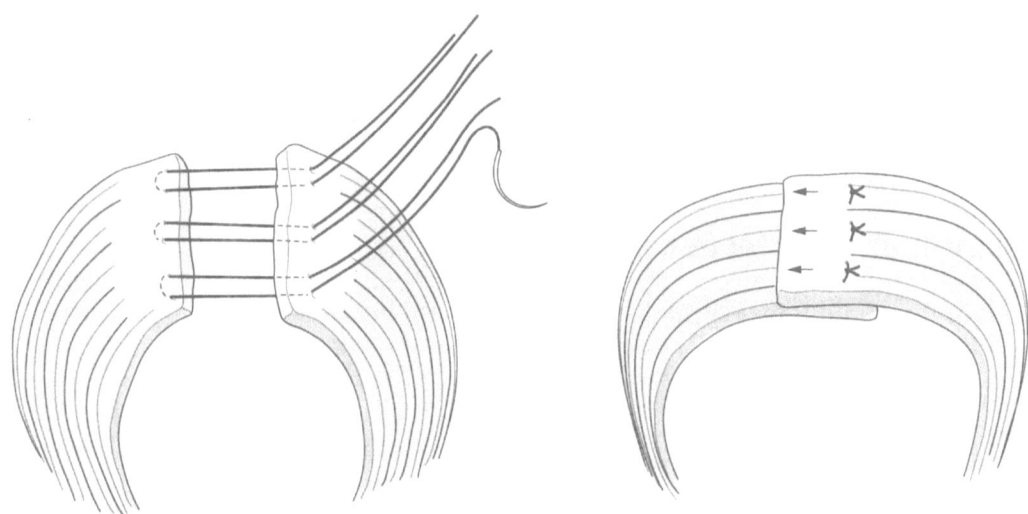

Figure 11.4 Technique of overlap repair of the external anal sphincter. As illustrated, the first suture is inserted about 1.5 cm from the torn edge of the muscle (open arrow) and carried through to within 0.5 cm of the edge of the other arm of external sphincter. A second row of sutures (small arrows) is inserted to attach the loose end of the overlapped muscle.[26] From Sultan AH, Monga AK, Kumar D, Stanton SL (1999) Primary repair of obstetric anal sphincter rupture using the overlap technique. Br J Obstet Gynaecol 106:318–23.

- Intravenous antibiotics (cefuroxime 1.5 g and metronidazole 500 mg) should be commenced intraoperatively and continued orally for 1 week. Although there are no randomized trials to substantiate benefit of this practice, the development of infection may jeopardize repair and lead to incontinence or fistula formation.
- As passage of a large bolus of hard stool may disrupt the repair, a stool softener (lactulose 10 ml three times daily) and a bulking agent such as

ispaghula husk (Fybogel, 1 sachet twice daily) is prescribed for at least 2 weeks postoperatively.

Follow-up and Management in Subsequent Pregnancy

All women should be warned of the possible sequelae of anal sphincter disruption and ideally they should all be assessed 6–12 weeks postpartum with anorectal physiology tests and anal ultrasound. If these facilities are unavailable locally, then certainly all symptomatic women should be referred to a specialist center for these investigations.

Symptomatic women with severe injuries should be offered a secondary sphincter repair and, if successful, subsequent pregnancies should be delivered by cesarean section. Women with mild symptoms should be managed with regulation of bowel action, dietary advice to avoid gas-producing foods, bulking agents, constipating agents such as loperamide and codeine phosphate, and biofeedback. Women in this group are also at risk of deterioration with a subsequent vaginal delivery and should therefore be offered cesarean section.

Tetzschner et al.[24] found that the frequency of anal incontinence increased from 17% at 3 months (n = 94) to 42% at 2–4 years post-partum (n = 72). Five of the 17 women who underwent a subsequent vaginal delivery were incontinent to flatus before delivery. Two of these five experienced an increase in frequency of flatus incontinence while in the remaining three symptoms remained unchanged. Only one (6%) of the 17 women developed anal incontinence (flatus only) de novo but none developed frank fecal incontinence following a subsequent vaginal delivery. This is important information for clinicians counselling women about the mode of delivery in a subsequent pregnancy.

Secondary Anal Sphincter Repair

Diagnosis of Anal Sphincter Injury

There are many causes of fecal incontinence (see Chapter 2), but the most frequent indications for secondary anal sphincter repair are obstetric trauma, accidental injury, and surgical division particularly following fistula surgery. The mechanisms that maintain continence are extremely complex and therefore a diagnosis based on the history alone can be misleading. In general, more than one investigation is usually required to provide global information regarding the mechanical integrity and function of the anal sphincter. Anorectal physiology tests and anal endosonography are therefore complementary and should be regarded an essential prerequisite before embarking on any incontinence surgery. A low anal sphincter pressure measurement may be due to either mechanical disruption, neuropathy or both, and likewise an occult anal sphincter defect may be an incidental finding.[1] Anal endosonography is now regarded as the gold standard for the accurate diagnosis of external and internal sphincter defects and has superseded concentric needle EMG mapping which is painful and cannot diagnose internal sphincter defects.[30]

Principles and Technique of Secondary Repair

- Preoperative bowel preparation is essential and various regimens are used. A frequently used preparation is sodium picosulfate (Picolax, Nordic) 10 mg taken at 8 a.m. and a second dose taken 6–8 hhours later. A low-residue diet is recommended for 2 days before the procedure. It is important to ensure that copious amounts of clear fluids are taken during the treatment as severe dehydration and resultant hypotension may occur, particularly in the elderly. Alternatively, a phosphate enema may produce dramatic results.

- A general or regional anesthetic is necessary and the patient is placed either in prone jackknife or lithotomy position. Gynecologists in general prefer the more familiar lithotomy position; colorectal surgeons prefer the prone jackknife position with the buttocks taped apart.

- A urinary catheter is inserted and intraoperative antibiotics such as cefuroxime and metronidazole are given at induction.

- As the perineum is rather vascular, some surgeons prefer to infiltrate the area with dilute adrenalin solution (1 in 200 000 or 300 000). However, infiltration can disturb the natural anatomical planes and cause distortion so some surgeons prefer to dissect using a cutting diathermy blade.

- For anterior defects, a circumferential skin incision is made anteriorly about 1 cm from the anal verge from 3 o'clock to 9 o'clock. Extension of the incision beyond this posteriorly is more likely to

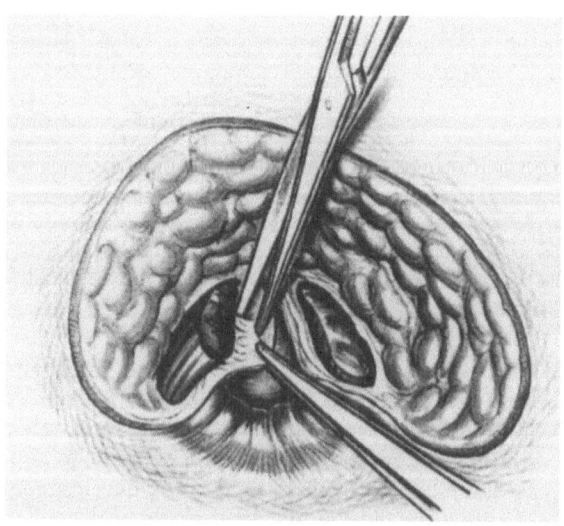

Figure 11.5 The ends of the external sphincter are mobilized and freed from the anal epithelium medially and the ischioanal fat laterally. The epithelium has been divided longitudinally to facilitate mobilization. (modified with permission[33]). Reprinted with permission from Mann & Glass (1997) *Surgical Treatment of Anal Incontinence* (2e), pp. 121–125.

be associated with injury to the branches of the pudendal nerve.[31] Anteriorly, the vaginal epithelium is mobilized by undermining and releasing scar tissue. With more severe injuries, the perineal muscles may be absent leaving only vaginal and anal epithelium with very little intervening tissue and in extreme cases when even the epithelium is absent a true cloaca is formed. In this situation the perineum needs to be reconstructed and other surgical options should be considered such as the layered method of repair, the Warren flap procedure or the Noble operation.[32]

• The outer periphery of the external sphincter is then easily recognized by its border adjacent to ischioanal and ischiorectal fat (Fig. 11.5). If muscle is not easily identifiable, a nerve or muscle stimulator may be useful. The scar tissue anterior to the anal mucosa is then divided longitudinally and grasped allowing mobilization between the anal epithelium and the inner aspect of the sphincter (Fig. 11.5). The epithelium is freed from the scarred muscle between 9 o'clock and 3 o'clock. If mobilization is difficult the epithelium can be divided longitudinally (Fig. 11.5) and then repaired with 3/0 nonabsorbable suture material such as polyglactin (vicryl) with either interrupted or continuous sutures (Fig. 11.6).

• Most texts state that it is not necessary to separate internal from external sphincter, or indeed to repair them separately.[7,33] Some surgeons routinely imbricate the internal sphincter whereas others perform a levatorplasty by plicating the levator ani muscle and a significant improvement in resting pressure and anal canal length has been demonstrated.[34] Briel et al.[35] performed an overlap repair with imbrication of the internal sphincter in 31 females and compared the results to 24 historical controls. They reported restoration of

continence in 68% compared to 63% although this was not significant. Despite this, there is good evidence to indicate that repair of isolated internal sphincter defects does improve continence. Meyenberger et al.[29] repaired isolated internal sphincter defects in 15 patients and reported excellent results in 67% and an improvement in 20%. It is therefore my routine practice to identify the internal sphincter and depending on the mobility and amount of scar tissue I will either approximate or overlap the internal sphincter ends using 2/0 polydioxanone (PDS).

• The external sphincter should also be mobilized on both surfaces but especially on its outer circumference just beyond its full width to a depth of 3–4 cm. With roughly equal amounts of scar tissue at the end of each arm of sphincter, an overlap repair as described by Parks and McPartlin[7] is performed. A suture is passed about 2–3 cm from the outer surface of the cut edge of the overlapping muscle and then passed from the outer surface of the leading edge (0.5–1 cm) of the other arm and then returned (Figs 11.4, 11.7). The sutures are held and tied only after a further one or two sets of similar horizontal mattress sutures have been inserted. A second set of sutures is then inserted to tack down the loose end of the overlapped muscle. For the sake of simplicity, only one set of sutures is shown in Figs 11.7 and 11.8. The repair should at least allow entry of the little finger which is held snugly by the anal sphincter. Mann and Glass[33] state that narrowing the anal canal to half its normal circumference is of no consequence as it is better to have a tight anal canal that can be dilated later than to have a repair that is too loose. In his original description Parks[7] used steel wire for this repair but, although effective, this can cause discomfort if it migrates.

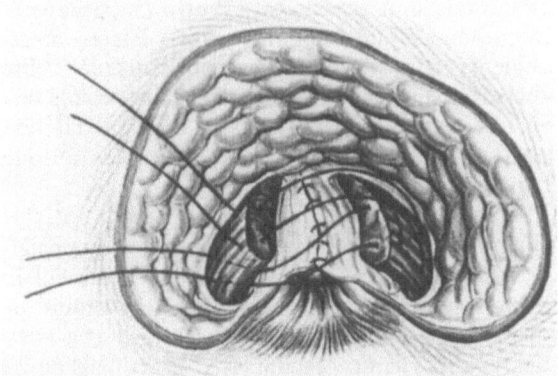

Figure 11.6 The anal epithelium has been repaired and two sets of sutures have been inserted into the sphincter for the overlap repair. Usually four or six sets of sutures are required, as shown in Figure 11.4 (modified with permission[33]) Reprinted with permission from Mann & Glass (1997) *Surgical Treatment of Anal Incontinence* (2e), pp. 121–125.

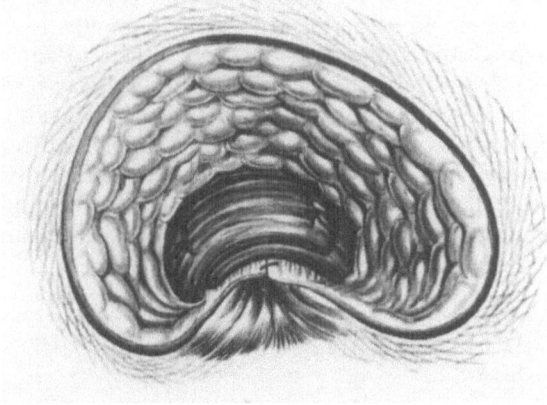

Figure 11.7 The final appearance of a successfully overlapped sphincter repair. (modified with permission[33]) Reprinted with permission from Mann & Glass (1997) *Surgical Treatment of Anal Incontinence* (2e), pp. 121–125.

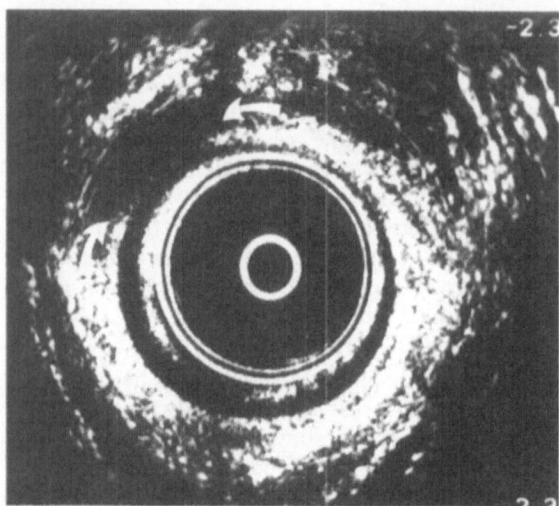

Figure 11.8 Anal endosonographic image demonstrating an external sphincter defect (between arrows) in a woman complaining of fecal incontinence-following an end-to-end repair. The arrows overlie the two retracted ends of the muscle.[26] Reprinted from Sultan et al (1999) Primary repair. In: Br J Obstet Gynaecol 106:318–23, with permission from Elsevier Science.

Nylon and prolene 2/0, both monofilament non-absorbable sutures, have now become popular but they can also migrate and cause discomfort and "stitch abscesses," necessitating removal. I therefore prefer the use of a monofilament delayed-absorbable suture such as PDS 2/0.

- The perineal skin can then be closed with interrupted 2/0 vicryl and a drain left in situ. However, skin closure is not essential and under no circumstances should the skin be closed under tension but rather just approximated in a "Y" fashion with the center left open to allow for drainage and heal with granulation tissue.

Timing of Repair

In general it is recommended that a secondary repair should be performed after 3–6 months have elapsed following a failed primary repair, to allow for edema and inflammation to settle.[32] Delay may enhance optimum viability of tissues by allowing time for return of adequate blood supply and re-innervation. However, others have shown that this delay is unnecessary and provided the wound appears to be clean with or without debridement, an earlier repair should be feasible.[28]

Role of Colostomy

There is no evidence that prior or concomitant colostomy improves functional outcome or healing following primary or secondary repair.[4,11,36] Colostomy should be reserved for selected patients and include some patients with Crohn's disease, recto-

vaginal fistulae, and possibly those undergoing recurrent sphincter repair.

Postoperative Management

The catheter and drain should be removed in the second postoperative day. Antibiotics should be continued for 3–5 days. Lactulose and fybogel should be prescribed for at least 2 weeks and some recommend a low-residue diet. A twice daily sitz bath is advised. It is absolutely essential that constipation is avoided at all costs, as fecal impaction requiring manual evacuation will invariably result in a breakdown of the repair. Nessim et al.[37] performed a prospective randomized controlled trial involving 54 patients undergoing anorectal reconstructive surgery. Group 1 was given a clear liquid diet, loperamide, and codeine phosphate while group 2 was allowed an unrestricted regular diet postoperatively. First bowel action occurred earlier in group 2 and fecal impaction occurred in 7%, compared to 26% in group 1. There was no difference in functional outcome.

Failed Secondary Sphincter Repair

There are many reasons for an unsuccessful outcome. Before the advent of anal ultrasound, inadequate preoperative assessment and poor patient selection were important reasons for failure. However, long-term studies have shown that although most patients improve after sphincter surgery, continence is rarely perfect and many deteriorate with time.[10] Associated factors such as aging, progression of pelvic neuropathy, and estrogen deficiency are all implicated. Some studies have shown that preoperative prolonged pudendal nerve motor latency measurements are associated with a poor outcome[11,38] but others found no such relationship.[4] It is possible that this test is not a sensitive measure of pudendal neuropathy, or that surgery itself contributes to long term deterioration.

Pinedo et al[39] have shown that a repeat anterior repair after failed sphincter repair following obstetric injury produces a significant improvement in continence scores in 58% and therefore should be considered before other procedures such as a postanal repair, dynamic graciloplasty, or artificial bowel sphincter (see Chapter 16). Biofeedback may improve the results of sphincter repair,[40] but long-term results are unknown. In one study of 20 postmenopausal women with fecal incontinence, 25% became continent after 6 months of hormone replacement therapy.[41]

References

1. Sultan AH, Kamm MA, Hudson CN, Thomas JM, Bartram CI (1993) Anal sphincter disruption during vaginal delivery. N Engl J Med 329: 1905–11.
2. Donnelly V, Fynes M, Campbell D et al. (1998) Obstetric events leading to anal sphincter damage. Obstet Gynecol 92: 955–961.
3. Chaliha C, Kalia V, Sultan AH, Monga AK, Stanton AL (1998) Anal function: effect of pregnancy and delivery. Neurourol Urodyn 17(4): 417–18.
4. Engel AF, Kamm MA, Sultan AH, Bartram CI, Nicholls RJ (1994) Anterior anal sphincter repair in patients with obstetric trauma. Br J Surg 81: 1231–34.
5. Blaisdell PC (1940) Repair of the incontinent sphincter ani. Surg Gynecol Obstet 70: 692–7.
6. Arnaud A, Sarles JC, Sielezneff I, Orsoni P, Jolly A (1991) Sphincter repair without overlapping for fecal incontinence. Dis Colon Rectum 34: 744–7.
7. Parks AG, McPartlin JF (1971) Late repairs of injuries of the anal sphincter. Proc R Soc Med 64: 1187–89.
8. Browning GGP, Motson RW (1984) Anal sphincter injury. Management and results of Parks sphincter repair. Ann Surg 199: 351–7.
9. Jorge JMN, Wexner SD (1993) Etiology and management of fecal incontinence. Dis Colon Rectum 36: 77–97.
10. Malouf AJ, Norton CS, Engel AF, Nicholls RJ, Kamm MA (2000) Long term results of overlapping anterior anal-sphincter repair for obstetric trauma. Lancet 355: 260–5.
11. Londonno-Schimmer EE, Garcia-Duperly R, Nicholls RJ et al. (1994) Overlapping anal sphincter repair for faecal incontinence due to sphincter trauma: five year follow-up functional results. Int J Colorect Dis 9: 110–13.
12. Sultan AH, Kamm MA, Hudson CN, Bartram CI (1994) Third degree obstetric anal sphincter tears: risk factors and outcome of primary repair. BMJ 308: 887–91.
13. Poen AC, Felt-Bersma RJF, Strijers RLM et al. (1998) Third-degree obstetric perineal tear: long-term clinical and functional results after primary repair. Br J Surg 85: 1433–8.
14. Sorensen SM, Bondesen H, Istre O, Vilmann P (1988) Perineal rupture following vaginal delivery. Acta Obstet Gynecol Scand 67: 315–18.
15. Hueston WJ (1996) Factors associated with the use of episiotomy during vaginal delivery. Obstet Gynecol 87: 1001–5.
16. Sultan AH, Kamm MA, Bartram CI, Hudson CN (1994) Perineal damage at delivery. Contemp Rev Obstet Gynaecol 6: 18–24.
17. Sultan AH, Kamm MA, Hudson CN (1995) Obstetric perineal tears: an audit of training. J Obstet Gynecol 15: 19–23.
18. Donald I (1979) Practical Obstetric Problems, 5th ed. Lloyd-Luke, London, p. 811.
19. Sultan AH (1999) Obstetrical perineal injury and anal incontinence. Clin Risk 5: 193–6.
20. Sultan AH (1997) Anal incontinence after childbirth. Curr Opin Obstet Gynecol 9: 320–4.
21. Gjessing H, Backe B, Sahlin Y (1998) Third degree obstetric tears; outcome after primary repair. Acta Obstet Gynecol Scand 77: 736–40.
22. Goffeng AR, Andersch B, Berndtsson I, Hulten L, Oresland T (1988) Objective methods cannot predict anal incontinence after primary repair of extensive anal tears. Acta Obstet Gynecol Scand 77: 439–43.
23. Kammerer-Doak DN, Wesol AB, Rogers RG, Dominguez CE, Dorin MH (1999) A prospective cohort study of women after primary repair of obstetric anal sphincter laceration. Am J Obstet Gynecol 181: 1317–23.
24. Tetzschner T, Sorensen M, Lose G, Christiansen J (1996) Anal and urinary incontinence in women with obstetric anal sphincter rupture. Br J Obstet Gynaecol 103: 1034–40.
25. Nielsen MB, Hauge C, Rasmussen OO, Pedersen JF, Christiansen J (1992) Anal endosonographic findings in the follow-up of primarily sutured sphincteric ruptures. Br J Surg 79: 104–6.
26. Sultan AH, Monga AK, Kumar D, Stanton SL (1999) Primary repair of obstetric anal sphincter rupture using the overlap technique. Br J Obstet Gynaecol 106: 318–23.
27. Fulsher RW, Fearl CL (1955) The third-degree laceration in modern obstetrics. Am J Obstet Gynecol 69(4): 786–93.
28. Hauth JC et al. (1986) Early repair of an external sphincter ani muscle and rectal mucosal dehiscence. Obstet Gynecol 67(6): 806–9.
29. Meyenberger C, Bertschinger P, Zala GF, Buchmann P (1996) Anal sphincter defects in fecal incontinence: correlation between endosonography and surgery. Endoscopy 28: 217–24.
30. Sultan AH, Kamm MA, Talbot IC, Nicholls RJ, Bartram CI (1994) Anal endosonography: Precision of identifying sphincter defects confirmed histologically. Br J Surg 81: 466–9.
31. Shafik A, Doss S (1999) Surgical anatomy of the somatic terminal innervation to the anal and urethral sphincters: role in anal and urethral surgery. J Urol 161: 85–9.
32. Wiskind AK, Thompson JD (1997) Fecal incontinence and rectovaginal fistulas. In: Rock JA, Thompson JA (eds) Te Linde's Operative Gynecology, J.B. Lippincott-Raven, Philadelphia, Pa., pp. 1218–23.
33. Mann CV, Glass RE (1997) Technique of anal sphincter repair. In: Mann CV, Glass RE (ed) Surgical Treatment of Anal Incontinence, 2nd ed. Springer, London, pp. 121–125.
34. Wexner SD, Marchetti F, Jagelman DG (1991) The role of sphincteroplasty for fecal incontinence reevaluated: a prospective physiologic and functional review. Dis Colon Rectum 34: 22–30.
35. Briel JW, Boer LM de, Hop WC, Schouten WR (1998) Clinical outcome of anterior overlapping external anal sphincter repair with internal anal sphincter imbrication. Dis Colon Rectum 41: 209–14.
36. Sitzler PJ, Thompson JP (1996) Overlap repair of damaged anal sphincter. A single surgeon's series. Dis Colon Rectum 39: 1356–60.
37. Nessim A, Wexner SD, Agachan F et al. (1999) Is bowel confinement necessary after anorectal reconstructive surgery? A prospective, randomized, surgeon-blinded trial. Dis Colon Rectum 42: 16–23.
38. Gilliland R, Altomare DF, Moreira H Jr et al. (1998) Pudendal neuropathy is predictive of failure following anterior overlapping sphincteroplasty. Dis Colon Rectum 41: 1516–22.
39. Pinedo G, Vaisey CJ, Nicholls RJ et al. (1999) Results of repeat anal sphincter repair. Br J Surg 86: 66–9.
40. Jensen LL, Lowry AC. (1997) Biofeedback improves functional outcome after sphincteroplasy. Dis Colon Rectum 40: 197–200.
41. Donnelly V, O'Connell PR, O'Herlihy C (1997) The influence of oestrogen replacement on faecal incontinence in postmenopausal women. Br J Obstet Gynaecol 104: 311–15.

Prolapse Surgery

12 Anterior Compartment

- make sure the shelf on which the bladder rests is intact, reconstructing that shelf if necessary
- treat the female pelvis as a unit.

In its classic formulation, anterior colporrhaphy has been performed as a midline surgical repair of the anterior vaginal wall for cystocele, frequently incorporating a Kelly urethrovesical plication for the treatment of concurrent stress urinary incontinence (Fig. 12.1).[2]

Anterior Colporrhaphy

Christopher J. Walshe and Lewis Wall

> I have been surprised many times in working out this subject to follow the logic of many of the operations recommended for the cure of cystocele. Everything as recommended except repair of the anatomic supports of the bladder. The problem of keeping the bladder in place is solved in *repairing the shelf on which it rests*. Otherwise I do not see how we can expect to cure cystocele. The point of great importance is that the pelvic organs are a *unit*. It will not do to repair one part and let the others go and expect to get a cure. There is no use in repairing a cystocele and leaving a relaxed perineum ...
> *George R. White*

Dr. White's clinical insight regarding reconstructive surgery on the anterior pelvic compartment is as true today as it was 90 years ago.[1] Two principles should govern the surgeon's approach to prolapse in this area:

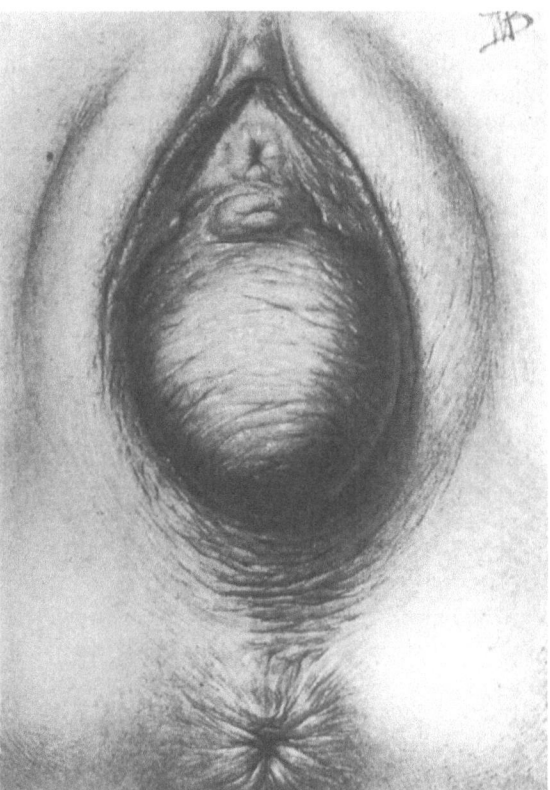

Figure 12.1 Massive anterior compartment failure resulting in large cystocele. From Kelly HA, Affections of the urethra and bladder. From: *Operative Gynecology*, New York, D. Appleton and Company, 1898.

Kennedy extended this concept to include a more sling-like support.[3] Since the original description of these procedures by Kelly and Kennedy, over 20 variations have been described in the medical literature.[4] In our opinion, anterior colporrhaphy is most useful as a treatment for cystocele in patients undergoing vaginal reconstructive surgery; but it is not a first-line treatment for patients with stress incontinence. The success of anterior colporrhaphy in the treatment of stress incontinence is highly variable, depends substantially on the skill of the operator, and compares unfavorably with other operations. The reported success rates for the cure of stress incontinence using anterior colporrhaphy ranges from 30% to 90%, and the best success rates have been obtained with a variation of the operation that closely resembles a transvaginal version of a Marshall–Marchetti–Krantz retropubic urethropexy.[5]

In recent years gynecologic surgeons have rediscovered key principles regarding the surgical reconstruction of the female pelvis and have expanded the applicability of these principles to modern operations. This has resulted in a shift of focus from a narrow, compartmentalized view of the pelvis to a more integrated, multidimensional, holistic approach. Anterior colporrhaphy will most often be useful as a technique for addressing one limited defect in pelvic support. The key philosophical point is that all defects of pelvic support must be identified and addressed at the time of reconstructive surgery. Pelvic support must be understood in terms of the dynamic interaction of all of its components. Successful correction of pelvic support defects requires that this concept be translated into effective surgical strategies in the operating room.

Surgical Anatomy of the Anterior Vagina

The anatomy of vaginal and bladder support is not complex. The most appealing contemporary techniques for surgical reconstruction in this area are based on the concept that anterior vaginal prolapse results from fascial defects or separations of the endopelvic fascia from its normal sites of attachment. These defects in turn produce various kinds of vaginal "hernias." The vagina has three primary layers, the surface epithelium (often erroneously referred to as "mucosa"), the underlying muscularis, and the controversial deep layer of vagina "fascia." Cullen Richardson refers to this latter layer as the "pubocervical fascia" (Fig. 12.2).[6] Kennedy referred to this layer as a "table on which the urethra rests in intimate relationship." Classic descriptions of operative techniques for anterior colporrhaphy refer to this layer as the "fascia," and the term "pubocervical fascia" will be used in this discussion when referring to the trapezoidal configuration of connective tissue that supports the anterior vaginal wall, bladder and urethra . Delancey has clearly described three principle levels of anatomic support for the vagina and the structural components that make up each level.[7] In Delancey's description, level II defects lead to cystoceles and level III defects lead to urethroceles. Durable support of the vagina depends upon ade-

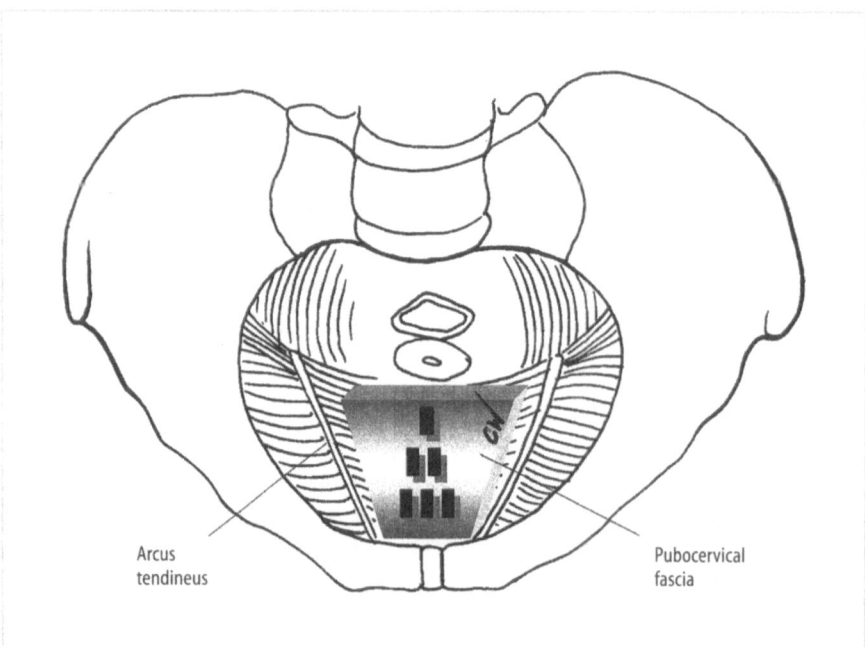

Arcus tendineus

Pubocervical fascia

Figure 12.2 "Trapezoidal" configuration of the pubocervical fascia bordered by the arcus tendineus fasciae pelvis as seen from above. Note bladder and urethra absent.

quate structural integrity of each of these levels, which are interrelated and which must be addressed at the time of surgical repair.

The pelvic fascia can be described as either parietal or visceral. These terms were coined by Derry[8] and have been used by other authors, such as Weber and Walters.[4] *Parietal fascia* is composed of regular collagen bands, covers the pelvic skeletal muscles, and attaches these muscles to the pelvic bones. *Visceral fascia* envelops the pelvic organs in dissectable planes and provides conduits for blood vessels, lymphatics, and nerves, while simultaneously permitting the movement and growth of pelvic organs. The collagen found in visceral fascia is less dense and less organized that found in parietal fascia.

In summary, the anatomical support of the vagina, bladder, and urethra ("the anterior pelvic compartment") includes the following structures:

- the levator ani sling
- the anterolateral attachments of the vagina to the arcus tendineus levator ani and the arcus tendineus fasciae pelvis
- the anterolateral musculofascial attachments of the urethra and the distal anterior vaginal wall to the pubic bone and to the arcus tendineus fascia pelvis
- the pubocervical fascia and the anterior vaginal wall
- the pericervical ring of fascia which is often disrupted after a hysterectomy, resulting in a hiatus
- the perineal body, posterior vaginal wall, and Denonvillier's fascia
- the perineal membrane.

The anterior vaginal wall is a trapezoid, and the pubocervical fascia is attached to other pelvic structures at multiple points (Fig. 12.3a–c). An important component of anterior vaginal support is action of the levator ani muscles, exerted through their connections with the endopelvic fascia. The upper two-thirds of the vagina is nearly horizontal, and is held in this position upon the levators through such lateral attachments. The lateral anterior vaginal sulci are attached through fibrous bridges to the condensed parietal fascia known as the white line or arcus tendineus fasciae pelvis. This arrangement stabilizes the vagina over the levator plate. The upper vagina is also supported by its connection to the uterosacral ligaments. At the time of hysterectomy, the pericervical connective tissue should be reapproximated to the vaginal cuff in order to maintain this support. The distal vagina is supported by the perineal membrane superiorly and the perineal body posteriorly.

The posterior vaginal wall is usually neglected in discussions concerning anterior vaginal wall support, but it must be kept in mind that both the anterior and posterior vaginal walls lie coapted over the levator muscles. Ultimately, these structures function as a unit, and all pelvic support defects should be identified and repaired at the time of surgery for optimum results. Similarly, anterior vaginal operations that elevate the anterior vagina will also elevate the posterior vagina, potentially worsening any posterior vaginal support defect that is not repaired concurrently.

Pathophysiology

"Cystocele" is really a support defect of the anterior vaginal wall. When this occurs, it results in a prolapse of the bladder caused by an anterior fascial defect (level II). "Urethrocele" is a similar condition resulting from a loss of urethral support from a similar fascial defect, most notably at the urethrovesical junction and distally along the urethra (levels II and III). What causes this weakening and subsequent prolapse of the anterior vaginal wall? It is generally believed that damage to the structures of pelvic support often occurs as the result of pregnancy and subsequent vaginal delivery. This occurs during delivery by distention of the supporting vaginal tissues beyond a certain critical point, combined with pressure, ischaemia, pudendal, and pelvic nerve injury[9,10] and shearing forces generated by the fetal head as it negotiates the tight fit of the pelvis through the mechanism of labor. This is thought to produce fascial breaks and muscle tears that result in the loss of both the active and passive supports to the pelvic organs. The effects of chronic diseases are then layered upon the trauma that results from vaginal birth. Hypoestrogenic states, vasculopathy, obesity, smoking, chronic obstructive pulmonary disease, chronic severe constipation, and diabetes all add to the weakened ability of the pelvic floor to support its burdens. If the individual woman has a genetic predisposition to prolapse in the form of abnormal collagen, the problem is likely to present earlier, progress more rapidly, and end in a more advanced state than is the case of women with stronger connective tissue. Over time, these injuries converge with the forces of gravity and the strains of daily physical activity to worsen the problem of pelvic organ prolapse.

Indications

Anterior colporrhaphy is one possible treatment for symptomatic prolapse of the anterior vagina. There are many manifestations of anterior vaginal prolapse, including voiding dysfunction, high residual urine volume, pelvic pressure, inguinal discomfort,

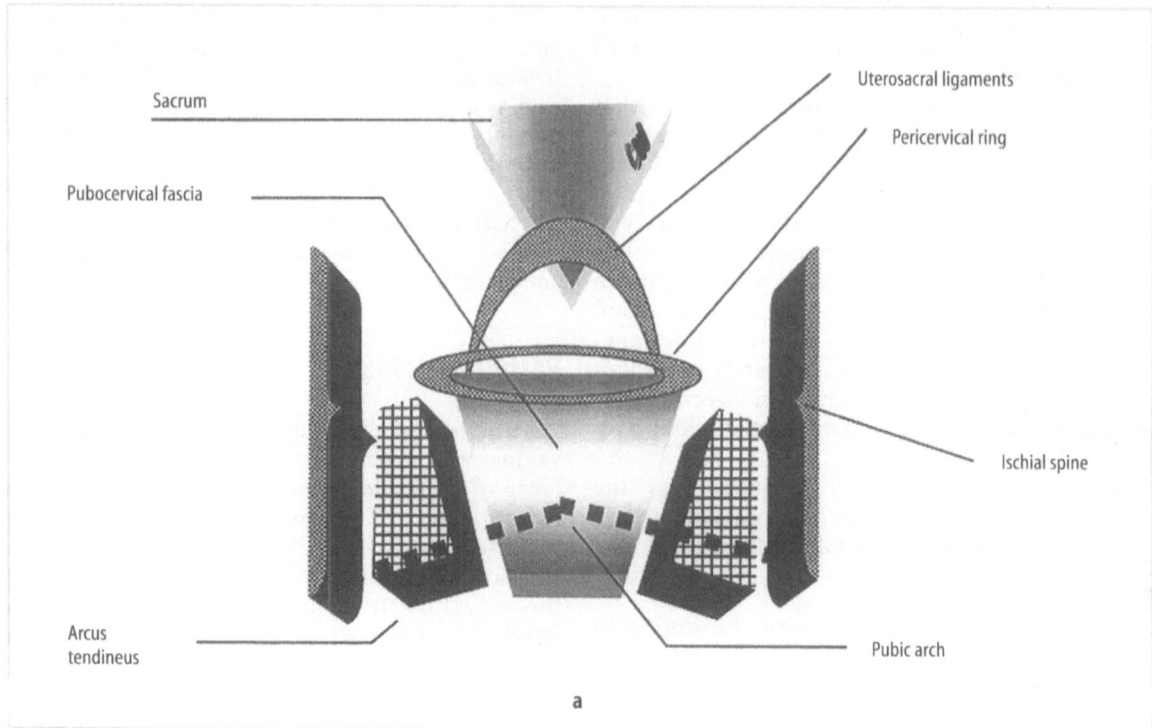

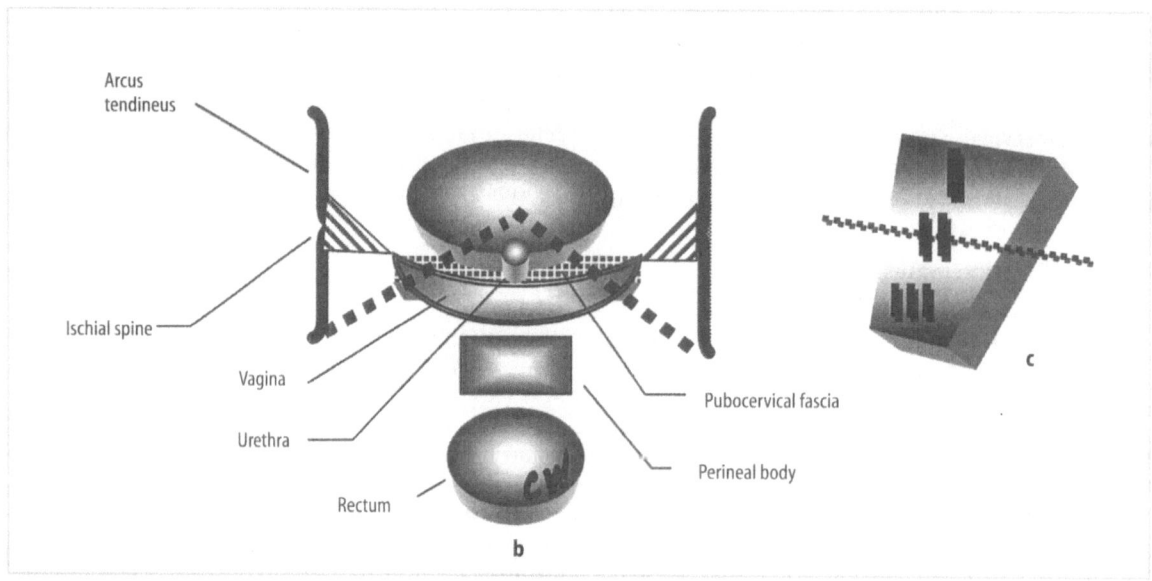

Figure 12.3 **a** Three-dimensional representation of the support structures of the "pubocervical" fascia. **b, c** Coronal view of the support structures of the pubocervical fascia at level II.

bulging of the anterior vaginal wall, recurrent cystitis, dyspareunia, urinary frequency, hesitancy, stress urinary incontinence. Unfortunately, other etiologies as well as anterior vaginal prolapse may produce many of these symptoms. The surgeon should always carefully exclude other causes of patient symptoms prior to performing an operation to cure them. Anterior colporrhaphy is used most appropriately as part of a comprehensive plan for pelvic reconstruction associated with specific types of prolapse involving the distal, middle and upper thirds of the anterior vaginal wall (levels I–III).

Surgical Principles of Anterior Vaginal Wall Reconstruction

A comprehensive and effective reconstruction of the anterior vaginal wall takes into account the many dimensions of support that affect this structure. Because stress urinary incontinence is often (but by no means always) associated with defects of anterior vaginal support, all patients with anterior vaginal prolapse should be examined with a full bladder under conditions of raised intraabdominal pressure. If urine loss is demonstrated in association with coughing or a Valsalva maneuver, further evaluation is necessary. If the prolapse is large, it should be reduced to unkink a compressed urethra and reveal latent stress incontinence that may manifest itself after surgical repair. Careful manoeuvres of this kind during the initial evaluation of the patient will insure that all relevant problems are addressed at the time of surgery.

Basic Principles

- All vaginal support defects should be corrected to insure the best possible surgical result.
- Vaginal surgeons must always be cognizant of female sexual functioning. Reconstructive vaginal operations must take into account the caliber, length, and orientation of the vagina in order to maintain satisfactory coital functioning postoperatively.
- In a woman standing erect, the vagina is nearly horizontal, and the suspensory mechanism of the vagina is engineered with this principle in mind. (Fig. 12.3a–c).
- Defects in the fascial support of the anterior vagina may be simple isolated defects, but multiple breaks may also occur. Such breaks may occur in any plane: apical, distal, sagittal, parasagittal, lateral, or coronal. Each defect should be identified and addressed separately during surgery.
- The anterior vaginal wall rests on the posterior vaginal wall; therefore, posterior vaginal wall defects can significantly affect anterior wall strength and function. Patients with an enlarged genital hiatus, rectocele, and attenuated perineal body should undergo reconstruction of these defects at the time of repair of the anterior vaginal defect. Correction of these posterior defects will help provide auxiliary support to the anterior vagina.
- Patients with a cystocele but no complaint of incontinence may, in some cases, develop stress incontinence after undergoing anterior colporrhaphy. In patients who can be shown to have latent stress incontinence after reduction of their prolapse, consideration should be given to performing a specific anti-incontinence procedure to address this problem.
- The integrity of the tissues of the anterior vaginal wall and endopelvic fascia is a critical variable if reconstructive surgery is to be both effective and long lasting. Although it is not currently the standard of care, consideration is increasingly being given to wholesale replacement of these tissue layers using tissue grafts or flaps or interposition of autologous or synthetic materials when extensive fascial defects exist. It may even be possible in the future to use allogenic tissue cultures from living human epidermal keratinocytes and dermal fibroblasts to replace damaged connective tissue. In addition to providing new graft tissue the keratinocytes and fibroblasts release potent cytokines, growth factors and matrix proteins that may promote the process of wound healing.[11]

Surgical Techniques

The patient should be placed in a high dorsal lithotomy position. Pelvic examination should then be performed prior to the operation to reassess the vaginal support defects. A weighted speculum should be placed in the vagina and the bladder drained by a urethral catheter.

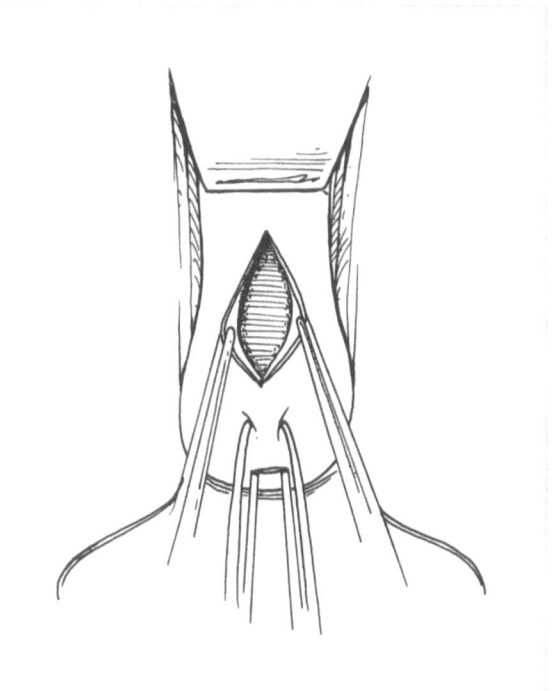

Figure 12.4 Anterior vaginal wall median longitudinal colpotomy incision. The vaginal wound edges are grasped and retracted by toothed clamps. The colpotomy is extended upward toward the urethral meatus. From: Reiffenswtuhl (1974) Vagina Operations of Surgical Anatomy and Techniques (2e) Lippincott Williams & Wilkins, pp. 133–137.

The traditional approach to anterior colporrhaphy utilizes a midline incision in the anterior vaginal wall. An incision is made through the full thickness of the vaginal epithelium to within 2 cm of the urethral meatus (Fig. 12.4). A scalpel or scissors (Metzenbaum or Strully) are used to undermine the full thickness of the anterior and lateral vaginal wall, exposing the underlying vesicovaginal space and fascia (Fig. 12.5). Care must be taken to avoid urethral injury during this part of the dissection. The lateral periurethral tissue contains the neurovascular supply to the urethra.[12] Denervation injury as the result of aggressive dissection may affect pelvic floor and urethral function adversely. As the anterior vaginal wall dissection progresses, the flaps raised are grasped along their margins with Pratt clamps (Fig. 12.5). The pubocervical fascia should remain attached to the exposed bladder base. The extent of dissection depends upon the size, number and character of the fascial defects. Exposure of the operative field can be facilitated using a vaginal ring retractor, freeing the surgeon's hands while providing excellent stable exposure.

More extensive dissection may be required when multiple fascial defects are encountered or if large isolated defects require tissue grafting. In such cases, the bladder base must be adequately mobilized all the way to the peritoneal reflection to ensure a good surgical result (Fig. 12.6).

Sharp dissection near the urethrovesical junction and urinary meatus is important because the bladder, urethra, and vagina are closely adherent in

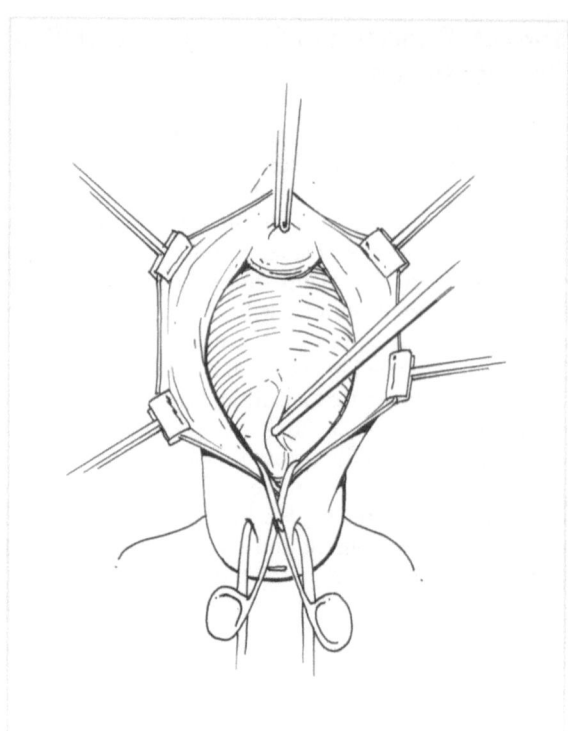

Figure 12.6 Wide extensive dissection of a large cystocele. The bladder is being mobilized from the cervix. From: Reiffenswtuhl (1974) Vagina Operations of Surgical Anatomy and Techniques (2e) Lippincott Williams & Wilkins, pp. 133–137.

this area. Lateral dissection can be carried out with scissors or scalpel initially and then followed by blunt dissection near the lateral margins. The bladder base, urethrovesical junction, and lateral fascial margins are now exposed for inspection. Excess vaginal tissue is incised (Fig. 12.7). At this point in the reconstruction an anti-incontinence procedure may be performed when indicated, i.e. transvaginal or transabdominal pubourethral sling or colposuspension. Some surgeons advocate placing a suburethral plication suture as an anti-incontinence procedure. Because of the unreliability of this operation we prefer a Burch colposuspension as described by Tanagho or a modified Goebell–Stoeckel–Frankenheim suburethral sling procedure, two procedures with a proven track record.[13,14] This method addresses coexistent level III defects, which can result in postoperative urinary incontinence if not addressed. (see Fig. 12.2) Level II defects are addressed by the plication of the pubocervical fascia and redundant tissue at the bladder base using interrupted vertical mattress sutures placed perpendicular to the midline to prevent attenuation of the urethral length. The use of 2-0 or 3-0 delayed-absorbable polyglycolic acid suture on an atraumatic needle is recommended (Figs 12.7, 12.8). Care should be exercised to avoid placing suture into the bladder. Lateral fascial (level II) defects can also be addressed with a unilateral or bilateral transvaginal

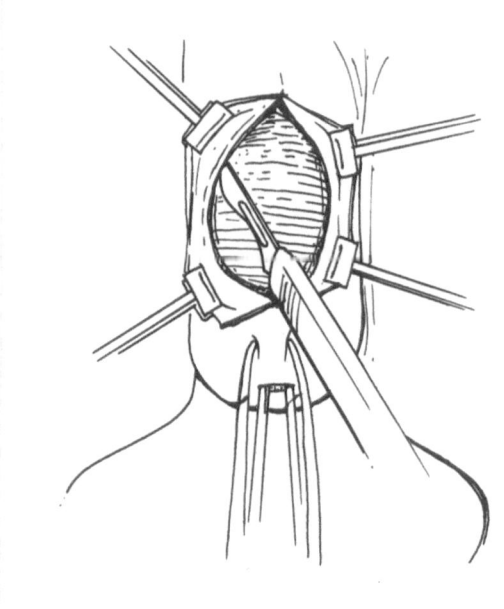

Figure 12.5 Extended colpotomy incision. Dissection of the vaginal wall on the right side. Traction on Pratt clamps fans out the vaginal tissue. From: Reiffenswtuhl (1974) Vagina Operations of Surgical Anatomy and Techniques (2e) Lippincott Williams & Wilkins, pp. 133–137.

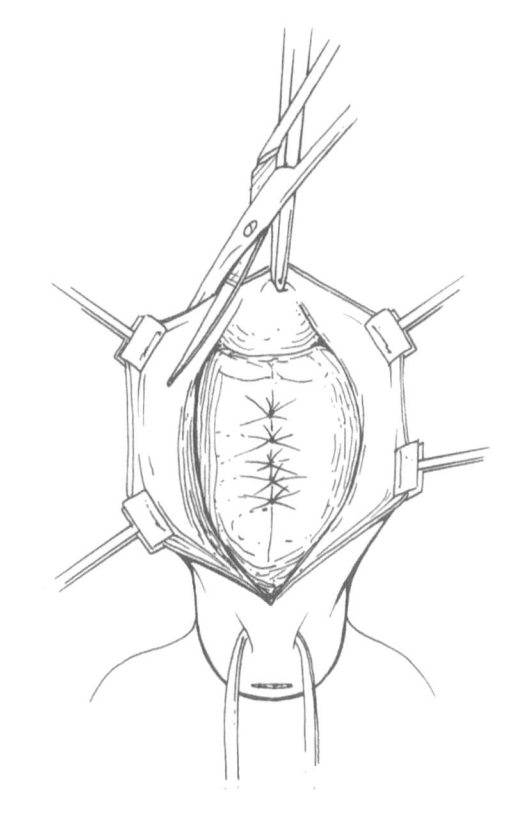

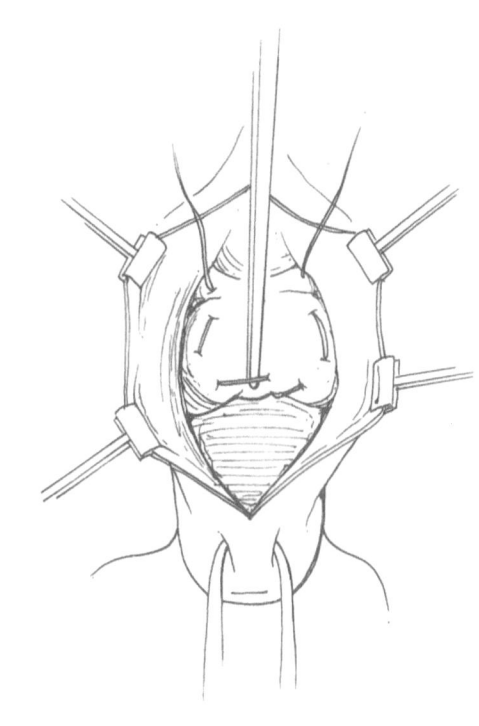

Figure 12.8 Pubocervical fascial plication stitch. Tissue forceps invaginate the fascia in the midline. From: Reiffenswtuhl (1974) Vagina Operations of Surgical Anatomy and Techniques (2e) Lippincott Williams & Wilkins, pp. 133–137.

Figure 12.7 Excess vaginal tissue is excised after midline plication of the pubocervical fascia. From: Reiffenswtuhl (1974) Vagina Operations of Surgical Anatomy and Techniques (2e) Lippincott Williams & Wilkins, pp. 133–137.

paravaginal defect repair as described by Shull.[15] The arcus tendineus fasciae pelvis and ischial spine can be easily palpated and visualized when proceeded by precise and meticulous dissection. The use of a surgical headlight will also facilitate the exposure of these essential surgical landmarks while avoiding injury to adjacent vital pelvic structures. Excess vaginal tissue may be resected, but care must be taken not to remove so much as to place the wound edges under tension when the incision is closed. This may result in vaginal stenosis or wound dehiscence, and require additional surgery at a later date. The edges of the vaginal incision are reapproximated longitudinally using a running 2-0 or 3-0 delayed-absorbable polyglycolic acid suture on an atraumatic needle (Fig. 12.9).

Large or Recurrent Anterior Compartment Defects

Recurrent and/or severe anterior compartment prolapse has been a significant challenge to the reconstructive pelvic surgeon since the early twentieth century. Attempted correction of such problems still results in a high failure rate and significant numbers of patients with recurrence.[16] Anterior compartment failure or recurrence rates as high as 30% have been reported.[16,17] Patients with large and or recurrent anterior compartment fascial defects as shown in Fig. 12.1 may need specially designed adjunctive procedures to achieve durable results. The fascia of the anterior compartment is not a true dense fascia and as a result may contribute to this problem.

Many different approaches to address this problem have been suggested using natural or synthetic materials to bolster the anterior vaginal wall. Zacharin placed a free graft of vaginal epithelium over the plicated anterior vaginal wall fascia.[18] Julian used polypropylene mesh to repair severe recurrent vaginal prolapse of the anterior midvaginal wall.[19] Bilateral bulbocavernosus grafts have also been employed to reinforce the pubocervical fascia. Wall and co-workers have described a sling using a pedicled rectus abdominis muscle flap.[20] Symmonds described the use of a full thickness labial flap to reconstruct the urethra and anterior vaginal wall.[21] Chesson et al. reported using a trapezoidal

168

Christopher J. Walshe and Lewis Wall

slough, postoperative urinary retention, and eight rectoceles. In addition, several of the patients in the study had complications with granulation tissue formation and subsequent dyspareunia related to graft erosion through the anterior vaginal wall. The complications were attributed to the pioneering nature of the procedure, failure to perform cystoscopy to check ureteric patency prior to securing the graft, and failure to reattach the superior aspect of the rectovaginal septum to the pubocervical fascia as a cause for recurrent enteroceles. The authors agree that more experience with this complex procedure is needed before it can be recommended for primary repair of anterior compartment prolapse.

Complications

Complications encountered following anterior colporrhaphy include urinary retention, detrusor instability; injury to the bladder, urethra or ureters; vesicovaginal fistula, decreased vaginal capacity or length, dyspareunia, sexual dysfunction, granulation tissue formation, mesh or graft erosion or migration, vaginal sloughing, incontinence, hematoma formation, vaginal wall cellulitis, graft rejection, mesh or graft infection, graft autolysis, and urethral diverticulum formation.

Results

No controlled, prospective randomized studies have been performed to date comparing the various reconstructive operations used in the anterior compartment. Many articles describe surgical techniques but fail to report outcomes in any meaningful way.[23] There are many operations of mainly histori-

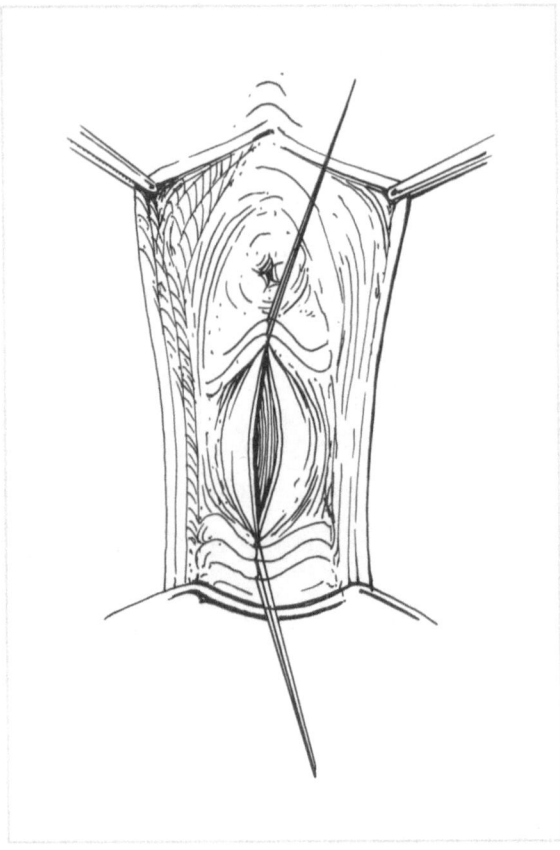

Figure 12.9 Closure of the anterior midline colpotomy incision using interrupted absorbable sutures. From: Reiffenswtuhl (1974) Vagina Operations of Surgical Anatomy and Techniques (2e) Lippincott Williams & Wilkins, pp. 133–137.

hammock composed of grafted tensor fascia lata suspended bilaterally from the arcus tendineus fasciae pelvis for correction of severe or recurrent anterior wall defects (Fig. 12.10).[22] They reported one anterior compartment failure and various complications including ureteric injury, partial graft

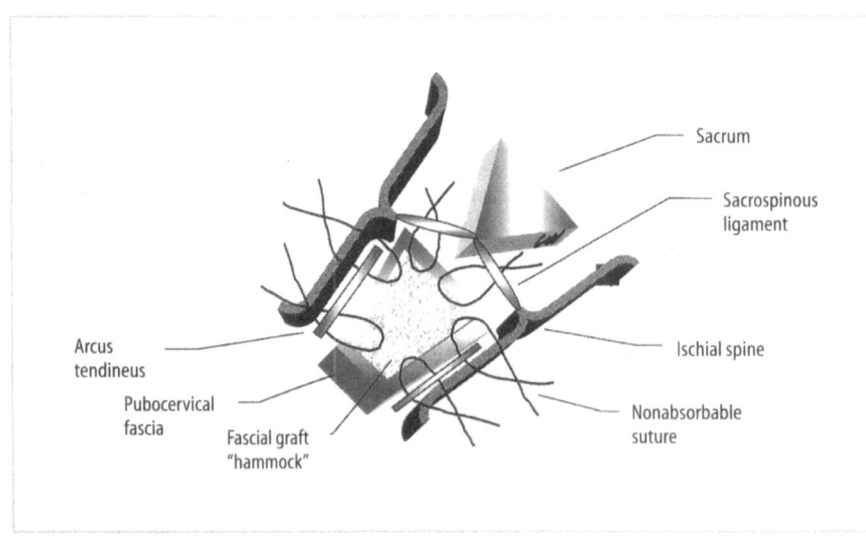

Figure 12.10 Three-dimensional representation of the transvaginal arcus to arcus "Hammock" surgical procedure. Indicated for extensive recurrent pubocervical fascial failures. Note the "marble"-textured tissue graft overlying the damaged pubocervical fasci.

cal significance that have limited applicability today: anterior colporrhaphy with trachelectomy, Manchester (Donald –Fothergill) operation,[24] the Watkins–Wertheim procedure which sutures the uterine fundus to the periosteum of the pubic rami,[25] transposition of the uterus – the Ocejo modification were the uterus is temporarily bivalved and the endometrium excised then the uterus is acutely anteverted and sutured to the anterior vaginal wall.[26]

Most contemporary studies of anterior vaginal reconstruction are observational studies with inadequate follow-up that suffer from lack of standardized definitions and measurements of outcome, with resultant bias. Are the defects described found in the clinic setting or under anesthesia? The discrepancy in findings can be large. Anterior compartment defects usually occur in association with other pelvic support defects requiring repair; isolated defects are rather rare. What works very well in one surgeon's hands may be a failure in another's, as a result of subtle and sometimes unrecognized

modifications in technique. Many patients have had more than one operation at presentation and some have had as many as four previous procedures.[18] Shull's data on sacrospinous ligament suspension indicate that some patients underwent as many as six different transvaginal pelvic reconstructive procedures concomitantly.[27] This results in a tangle of potential combinations of surgical procedures that varies with the training and expertise of the surgeons involved. Weber and Walters have attempted to summarize this data in table format reporting recurrence rates after various surgical procedures used for anterior vaginal wall prolapse.[4] (Table 12.1)

Summary

Isolated pelvic support defects are very rare. Separate discussion of anterior colporrhaphy should not lead the reader to consider this operation in isolation, but rather as one of a number of different procedures that may be used together to address the surgical reconstruction of the female pelvis as a single functional unit. The clinician must evaluate all aspects of pelvic support prior to undertaking surgical repair and should attempt to identify and address all support defects simultaneously. Anterior colporrhaphy in its many guises is primarily an operation to correct symptomatic anterior vaginal wall prolapse. Its role in the treatment of stress incontinence is limited (if not anachronistic).

Vaginal and Abdominal Paravaginal Repair

Alfred E. Bent and Aileen M.K. Yee

The standard surgical approach to the cystocele has been the anterior colporrhaphy with the reported recurrence rate of 45–49%.[28,29] More recently Richardson[30] has brought attention to the paravaginal repair which was first described by White in 1909.[1] The paravaginal repair forces the pelvic surgeon to re-examine the paradigm of anterior compartment support and to be more attentive to accurate diagnosis of site-specific defects with the overall goal of restoring normal anatomy and function

Indications

The bladder is supported by a hammock of endopelvic fascia attached laterally to the pelvic sidewall at the arcus tendineus fascia pelvis, otherwise

Table 12.1. Reported recurrence after different surgical procedures for anterior vaginal prolapse (adapted from Weber and Walters[4])

Author		Recurrence	Follow-up (years)
Anterior colporrhaphy			
Goff	Vaginal flap	2/55 (4%)	1–8
Goff	Vaginal excision	2/31 (6%)	1–8
Moore		0/9	0.5–1.5
Friedman		0/4	2–4
Stanton		8/54 (15%)	up to 2
Macer		22/109 (20%)	5–20
Walter		0/86	1–2.5 (average 1.2)
Porges		10/388 (3%)	1–20 (average 2.6)
Anterior colporrhaphy with sacrospinous ligament suspension			
Morley		16/71 (22%)	1–11 (average 4.3)
Shull		20/81 (25%)	2–5
Holley		33/66 (92%)	1.2–6.6
Abdominal cystocele repair			
Masters		0/25	1–3.5
Speirs		2/40 (5%)	up to 4
Macer		6/76 (8%)	5–20
Weinberg		0/96	2–10
Rosing		0/9	up to 4
Retropubic paravaginal repair			
Goetsch		1/7 (14%)	up to 2
Richardson		2/60 (3%)	0.25–4 (average 1.7)
Shull		8/149 (5%)	0.5–4
Richardson		10/213 (5%)	2–8
Bladder needle suspension			
Gardy		3/58 (5%)	0.75–5 (average 2)
Raz		2/107 (2%)	0.5–5 (average 2)
Raz		5/50 (10%)	0.5–5.3 (average 2.8)
Miyazaki		13/22 (59%)	3.5–4
Sadoughi		1/26 (4%)	0.5–3 (average 1.25)
Vaginal paravaginal repair			
Shull		4/56 (7%)	0.1–5.6 (average 1.6)

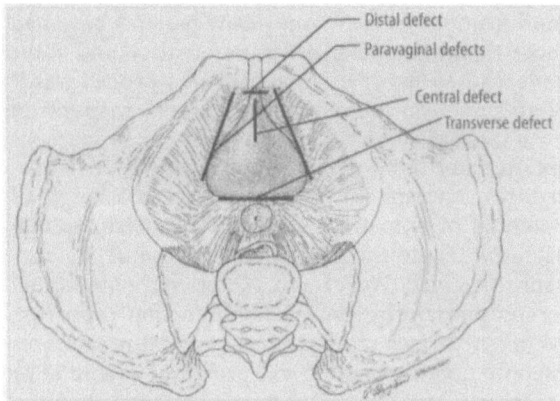

Figure 12.11 Four sites where anterior wall defects may occur. From Richardson AC. Paravaginal repair. In: Gershenson DM, AronsonMP (ed). *Operative Techniques in Gynecological Surgery*. W.B. Saunders, Philadelphia, p. 70, 1996, with permission.

known as the white line.[30] The paravaginal repair is indicated for the repair of a cystocele that has developed as a result of a detachment of the anterior pubocervical fascia from the white line. The cephalad support of this hammock is the pericervical ring. The uterosacral and cardinal ligaments also come together at the pericervical ring. Distally the hammock is attached to the urogenital diaphragm. A central defect occurs if there is a break or attenuation of the pubocervical hammock itself (Fig. 12.11). It is in this population that the traditional anterior colporrhaphy is indicated. The most commonly observed fascial defect is the lateral or paravaginal defect accounting for 75–85% of cystoceles.[31,32] The

paravaginal defect is unilateral in 53–75% and bilateral in 25–47%.[30,33,34] If unilateral defects are found, the majority will be right unilateral defects.[30,34] It is hypothesized that the sigmoid colon is of some protective value in making isolated left lateral defects less likely. When combined defects of anterior endopelvic fascia exists, surgical procedures specific to each defect must be performed in order to properly address all facets of the cystocele.

Clinically if there is descent of the anterior vaginal wall accentuated when the patient performs a Valsalva maneuver, a cystocele is present. The job of the pelvic surgeon is to diagnose the specific defect in the endopelvic support. With the patient in lithotomy position, the open arms of a ring forceps or Baden vaginal wall analyzer are placed in the lateral vaginal fornices mimicking the anatomical path of the white line. The anterior wall is gently supported as the patient is asked to perform a Valsalva maneuver. If the cystocele is thus reduced, the patient has a paravaginal defect (Fig. 12.12). Unilateral paravaginal defects can be identified by supporting one lateral fornix at a time. If support to that side effectively reduces the cystocele, the fascial detachment is said to predominate from that side. Likewise the ring forceps can be placed along the midline of the anterior vaginal wall and gentle elevation applied. With lateral cystoceles, the prolapsed tissue will bulge around the midline support, whereas central defect will be reduced. The rugation of the anterior vaginal mucosa persists in lateral cystoceles. The vaginal mucosa overlying the cystocele that result from central defects or detachment from the pericervical ring is smoother in appearance.

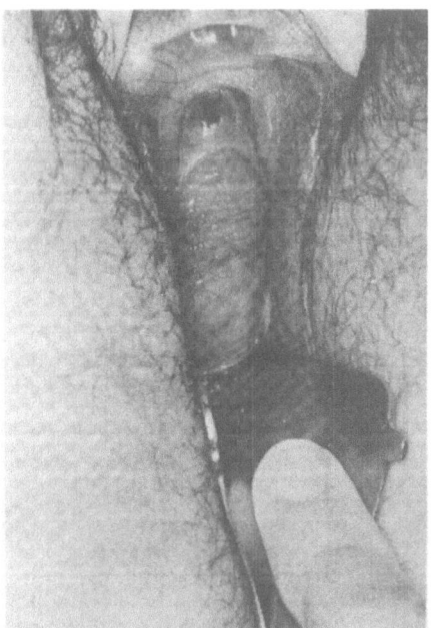

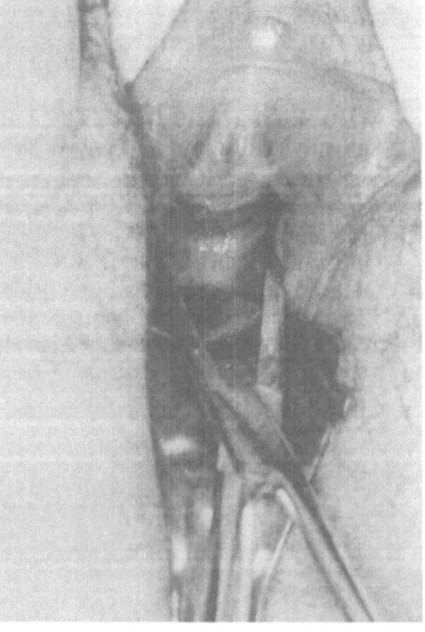

Figure 12.12 Clinical assessment of a patient for a paravaginal defect. **a** As the patient performs a Valsalva maneuver, an anterior defect is identified. Note that the rotation of the anterior vaginal wall is apparent. **b** Gentle upward traction with a ring forceps applied along the path of the fascial white line restores normal anatomy to the anterior compartment. From: Shull BL Clinical evaluation of women with pelvic support defects. *Clin Obstet Gynecol* 1993;36(4):945, with permission.

The paravaginal repair should not be considered as an anti-incontinence procedure. Although there are several retrospective studies that quote 92–97%[30,35] of patients achieving a satisfactory degree of continence, Colombo in the only published randomized prospective study reports objective cure rates of 61%.[36]

Technique

The paravaginal repair can be accomplished via any route in which the retropubic space can be accessed. The paravaginal repair has been described via the open, laparoscopic, and vaginal approaches. The route of repair is dictated by other concomitant procedures, patient factors, (i.e. body habitus, previous surgeries, and overall health) as well as the surgeon's experience.

Open Paravaginal Repair

At the start of the surgery, a Foley catheter is placed to drain the bladder and to aid in the identification of the urethrovesical junction. The skin and fascial incision is based on other concomitant surgical procedures. If the paravaginal repair is the only procedure to be performed, it can be accomplished through a Pfannenstiel or mini-lap incision. The bellies of the rectus muscles are divided at midline and the retropubic space is developed. Using blunt dissection the index and middle finger are swept along the inferior aspect of the superior pubic rami. The obturator notch and neurovascular bundles should be identified (Fig. 12.13). Dissection into the space of Retzius should be medial to this landmark.

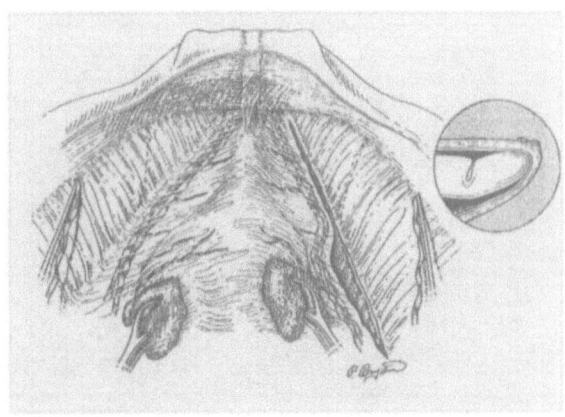

Figure 12.14 Once the space of Retzius is developed, gentle medial retraction of the bladder aids in the identification of the fascial white line defect. Engorged vessels often exist along the lateral vaginal fornices. From: Richardson AC. Paravaginal repair. In: Gershenson DM, Aronson MP (ed). *Operative Techniques in Gynecological Surgery.* WB Saunders, Philadelphia, 1996 p. 71, with permission.

The ischial spine is a key landmark as the white line originates from this point. A self-retaining retractor can then be placed. If a mini-lap incision is used, a curved Deaver or malleable retractor can be used to gain access. In addition long instruments and either a lighted suction irrigator or head lamp may be helpful. The surgeon's nondominant hand is placed in the vagina to elevate and to put on stretch the detached remnants of the pubocervical fascial attachment. The preperitoneal fat should be bluntly swept aside until the break in the fascial white line is identified (Fig. 12.14). Often engorged vessels will be encountered in the lateral vaginal fornices. The fascial white line can be split such that remnants

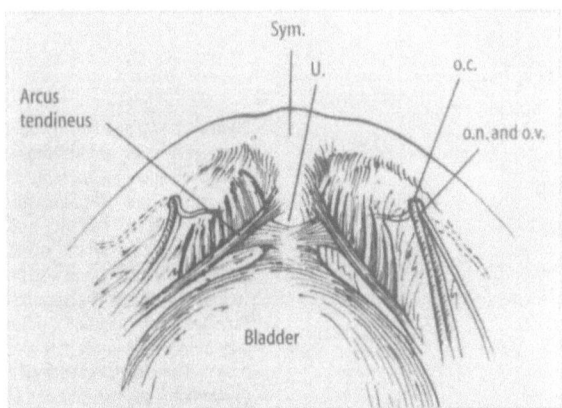

Figure 12.13 The arcus tendineus extends from the inferior margin of the pubic symphyasis (sym) to the ischial spine and is inferior to the path of the obturator nerve and vessels. o.c., obturator canal; o.n., obturator nerve; o.v., obturator vessels; u, urethra. From: Pillai-Allen A, Benson IT. Cystocele. In: Brubaker LT, Saclarides TI (ed) *Female Pelvic Floor: Disorders of Function and Support.* FA Davis, Philadelphia, 1996 p. 272, with permission.

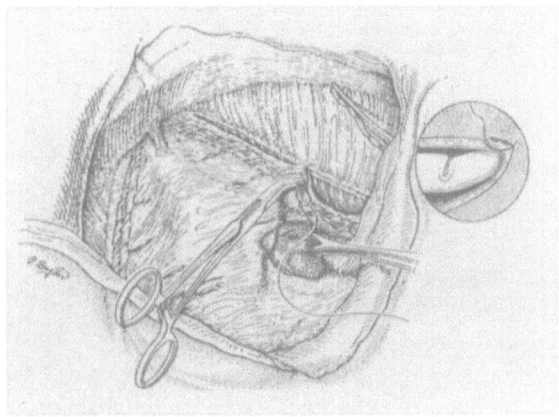

Figure 12.15 With the surgeon's nondominant hand in the vagina, the pubocervical fascia can be elevated to its proper anatomical position. The vaginal stitch should incorporate the pubocervical fascia and vaginal muscularis but be short of the vaginal mucosa. Prominent vessels in the lateral fornices should be either avoided or encircled. The suture is then passed through the condensation of the obturator internus fascia that marks the detachment of the white line. From: Richardson AC. Paravaginal repair. In: Gershenson DM, Aronson MP (ed). *Operative Techniques in Gynecological Surgery.* WB Saunders, Philadelphia, 1996, p. 72, with permission.

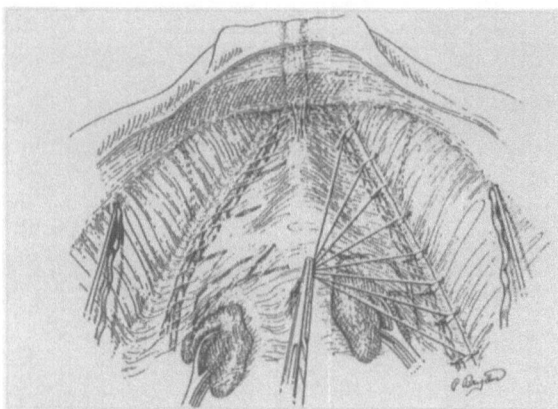

Figure 12.16 The first stitch is typically placed 1 cm distal to the ischial spine. Each subsequent suture is 1 cm distal to the previous. The repair is complete when the white line is reattached along its entire length. From: Richardson AC. Paravaginal repair. In: Gershenson DM, Aronson MP (ed). Operative Techniques in Gynecological Surgery. WB Saunders, Philadelphia, 1996, p. 72, with permission.

exist on both the pelvic sidewall and the pubocervical fascia of the vagina. The white line can also exist entirely on the pelvic sidewall or entirely on the vaginal side. In the latter instance, it may be difficult to judge where the pelvic side wall sutures should be placed. One then needs to keep in mind that anatomically the white line runs from the ischial spine to the pubic symphysis. The assistant helps retract the bladder medially. Permanent sutures are utilized. The first suture is placed along the pelvic sidewall through the white line at or approximately 1 cm distal to the ischial spine. The vaginal finger may be moved medially to better expose the white line. With a finger elevating the vaginal tissues, the bladder is gently swept medial to expose the glistening pubocervical fascia. The suture is then passed through the lateral edge of the pubocervical fascia at its most cephalad point (Figure 12.15). Each subsequent suture is placed 1 cm distal to the previous (Fig. 12.16). The stitch at the level of the urethrovesical junction is described by Richardson as the

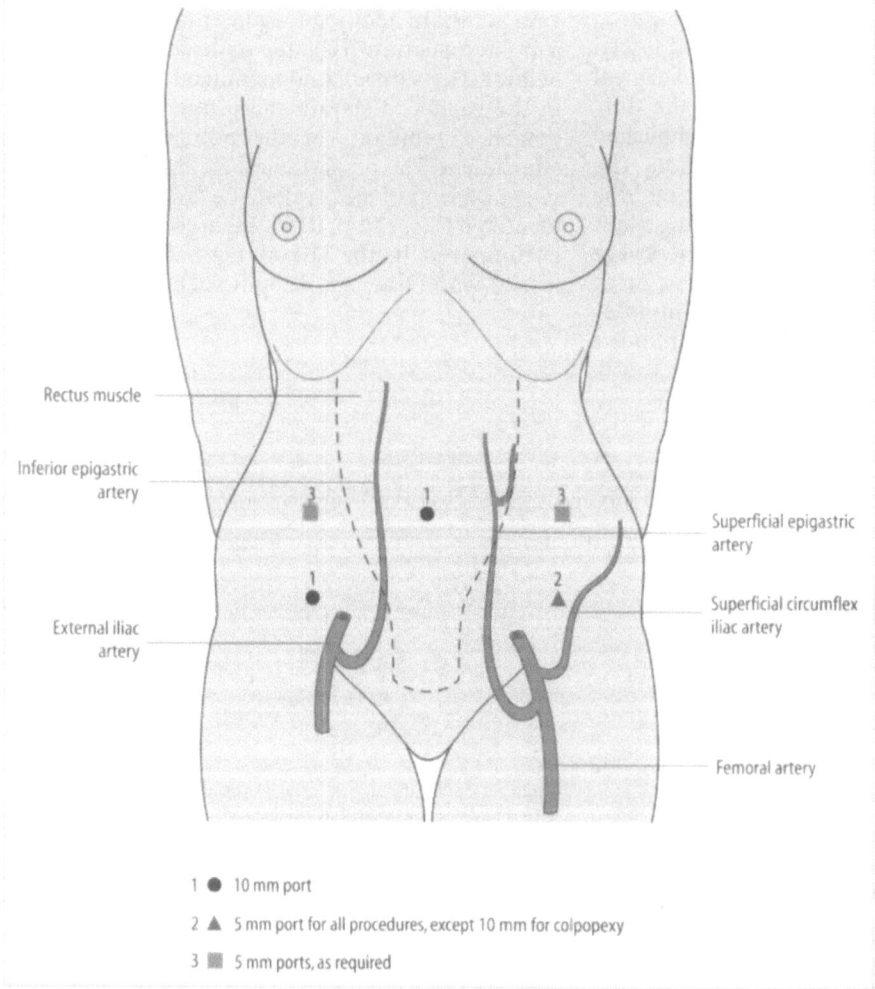

Rectus muscle

Inferior epigastric artery

Superficial epigastric artery

Superficial circumflex iliac artery

External iliac artery

Femoral artery

1 ● 10 mm port

2 ▲ 5 mm port for all procedures, except 10 mm for colpopexy

3 ■ 5 mm ports, as required

Figure 12.17 For a laparoscopic paravaginal repair, an infraumbilical and left and right lower quadrant ports are needed. The infraumbilical port is 10 mm in diameter. One of the other lower quadrant ports must also be 10 mm in diameter to accommodate the needle. Additional ports may be needed on the left and right mid-abdomen, especially if a concomitant vault suspension is performed. The additional ports are 5 mm in diameter. From: Hurd WW et al. The location of abdominal wall blood vessels in relationship to abdominal landmarks apparent at laparoscopy. *Am J Obstet Gynecol* 1994; 171: 642–6, with permission.

"key stitch" and serves to stabilize the bladder neck.[30] Cystoscopy is performed at the completion of the paravaginal repair to verify that the bladder mucosa is intact and free of inadvertently placed sutures, and that both ureters are patent. Drains are not needed in the retropubic space. Normal voiding typically occurs within the first postoperative day.[33]

Laparoscopic Paravaginal Route

The paravaginal repair can be accomplished laparoscopically. The retropubic space can be entered via the extraperitoneal route using a laparoscopic balloon or via the intraperitoneal route. The intraperitoneal route allows for other pelvic defects to be concomitantly addressed. A three-way Foley catheter is inserted at the start of the case. Trocars are introduced infraumbilically, at the left and right lower quadrants. Ten millimeter trocars are utilized at the infraumbilical and midline ports in order to accommodate the laparoscope. In addition, one of the lower quadrant ports also should be 10 mm in diameter in order to accommodate the needle (Fig. 12.17). For the intraperitoneal route, the bladder is filled to 250 ml to delineate the bladder dome. The peritoneum is incised just cephalad to the bladder dome and extended laterally to or just beyond the obliterated umbilical vein. The bladder is then drained and the retropubic space is developed using blunt and sharp dissection. A 2.0 Ethibond (Ethicon, NJ) suture on an SH needle passes easily down the 10 mm port. Identify the ischial spine with the vaginal finger. Suturing the pubocervical fascia and white line may be accomplished from either side. It is often easier to suture the pubocervical fascia from a port on the contralateral side and to approach the bite along the pelvic side wall from the ipsilateral port. When suturing the white line, move the vaginal finger medially to open access into the paravaginal space. When suturing the pubocervical fasica, firmly extend the vaginal finger superiorly and cephalad. An endokitner may be utilized to mobilize the bladder medial and to expose the pubocervial fascia. As in the open paravaginal repair, each subsequent suture is placed 1 cm distal to the previous.

Vaginal Paravaginal Repair

A marking suture is placed bilaterally along the lateral fornices at the level of the urethrovesical junction and at the vaginal apex if a hysterectomy has previously been performed. A midline incision on the anterior vaginal mucosa is made from vaginal apex to 1 cm distal to the urethrovesical junction. The vaginal mucosa is bluntly dissected off the

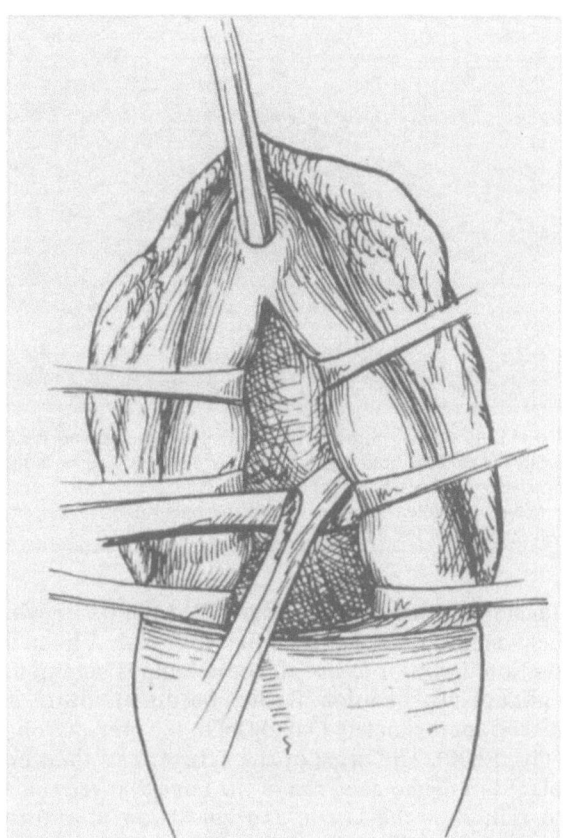

Figure 12.18 In the vaginal paravaginal repair, a midline incision is made from the vaginal apex to approximately 1 cm distal to the urethra meatus. The vaginal mucosa is dissected off the anterior pubocervical fascia. Remnants of pubocervical fascia to the white line are also dissected free and the retropubic space entered. From: Pillai-Ailen A, Benson IT. Cystocele. In: Brubaker LT, Saclarides TI (ed) *Female Pelvic Floor: Disorders of Function and Support.* FA Davis, Philadelphia, 1996, p. 272, with permission.

bladder and supporting pubocervical fascia. The dissection is carried out to the lateral vaginal fornix (Fig. 12.18). A Lone Star self-retaining retractor (model 3307, Lone Star Medical Products, Houston, TX) can be used to retract the vaginal mucosa. The retropubic space is entered at the level of the urethrovesical junction. The remnant of the attached pubocervical fascia is bluntly taken to the white line down to its origin at the ischial spine. Once the retropubic space has been entered, the obturator notch and neurovascular bundle can be palpated (Fig. 12.19). Damage to the obturator neurovascular bundle can occur if retractors in the retropubic space are allowed to drift too far ventrally. The pudendal vessels and nerves pass 1 cm lateral to the spine and can also be potentially damaged by overzealous dissection of the white line at its origin. A Breisky Navratil retractor is placed in the enlarged paravaginal defect. A suture is passed through the white line and obturator fascia with the first suture approximately 1 cm distal to the spine.

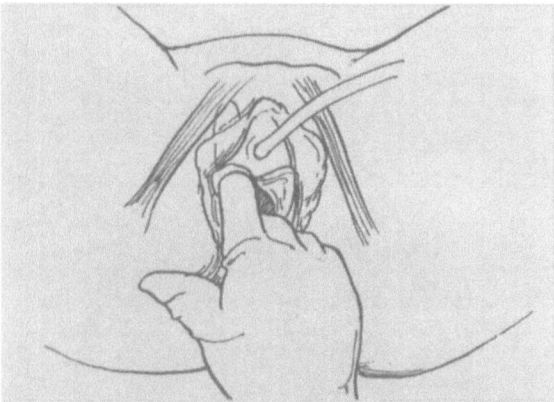

Figure 12.19 Once the space of Retzius is entered, the obturator notch is palpated. The obturator notch and neurovascular bundle is superior to the detached remnants of the fascial white line. From: Pillai-Allen A, Benson IT. Cystocele. In: Brubaker LT, Saclarides TI (ed) *Female Pelvic Floor: Disorders of Function and Support.* FA Davis, Philadelphia, 1996, p. 272, with permission.

Tension on this suture placed 90° to the tissue will help delineate the course of the white line. A lighted suction/ irrigator or use of a head lamp is helpful to enhance visualization. Each subsequent suture is placed approximately 1 cm distal to the previous one (Fig. 12.20). The arms of the sutures can then be placed in the notched rim of the Lone Star retractor to minimize the tangle and confusion of suture arms. Once all the sutures along the white line of the pelvic sidewall have been placed, the sutures are then passed through the lateral edge of pubocervical fascia and then through the vaginal wall just short of the mucosa. The marking sutures at the apex and urethrovesical junction are helpful in reattaching the vaginal mucosa appropriately.

Because of the potential neurological and structural damage that may occur in breaking down the pubocervial fascia remants,[37] we have utilized a modified approach to the vaginal paravaginal repair. The vaginal mucosa is disected off the pubocervical fascia and the paravaginal defect is exposed. Without breaking through the attachment of the pubocervical remnant to the white line, a bite is taken along the obturator fascia and white line at the point where the pubocervical fascia remnants attaches to the pelvic side wall. Intact pubocervial fascia is identified and the suture is then passed through the lateral margins. Acting as a natural mesh, cadaveric fascia or Alloderm (Life Cell Corp., Woodlands, TX) is also incorporated into the repair, reinforcing the pubocervical hammock. A trapezoid piece of Alloderm is suspended in sterile saline and dyed suture is passed though the four corners to aid in handling of the tissue. The mesh is oriented such that the base of the trapezoid is the most cephalad. The suture is then passed through the edges of the mesh and then through the vaginal wall just short of the mucosa. The base of the mesh is also attached to the pubocervial fascial ring. As in all paravaginal repairs, the most cephalad stitch is placed 1 cm from the ischial spine and each subsequent suture is placed 1 cm distal to the previous one. It is often easier to complete passing all of the sutures through one side of the pelvic side wall and pubocervical fascia before incorporating the mesh (Figs 12.21, 12.22).

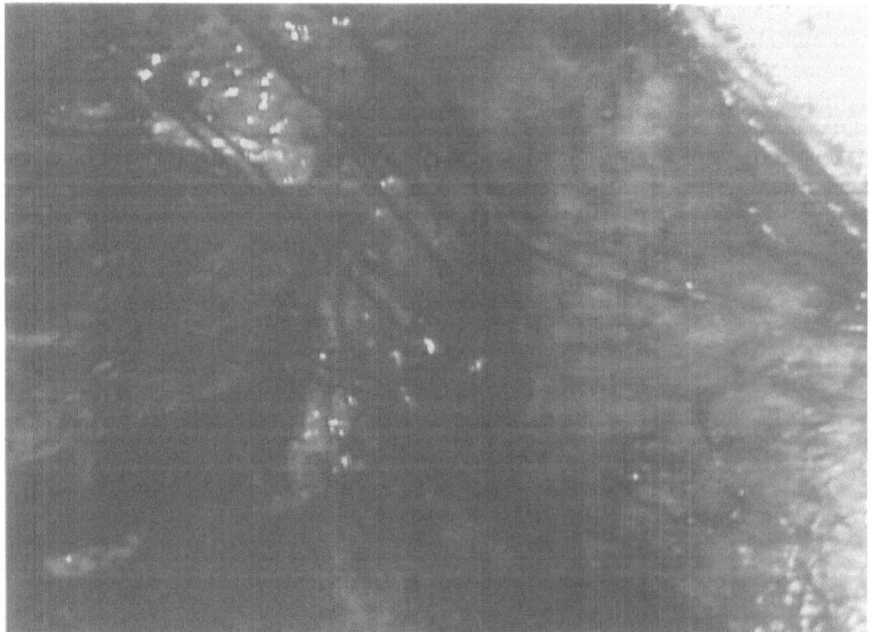

Figure 12.20 Permanent suture is passed through the obturator internus fascia at the level of the detached white line, through the edge of the anterior pubocervical fascia. The vaginal wall is then incorporated. The sutures are placed along the length of the fascial white line spaced at 1cm intervals.

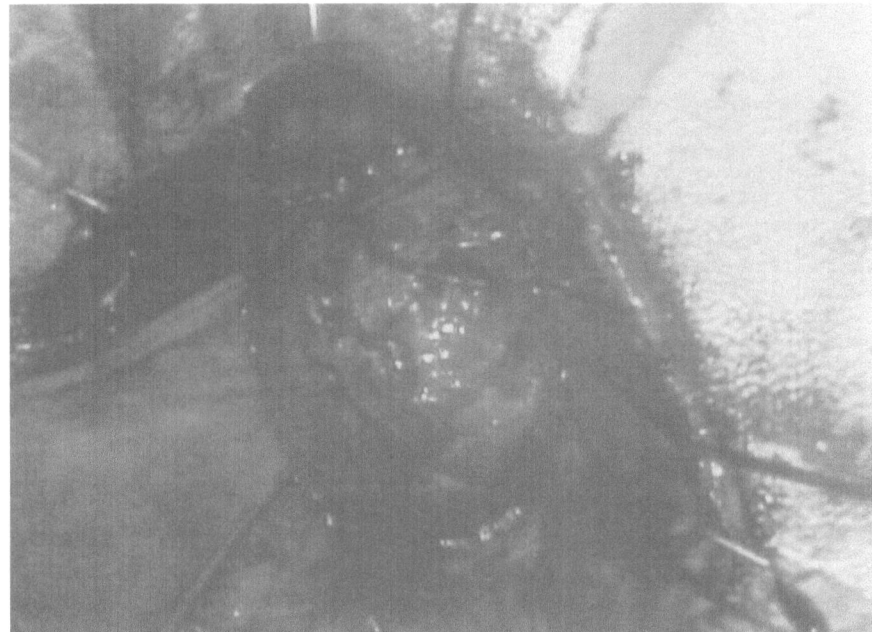

Figure 12.21 In a modified technique of the vaginal paravaginal repair, the pubocervical remnants are not detached from the white line. Permanent suture is used to approximate the white line defect but, in addition, a piece of donor fascia is incorporated in the repair.

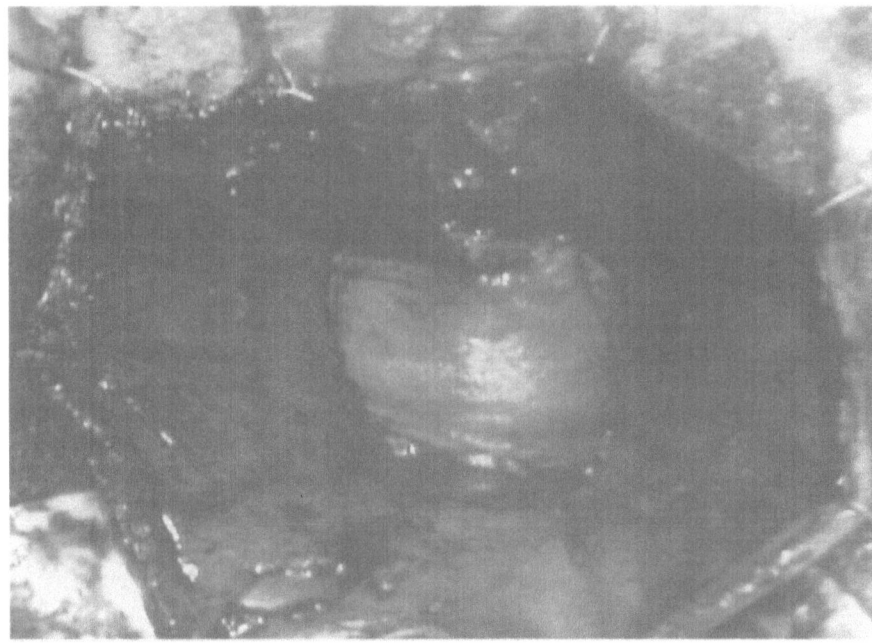

Figure 12.22 The donor fascia is attached bilaterally to the white line and provides additional support to the existing pubocervical fascia. The vaginal muscularis layer is then also incorporated.

Complications

In gaining access into the retropubic space, the obturator neurovascualr bundle exists ventral to the white line. Dissection should be limited to the medial aspect of the obturator neurovascular bundle. Anatomically there are few structures along the pelvic side wall portion of the white line that contribute to complications. Cadaver dissection of tissues underlying and adjacent to the white line reveals that there are no neurovascular structures along the white line, obturator fascia, or levators that precludes taking a full bite of tissue.[38] Prominent vessels typically exist along the lateral vaginal sulcus. Good surgical technique should be utilized in exposure and placement of sutures in the lateral margins of the pubocervical fascia. In performing

Table 12.2. Complications

Author	N	Route	Other procedures	Follow-up (months) Mean	Range	Time to normal voiding	De-novo DI (%)	Other area of prolapse	Infection	Transfusion	Other complications
Richardson[30]	60	Abd.[a]	Yes	20	3–48	93% by 3 days	0	–	–	–	
Richardson[33]	283	Abd.	Yes	–	48–96	73% on day of surgery, 100% prior to discharge	0	–	<6%	0%	
Shull[35]	149	Abd.	Yes	–	98%>6mo 80%>18mo 62%>30mo 49%>48mo	4 days(mean time to void)	6	5% enterocele Pulm. emboli 1.3% 6 % cuff prolapse	2 % wound infection 11 % cystitis		
Colombo[36]	18	Abd.	No	28	12–36	94% prior to discharge	0	0% enterocele 0% rectocele	–	0%	–
Ostrzenski[34]	28	Lsc.[b]	No		minimum 24	100% on day of surgery	–	–	0%	0%	–
Shull[15]	63	Vag.[c]	Yes	19.2	1.5–63.2	–		2% cuff 7% enterocele	4% pneumonia 2% cystitis	0%	Transient femoral N. paresis 1.6% exacerbation of sciatica 1.6%

Abd., abdominal; Lsc., laparoscopic; Vag., vaginal.

the vaginal paravaginal repair, blunt dissection through the lateral remnants of the pubocervical attachments may disrupt these vessels. Identification and ligation of these vessels may be required. Cystoscopy is recommended to verify that no permanent sutures compromise the bladder or ureter. Kinking of the ureter is less likely as the sutures on the pubocervical fascia are more lateral when compared to the Burch or Marshall–Marchetti–Krantz procedure.

Unlike procedures that create a compensatory distortion of normal anatomy, the paravaginal repair typically does not lead to postoperative problems of de-novo detrusor instability or long-term urinary retention. Published data reporting objective outcomes and complications of the paravaginal repair are scarce. A review of the literature revealed several articles that comment on complications (Table 12.2). Shull reports a de-novo detrusor instability rate of 6%. However, he performed concomitant surgeries along with the paravaginal repair, including anterior wedge resections. In addition, a modified paravaginal repair was performed where the suture arms were passed through the ileopectineal (Cooper's) ligament after the white line was reapproximated.[15] There have been no reports of prolonged urinary retention or obstruction following a paravaginal repair.[15,30,33,34,36] The vast majority void adequately within the first postoperative day, making a suprapubic catheter unnecessary.[33]

The Burch procedure is known to carry a 10% risk of a subsequent enterocele.[13] As the paravaginal repair restores normal anatomy, theoretically the risk of developing an enterocele or cuff prolapse should not be significantly increased above its baseline incidence. Three articles report that subsequent development of an enterocele and vaginal cuff prolapse is 5–7% and 0–7% respectively.[15,35,36] Colombo did not have any enteroceles develop after a paravaginal repair, but a prophylactic culdoplasty was performed if the surgeon felt it was warranted.

Results

Much of the data regarding the paravaginal repair focuses on the correction of stress urinary incontinence rather than the resolution of anterior vaginal vault prolapse as the outcome measure. Although there are several retrospective and prospective studies that report the failure rate of the paravaginal repair as anti-incontinence procedure to be 0–7%,[30,33,34] the only prospective randomized study comparing the paravaginal repair to the Burch shows the objective cure rate for the paravaginal repair to be 61% vs. 100% for the Burch procedure (Table 12.3).[36] An isolated paravaginal repair is not recommended as a procedure for stress incontinence.

The recurrence rate for a cystocele is reported to be 5–50%. This rate may be a function of route of surgery with greater recurrence rates following a vaginal paravaginal repair. Caputo reports that in a series of 60 patients in whom a vaginal paravaginal repair was performed, 50% had recurrence of anterior vaginal wall prolapse.[39] The majority of the recurrent cystoceles, however, were central in nature. The authors surmise that the recurrent cystocele was a result of neurological damage that may have occurred in the dissection needed to perform the repair from the vaginal route. The structural as well as vascular integrity of the pubocervical fascial hammock may likewise be compromised in the dissection.

References

1. White GR (1909) Cystocele. JAMA 853: 1707–10.
2. Kelly HA (1913) Incontinence of urine in women. Urol Cutan Rev 17: 291.
3. Kennedy WT (1937) Incontinence of urine in the female, the urethral sphincter mechanism, damage of function, and restoration of control. Am J Obstet Gynecol 34: 576–89.

Table 12.3. Outcome (all figures are percentages)

Author	Subjective cure of stress incontinence			Objective cure of stress incontinence	Return of cystocele
	Cured	Satisfaction improved	Failed		
Richardson[30]	83	8.3	3	–	–
Richardson[33]	81	6.4	4	–	–
Shull[35]	–	–	3	–	5.4
Colombo[36]	72	6	22	61	39
Ostrzenski[34]	–	–	–	93	–
Shull[15]	–	–	–	–	12.5 (cystourethrocele) 27 (cystocele)

Abd., abdominal; Lsc., laparoscopic; Vag., vaginal

4. Weber AM, Walters MD (1997) Anterior vaginal prolapse: review of anatomy and techniques of surgical repair. Obstet Gynecol 89: 311–18.
5. Fantl JA, Newman DK, Colling J et al. (1996) Urinary Incontinence in Adults: Acute and chronic management. Clinical Practice Guideline, no. 2. AHCPR publication no. 96–0682. US Department of Health and Human Services, Public Health Service, Agency for Health Care Policy and Research, Rockville, MD.
6. Richardson AC (1996) Paravaginal repair. Oper Tech Gynecol Surg 1: 66–75.
7. Delancey JOL (1992) Anatomic aspects of vaginal eversion after hysterectomy. Am J Obstet Gynecol 166: 1717–28.
8. Derry DE (1907) On the real nature of the so-called "pelvic fascia." J Anat 42: 7–11.
9. Norton PA (1993) Pelvic floor disorders: The role of fascia and ligaments. Clin Obstet Gynecol 36: 926–38.
10. Smith ARB, Hosker GL, Warrell DW (1989) The role of partial denervation of the pelvic floor in the aetiology of genitourinary prolapse and stress incontinence of urine. A neurophysiological study. Br J Obstet Gynaecol 96: 24–8.
11. Wilkins LM, Watson SR, Prosky SJ et al. (1994) Development of a bilayered living skin construct for clinical applications. Biotechnol Bioeng 43: 747–56.
12. Zivkovic F, Tamussino K, George R et al. (1996) Long-term effects of vaginal dissection on the innervation of the striated urethral sphincter. Obstet Gynecol 87: 257–60.
13. Burch J (1961) Urethrovaginal fixation to Cooper's ligament for correction of stress urinary incontinence, cystocele and prolapse. Am J Obstet Gynecol 81: 281–90.
14. Wheeless CR, Wharton LR, Dorsey JH et al. (1977) The Goebell-Stoeckel operation for universal cases of urinary incontinence. Am J Obstet Gynecol 128: 546–9.
15. Shull BL, Benn SJ, Kuehl TJ (1994) Surgical management of prolapse of the anterior vaginal segment: An analysis of support defects, operative morbidity, and anatomic outcome. Am J Obstet Gynecol 171: 1429–39.
16. Podratz KC (1998) Gynecologic surgery: An imperiled ballet. Am J Obstet Gynecol 178: 1229–34.
17. Morley GW, Delancey JOL (1988) Sacrospinous ligament fixation for eversion of the vagina. Am J Obstet Gynecol 158: 872–81.
18. Zacharin RF (1992) Free full-thickness vaginal epithelium graft in correction of recurrent genital prolapse. Aust N Z J Obstet Gynaecol 32: 146–8.
19. Julian TM (1996) The efficacy of Marlex mesh in the repair of severe, recurrent vaginal prolapse of the anterior mid-vaginal wall. Am J Obstet Gynecol 175: 1472–75.
20. Wall LL, Copas P, Galloway NTM (1996) A pedicled rectus abdominis muscle-flap sling for the treatment of complicated stress urinary incontinence. Am J Obstet Gynecol 175: 1460–6.
21. Symmonds RE (1969) Loss of the urethral floor with total urinary incontinence: a technique for urethral reconstruction. Am J Obstet Gynecol 103: 665.
22. Chesson RR, Schlossberg SM, Elkins TE et al. (1999) The use of fascia lata graft for correction of severe or recurrent anterior vaginal wall defects. J Pelvic Surg 5: 96–103.
23. Wall LL, Versi E, Norton PA, Bump RC (1998) Evaluating the outcome of surgery for pelvic organ prolapse. Am J Obstet Gynecol 178: 877–9.
24. Fothergill WE (1915) Anterior colporrhaphy and its combination with amputation of the cervix as a single operation. J Obstet Gynaecol Br Emp 27: 146–7.
25. Watkins TJ (1906) Treatment of cases of extensive cystocele and uterine prolapse. Surg Gynecol Obstet 2: 659–67.
26. Nichols DH, Randall CL (1996) Vaginal Surgery, 4th ed. Williams & Wilkins, Baltimore, Md., pp. 458.
27. Shull BL, Capen CV, Riggs MW et al. (1992) Preoperative and postoperative analysis of site-specific pelvic support defects in 81 women treated with sacrospinous ligament suspension and pelvic reconstruction. Am J Obstet Gynecol 166: 1764–71.
28. Baden WF, Walker T (1987) Urinary stress incontinence: Evaluation of the paravaginal repair. Fem Patient 2: 89
29. Stanton SL, Tanagho EA (1980) Preface. In: Stanton SL, Tanagho EA (eds) Surgery of Female Incontinence. Springer, New York.
30. Richardson AC, Lyons JB, Williams NL (1976) A new look at pelvic relaxation. Am J Obstet Gynecol 126: 568.
31. Richardson AC (1992) Cystocele: paravaginal repair. In Benson JT (Ed). Female pelvic floor disorders: investigation and management. Norton Medical Books, New York, pp. 280–287.
32. Youngblood JP (1993) Paravaginal repair for cystourethrocele. Clin Obstet Gynecol 36(4): 960–6.
33. Richardson AC, Edmonds PB, Williams NL (1981) Treatment of stress urinary incontinence due to paravaginal fascial defect. Obstet Gynecol 57: 357–62.
34. Ostrzenski A (1998) Genuine stress urinary incontinence in women: New laparoscopic paravaginal reconstruction. J Reprod Med 43: 477–82.
35. Shull BL, Baden WF (1989) A six-year experience with paravaginal defect repair for stress urinary incontinence. Am J Obstet Gynecol 160: 1432–40.
36. Colombo M, Milani R, Vitobello D, Maggioni A (1996) A randomized comparison of burch colposuspension and abdominal paravaginal defect repair for female stress urinary incontinence. Am J Obstet Gynecol 175: 78–84.
37. Benson JT, McClellan E (1993) The effect of vaginal disection on the pudendal nerve. Obstet Gynecol 82: 387.
38. Scotti RJ, Garely AD, Greston WM, Flora RF, Olson TR (1998) Paravaginal repair of lateral vaginal wall defects by fixation to the ischial periosteum and obturator membrane. Am J Obstet Gynecol 179: 1436–45.
39. Caputo RM, Benson JT (1993) Vaginal paravaginal repair with mesh placement for cystocele. American Urogynecologic Society Annual Meeting, 1993, San Antonio, TX.

13 Middle Compartment

Endofascial Reconstruction of Vaginal Vault Prolapse: the Levator Myorraphy

Gary E. Lemack and Philippe E. Zimmern

Proper repair of vaginal vault prolapse, whether occurring in conjunction with uterine prolapse or years after hysterectomy, will restore vaginal position, axis, and function. Conservative measures, such as pessaries or colpocleisis may be useful in a small subset of women who are not surgical candidates, but are not likely to be appropriate in most active women presenting for evaluation. Surgical procedures offer the best hope of a permanent correction, and several techniques have been described, both abdominal and vaginal.[1,2]

Vaginal approaches offer the advantage of minimizing postoperative pain, and reducing the morbidity

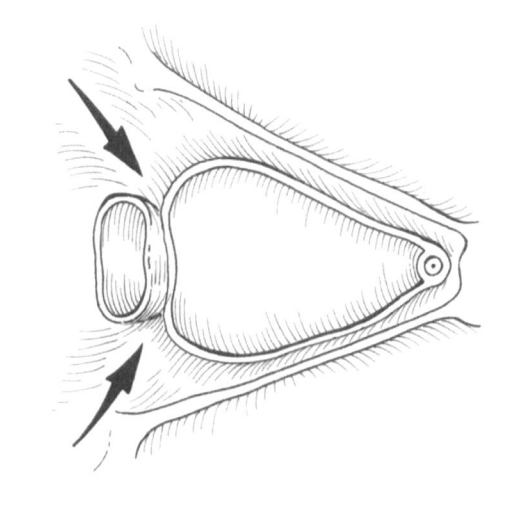

Figure 13.1 Transverse image through normal vagina. Arrows denote edges of levator fascia which weaken with prolapse, and which are joined across the midline to anchor the vagina during repair.

associated with open abdominal procedures, while being equally efficacious. Though several authors have advocated sacrospinalis fixation,[3,4] we feel that the inherent dangers associated with possible damage to the adjacent vascular and neural structures make it a less favored approach. Additionally, the altered vaginal axis, and well-described risk of secondary cystocele formation, caused us to search for an alternative approach. For these reasons, one of the authors (PZ), 10 years ago, developed a straightforward technique of using the levator shelf to both recreate the pelvic floor and to anchor the upper vagina (Fig. 13.1), and we have been using it for vault repair and prevention of enterocele recurrence since that time. The principles of this repair are based on an understanding of defects in the pelvic floor that have been addressed in previously described abdominal levator repairs for incontinence.[5]

Preoperative Evaluation

After performing a thorough history (with particular attention to previous attempts at repair) and physical examination, urinalysis, noninvasive flow rate, and postvoid residual tests are performed. It is currently our practice to perform urodynamics both with and then without a vaginal pack to reduce the associated cystocele which is frequently present. Although there is still controversy over the role of urodynamics in this situation, recent evidence suggests that correction of the prolapse during urodynamics, whether with vaginal pack or pessary, may affect both pressure–flow relationship during

voiding and the presence or absence of incontinence during testing.[6] This information may be helpful with further surgical decision making at the time of repair.

Since physical examination in the supine position may underestimate the degree of prolapse present (Fig. 13.2), we always obtain a standing voiding cystourethrogram (VCUG) before proceeding with surgical correction. This study is performed largely from a lateral view both with and without straining, and with and without a Foley catheter.[7] The VCUG gives information about the presence and extent (central and/or lateral defects) of cystocele, degree of urethral hypermobility, amount of postvoid residual, presence of bladder wall damage, and presence or absence of vesico-ureteral reflux. We also obtain a renal sonogram to assess for upper tract dilation that could be caused by exteriorization of a ureterovesical junction associated with a large cystocele. If hydronephrosis is present we usually obtain an intravenous pyelogram to better delineate the course of the ureters and pass a ureteral stent at the time of repair to help to avoid inadvertent injury. Finally, if the patient is noted to have an atrophic or ulcerated vagina, she is given vaginal estrogen cream to administer topically, which may enhance wound healing postoperatively.

The overall goals of the procedure depend on the clinical scenario. When uterine prolapse is present, the levator myorrhaphy is coupled with vaginal hysterectomy, vault fixation, and enterocele repair. A pelvic ultrasound is obtained preoperatively to evaluate the uterus and ovaries for size and other potential abnormalities that could affect the technique

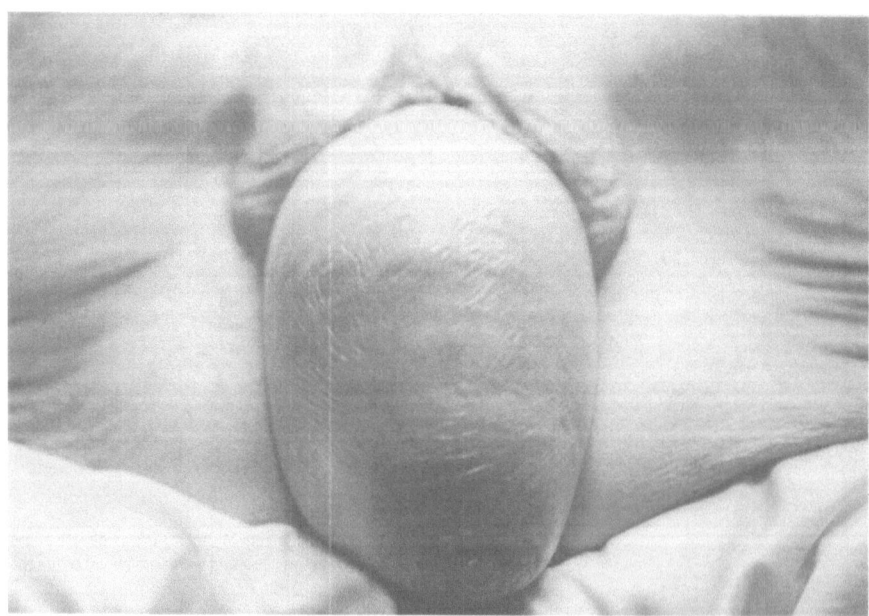

Figure 13.2 Complete uterine and bladder prolapse. Note location of cervix.

of hysterectomy. If the uterus has already been removed, vault fixation and enterocele repair are carried out. When an associated mild to moderate cystocele is present, an anterior vaginal wall suspension which anchors the upper vagina to the cardinal ligaments bilaterally is also performed. By closing the enterocele sac, recreating a strong levator plate, and anchoring the upper vagina to that plate, a normal vaginal cavity with an adequate posterior axis is restored. Since good visibility is present throughout the case, no special dissection or equipment is required, and the technique is easily taught, we feel that is the optimal treatment for vaginal vault or uterine prolapse.

Technique of Vault Prolapse Repair after Hysterectomy

Patients are normally administered general anesthesia and given intravenous antibiotics (cefazolin and gentamicin) at the start of the procedure. Pneumatic compression stockings are applied and the patient is placed in the lithotomy position, using either candy cane or Allen stirrups. The legs should be positioned fairly high, but care should be taken not to overextend or overflex them, and all joints are well padded. The perineum and suprapubic areas are shaved completely, since an associated bladder neck suspension is often also required. A critical step is the placement of a rectal pack (vaginal pack soaked with providone iodine and surgical lubricant), which is inserted after the vagina, perineum, and lower abdomen have been prepped.

After placing the patient in Trendelenburg position, a Scott retractor is placed, exposing the vaginal bulge over the prolapsed vault, which normally represents the position of the enterocele. Generally, panendoscopy is carried out, noting the position of the ureters, and examining for bladder wall changes (trabeculations, diverticuli). If either a ureteral stent, or suprapubic tube is required (for large prolapses it is our practice to place a suprapubic tube at this point using a Lowsley retractor) it is done at this point.[8] A urethral catheter is then placed, leaving the bladder on drainage during the entire case. Two sutures are placed at the fornices of the vaginal vault for identification at the conclusion of the case, and the dimensions of the reduced vagina are measured. We normally place a weighted speculum at this point, but because of foreshortening associated with the prolapse, it may not be able to be placed until later in the case.

After infiltrating the incision line with sterile saline, a midline incision is made overlying the area of prolapse extending from the vault as far distally as the associated rectocele is appreciated. Occasionally, if there is a large ulcerated area on the vaginal wall, this area will be excised superficially at the beginning of the procedure to insure it is not incorporated in the closure. If there is any suspicion of its appearance, it is sent to pathology for frozen section analysis. Vaginal flaps are developed on both sides of the original incision, reapplying the hooks of the Scott retractor periodically to provide enhanced exposure. Often, a Deaver will be required to retract the bladder superiorly during this dissection.

After the vaginal flaps have been created and the dissection continued to the vaginal apex, the enterocele sac can be identified. It may be difficult to differentiate the enterocele sac from a large cystocele, and in these cases either a Van Buren sound or cystoscope placed into the bladder may aid in differentiating between the two. The peritoneal cavity is entered and small laparotomy pads are positioned to displace the bowels superiorly. Placing the patient in a more exaggerated Trendelenburg position may enhance exposure by allowing the peritoneal contents to gravitate away from the operative field. The levator musculature can then be identified bilaterally along the pelvic sidewall, just lateral to the

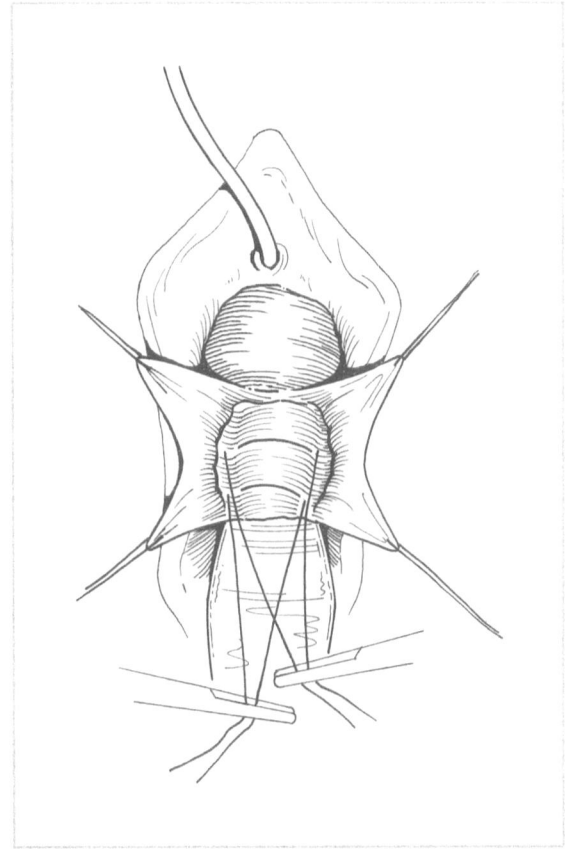

Figure 13.3 Placement of levator sutures. Two #1 absorbable sutures are placed intraperitoneally into the body of the levator muscles. The sutures are left on stay clamps until the enterocele closure is complete. Note bulging rectum (pack is within the rectal lumen) below these sutures.

rectum which can easily be appreciated by the presence of the pre-placed rectal pack. A #1 absorbable suture is then placed into the levator musculature (which is covered by a thin layer of peritoneum), approximately 3 cm above the junction of the levator with the rectum, coming out just above the rectum within the body of the levator. This suture should be placed fairly deep into the body of the muscle, and then the same suture is used to secure the levator muscle on the contralateral side (Fig. 13.3). This suture will later be tied across the midline to accomplish the levator myorraphy. It should then be possible to rock the entire pelvis by tugging firmly on this suture. Another suture, similarly positioned into the body of the levator, is then placed 1 cm proximal to the last suture. Both are left on stay clamps until the next step, the closure of the enterocele sac, is accomplished.

Before securing these sutures each across the midline and completing the levator myorraphy, a #1 PDS purse-string suture is placed circumferentially to close the peritoneal cavity, taking care to remain superficial particularly along the peritoneal surface of the posterior bladder. The landmarks used for enterocele closure are prerectal

fascia posteriorly, pelvic sidewall laterally (taking care to avoid the ovarian vessels which loom very close below the peritoneal surface), and peritoneal surface over the posterior bladder wall anteriorly (Fig. 13.4). One should take care to leave the ovaries within the peritoneal cavity if present and not easily reached to be removed during hysterectomy. This purse-string suture is placed above the levator sutures, so not to include them into the peritoneal cavity closure. After the peritoneal packs are removed and the PDS purse-string suture cinched down, indigo carmine is administered intravenously and cystoscopy is carried out to insure ureteral patency. Any redundant portion of the enterocele sac is excised.

The two pre-placed levator sutures are then tied sequentially across the midline (Fig. 13.5) and final cystoscopic examination is performed. A strong, gushing efflux should be seen from both ureters. If there is any doubt as to their patency, the levator suture may need to be cut and replaced. If there is persistent decreased flow (no flow or very sluggish), then retrograde pyelograms and/or stenting may be

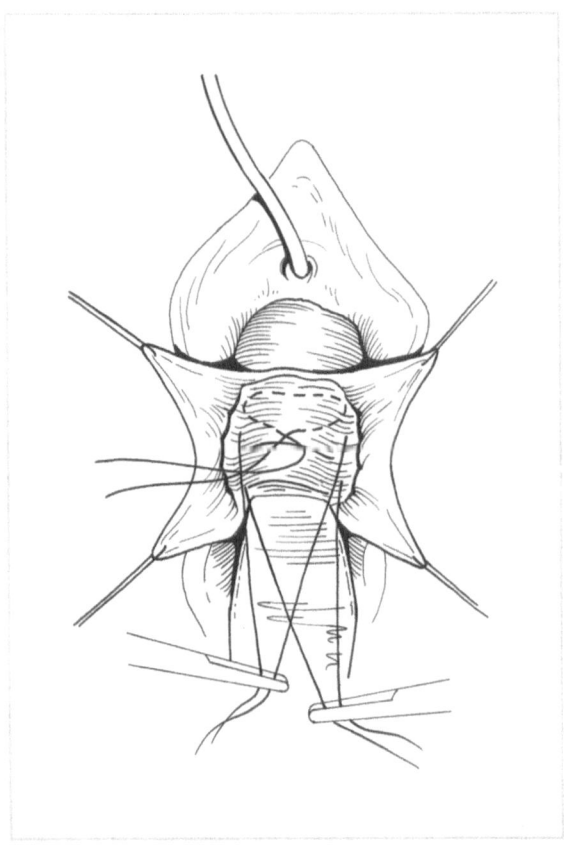

Figure 13.4 Purse string closure of enterocele sac. Care is taken to remain superficial to avoid ovarian vessels (laterally), bladder or ureteral injury (superiorly) and rectal injury (posteriorly).

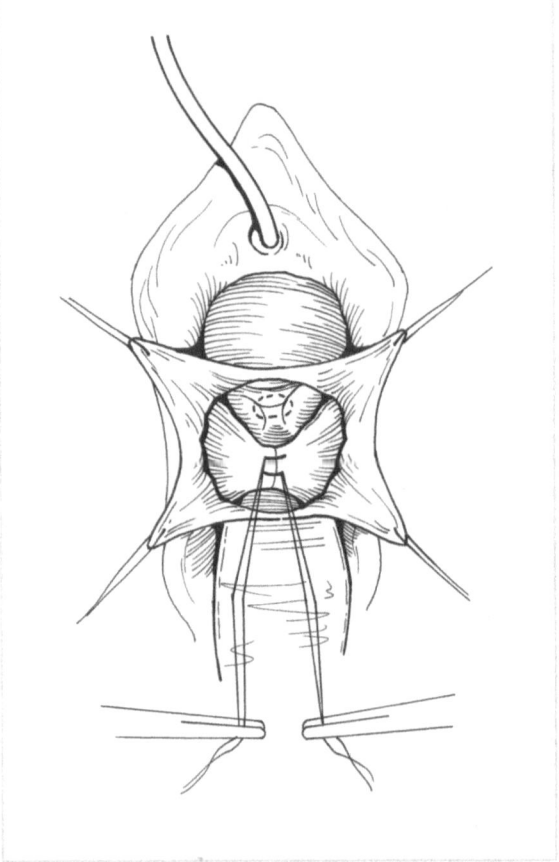

Figure 13.5 After closing the enterocele sac, the levator sutures are tied across the midline and tagged. Cystoscopy must be done at that stage to ensure ureteral patency.

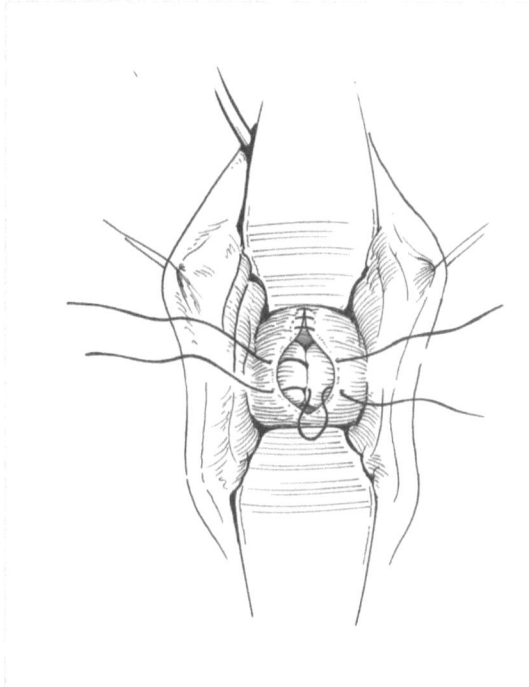

Figure 13.6 Once tied across the midline, the levator sutures are transfixed to the upper vagina to provide direct tissue apposition of the vaginal vault to the rebuilt levator plate.

required to assure ureteral patency. The levator sutures (proximal and distal) are then tagged with a hemostat. If the patient is sexually active, one should insure at this point that there is not excessive tightening of the upper vaginal segment by inserting 2–3 fingers into the vaginal cavity. If this is the case,

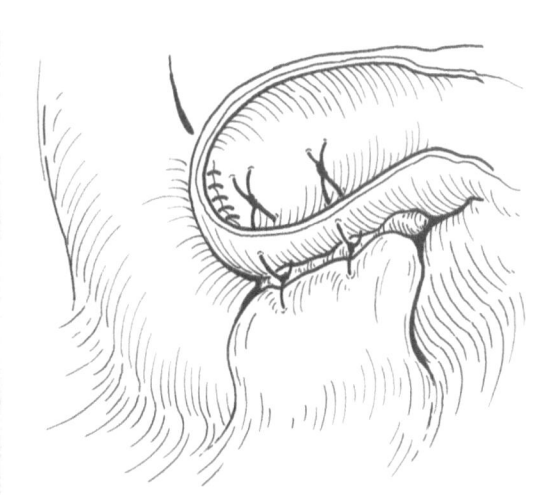

Figure 13.7 Sagittal view showing upper vagina transfixed to the recreated levator plate at conclusion of procedure.

usually the more distal of the levator sutures can be removed without jeopardizing the strength of the repair.

Before closing the mucosal edges at the vaginal apex, one end of each of the proximal and distal levator myorraphy sutures from one side is threaded on a #6 curved Mayo needle and is transfixed at the new vaginal apex from the inside out, separated by approximately 1 cm from each other (Fig. 13.6). The same process is carried out on the other side with one end taken from the more proximal of the levator sutures, and one from the more distal of the two. The former proximal and distal levator sutures are then secured to one another, thereby firmly anchoring the upper vagina to the newly created levator plate (Fig. 13.7).

If an anterior repair or anti-incontinence procedure is required, it can now be carried out, followed by a rectocele repair if indicated. After completion, an antibiotic-soaked vaginal pack is placed, and a Foley urethral catheter (and suprapubic tube if placed earlier) is left to drainage. The vaginal pack and urethral catheter are left in place for 24–48 hours and removed. Residuals are checked by ultrasound or suprapubic tube. If residuals are >100 ml, clean catheterization is performed, or, if a suprapubic tube had been placed, the tube is opened and residuals recorded until less than 100 ml (generally less than 5 days).

Results and Complications

The major complications associated with any repair of vaginal prolapse include hemorrhage requiring transfusion, ureteral injury, rectal injury, rectal pain upon defecation, vaginal narrowing affecting sexual function, and prolapse recurrence. In our hands, the risk of significant bleeding has been nil, with only 2 patients requiring transfusion over a 10 year period of performing this procedure in over 120 patients. We had one patient with bilateral ureteral obstruction who was noted to be anuric in the recovery room. She was taken back to the operating room where removal of the levator sutures resulted in prompt return of bilateral ureteral flow. The sutures were repositioned with ureteral stents in place, and the patient had no further complications. One patient was noted to have flank pain and unilateral hydronephosis after repair (Fig. 13.8), which permanently resolved after 3 months of ureteral stenting. We have had 5 cases where ureteral drainage was noted to decrease intraoperatively after tying one of the levator myorraphy sutures. Prompt return of urine flow was observed after removing one of the sutures. Secondary anterior enterocele formation has been noted in two asymptomatic patients postoperatively, neither of whom has

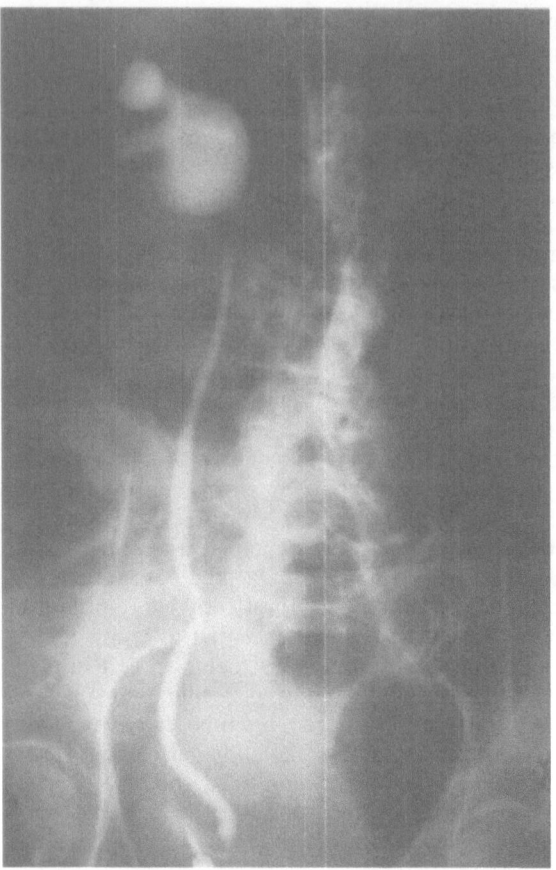

Figure 13.8 Retrograde pyelogram from woman with right flank pain after levator myorraphy. Note patency of ureter, but medial deviation of distal ureter away from position of orifice (at cone tip catheter). After 3 months of stenting, follow-up IVP revealed no ureteral obstruction and a normal ureteric course with no further deviation.

required revision or sacrocolpopexy as yet. Rectal pain is uncommon, but when present usually subsides within 4–6 weeks after the procedure and is best treated with stool softeners and warm sitz baths. Finally, though sexual function may not be a priority in most of the elderly patients undergoing prolapse surgery,[9] it is important to many and we are currently in the process of evaluating sexual function using a newly developed questionnaire.

Sacrohysteropexy and Sacrocolpopexy

Kaven Baessler, Elad Leron, and Stuart L. Stanton

The aim of pelvic reconstructive surgery is to correct prolapse, maintain urinary and fecal continence and to preserve coital and reproductive function if desired. Difficulties and dissatisfaction with vaginal correction of prolapse, particularly enterocele and recurrent pelvic organ prolapse, and frequent loss of vaginal function associated with vaginal procedures, have led gynecologic surgeons to develop an abdominal prolapse operation.[10,11]

Arthure and Savage were the first to publish data on direct fixation of the uterus or vaginal vault to the sacral promontory using silk sutures, thus avoiding inadequate supportive tissue and vaginal scarring.[12] Embrey used fascia lata to attach the vaginal vault to the sacrum.[13] In 1962 Lane interposed a synthetic graft, with "satisfactory" results.[14] Later, macroporous mesh (type I: Marlex, Prolene), totally microporous mesh (type II: Gore-Tex) and macroporous mesh with multifilamentous components (type III: Teflon, Mersilene, Dacron) was used. Type I mesh allows bacteria and macrophages to infiltrate, and an infection is extremely unlikely. When it occurs, it may be treated successfully by antibiotics without mesh removal. In type III mesh one component is microporous or multifilamentous admitting bacteria but not macrophages contributing to the development of an infection. Type II mesh deters penetration of macrophages completely,[15] but has the advantage that there is no fibroplasia or angiogenesis to cause intestinal adhesions. Because of the risk of infection and mesh rejection some clinicians use homologeous material such as fascia lata or rectus sheath.

Uterine preserving surgery for significant uterine prolapse has included sacrohysteropexy using silk sutures described by Arthure and Savage in 1957,[12] fixation of the uterus to the undersurface of the abdominal wall,[16] transvaginal uterosacral ligament fixation to the sacrospinous ligament,[17] and laparoscopic uterine suspension by suturing the round ligaments to the rectus sheath.[18]

Indications

Sacrohysteropexy

Significant uterine prolapse in women in their reproductive years may occur in parous women but also in young nulliparous women, virgins, and women with congenital anomalies (e.g. bladder exstrophy). Those women may wish to remain fertile. Sacrohysteropexy was designed to treat uterine prolapse. The use of synthetic mesh to attach the uterus to the sacrum provides durable support. Concomitant pelvic organ prolapse like cystourethrocele or rectocele can be addressed separately.

The indication for surgical correction of uterine prolapse by preserving the uterus is failure of conservative treatment in a young woman who has not completed her family or if the woman refuses hysterectomy and wishes to retain her uterus.

Sacrocolpopexy

Initially, a woman with symptomatic vault prolapse has to decide whether she wishes to undergo conservative or surgical treatment. Several operations are available and the patient should be included in the discussion of risks and benefits. If there are no contraindications for a specific approach, the final decision is the patient's but the surgeon's success rate must also be considered. Medical problems, which limit general or regional anesthesia, will not be discussed here but need to be covered in the risk-benefit estimate. Table 13.1 gives an overview of indications and advantages of sacrocolpopexy.

The advantages of an abdominal procedure are that further scarring, shortening, and narrowing of the vagina are avoided. Furthermore, there is no additional damage to the perineal and pudendal nerve, which could result in neuropathy.[19] If additional abdominal surgery (e.g. colposuspension, ovarian cystectomy) is needed, the abdominal route is more convenient. However, adhesions, previous mesh hernia repair or rectopexy might make it technically more difficult.

The disadvantage of the traditional abdominal sacrocolpopexy is that it only addresses prolapse of the middle compartment. To repair support defects in the anterior compartment, a colposuspension can be added in patients with stress incontinence

Table 13.1. Indications and advantages of sacrocolpopexy

Indications

Recurrent vaginal vault prolapse

Contraindications for vaginal surgery

Woman's choice

Reduced vaginal capacity

Descending perineum syndrome

Concurrent abdominal surgery (e.g. colposuspension)

Desire to maintain sexual function

Chronic pelvic floor stress

Connective tissue diseases

Obesity

Advantages

Inadequate tissue is avoided and substituted with indestructible mesh

Best long-term success rates (90–100%)

No vaginal incision, so no shortening, scarring, narrowing of vagina, so no damage to perineal and pudendal nerve

Additional pelvic floor support defects can be addressed transabdominally

due to urethral sphincter incompetence. Extension of the mesh on to the anterior vaginal wall can also correct anterior vaginal wall support defects.

Simultaneous correction of vault prolapse and rectocele has been described by Villet et al.[20] and more recently by Cundiff et al.[21] The technique involved dissection of the rectum from the posterior vaginal wall and insertion of a mesh down to and sutured to the perineal body and vault and then to the anterior longitudinal ligament over the sacrum. Cundiff et al.[21] claimed that perineal descent can be corrected by attachment of the mesh to the perineal body. The paper gave no long-term follow-up and the objective evidence was rather sparse. Abdominal sacrocolpopex with mesh interposition (SCMI) would therefore be indicated in women with vaginal vault prolapse and marked perineal descent or descending perineum syndrome.

Sacrocolpopexy was performed initially in women with posthysterectomy vaginal vault prolapse who wanted to preserve coital function. Along with modifications and improvements in technique and material, indications have changed. Due to an extended life expectancy the incidence of primary and recurrent pelvic organ prolapse has increased. Good general socioeconomic conditions and HRT contribute to an increasing number of very fit and active women who will seek medical help when incontinence and prolapse interfere with their quality of life. Symmonds and colleagues stated in 1981 that postoperative assessment of sexual function is almost impossible, because many women have died, lost libido, are widowed, or their partners have medical problems or lost interest.[11] One-third of the patients over 60 years old and 12% of those over 70 years old attending our urogynecology clinic are sexually active.[22] Drugs such as sildenafil (Viagra) will increase this expectation. Future coitus has therefore always to be considered even if the woman is not currently sexually active and gynecologic surgeons have to choose prolapse operations very carefully.

When choosing an operation coexisting factors should be considered. Congenital or acquired connective tissue weakness and chronic pelvic floor stress, which includes chronic bronchitis, asthma, slow-transit constipation associated with excessive defecation straining, and occupational heavy lifting, might predispose to failure. These women should undergo the surgery, which offers the best anatomic and functional success rate.

The use of inorganic mesh may aggravate autoimmune disease. Heterologous material should probably not be used in HIV-positive women or in chronically immunosuppressed patients. In theses cases autogenous fascia lata or rectus sheath would be a safer option.

Preoperative Assessment and Management

History

A careful history, preferably using a standardized pre- and postoperative questionnaire to include prolapse, bladder and bowel symptoms, and sexual function is essential. Of particular importance is the presence of urinary and fecal incontinence.

Examination

Preoperative assessment should include a lumbosacral neurological examination. Several classifications can be used to stage pelvic organ prolapse. The International Continence Society (ICS) has recommended a quantitative standardization system to enable inter and intra-individual comparison.[23] This system provides quantitative information on the extent of prolapse of the anterior, posterior and middle compartments of the vagina. A rectal examination is carried out to determine the size and exact location of a rectocele and defects in the endopelvic fascia. Bimanual palpation is performed to detect an enterocele.[23]

Urodynamic Assessment

Preoperatively, a full urodynamic assessment including a urinary diary should be performed. A normal cystometrogram without reduction of the prolapse does not exclude stress incontinence due to urethral sphincter incompetence after restoration of pelvic anatomy. A cough stress test with the prolapse reduced should therefore be included. In recurrent stress incontinence or previous vaginal prolapse surgery, urethral pressure profiles at rest and during stress (coughing) as well as bladder neck ultrasound may give more information on the urethral sphincter and its support.

Imaging studies such as perineal ultrasound, pelvic fluoroscopy and videocystourethrography may be required to substantiate findings detected at vaginal examination and to define the prolapse. Isotope defecography will give data on bowel emptying. Ideally, all pelvic floor support defects should be addressed during one operation (Table 13.2).

Preoperative Management

The procedure and its risks and complications have to be explained thoroughly to the patient, although sometimes the extent of dissection in secondary surgery may be unknown beforehand. Although anatomic results of abdominal sacrocolpopexy are well described, there is scarce prospective data on functional outcome regarding bowel and sexual function. The patient should be told that a good anatomic restoration does not necessarily correlate with restoration of normal function. Good estrogenization might be an advantage, but also increases blood loss. HRT is not routinely recommended before the operation but should be administered postoperatively.

Prophylaxis for thrombosis and pulmonary embolism consists of compression stockings, early mobilization and heparin 5000 IU twice daily if the patient has not experienced heparin-induced thrombocytopenia (HIT I or II). It is started preoperatively and continued until the patient is fully ambulant.

In most primary cases, bowel preparation with a small enema or glycerine suppositories are adequate. In secondary operations, oral bowel preparation (e.g. bisacodyl [Fleet] 45 ml twice starting the day before operation) might be advisable, particularly if adhesions are expected. Two hours before surgery a single dose of metronidazole 1 g is given per rectum to cover anaerobic bacteria and a broadspectrum antibiotic (e.g. cephradine 1 g) is given at the time of induction.

Technique

The following descriptions are the senior author's techniques. In addition, the available literature is reviewed.

Positioning of the Patient, Additional Operations, and Incision

The patient is put in the lithotomy Trendelenburg position with the legs in stirrups slightly apart and flexed so that the assistant can stand comfortably between them. Care should be taken to avoid pressure points and particularly damage to the peroneal nerve. The patient's buttocks should protrude at

Table 13.2 Pelvic floor support defects and its abdominal correction

Compartment	Pathology	Operation
Anterior	Cystourethrocele	Anterior mesh extension
	Cystourethrocele + USI	Colposuspension
	Paravaginal support defects	Paravaginal defect repair
	High cystocele	Anterior mesh extension
	Anterior enterocele	Anterior mesh extension
Middle	Vault prolapse/enterocele	Abdominal sacrocolpopexy
Posterior	Rectocele	Posterior mesh interposition
	Posterior enterocele	Posterior mesh interposition

USI, urethral sphincter incompetence.

least 5 cm off the operation table to guarantee maximum anterior elevation of the vagina using an obturator.

If a colposuspension or tension-free vaginal tape operation (TVT) is planned, it is carried out first to avoid unnecessary tension by the sacrohysteropexy or sacrocolpopexy on the anterior vaginal wall which may lead to persistence or sometimes development of urethral sphincter incompetence.

A Pfannenstiel incision is preferred, but in short obese women best access is obtained by a subumbilical midline incision.

Sacrohysteropexy

The sacrohysteropexy is performed under general or spinal anaesthesia. Uterine holding forceps elevate the uterus. A sterile piece of Teflon mesh (Bard Europe, London, UK) 20 cm x 4 cm is bifurcated to produce a Y shaped graft (Fig. 13.9). Each broad ligament at the level of the cervico-uterine junction (CUJ) is perforated through an avascular area using diathermy and scissor dissection. The vesico-uterine peritoneum is incised and the bladder dissected distally for a distance of 1–2 cm. One limb of the bifurcated mesh is introduced through this lumen and sutured to the anterior CUJ using no. 1 polybutylate coated polyethylene suture on a J needle (Ethibond, Ethicon Ltd., Edinburgh, UK) (Fig. 13.10). This was repeated on the other side. The mesh was then sutured to the posterior CUJ. The arms of the bifurcated mesh are not sutured together anteriorly to avoid constriction and to allow distension during potential pregnancy and delivery.

Sacrocolpopexy

The abdominal sacrocolpopexy can be performed either open or laparoscopically. The laparoscopic

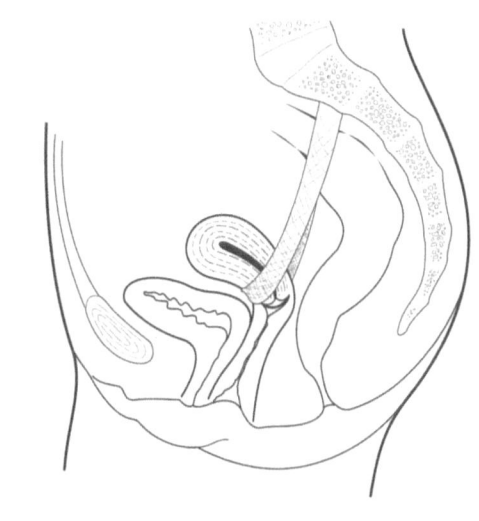

Figure 13.10 Bifurcated mesh in position for sacrohysteropexy

technique follows the principles of open sacrocolpopexy. Its success rate seems to be equally good,[24,25] although long-term follow up is not available yet. Apart from a shorter hospital stay there might be the technical advantage of easier dissection in the pouch of Douglas because of better access.

Open sacrocolpopexy (which is the choice of the senior author) is usually performed under general anesthesia, but epidural or spinal anesthesia might be used. Mean operation time including additional procedures varies from 89 min to 269 min.[26-33]

After placing the self-retaining ring retractor and packing away the bowel an obturator is inserted into the vagina to identify the vaginal apex and to facilitate attachment of the mesh to the vault. For a posterior mesh interposition to correct a rectocele and perineal descent the obturator has to be elevated as much as possible to give good access to the pouch of Douglas. The rectum is dissected off the vagina keeping close to the posterior vaginal wall using a combination of sharp and blunt dissection with prophylactic diathermy of vessels (Fig. 13.11). Dissection is carried out down to the perineal body, the level of dissection being checked with the surgeon's hand at the distal point of dissection and the other hand flat on the perineum. At the level of the perineal body the dissection becomes more difficult because of its dense connective tissue. Polytretrafluoethylene (PTFE, Teflon, Bard Inc.) mesh 20 cm × 4 cm is used and cut to the required length. The mesh is sutured with a nonabsorbable suture (No. 1 Ethibond, Ethicon Ltd, Edinburgh, UK) to the posterior vaginal wall as far laterally as possible on either side. Deep bites are taken but not through the

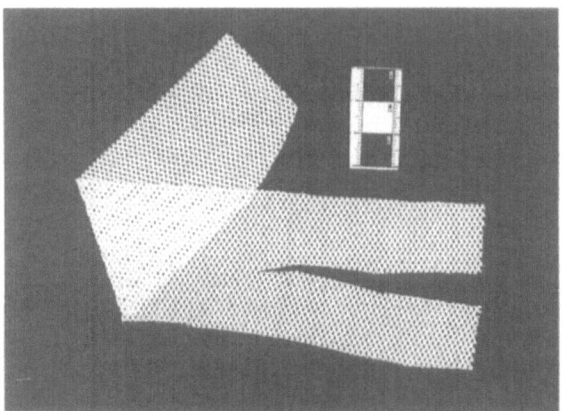

Figure 13.9 Bifurcated Y-shaped mesh for sacrohysteropexy

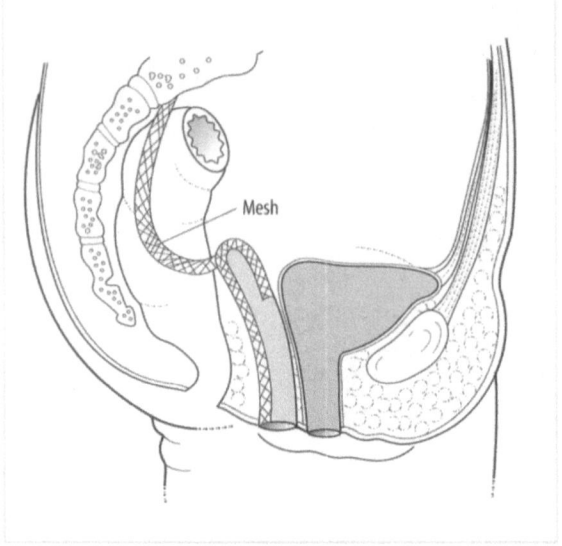
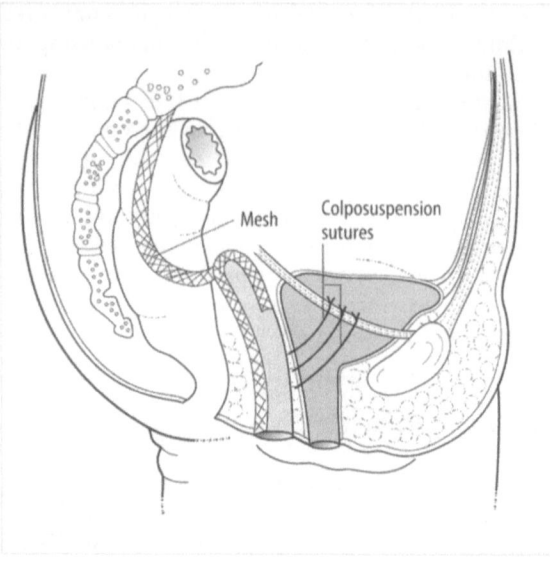

a   b

Figure 13.11 Sacrocolpopexy with anterior and posterior mesh extensions. Two separate meshes are used. Without (**a**) and with (**b**) colposuspension.

entire thickness of the vagina. Two to three further sutures are inserted on either side of the mesh up the vaginal wall until the vault is reached. A Finochietto needle holder is helpful in placing the sutures.

If there is a significant cystocele without incontinence and an incontinence operation is not required, a separate mesh can be sutured to the anterior vaginal wall. The bladder is sharply dissected off the appropriate area and the mesh is attached to the anterior vaginal wall. This piece is then also sutured to the mesh already fixed to the posterior vaginal wall. Care is taken to avoid too extensive a dissection anteriorly because the effects on bladder function have not been assessed comprehensively. It is important to avoid circumferentially enclosing the vagina with the mesh, which may potentially constrict its caliber and lead to dyspareunia.

Dissection of the Sacral Area

The rectosigmoid is bluntly displaced to the left side using a swab on a holder. After careful palpation a longitudinal midline incision in the peritoneum is made beginning over S1 or S2. It is continued to the edge of the dissected posterior vaginal wall peritoneum creating peritoneal flaps either side which will later be sutured together to peritonealize the mesh. The presacral areola tissue is dissected off the sacrum until the anterior longitudinal ligament is visible over an area of approximately 1.5 cm × 1.5 cm. Blunt and sharp dissection with

prophylactic diathermy is utilised. Care is taken to avoid the sacral vessels. Two Ethibond no. 1 sutures are secured in the anterior longitudinal sacral ligament.

A proximal attachment at S1 or S2 is usually preferred because it is more accessible and any bleeding can be easily reached, although a more distal sacral fixation results in a more physiological, almost horizontal, vaginal axis. To arrest hemorrhage in this area diathermy, local compression, additional sutures or thumb tacks may be used.[34]

Vaginal Vault Fixation

The length of the mesh has to be adjusted without tension, taking into account that it may shrink by 20%[15] and that it is peritonealized by laying it on the curve of the sacrum. Excessive mesh is trimmed and it is then attached to the sacrum. The mesh is then completely covered with peritoneum to prevent subsequent bowel adhesion or strangulation.

Closure of Abdomen

If a colposuspension has been performed, the parietal peritoneum is closed and a suprapubic catheter inserted. A redivac drain may be required in the pouch of Douglas and in the retropubic space. If there is no suprapubic catheter, a 14 Charriere urethral Foley catheter is used for 24–48 hours.

Secondary Abdominal Sacrocolpopexy

Recurrent vaginal vault prolapse or enterocele after abdominal sacrocolpopexy is rare. In these cases the mesh has usually come off the vagina and is still attached to the sacrum. Detachment of the sacral sutures is less common. Provided the old mesh is still firmly attached at its other end, a new mesh may be attached to it. Removal of the original mesh can be very difficult and potentially hazardous to ureter and bowel. If it does not represent a risk of bowel obstruction, it can be left in place.

Postoperative Management

Drains and urethral catheters should be removed within 24 hours as appropriate. When a colposuspension was performed the routine suprapubic catheter regime is applied. The suprapubic catheter is clamped at the second postoperative day and can be removed when the patient has voided > 200 ml with a residual of < 200 ml in the evening and on the following morning. Mobilization starts on the first postoperative day. The patient is advised to avoid heavy lifting at least for 2 months. Otherwise the patient is encouraged to walk as much as she wants, but to avoid formal exercise and sexual intercourse until after the routine follow-up at 6 weeks.

Complications

Complications of sacrohysteropexy and sacrocolpopexy are uncommon. Specific complications related to abdominal sacrocolpopexy are listed in Table 13.3. Erosion and infection of the mesh occurs in approximately 4.5% of patients irrespective of the synthetic mesh material used [10,21,26–29,33,35–43,47,55] (Table 13.3). Erosion of the nonabsorbable suture material frequently seems to precede erosion of the mesh.[27] Symptoms include increased vaginal discharge, which may or may not be offensive, vaginal bleeding, and occasionally dyspareunia for the woman and/or her partner. Suture erosions seem to remain asymptomatic.[41] If type I mesh had been used (Dacron, Marlex, Prolene), removal of the mesh is not necessary because the macroporous material allows macrophages to pass.[15] Therefore treatment with antibiotics and trimming and covering of the mesh may be sufficient. Infected type II mesh (microporous material: Gore-Tex) has to be removed completely. In type III mesh infections (combination of multifilament and macroporous components: Teflon, Mersilene) partial removal of the mesh with re-closure of the refreshed vaginal skin edges is recommended.

Mesh rejection had been associated with a concomitant hysterectomy.[43] However, a prospective study with 235 patients showed that hysterectomy at the time of abdominal sacrocolpopexy did not increase the risk of febrile morbidity.[44] Timmons and Addison reported on one vesical mesh erosion, which led to recurrent urinary tract infections. The mesh had to be removed transabdominally.[38] Another mesh erosion has been described by Patsner[45] 2 months after sacrocolpopexy with a monofilament polypropylene mesh and prolene sutures. The patient complained of hematuria. Cystoscopy revealed mesh erosion into the bladder, which had to be openly excised after two unsuccessful cystoscopic removals. There have been no reports of mesh erosion into the rectum, which might be an issue, when the mesh is placed between vagina and rectum.

To prevent late infection of the mesh, McLelland (personal communication, 1999) suggested treating the mesh similarly to artificial heart valves and giving prophylactic antibiotics for any invasive operations. Drutz observed a retropubic abscess and removed the mesh completely.[46]

Postoperative pain or discomfort in the sacral area is rare, and coincidental orthopedic diseases are often present.[47–49] Two cases of lumbosacral osteomyelitis after abdominal sacrocolpopexy were recently reported by Weidner et al.[50] One patient developed low back pain 5 years postoperatively, the other patient 4 months later. MRI is the method of choice to detect osteomyelitis. Six more cases of osteomyelitis have been reported by rheumatologists.[51,52] Enteroceles have been found behind the mesh[53] and an obstructive ileus has been reported in up to 4% of patients.[54,55] Peritoneal-

Table 13.3. Sacrocolpopexy-related observed complications

Complication	Observed cases	Number of operated patients	%	References
Synthetic mesh erosion/infection	45	1006	4.5	10, 21, 26–29, 33, 35–43, 47, 55
Blood loss >500 ml	41	690	5.9	26, 29, 30, 33, 37, 39, 49, 55, 59, 64, 66
Obstructive ileus	11	392	2.8	30, 54, 55, 59
Adynamic ileus	15	552	2.7	27, 28, 33, 36, 39, 41, 49, 59, 63, 66
Pelvic hematoma	3	166	1.8	28, 30, 55

ization of the mesh is therefore emphasized to avoid both of these.

Results

Restoration of Anatomy

Sacrohysteropexy

In our own series of 13 patients employing the technique described above, no recurrent uterine prolapse has occurred during a follow up period of 1–3 years.[56] Other authors used Gore-Tex[27,57] and Mersilene[58] with no failures over a long-term follow-up of 1–5 years. Direct sacral attachment of the uterus using silk sutures resulted in a failure rate of 10% in 49 women.[12]

The effect of vaginal delivery after sacrohysteropexy seems to be unknown and has not been described.[12,56,58] One woman underwent caesarean section during which the sling was found to be intact and at routine follow-up postpartum the cervix was in a normal position.[58]

Sacrocolpopexy

Success of abdominal sacrocolpopexy is not consistently defined, but authors usually refer to the anatomic restoration of the vaginal vault. Success rates range between 77.8% and 100% when synthetic mesh and nonabsorbable suture material are used.[10,11,22,26,27,30,37,39,43,57,59-65] Autologous and homologous material such as dura mater, fascia lata and rectus sheath have also successfully been used in a smaller number of prolapse patients.[13,28,33,48,61,62,66] Direct attachment of the vagina to the sacrum without interposing mesh has not been satisfactory. There were 12 failures out of 58 notified cases (20.7%).[12,26,28,43,46,61,67]

Anterior Compartment

The incidence of anterior vaginal wall prolapse after abdominal sacrocolpopexy ranges between 8% and 30%.[28,31,32,39,57,60,61,63,68] It is difficult to estimate because of additional procedures carried out at the same time. There seems to be a high recurrence rate of cystoceles despite anterior colporrhaphy[33] or paravaginal defect repair and/or Burch colposuspension (30%).[68] In our own series of 22 women who underwent concomitant Burch colposuspension for urethral sphincter incompetence and grade 1–3 prolapse of the anterior vaginal wall, 8 women (18%) developed an asymptomatic grade 1 high cystocele

(ICS prolapse staging Aa –3 or –2, Ba –2 to –1.5) and one woman had a grade 2 cystocele postoperatively (Ba –0.5).[22]

Two anterior enteroceles have been reported.[60,69] A first-degree cystocele recurred in three out of seven patients after sacrohysteropexy.[57]

Posterior Compartment

The occurrence of rectoceles after abdominal sacrocolpopexy has infrequently been reported. The incidence ranges between 2 and 13%, without considering length of follow-up and prolapse staging.[26,28-31,37,39,60] Early observations of sacrocolpopexy with mesh interposition down to the perineal body 4–24 weeks postoperatively suggested cure of the rectoceles.[21] However, we found that, at a mean follow up of 22 months (range 12–40 months), the mesh had become detached from the perineal body in 11 of 44 women (25%). It was felt 3–5 cm above the hymen. The more the mesh had come off the perineal body, the higher the stage of posterior vaginal wall prolapse ($R^2 = 0.45$, $p < 0.001$). The incidence of postoperative posterior vaginal wall prolapse was not higher in the group of 22 women who had received concomitant Burch colposuspension for stress urinary incontinence.[22]

Posterior enteroceles behind the suspending mesh have been observed[53,59] and obliteration of the pouch of Douglas is generally recommended. However, on reviewing the available literature, there seems to be no considerably higher incidence of enteroceles in women who did not undergo any form of pouch of Douglas obliteration.

Restoration of Function

Pelvic organ prolapse of any vaginal site can lead to a number of symptoms such as feeling of a lump, walking difficulties, vaginal pain, backache, dyspareunia, feeling of "slackness" during intercourse, and voiding difficulties. Specific symptoms related to insufficient support of the anterior vaginal wall are stress urinary incontinence and voiding difficulties. Typical symptoms attributable to posterior vaginal wall prolapse are incomplete bowel emptying, need to strain excessively, digitation during defecation, rectal pain and bleeding, and feeling a lump in the vagina during defecation. Restoration of normal function is one goal of pelvic reconstructive surgery.

Sexual Function

Disturbed sexual function such as dyspareunia and "slackness" at intercourse are common symptoms of pelvic organ prolapse. There are limited controlled data available on sexual function after sacrocolpopexy. Comments like "normal sexual life," "normal coitus," or "functional vagina" can be read in various papers. The only symptom investigated seems to be dyspareunia, which usually improves after fixation of the prolapse.[22,28,37,70] Given et al. measured the vaginal length pre- and postoperatively and attributed it to adequate sexual function. Vaginal length was best maintained by abdominal sacrocolpopexy compared to sacrospinous ligament fixation.[71]

Anterior Compartment

The effect of abdominal sacrocolpopexy on function of the anterior compartment has been well described. There is a high risk of recurrent stress incontinence due to urethral sphincter incompetence in up to 36% of patients despite retropubic or colpopexy surgery.[29,33,49,59] Virtanen et al. reported de-novo stress incontinence in 18% of their patients.[28] Straightening the urethro-vesical angle is thought to contribute to the development of stress incontinence. Preoperative urodynamic evaluation with the prolapse reduced detects women at risk and a concomitant colposuspension accordingly decreases the postoperative incidence of stress incontinence.[22,68,72]

In 22 women complaining of stress incontinence, we found a subjective success rate of colposuspension in conjunction with sacrocolpopexy of 73%. Postoperatively, 6 of the women complained of persistent but improved stress incontinence: 5 of them had had previous bladder neck surgery. In 22 women without preoperative urethral sphincter incompetence even with the prolapse reduced and who did not undergo Burch colposuspension, stress urinary incontinence recurred in 2 women, both of whom had had previous bladder neck surgery for urethral sphincter incompetence. We therefore do not believe that every woman needs a concomitant prophylactic colposuspension but it should be performed in selected cases with preoperatively proven urethral sphincter incompetence.[22] Patients with previous successful continence surgery should be carefully assessed to confirm cure before sacrocolpopexy.

Posterior Compartment

The effect of abdominal sacrocolpopexy on function of the posterior compartment has been rather neglected. Constipation and difficult rectal emptying after abdominal sacrocolpopexy have been described by several authors, although definitions and data have been inconsistent.[21,28–30, 57,63] Constipation is a known sequel to rectopexy procedures resulting from denervation after rectal dissection and division of the lateral ligament.[73] Presacral and rectosigmoid dissection during abdominal sacrocolpopexy should therefore be minimized. In our series of 44 women assessed with a standardized questionnaire pre- and postoperatively, de-novo incomplete defecation occurred in 4 women (9%). In order to achieve complete defecation, 2 of them had to strain, 1 woman had to digitate transvaginally and perineally. Five women reported persistent and 3 worsening difficulties in bowel emptying, whereas symptoms improved in 4 women. In 7 of these 16 women, postoperative bowel symptoms were not attributable to a rectocele. Perineal descent or constipation due to denervation might explain this phenomenon. A comparison of 22 women who underwent concomitant Burch colposuspension and 22 women without colposuspension revealed no adverse effect of Burch colposuspension on anatomy and function of the posterior compartment.[22]

Conclusion

With abdominal sacrohysteropexy it is possible to comply with the woman's wish to retain the uterus and accomplish good anatomic long-term results. However, there is limited data available on functional outcome, and experience with subsequent pregnancy and delivery is scarce. Sacrohysteropexy remains an effective operation for uterine prolapse.

Sacrocolpopexy employing autologous, heterologous or synthetic material to attach the vaginal vault to the sacrum is an efficient and safe operation in terms of anatomic long-term results. Restoration of normal bladder function can be achieved with a concomitant Burch colposuspension if urethral sphincter incompetence is present with or without the prolapse reduced. However, restoration of normal bladder, bowel, and sexual function does not always correlate with anatomic outcome. Mesh detachment from the perineal body is a cause for concern and the technique needs to be adapted to minimize this.

Key Points

- Sacrohysteropexy can effectively treat uterine prolapse if the patients wishes to retain her uterus
- Sacrocolpopexy is effective in curing vaginal vault prolapse with excellent long-term results
- Preoperative urodynamic studies should be performed with and without the prolapse reduced

- Concomitant colposuspension usually but not always cures urethral sphincter incompetence
- Posterior mesh interposition corrects concomitant rectoceles if the mesh does not become detached from the perineal body
- Complications are rare
- Hemorrhage from presacral vessels can be stopped by pressure, figures of eight or thumb tacks
- Mesh erosion may be treated conservatively depending on the mesh material

Sacrospinous Fixation According to Richter

Brigitte Fatton and Bernard Jacquetin

The first description of vaginal vault fixation to the sacrospinous ligament is credited to Zweifel in 1892.[74] Since then, the technique has evolved and continues to be popular throughout the world. Except for two cases reported by Miller in 1927,[75] expansion of the technique remained limited until 1951 when Amreich[76] reactivated interest in the sacrospinalis fixation, initially through a transacral approach, then transvaginally. However, despite a resurgence of interest in the procedure, it remained a technically difficult operation. True expansion of the technique really dates to Richter in 1968,[77] followed by Nichols in the United States in 1971,[78] and Dargent in France. In 1986, the latter reported a personal series of 133 cases which were followed up to 6 years.[79] Since 1985, our department has routinely performed sacrospinalis fixation, with over 1200 cases of bilateral suspensions performed thus far, and open sacrocolpoplexy is currently an exceptional indication in our practice. The sacrospinous fixation according to Richter is a reliable operation with limited morbidity and good long-term data. It should be part of the armamentarium of all vaginal surgeons.

Technique

Goal of the Surgery

According to Amreich's description, the sacrospinous fixation is the most physiologic procedure capable of repositioning the vaginal canal over the levator muscles, thus mimicking "the natural support." Orientation of the upper vaginal axis is towards S2–3. Thus, during increases in abdominal pressure, the vagina is compressed over the levator plate, which prevents its sliding inside the urogenital hiatus. This normal anatomic position must be re-established to adequately correct or prevent vaginal vault prolapse. Although the sacrospinalis fixation procedure re-establishes a slightly more posterior vault fixation, it provides a more anatomical result than the classical sacrocolpopexy to the promontory, which tends to verticalize the vagina. Such verticalization exposes the vagina to secondary pelvic floor herniations such as enterocele or rectocele. Although the original operation was unilateral, we prefer to perform it bilaterally to maintain the vagina in a more midline position.[80,81]

Perioperative Care

Hormonal therapy for a few months prior to the procedure is strongly recommended, along with removal of any pessary, to promote a healthier vaginal wall. Prior to surgery, vaginal douching, an enema, and complete shaving of the pubis and perineal areas is recommended. Antibiotic coverage is also recommended as long as a urinary drainage system remains in place.

Instrumentation

The following instruments are necessary to perform the procedure.

- Breisky valves, which are long and narrow, allow maximal exposure of the sacrospinous ligament. Some valves are equipped with an end- or side-light to facilitate anatomic recognition of the ligament. A median valve is also needed to protect the rectum.
- Allis clamps are optimal to gently hold and grasp the vaginal wall.
- A long-needle holder is required to secure a strong bite in the ligament.

Bilateral Sacrospinous Fixation of the Vaginal Vault Prolapse after Hysterectomy

Step 1

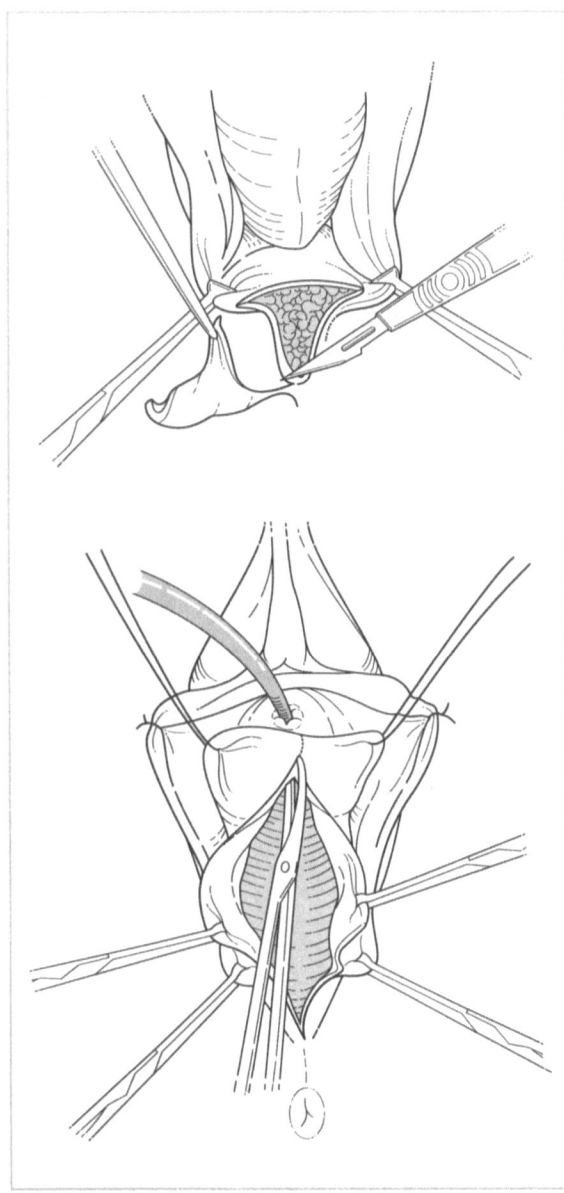

Figure 13.12 Perineal incision (**a**) followed by a long posterior midline incision all the way up to the vault (**b**). After excising a low, limited posterior vaginal wall triangle, two vaginal flaps are separated from the peri- and para-rectal tissues all the way up to the vault. Two stay sutures have been positioned at each vaginal vault apex.

The patient is placed in the high lithotomy position. Two assistants are usually present to hold valves and to facilitate exposure of the ligament. Stay sutures are placed at each vaginal apex, corresponding to the former insertion of the uterosacral and cardinal ligaments. Due to the redundancy of the prolapsed vaginal wall and a tendency for the posterior vaginal wall to be longer than the anterior vaginal wall, a new vaginal vault should be defined. Therefore, the optimal point for this new location is determined by moving the future vaginal apex to the ischial tuberosities bilaterally, then using this landmark to anchor the sacrospinous ligament.

Step 2

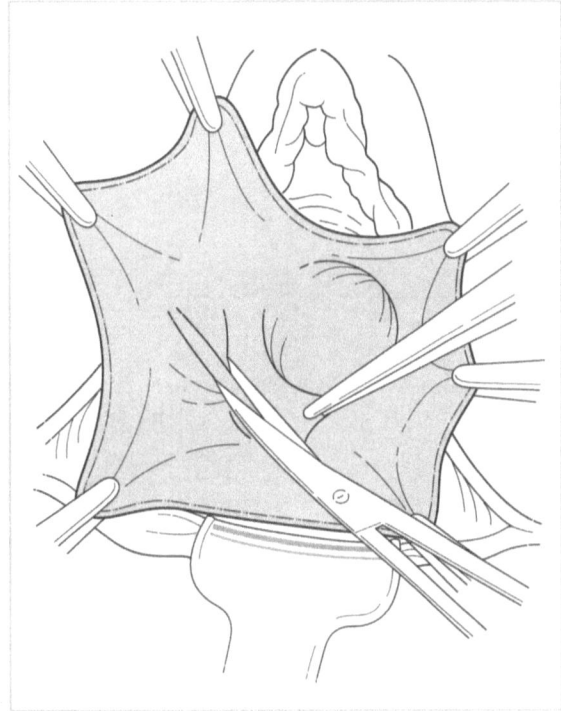

Figure 13.13 The para-rectal space is widely exposed.

The posterior fourchette is incised transversely, between two Kocher clamps, and a small, cutaneous triangular section is excised with the apex of the triangle towards the perineum. This incision allows the central tendon of the perineum to be rebuilt later. In sexually active patients, it is critical to avoid excessive excision, which can produce introital dyspareunia.

Step 3

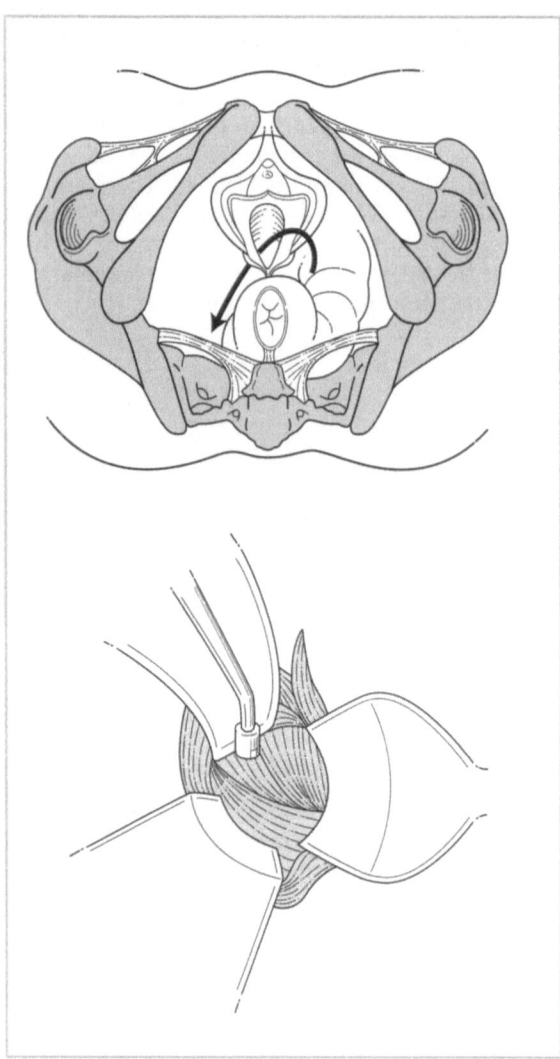

Figure 13.14 Dissection plan towards the sacrospinalis ligament.

The posterior vaginal wall is incised from the perineal incision to approximately 2 cm short of the urethral meatus. Two vaginal flaps are created bilaterally. These flaps are held by Allis clamps, and hemostasis is performed by electric cautery or bipolar scissors when available.

Step 4

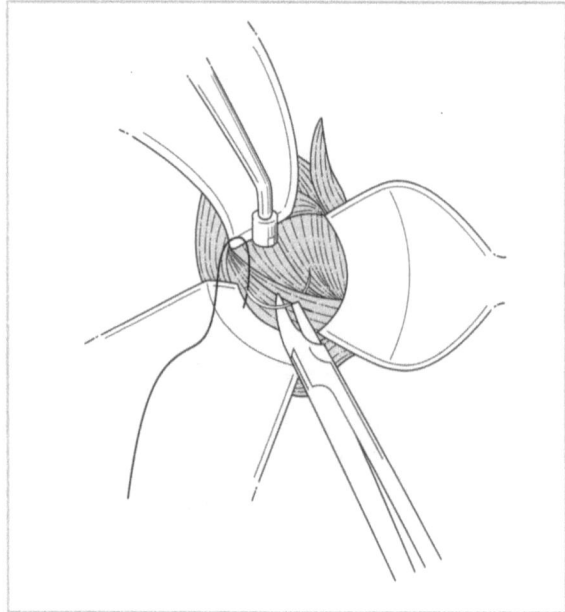

Figure 13.15 Three valves are positioned to expose the sacrospinalis ligament, which is then secured under direct visual control.

The peritoneal sac is opened, and any bowel loops or adhesions in the Douglas pouch are freed. After being dissected, the sac is excised, and the peritoneum is closed with a running absorbable suture. During that step, the Tredelenburg position is recommended along with a large vaginal pack to protect the bowel.

Step 5

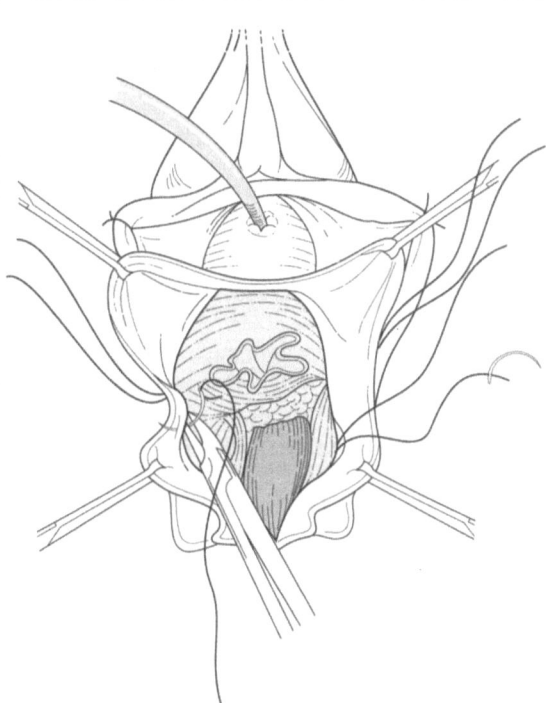

Figure 13.16 The same non-absorbable suture used to secure the sacrospinalis ligament is then passed through the initially identified vaginal vault apex at the location of the uterosacral ligament insertion.

Pararectal spaces are entered bilaterally with blunt or sharp dissection, which is extended to the ischial tuberosities. Three vaginal retractors or valves are then used. One is placed medially to protect the rectum, one superiorly to retract the peritoneum, and one laterally to protect the levator muscles. During dissection of the pararectal space, it is important that the dissection remains lateral, away from the pararectal fat, to avoid dissecting into the levator plane, which could lead to weakening of the muscle and possible bleeding.

Step 6

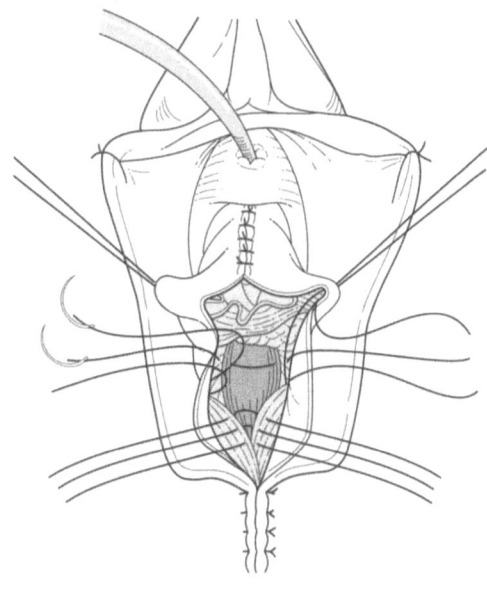

Figure 13.17 Transversal closure of the vaginal vault, care being taken to avoid a high compression of the rectum, possibly causing defecation difficulties. Then closure of the posterior midline incision after colpectomy, although limited in sexually active patients.

With proper retraction, the coccygeus muscle covering the sacrospinous ligament is exposed. The sacrospinalis ligament is secured with a no. 1 prolene (26 mm needle) halfway between the sacrum, medially, and the ischial tuberosity, laterally. Next, the suture is passed through the vaginal wall at the previously identified site for the future cuff. A similar procedure is performed on the opposite side. Then, the vaginal cuff is closed transversely to avoid narrowing the upper vagina and compressing the rectum, which leads to defecation difficulties. This transversal closure of the vaginal vault is performed with a running absorbable suture (2/0 Vicryl). A high levator myorraphy is then performed, recognizing the risk of possibly inducing dyspareunia if the sutures are too tight or placed too high beneath the posterior vaginal wall. We normally place three or four sutures of no. 1 PDS or Vicryl (36 or 48 mm needle) and then control the integrity of the rectum by digital rectal examination prior to tying the myorraphy sutures. This is certainly the most difficult part of the procedure for two reasons

- the sacrospinalis fixation sutures must remain loose preventing the vaginal apices to be tied directly over the sacrospinous ligament
- excessive traction on the cuff might pull down the anterior compartment resulting in secondary cystocele.

Once the sacrospinous fixation sutures are tied and the levator myorraphy is completed, the anterior and posterior vaginal incisions are closed with running absorbable sutures. Next, the perineorraphy is performed systematically to rebuild the central tendon of the perineum.

Technical Modifications

Unilateral Fixation

A unilateral fixation of the vaginal fornix directly into the sacrospinalis ligament can be performed with a permanent suture but will lead to a distorted vaginal cavity towards one side. This lateral deviation may lead to secondary enterocele and/or cystocele.

Bilateral Fixation Using Two Posterior Vaginal Wall Strips

In the case of a large prolapse, the sacrospinalis fixation cannot use uterosacral ligaments for support since those ligaments are loose or sometimes cannot be reliably identified. The quality of support therefore depends on the attachment of each vaginal fornix, which, given the obvious weakness of the vaginal wall tissue, puts the repair at risk. To broaden the vaginal anchoring and reduce the risk of pull-through, two, large, posterior vaginal strips coming from the excess posterior vaginal wall tissue at each apex can be secured to the sacrospinalis fixation sutures. This maneuver allows direct apposition of the vaginal strip to each ligament and diminishes tension on the sutures themselves. This modification has been described as a posterior vaginal wall "Bologna" repair.

Fixation Anterior to the Sacrospinalis Ligament

Some authors recommend securing the vagina to the ileococcygeous fascia. This procedure has the advantage of avoiding risk of sciatic nerve or pudendal vessel injuries, two known dramatic complications of the sacrospinalis fixation procedure. In addition, fixing the vagina more anteriorly might prevent development of an enterocele or cystocele secondarily. However, such a muscular attachment may diminish the long-term durability of the results.

Enterocele Closure

Richter describes a complete closure of the Douglas pouch that might be a more definitive procedure than the simple purse-string closure usually performed by these authors. However, the complexity of the Richter technique may not be necessary for all cases. In the case of a large enterocele, we recommend two purse-string closures, one on top of the other.

Sacrospinalis Fixation with Uterine Preservation

For years we have performed a unilateral sacrospinalis fixation for uterine preservation in young women with uterine prolapse but persistent desire for pregnancy, with good anatomic results.[82,83] However, persistent dyspareunia at the site where the uterine isthmus had been secured to the uterosacral ligament has been reported postoperatively in up to 15% of patients. Bilateral fixation can lead to significant constipation as a result of the cervix's direct compression on the rectum. Since 1994, a posterior vaginal strip, based on the posterior aspect of the cervix, has been anchored to the sacrospinous ligament. This restores support without inducing dyspareunia.

Specialized Instruments

Several instruments have been designed to grasp the ligament, including the Deschamps needle,[78] the Miya Hook,[84] and different stapling devices or needle drivers.[85–88] Our most recent modification uses the Endostitch laparoscopic device,[89] which by finger palpation, with a limited dissection of the ligament itself, allows placement of a strong nonabsorbable suture through the ligament. The Endostitch is a 36 cm clamp equipped with a needle that is connected to a Surgidac 0 suture. Transfer of the needle at the extremity of the jaws of the clamp facilitates good grasp of the ligament under direct fingertip control.

Results

Intraoperative Complications

Although rare, vascular complications are the most dreaded. Injuries to the pudendal venous plexus, perirectal veins, or internal pudendal artery have been reported during this operation.[90,91] However, even large series describe no more than a 2% blood transfusion rate.[92] Selective embolization may be necessary when transvaginal control with packing and vaginal compression does not control bleeding. Since we started using the Endostitch modification, no hemorrhagic complications have been reported despite our exposure to less experienced surgeons learning the technique. Although bladder or rectal injuries have only been reported between 3.6 and 4.5%,[92] the major risk is not to recognize them at the

Table 13.4. Anatomic results of largest series since Richter (1981)

Authors	Year	Follow-up	N	Success rate	Outcome measure
Richter[101]	1981	1–10 y	81	70%	Objective
Nichols[a][102]	1982	>2 y	163	97%	
Morley and Delancey[103]	1988	1 mo–11 y	92	82%	Subjective Objective
Brown[104]	1989	8–21 mo	11	91%	Objective
Kettel and Herbertson[105]	1989		31	81%	Subjective Objective
Cruikshank[106]	1990	8 mo–3;2 y	48	83%	Objective
Monk[107]	1991	1 mo–8;6 y	61	85%	Objective
Backer[108]	1992	?	51	94%	Objective
Heinonen[109]	1992	6 m0–5;6 y	22	86%	Objective
Imparato[a][110]	1992	?	155	90%	Objective
Shull[111]	1992	2–5 y	81	65%	Objective
Kaminski[112]	1993	?	23	87%	Objective
Ohana[a][93]	1993	6–78	145	91%	Objective
Carey[113]	1994	2 mo–1 y	63	73%	Objective
Holley[114]	1995	15–79 mo	36	8%	Objective
Sauer[115]	1995	4–26 mo	24	63%	Objective
Peters[116]	1995	48 mo	30	77%	Subjective Objective
Elkins[117]	1995	3–6 mo	14	86%	Objective
Pasley[a][118]	1995	6–83 mo	144	94%	Subjective Objective
Penalver[119]	1998	18–78 mo	160	85%	Objective

Except for the series of Nichols, Imparato, Ohana, and Pasley ([a]) which focus primarily on vaginal vault fixation, the success rates (%) reflect all aspects of pelvic floor reconstruction.

time of the procedure. In our series none of these complications have ever occurred.

Anatomic Results

On the basis of a large literature review, it seems that the success rate for the sacrospinalis fixation procedure is around 82%, with follow-ups ranging from 1 month to 10 years.[92] The experience of our unit is reported by Ohana[93] and Mansoor[94] with a correction of vaginal vault prolapse in 91% of the cases. Reported series are very inhomogeneous, and outcome measures are not well standardized (Table 13.4). Secondary cystocele ranges from 5% to 25%, with only 8% being symptomatic and requiring surgical correction (Table 13.5). This risk increases when a Burch colposuspension is performed concomitantly. When the vaginal cuff is well supported and the urethrovesical junction is fixed, the only remaining weak area in the anterior vaginal wall is in the mid to upper vagina, and this is where cystoceles are likely to occur.

Table 13.5. Comparative results of unilateral versus bilateral sacrospinalis fixation according to Mansoor et al.[94]

	SSF unilateral	SSF bilateral	Total
N	54	96	150
Date	1985–1989	1988–1990	
Lost to follow-up	3	2	5
Success	40/51 = 78.4%	92/94 = 97.8%	132/145 = 91%
Failure	11/51 = 21.6%	2/94 = 2.2%	13/145 = 9%

Postoperative Complications

Pain

Temporary gluteal or pericoccygeal pain occurs in 3% and 4.5% of patients, respectively, but tends to disappear within 3–6 months after surgery. Fortunately, lasting pain involving the sciatic nerve is rare. Among 800 sacrospinalis fixations performed in our department between June 1995 and December 1996, 4.5% of pain related to the sacrospinalis fixation was noted.[95] Pain originated in the gluteal

Table 13.6. Sexual activity (SA) results of sacrospinalis fixation

Authors	Year	N	Preop SA	Postop SA	SA		
					Same	Better	Worse
Richter and Albright[101]	1981	71	?		25 – Not SA 38 – same SA 8 – dyspareunia (narrow vagina)		
Ohana[a 93]		150	69	59	26	11	8
Heinonen[109]	1992	22	?	3	No sexual dysfunction		
Jacquetin and Fatton[b 83,120]	1996	39 (<40 y)	39	39	21 (54%)	12 (31%)	6 (15%)
Holley[121]	1996	36	17	16	7	3	6 narrow
Paraiso[122]	1996	243	163	163	Sexual dysfunction pre-op: 30.6% Sexual dsyfunction post-op: 20.2%		

[a] 10 are not SA postoperatively, 5 by lack of partner, 2 by fear of recurrence, and 3 because of dyspareunia (narrow vagina).
[b] Uterine preservation.

nerve in 41% of the cases, the pudendal nerve in 30%, the sciatic nerve in 14%, and vagina, causing dyspareunia in only 14% of the cases. Only 8 patients, 1% of the overall population, had persistent pain. Despite rather minimally invasive procedures, including the Endostitch variant described above, it is not likely that a totally pain-free procedure will ever be achieved considering the variability of the nerve terminals in this region.[91,96]

Dyspareunia

Limited data has been published on sexual function following vaginal surgery for prolapse (Table 13.6). In our own prospective study involving sexually active women less than 55 years old,[97-99] we found similar vaginal lengths comparing vaginal sacrospinalis fixation to abdominal mesh sacrocolpopexy (10.12 cm versus 10.32 cm), and similar vaginal caliber (Hegar dilator #30). Also, both groups responded similarly to sexual parameters (sexual drive, frequency of intercourse, quality of intercourse). These good results stem from surgeons experienced in vaginal surgery having learned to avoid excessive tension on posterior myorraphy and having carefully excised the redundant prolapsed vaginal wall. Although similar in our study, vaginal length is generally longer when an abdominal approach is selected.[100] But length did not correlate with sexual satisfaction.

Urinary Incontinence

The effect of a sacrospinalis fixation on unmasking incontinence is difficult to evaluate because the procedure is generally associated with cure of stress urinary incontinence, either present or potential. It is, however, agreed that the sacrospinalis fixation,

which brings the vaginal wall posteriorly over the levator plane, exposes more the anterior vaginal wall to intra-abdominal pressure changes. These may lead to sphincteric insufficiency or urethral hypermobility. Preoperative assessment with reduction of the prolapse with a gauze or a pessary is commonly used in urodynamic centers to detect latent stress incontinence. Overall, the exact effect of the sacrospinalis fixation on incontinence remains difficult to evaluate.

Future Perspectives

Several issues related to sacrospinalis fixation remain incompletely answered. Some of these issues have been debated in this chapter including the unilateral versus bilateral sacrospinalis fixation; the standard suturing procedures against the more recent Endostitch securement of the sacrospinalis fixation under finger guidance; outcome comparison between abdominal sacrocolpopexy and vaginal sacrospinalis fixation in terms of secondary prolapse (cystocele more common for the sacrospinalis fixation, rectocele more common for the open mesh sacrocolpopexy), and lastly, development of more objective outcome measures to provide reliable comparisons between series.

Conclusion

The sacrospinalis ligament fixation is a safe, reliable method to correct vault prolapse after hysterectomy. We also perform this operation preventively when the cervix drops to the level of the introitus under anesthesia. Its ease of performance and limited morbidity permit securing the vaginal vault after completion of a vaginal hysterectomy. Our long-term anatomical and functional results are acceptable even in younger patients. Until better techniques to repair anterior vaginal laxity are developed, the vaginal approach remains in competition with its abdominal counterpart, the abdominal sacrocolpopexy.

Iliococcygeus Hitch

Peter L. Dwyer and Steven E. Schraffordt

Vaginal vault prolapse is a common problem after hysterectomy; the incidence varies between 0.2% and 43%,[123] with most reports in the order of less than 5%.[124-127] The most effective method of supporting the upper vagina, either at the time of hysterectomy for uterovaginal prolapse or in the treatment of post-hysterectomy vault prolapse, is still debated. The vagina can be narrowed significantly by anterior and posterior colporrhaphy with vaginal mucosa excision to prevent the upper vagina telescoping downwards, but to the detriment of sexual function. In 1956 McCall[128] described the posterior culdoplasty where sutures were placed through the vagina, uterosacral ligaments, and peritoneum to close the cul-de-sac and support the vaginal vault. This procedure, with its numerous modifications[129,130] uses the cardinal/uterosacral complex to prevent or treat posthysterectomy vault prolapse. However, if these ligaments are absent or of poor quality, or the prolapse is of such severity that the vaginal apex is not pulled back into the upper vagina, other options are necessary for an effective surgical outcome. The vaginal apex can be attached to the pelvis either directly by suturing or indirectly by using autologous or synthetic material. The two sites in most common use today for transvaginal suture fixation of the vaginal apex are the sacrospinous ligament and iliococcygeal fascia. This chapter reviews the indications, surgical technique, and results of iliococcygeal fixation.

Anatomy

Surgical anatomy is covered in Chapter 1, but the anatomy of particular relevance to iliococcygeal fixation is reviewed here.

The muscular and fascioligamentous elements of the pelvic floor support the pelvic viscera and act as a platform against which the upper vagina and uterus are compressed with rises in abdominal pressure. The pubococcygeus muscles originate from the inner aspect of the pubis and anterior portion of the arcus tendineus fascia pelvis to form the medial part of the levator ani before inserting into the anococcygeal raphe and sacrum; the iliococcygeal muscles arise from the posterior arcus tendineous (tendinous arch) and ischial spine and insert into the lateral coccyx and sacrum. The upper vagina is also suspended to the lateral pelvic side wall by the fibromuscular paracolpos which is the inferior extension of cardinal and uterosacral ligaments.[131] The mid vagina lies close to the pelvic side wall and is attached laterally by the superior fascia of the levator ani to the pelvis along the arcus tendineous fasciae pelvis which runs from the ischial spines posteriorly to the posterior aspect of the symphysis pubis (Fig. 13.18). These

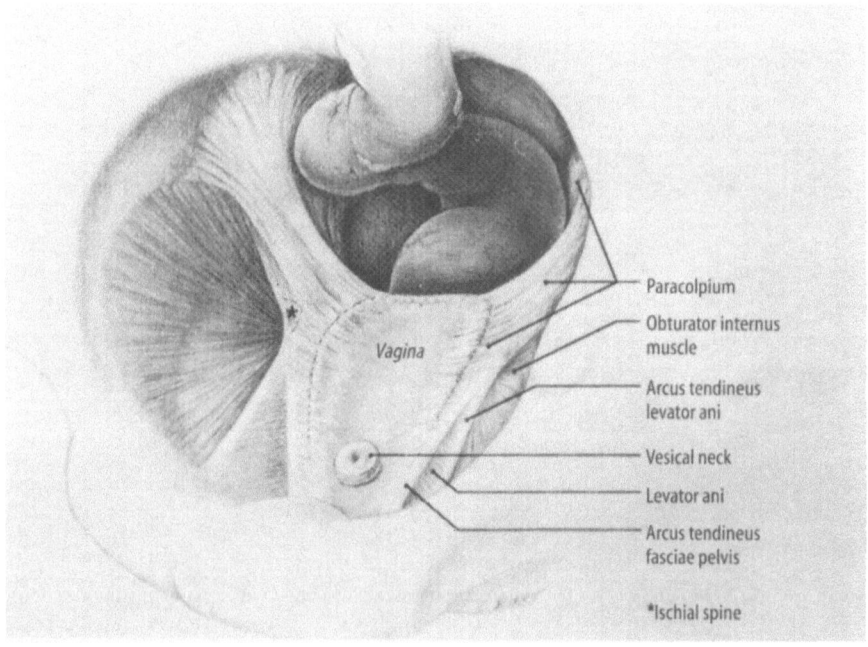

Paracolpium

Obturator internus muscle

Vagina

Arcus tendineus levator ani

Vesical neck

Levator ani

Arcus tendineus fasciae pelvis

*Ischial spine

Figure 13.18 The vagina and supporting structured drawn from a dissection of 56-year-old cadaver. The bladder has been removed above bladder neck. Note the closeness of the vagina to the ischial spine. From De Lancey.[131]

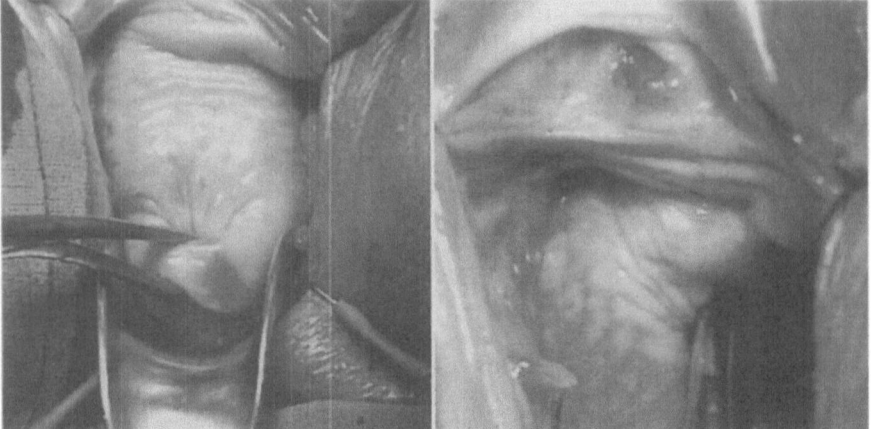

Figure 13.19 Woman with a grade 3 uterocervical prolapse and midline cystocele (**a**). In (**b**) the cervix is supported with a volsellum to reveal good lateral vaginal support and well-formed paravaginal gutters.

lateral supports are evident on speculum examination as paravaginal gutters with the upper aspect in close proximity to the ischial spine (Fig. 13.19b). The levator ani muscles provides the predominant active support to the pelvic floor[132] with the pelvic fascia and ligaments providing passive stabilization to prevent excessive movement. Once there is significant damage to the musculature either from a congenital (e.g. spina bifida) or acquired cause (e.g. childbirth, aging), loss of support will occur.

The anatomy relevant to iliococcygeal fixation is shown in Fig. 13.20. The obturator fascia which gives attachment to the levator ani muscles has been removed to reveal the underlying vessels, nerves and obturator internus muscle. Anterior and left of the Miya hook is the inferior vesical artery and the obturator nerve and artery which lies on the obturator internus before passing into the obturator foramen. The inferior gluteal artery can be seen posterior to the

sacrospinous ligament and is the most likely cause of severe hemorrhage secondary to misplaced suturing, careless retraction or overaggressive denudation of the sacrospinous ligament.[133] The pudendal nerve and accompanying vessels are relatively more protected beneath the ischial spine and sacrospinous ligament. The pudendal nerve then passes through Alcock's canal on the lateral wall of the ischiorectal fossa. The sciatic nerve and the posterior femoral cutaneous nerve leave the pelvis through the greater sciatic foramen between the pyriformis and the sacrospinous ligament.

In 1963 Inmon[134] discussed the pathogenesis of vaginal vault prolapse and reviewed the technique of vaginal hysterectomy and posthysterectomy vaginal prolapse repair. He also described the bilateral suspension of the vaginal cuff to the iliococcygeal fascia which he used in three patients with vaginal prolapse following hysterectomy where he was unable to iden-

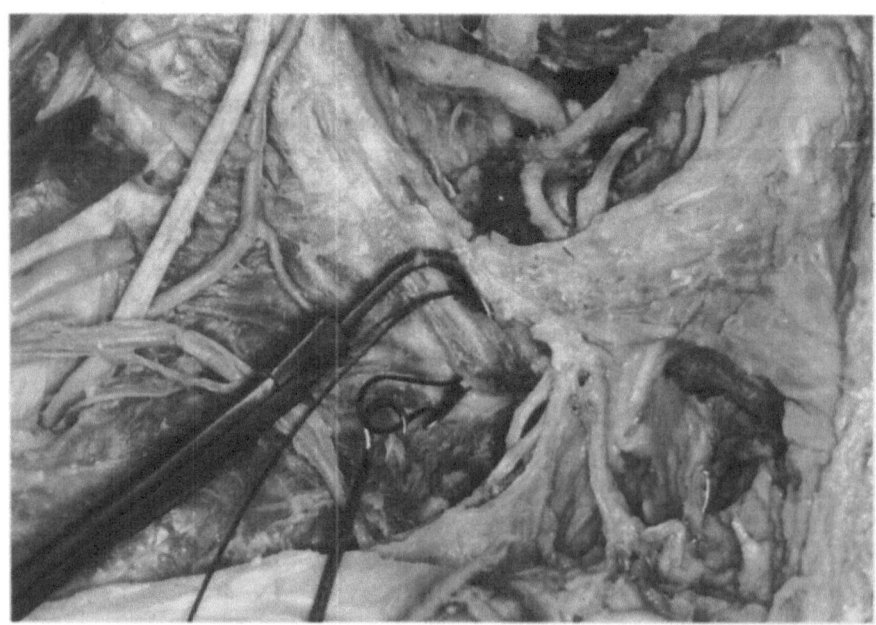

Figure 13.20 Lateral pelvic wall showing placement of iliococcygeal suture with Miya hook and nerve hook retrieval. The position of the ischial spine is marked with a dark pin.

tify uterosacral ligaments. Since then Shull et al.[135] and Meeks et al.[136] have reported their experience of iliococcygeal fixation for vaginal vault prolapse with excellent medium- to long-term results.

Indications

Iliococcygeal fixation, like the sacrospinous fixation, is an adjunctive procedure to provide extra support to the vaginal apex and upper vagina. This procedure is performed with vaginal repair of all other defects using appropriate procedures such as the anterior and posterior colporrhaphy, enterocele repair and the McCall procedure. Co-existing genuine stress incontinence with vaginal vault prolapse will require surgery which effectively treats both problems.

Indications for iliococcygeal fixation procedure are posthysterectomy vault prolapse or uterine prolapse where the upper vagina is detached from its fascial supports to the ischal spine. Iliococcygeal fixation of the vaginal cuff at the time of vaginal hysterectomy will provide better vaginal depth and support when the McCall procedure is unable to restore the apex to the upper vagina.

Operative Technique

Inmon's original description[134] and illustration (Fig. 13.21) provide a clear picture of this procedure and cannot be improved today:

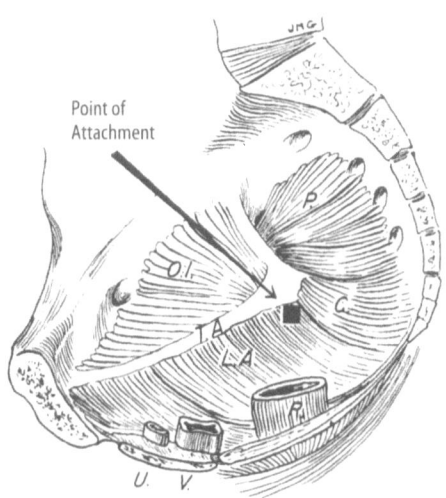

Point of Attachment

to avoid an abdominal approach in the absence of uterosacral ligaments, the lateral angles of the vagina may be attached to the fascia overlying the iliococcygei (Fig. 13.20). A chromic 1 suture begins in the left lateral angle of the vaginal cuff, enters the iliococcygeus below the ischial spine and is brought back through the cuff and tied. In like manner the right lateral angle of the vaginal cuff is attached to the right iliococcygeus.

Modifications to this procedure since 1963 have only been minor.[135,136]

In women with posthysterectomy vaginal eversion, a midline vertical incision is made the full length of the vaginal prolapse from just beneath the urethra to the perineum. If the anterior vaginal wall has good support on pre- and intraoperative assessment, a smaller incision over the posterior and vault prolapse would be made. Little or no vaginal mucosa needs to be excised as the upper vagina is fixed bilaterally to maintain good vaginal length and caliber. The ischial spines can be approached through either an anterior or posterior vaginal wall incision. The rectum, any enterocele sac and bladder are freed from the vagina with sharp and blunt dissection which is carried laterally up the pelvic side wall to the ischial spines. The prominent ischial spines are easily palpated; the coccygeal and sacrospinous ligament complex can be identified running posterio-medially from the spines and the iliococcygeal fascia covering the muscle anteriorly. Any midline pubo-cervical or rectovaginal fascial defect should be repaired. If an enterocele sac is identified, it is opened and the peritoneum is closed with a high purse-string suture of 2/0 PDS which is sutured to any remnant of the uterosacral or cardinal ligaments. These sutures are left long to close the vaginal vault and to provide further apical support. A 1 PDS suture (polydioxonane suture, Ethicon) is then placed into the iliocooccygeal fascia anterior to the ischial spine using a Miya hook (Fig. 13.14) similar to the techique described by Miyazaki for sacrospinous fixation;[137] suture placement is determined by palpation with adequate suture anchorage confirmed by traction. The 1 PDS suture is retrieved by a nerve hook and then passed through the full thickness of the lateral vaginal wall at the junction of the upper one-third and middle two-thirds. This is then repeated on the other side. The position for suture placement can also be marked preoperatively by resting the vagina against the ischial spine. The suspension sutures are tied over the vaginal mucosa once the anterior and posterior colpoperineorrhaphy have been completed and epithelium closed. If nonabsorbable suture material is used, the suture should be passed subepithelially to avoid vaginal exposure and suture granuloma.

Prophylactic antibiotics are administered preoperatively. Postoperatively routine cystourethroscopy is performed to exclude urinary tract injury and to insert a suprapubic bladder catheter.[138] A vaginal pack is inserted into the vagina for 24 hours postoperatively.

Results and Complications

In Inmon's initial report of 3 cases, all achieved a good surgical outcome.[134] Shull et al.[135] reported on 40 women who had bilateral iliococcygeal fixation, 30 for posthysterectomy vaginal vault prolapse and 10 for uterine prolapse. Two women developed recurrent vault prolapse, 4 patients developed anterior wall prolapse (≥ grade 2) and 2 posterior wall prolapse. One patient with vault prolapse was asymptomatic, the other required further surgery and was successfully treated with a sacrospinous colpopexy. In the Meeks et al. series of 110 women,[136] two-thirds had posthysterectomy vaginal vault prolapse and a third had uterine prolapse. There were only 4 failures, all having recurrent prolapse of the anterior vaginal wall. No comment was made in either study on other aspects of pelvic floor function such as sexual, urinary, and bowel function.

Maher et al.[137] evaluated 128 women who had surgery for symptomatic vaginal vault prolapse in our department between January 1994 and June 1998; 78 had undergone sacrospinous fixation and 50 had iliococcygeal fixation. From these 128 women, 36 pairs were matched for 8 or more of 10 criteria for age, parity, body mass index, menopause, previous prolapse or incontinence surgery, constipation, sexual activity, grade of prolapse, stress incontinence, and length of follow-up. Concomitant surgery is shown in Table 13.7; one of the 36 women in each group had a vaginal hysterectomy for uterocervical prolapse as well as cuff fixation. The mean length of postoperative review was 21 months in the iliococcygeal group and 19 months for the sacrospinous group (p = 0.52) and mean ages were 64 and 67 years (p = 0.08). Thirty-one of 36 women in the iliococcygeal group and 32 of 36 in the sacrospinous group had no symptoms of prolapse when assessed by an

independent nurse reviewer who was blinded to their previous surgery. Patient's satisfaction with surgery was recorded on a visual analogue scale (0–100); the mean postoperative satisfaction rate was 78/100 (iliococcygeal) and 91/100 (sacrospinous) (p = 0.1). One woman, who had an excellent anatomical result at 2 years review following iliococcygeal, rated the surgery as highly unsatisfactory due to buttock pain that lasted 3 months. Vaginal examination was performed by both assessors; if assessment differed the highest grade of prolapse was assigned. Seventeen of 36 in the iliococcygeal group and 12 of 36 who had sacrospinous fixation were assessed as having "prolapse" to or beyond the mid vagina. The anterior vaginal wall was the commonest site of recurrence occurring in 12 and 9 women who had iliococcygeal and sacrospinous fixation respectively. Only one woman who had a iliococcygeal fixation required further surgery (abdominal sacrocolpopexy) for recurrent vaginal prolapse. Another woman in the sacrospinous group underwent a Fenton's repair for superficial dyspareunia. No other women in either group required further surgery for symptomatic prolapse.

In the Meeks et al. series[136] there were 4 intraoperative complications, 1 rectal and 1 bladder perforation and 2 patients required transfusion secondary to hemorrhage. Two patients developed a cuff abscess which required surgical drainage. There were no bladder or bowel injuries in Shull's series[135] or ours.[139] The incidence of blood transfusion (1/36) was similar in our iliococcygeal and sacrospinous fixation groups, as was the operating time, hospital stay, and return to normal voiding (5.5 days).

Gluteal pain has been reported following the sacrospinous fixation but not following the iliococcygeal fixation. Cruikshank et al.[127] found 20 of 135 women (15%) experienced of gluteal pain on the side of the sacrospinous fixation which resolved spontaneously by 6 weeks in all cases. They considered this was caused by dissection in the perirectal space, although Sze and Karram[129] thought that it was due to injury to nerves in the coccygeal sacrospinous ligament complex. We found that the incidence of gluteal pain following iliococcygeal fixation was 19%, similar to the sacrospinous group (14%) (p = 0.1). This resolved spontaneously in all cases by 2–3 months. Consequently, we believe that muscular injury secondary to suture fixation is a more likely cause.

Sacrospinous and iliococcygeal fixation were equally effective for vaginal vault prolapse in our series with a similar rate of recurrent prolapse and complications. Anterior vaginal wall prolapse is the most difficult area to provide long-term support in women with vaginal eversion and is the commonest site of failure after both transvaginal and abdominal vault fixation procedures.[140] The similar incidence of

Table 13.7. Concomitant surgery with iliococcygeal or sacrospinalis fixation. From Maher et al.[139]

Procedure	Iliococcygeal	Sacrospinous
n = 36 (%)	n = 36 (%)	
Anterior colporrhaphy	26 (72)	29 (81)
Posterior colporrhaphy	36 (100)	36 (100)
Enterocele	18 (50)	21 (58)
Vaginal hysterectomy	1	1
Colposuspension	2	1
Anal sphincter repair	0	1

postoperative cystocele in our series was surprising. The iliococcygeal fixation sutures are bilateral and anterior to the unilaterally placed sacrospinous sutures which should give better support to the anterior wall and a more horizontal vaginal axis.

Barlow et al.[141] in a community survey of British women of a similar age indicated that 50% of women over 50 years with a partner are sexually active and the prevalence of dyspareunia was 12%. The percentage of women sexually active preoperatively in our study was 54%, and did not change significantly postoperatively in the iliococcygeal (21/21) or sacrospinous (18/20) groups. The incidence of dyspareunia postoperatively was not significantly different in the two groups (14% vs 10%). In a study by Given et al.[142] the sacrospinous vault suspension did not reduce vaginal length or interfere with coital function in a group of sexually active women compared to matched controls. Maintaining the option of sexual activity is important in many women, although where coitus is no longer desirable, more extensive mucosal excision or colpocleisis may be appropriate. In vaginal repair using the modified McCall procedure the vagina is frequently reduced to 1 fingerbreadth diameter.[126,130] Webb et al.[130] reviewed a large series of 693 women who underwent primary repair of vaginal vault prolapse using this procedure. The patient's age at surgery (66 years) and satisfaction with surgery (82%) were similar to our series; 29% stated that they were sexually active postoperatively and 22% had dyspareunia.

The presence of stress incontinence with vaginal vault prolapse is not uncommon and presents a double challenge. The Burch colposuspension has been reported to predispose to the development of vault and posterior wall prolapse, which would make a sling procedure more appropriate for these patients. Newer sling procedures using cadaveric tissue or prolene mesh are predominantly vaginal procedures and may prove equally effective without leading to prolapse. For transvaginal repair of vault prolapse we prefer iliococcygeal rather than sacrospinous fixation as there is less posterior traction on the anterior vaginal wall which may compromise the continence mechanism.

One modification we have made to try to improve our transvaginal results is the use of prolene mesh. In women with vault and high cystocele, a strip of prolene mesh (2 cm × 10 cm) is placed under the bladder base and on to the iliococcygeal fascia bilaterally, to give good vault and upper anterior vaginal wall support. For vault and posterior wall prolapse the prolene mesh is cut in a Y shape, each upper arm is placed on to the ipsilateral sacrospinous ligament and the lower arm over the posterior vaginal wall. To date, results of this modification of the transvaginal fixation procedures have been good with no mesh complications.

Conclusion

A pelvic surgeon requires the flexibility and skill to vary the surgical approach (vaginal or abdominal) to the repair of complex prolapse to suit the patient's clinical situation, and anatomical and functional defects. Transvaginal repair of prolapse does have many advantages over the abdominal approach. All fascial defects can be repaired without the need for abdominal surgery, which at times can be extremely difficult in the presence of dense adhesions from previous pelvic surgery. The iliococcygeal suspension fixes the vagina anterior to the ischial spine and is indicated in women with uterovaginal or vault prolapse where there is complete detachment of the vagina from their normal supports.

The place of the sacrospinous fixation is for the patient with a posterior enterocele where the vaginal vault has good support. In the sacrocolpopexy, synthetic mesh is fixed to the anterior and posterior vaginal walls which is then attached to the anterior sacrum. Comparative studies have shown a better anatomical and functional outcome with the abdominal route rather than the vaginal route presumably because the mesh gives stronger, broader and more permanent attachment of the vagina to the pelvis.[21]

Vaginal Hysterectomy

Andrew C. Steele and Mickey Karram

Historical Perspective

Vaginal hysterectomy is one of the oldest surgical procedures, initially described at the time of Hippocrates (5th century BCE) for prolapse and later for carcinoma of the cervix. It was popularized by William Freund in 1878 in Germany and later improved by Doyen and Pean in France. Vaginal hysterectomy for cervical cancer in a prolapsed uterus was performed as early as 1813 by Langenbeck. Between 1813 and 1861, the indications for vaginal hysterectomy included cervical cancer and uterine gangrene. In 1829 John Warren of Harvard University performed the first documented vaginal hysterectomy, and in 1861 Choppin in New Orleans performed a vaginal hysterectomy specifically for prolapse. However, during the late 1800s the advancement of the technique was delayed by the emphasis on the less morbid vaginal obliterative procedures. LeFort in 1877 and Donald in 1888, reported procedures still in use today – the LeFort and Manchester procedures.[143]

With improvements in anesthesia and surgical techniques, the safety and hence the feasibility of performing vaginal hysterectomies led to a boom in descriptions of the technique. In 1934, Heaney[144] had performed 565 vaginal hysterectomies and described his technique; the soundness of his approach is demonstrated by the fact that this is still one of the most common techniques for vaginal hysterectomy.

Indications for Vaginal Hysterectomy

Abdominal and vaginal hysterectomies share common indications. However, there are several reasons why the gynecologic surgeon must be aware of both the indications for a hysterectomy as well as the intervening steps that should occur before a patient is considered a hysterectomy candidate. First, newer medications such as the GnRH agonists have provided effective therapy for some patients who would otherwise have required hysterectomy. Second, modern minimally invasive surgical techniques such as endometrial ablation and endoscopic electrocoagulation of myomas have added a new level of treatment options for the gynecologic surgeon.

Leiomyomata

The most common indication for hysterectomy in many countries continues to be that of the leiomyomatous, or fibroid, uterus, particularly when the fibroid uterus demonstrates rapid growth, when fibroids become symptomatic, or when significant uterine enlargement occurs postmenopausally.[145] Young women who want to conceive and women in the perimenopause who could reasonably expect resolution of their symptoms with the diminishing hormone output of the menopause should consider minimally invasive techniques before hysterectomy.

Chronic Pelvic Pain

Pelvic pain may be an indication for hysterectomy. Conditions such as adenomyosis or endometriosis should first be treated with conservative therapies. These include the use of nonsteroidal antiinflammatory agents as well as hormonal therapy. Other sources of the patient's pain, such as the gastrointestinal tract, the urinary tract, and the musculoskeletal system, should be evaluated and ruled out before proceeding with hysterectomy. If a hormonally sensitive condition (such as endometriosis or adenomyosis) is believed to be the cause of the patient's pain, then a trial of a GnRH agonist may be warranted as a diagnostic as well as therapeutic measure. If the pseudo-menopause induced by the GnRH agonist fails to relieve chronic pain attributed to endometriosis or adenomyosis, then a hysterectomy may be an inappropriate treatment option. An antidepressant medication as well as psychological counseling may be prudent before hysterectomy for chronic pelvic pain, and the patient should be aware that the procedure may not relieve her pain.

Dysfunctional Uterine Bleeding

After ruling out other causes of uterine bleeding such as cancer, fibroids, and endometrial polyps, the clinician treating abnormal uterine bleeding must consider that the bleeding is related to hormonal causes, a process termed dysfunctional uterine bleeding. Management with estrogenic and progestogenic compounds is the least invasive first step, but a proportion of women may fail or not tolerate these therapies. The decision to progress on to more aggressive surgical methods for control of bleeding would then be based on the degree of hemorrhage and the age and desires of the patient. Minimally invasive techniques for the control of menorrhagia include endometrial ablation by means of rollerballs, lasers, or balloons. In a recent randomized control trial of endometrial ablation versus hysterectomy, an approach including an initial attempt at ablation appeared superior to proceeding directly to hysterectomy. Performing an ablation as an initial step enabled 76% of women with dysfunctional bleeding were able to avoid hysterectomy and its associated morbidity.[146] For women in the perimenopause, even a few years' relief from abnormal bleeding may take them to the menopause and a natural end to their periods. The subgroup of women for whom conservative therapy does not work would then be considered candidates for hysterectomy.

Pelvic Organ Prolapse

Pelvic organ prolapse, with or without uterine prolapse, is an indication for hysterectomy. In some young women with pelvic organ prolapse who desire to preserve their fertility, a uterine conserving repair may be indicated. Kovac and Cruikshank described successful pregnancies and vaginal deliveries in 5 of 19 patients treated by a sacrospinous uterosacral fixation technique.[147] However, for the majority of women, the uterus should be removed for several reasons. First, the understanding of prolapse suggests that causation is based on the presence of global defects in the pelvic supportive tissue structures. Failure to recognize and repair all defects in prolapse support only leads to re-operation at a later time. Second, cervical elongation may develop when a cystocele or rectocele are repaired but the uterus is left in situ.

Although there are no randomized trials in the literature discussing the need for hysterectomy at the time of anti-incontinence surgery, a small prospective study by Langer suggested that patients who underwent urethropexy had no difference in incontinence cure rates if they underwent a concomitant hysterectomy.[148]

Other Indications

Other indications for hysterectomy include cervical intraepithelial neoplasia (CIN) and adenomatous hyperplasia. Most CIN may be treated by techniques such as loop electrode excision, cryosurgery, and conization, but some patients with multifocal severe disease who have completed childbearing may desire hysterectomy, especially if the CIN is recurrent. Obviously, many malignant conditions of the abdomen and pelvis may necessitate hysterectomy; however, that discussion is beyond the scope of this chapter.

Choosing the Route of Hysterectomy

With the advent of laparoscopic hysterectomy and laparoscopic assisted vaginal hysterectomy, the gynecologist today is faced with a choice of routes for removal of the uterus and adnexa. A great deal of literature has been published on the indications for choosing the route of removal of the uterus.

Vaginal hysterectomy provides clear benefits over abdominal hysterectomy in regards to operating room time and overall recovery. Operating room time may be decreased by 50% in patients undergoing a vaginal hysterectomy rather than an abdominal hysterectomy.[149] Dorsey et al. reported average hospital stays as 2.9 days in the group undergoing vaginal hysterectomy compared with 3.9 days in the group undergoing abdominal hysterectomy. In this study, the vaginal hysterectomy group was found to have mean facility charges of £1947 ($3116), compared with £2471 ($3954) for the abdominal group and £3071 ($4914) for the laparoscopically assisted group.[150]

Vaginal hysterectomy appears to be underutilized when compared with abdominal or laparoscopically assisted hysterectomy. In a study on hysterectomies done at one large teaching hospital in 1992–93, 6.6% of all abdominal hysterectomies and 16.7% of all laparoscopically assisted vaginal hysterectomies lacked a clear indication over a simple vaginal hysterectomy.[151] Davies found that 76% of the patients undergoing hysterectomy at the Royal Free Hospital in London had no contraindication to vaginal hysterectomy; however, only 19% of all hysterectomies were performed vaginally.[152]

Laparoscopically assisted vaginal hysterectomy is superior to abdominal hysterectomy. However, when compared to vaginal hysterectomy there appears to be little benefit to the laparoscopic route.[153] In a randomized trial of laparoscopically assisted versus traditional vaginal hysterectomy, Summitt et al. found no benefit to the addition of the laparoscopic portion of the procedure, other than to nearly double the costs.[154] Although there is a clear place for laparoscopic hysterectomy, such as in women with adnexal disease, most women should be considered candidates for vaginal hysterectomy.

The primary contraindication to the vaginal approach is malignant disease requiring upper abdominal debulking. Many other conditions felt to be relative contraindications to vaginal hysterectomy have in fact proved to be amenable to this approach. For instance, many surgeons defer vaginal hysterectomy in the patient with an enlarged uterus. Although there is no specific upper limit of normal size above which a vaginal hysterectomy should be attempted, many gynecologists limit vaginal hysterectomies to patients with uteri less than 12 weeks' size. However, uterine size alone is not a contraindication to vaginal hysterectomy. Kovac has described his results utilizing intramyometrial coring to remove myomatous and other enlarged uteri. His impressive series of 575 patients undergoing intramyometrial coring demonstrated no difference in outcomes, including blood loss, when compared with vaginal hysterectomies.[155] Hoffman et al. compared morcellation with abdominal hysterectomy and found that blood loss, operating time, and time till discharge was significantly less in patients undergoing morcellation.[156] Pelosi and Pelosi[157] have reported the vaginal removal of a 2003 g uterus, which clearly suggests that uterine size should not contraindicate vaginal hysterectomy.

Similarly, a previous cesarean section should not prohibit a vaginal hysterectomy. Unger and Meeks found that a history of a prior cesarean section did not significantly affect the complication rate of vaginal hysterectomies performed for various indications, including prolapse.[158] Further, they failed to find an association between number of prior cesareans and increasing complications during vaginal hysterectomy.

Ultimately, the patient's informed preference, the surgeon's comfort level with various procedures, and the underlying disease process must guide the gynecologist in choosing the most appropriate route for hysterectomy.

Technique

The technique of vaginal hysterectomy begins with patient positioning. The patient should be placed in the dorsal lithotomy position with her feet in long vertical (candy cane) stirrups (Fig. 13.22). We have found that Allen stirrups provide inadequate room within the operative field for the surgeon and two assistants necessary for vaginal surgery. Care should be taken to avoid hyperextension at the hip. The lateral aspects of the legs should be clear of the stirrup to avoid pressure on the peroneal nerve.

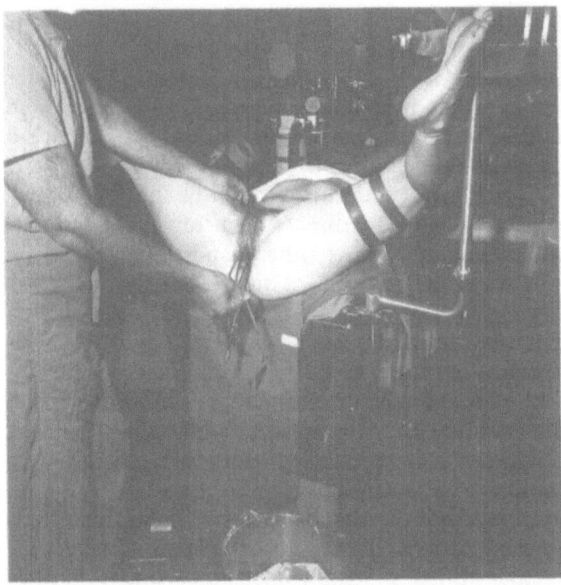

Figure 13.22 Vertical poles will support the patient's legs and allow the surgeon and two assistants to sit and operate comfortably. The scrub nurse stands behind or to the side of the surgeon.

Examination under anesthesia is an important first step in the surgical procedure. The degree of uterine decensus, the width of the vaginal outlet, and the presence or absence of pelvic pathology should all be assessed.

The patient is then prepped and draped and her bladder drained. Vasoconstrictors such as pitressin (2 units in 50 ml of normal saline), neosynephrine, or epinephrine may be injected if no medical contraindication, such as hypertension or heart disease, contraindicates their use. We prefer using a prepared solution of either 1 or 2% xylocaine or 0.5% bupivacaine with 1 : 200 000 of epinephrine. Use of these readymade solutions negates the need for mixing in the operating suite and provides some pre-emptive analgesia at the surgical site. The surgeon should remember that the maximum amount of xylocaine with epinephrine used should not exceed 7 mg/kg or 500 mg total in the healthy adult, and bupivacaine with epinephrine should generally not exceed 225 mg. These total doses should be adjusted downward for elderly or debilitated patients but this should present no problem since only around 5–10 ml of injection is required during the procedure. Should a medical contraindication to the use of vasopressors be present, injectable saline provides the benefits of hydrodistension without the cardiovascular risks.

The initial incision begins circumferentially at the reflection of the vaginal mucosa onto the cervix. We prefer to incise in a posterior to anterior direction through the full thickness of the vaginal mucosa. Although a scalpel is appropriate, electrocautery is the preferred method for incision since it provides

some hemostasis. Using a low cutting current with a low blend of coagulation minimizes charring. A plane between the mucosa of the vagina and the underlying cervical stroma may be located utilizing sharp dissection. The bladder must be mobilized off the cervix in the midline. Once the bladder has been displaced enough to allow clamping of the uterosacral ligaments, we proceed along the posterior aspect of the uterus. The posterior cul-de-sac is entered sharply, as close to the reflection of the parietal peritoneum onto the cervix as possible. After placing a weighted vaginal retractor into the cul-de-sac, the bilateral uterosacral ligaments are identified and clamped individually using a crushing clamp such as a Heaney. The uterosacral ligament should be clamped as close to its insertion into the uterus as possible (Fig. 13.23a,b). The pedicle should be ligated proximal to the clamp, with care taken to include the entire pedicle in the ligature. We prefer a 2–0 delayed-absorbable synthetic suture for all our uterine pedicles. After ligating and cutting the uterosacral, the sutures should be tagged for later identification of the ligament. It is prudent to perform a digital examination of the adnexa at this time, as the occasional adnexal mass not detected on preoperative evaluation may lead the surgeon to consider conversion to an abdominal approach.

At this point an attempt should be made to enter into the anterior cul-de-sac. Initially, resistance may be encountered at the attachment of the endopelvic fascia to the anterior cervix. Once through this, the plane between the bladder and the cervix becomes readily apparent. Further mobilization is done by careful sharp dissection in the plane between the endopelvic fascia and the cervical stroma. This dissection should remain in the midline, as the lateral bladder pillars tend to be quite vascular (Fig. 13.24). A Heaney retractor is then placed, exposing the anterior peritoneal fold. This serves to expose the operative field more fully, to elevate the bladder away from the area of dissection, and to distance the ureters from the operative site. The peritoneal fold is grasped with toothed pick-ups and entered sharply. Once the anterior cul-de-sac is entered, the bladder can be elevated out of the operative field using a Heaney retractor inserted into the peritoneal cavity between the bladder and the cervix.

Much time and frustration can be avoided by not rushing to get into the anterior cul-de-sac. It is more prudent to take several pedicles posteriorly rather than struggling with the anterior entry. Once mobilized in this manner, the difficult anterior entry can be facilitated by hooking a finger around the fundus to identify the anterior peritoneum.

The hysterectomy proceeds with the cardinal ligament being clamped at its insertion into the uterine isthmus. When both the anterior and posterior parietal peritoneum can be included in a single

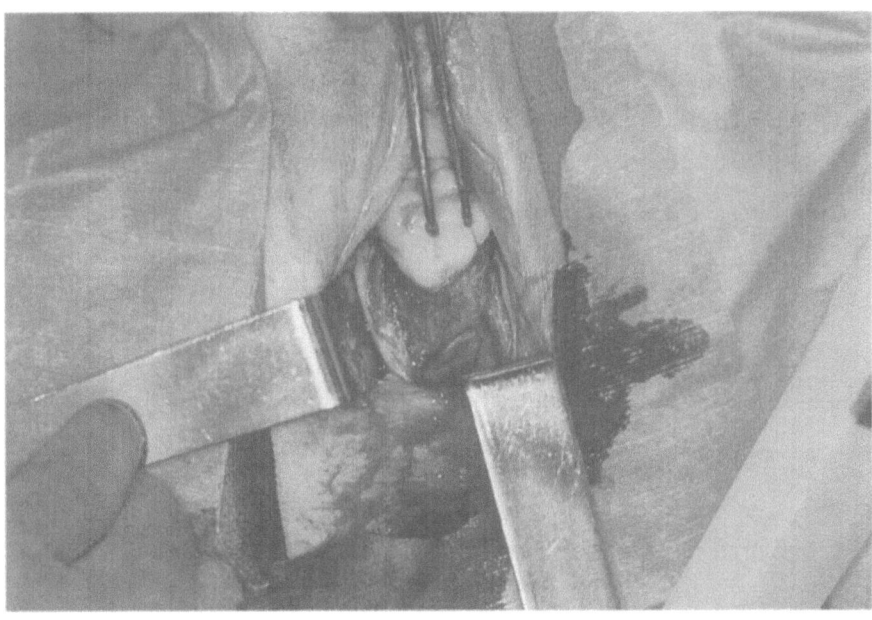

Figure 13.23 a The posterior cul-de-sac is entered. **b** The uterosacral is clamped close to its insertion into the cervical stroma. Part b reprinted with permission from Baggish and Karram (2001) Atlas of Pelvic Anatomy and Gynaecologic Surgery. WB Saunders Co., 353.

a

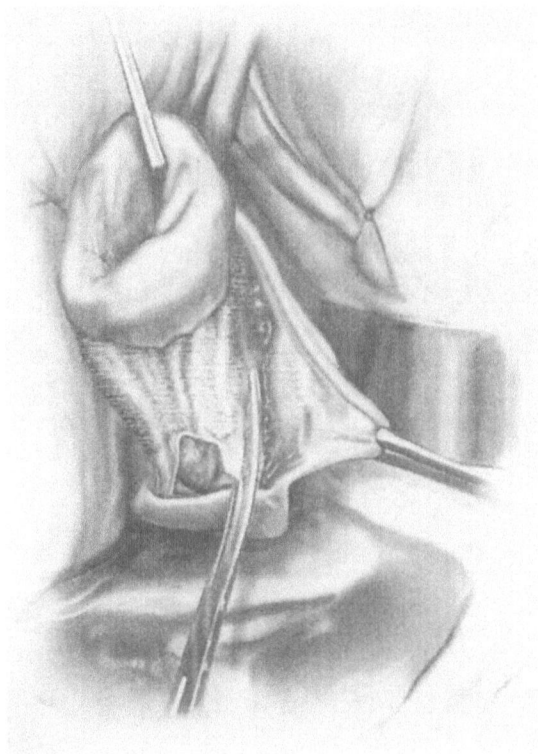

b

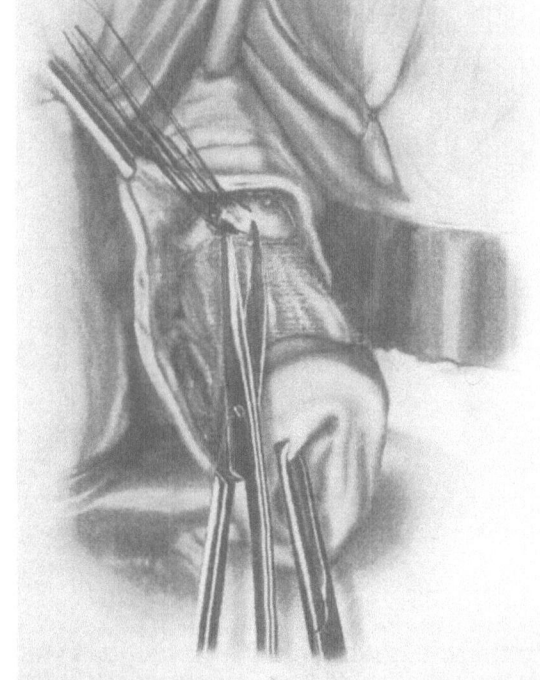

Figure 13.24 The vesico-uterine peritoneal fold is sharply incised. Reprinted with permission from Baggish and Karram (2001) Atlas of Pelvic Anatomy and Gynaecologic Surgery. WB Saunders Co., 354.

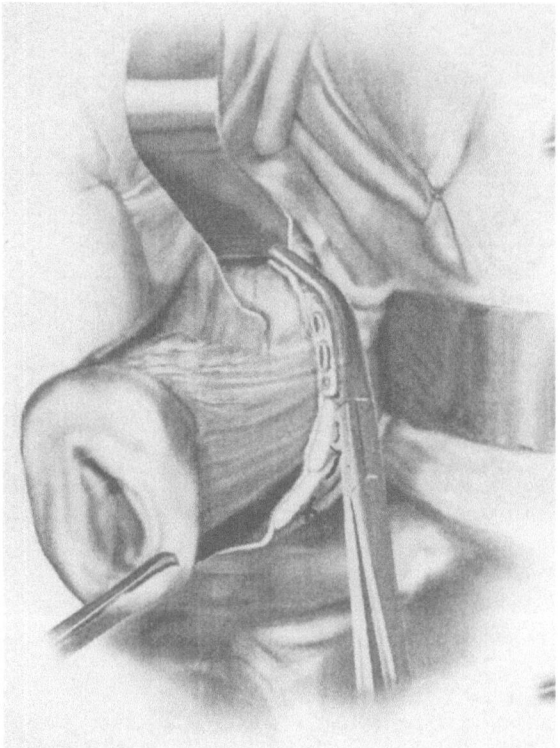

a

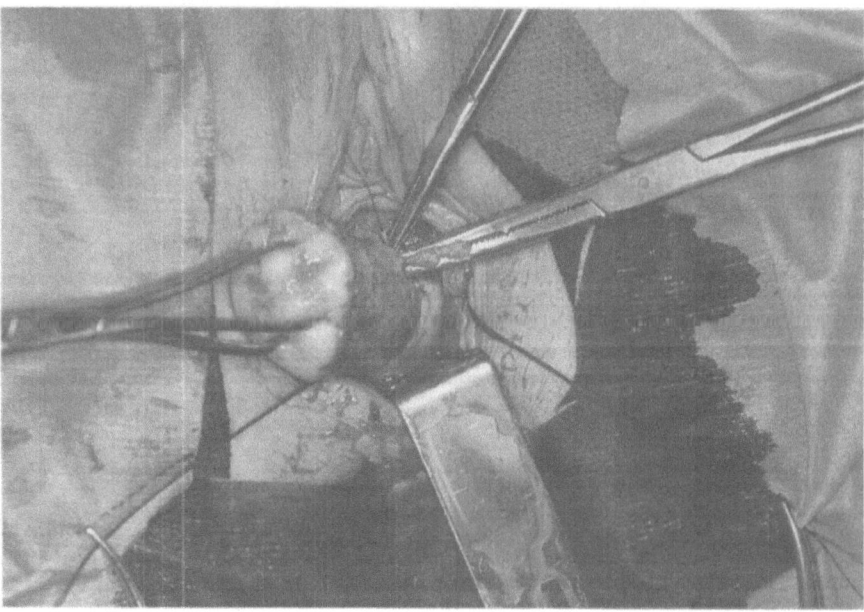

b

Figure 13.25 a The vessels are located when the anterior and posterior leaves of the broad ligament can be included in a single clamp. **b** The surgical needle should be passed close to the tip of the clamp. Care should be taken to avoid transfixing the vessels with the needle as this may lead to an ascending hematoma.
Part a reprinted with permission from Baggish and Karram (2001) Atlas of Pelvic Anatomy and Gynaecologic Surgery. WB Saunders Co., 356.

clamp, the uterine vessels are generally found to be included in the pedicle (Figure13.25a,b).

The remaining broad ligament should be serially clamped with a crushing clamp. Transfixion suture ligatures should be used to secure each pedicle. This process may be carried bilaterally to the top of the uterus. Alternately, the uterus may be rotated 180° by grasping the fundus with a single toothed or thyroid tenaculum, and applying gentle outward traction. This provides access to the top of the broad ligament and also compresses the remaining tissue together, providing a smaller pedicle (Fig. 13.26). Care should be taken at this point to avoid taking too large "bites", as this may lead to slippage of tissue and bleeding which is difficult to control. Also, any downward traction should be gentle, as only a small amount of tissue remains to support the uterus and evulsion of this last pedicle is possible.

Another technique for securing this final pedicle involves passing a free ligature around the pedicle; the Deschamps ligature carrier is especially helpful for this. When this free ligature is tied down, the pedicle becomes more readily managed with clamps.

Irrigation and inspection of the pedicles should be performed. In our experience, the most common site of hemorrhage is the posterior colpotomy incision. The uterine specimen should also be inspected and bivalved to allow fixation of the endometrial tissue in formalin.

The adnexa should always be inspected. The techniques for performing vaginal oophorectomy, when indicated, are described in the next section. Although it is helpful to perform a purse-string closure of the peritoneum in order to exteriorize the vascular pedicles, this is less important than assuring closure of the defect created in the endopelvic fascia by the hysterectomy.

The cul-de-sac should be routinely evaluated to determine the presence of an enterocele. A culdoplasty of some sort should be routinely considered in all cases. A McCall's-type culdoplasty begins by passing a delayed-absorbable suture through the posterior vaginal cuff from the vagina into the peritoneal cavity. The suture is then passed through the ipsilateral uterosacral ligament as cephalad as is feasible. The suture is then used to take "skimming" bites of tissue over the posterior parietal peritoneum and the serosa of the sigmoid. It is passed through the contralateral uterosacral and then brought back out into the vagina. This procedure can be repeated with a series of sutures. After closure of the vaginal cuff, the culdoplasty sutures are tied down, approximating the uterosacral ligaments, posterior parietal peritoneum, and vaginal cuff, and elevating the cuff.

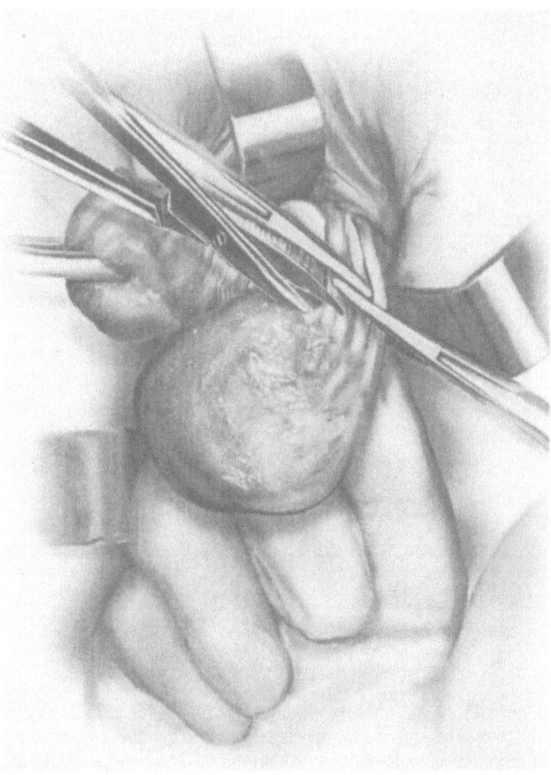

Figure 13.26 The uterine fundus may be inverted and delivered to facilitate access to the upper pedicles. Reprinted with permission from Baggish and Karram (2001) Atlas of Pelvic Anatomy and Gynaecologic Surgery. WB Saunders Co., 357.

Another technique involves the suspension of the vagina to the uterosacral ligaments with a fascial reconstruction. This allows a restoration of the continuity of the pubocervical and rectovaginal fascia. The uterosacral ligaments, which were tagged bilaterally at the start of the procedure, are identified. The ureter is identified on the lateral sidewalls. Interrupted sutures of permanent monofilament suture are passed through one uterosacral at the level of the ischial spine. Numerous superficial bites are then taken through the posterior parietal peritoneum and serosa of the sigmoid colon. The suture is then passed through the opposite uterosacral ligament (Fig. 13.27a). Two or three sutures are passed in this fashion and then tied across the midline. This creates a durable ridge of tissue high up in the hollow of the sacrum. Delayed-absorbable sutures are then passed through the posterior vaginal mucosa, the posterior endopelvic fascia, and into the uterosacral ledge. The sutures are then passed through the endopelvic fascia anteriorly and brought out through the vagina (Fig. 13.27b). Four to five sutures are passed in this manner from one corner of the vaginal incision to the other. When tied down, these sutures effectively close the fascial defect as well as support the vagina on the uterosacral ridge (Fig. 13.28a,b). Interrupted delayed-absorbable

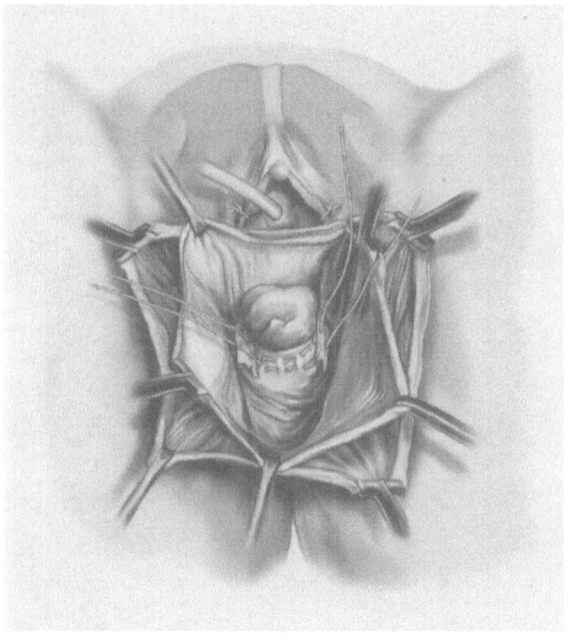 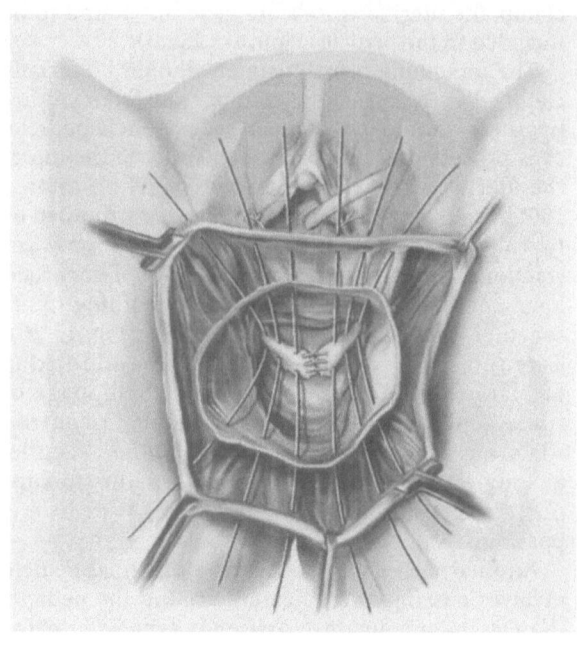

a   b

Figure 13.27 a Permanent monofilament sutures are passed through one uterosacral ligament, skimmed across sigmoid serosa, and passed through the contralateral uterosacral. **b** Delayed-absorbable sutures are passed through the posterior endopelvic fascia, into the uterosacral ridge, and out through the anterior endopelvic fascia. Reprinted with permission from Walters and Karram, Urogynecology and Reconstructive Pelvic Surgery (2e), Mosby, 246.

sutures may be used to close any defects in the vaginal mucosa. The surgeon should be careful at this point to only re-approximate the vaginal mucosa in order to prevent vaginal shortening.

Managing the Adnexa

An important adjunctive procedure for the surgeon performing vaginal hysterectomies is adnexectomy.

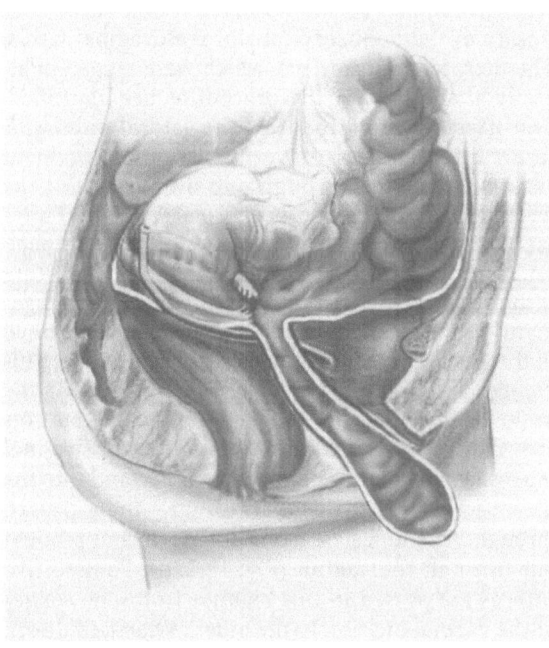 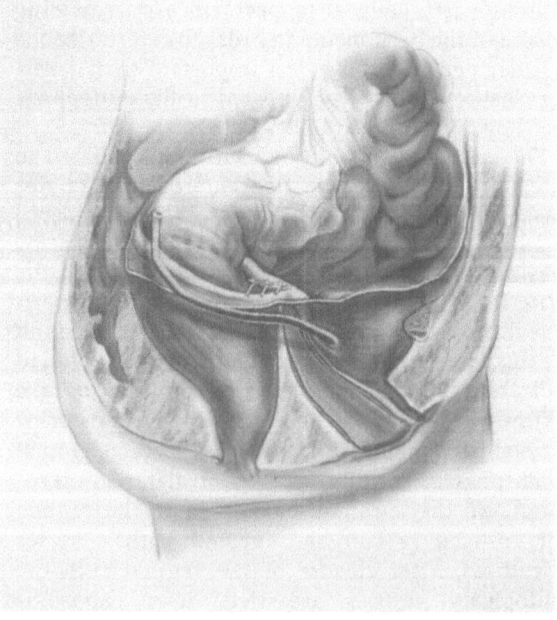

a   b

Figure 13.28 a Pelvis with large enterocele. **b** Following excision of the enterocele sac, the vaginal vault is suspended to the uterosacral ligaments. Note the continuity of the pubocervical and rectovaginal fascias. Reprinted with permission from Walters and Karram, Urogynecology and Reconstructive Pelvic Surgery (2e), Mosby, 252.

The procedure begins by locating the adnexa. Utilizing suture tags to provide gentle traction to the round ligaments will aid in visualization of the tube and ovary. Next, the ovary and tube are grasped with a Babcock clamp. The location of the ureter must be identified and its course noted to be well clear of the operative field. The infundibulopelvic ligament with its associated ovarian vessels is then clamped across utilizing a curved clamp. A curved Heaney clamp may be utilized for this, but the Satinsky vascular clamp is actually ideal for the procedure. The tissue is then cut and the pedicle suture ligated with 2-0 delayed-absorbable synthetic sutures. We place an initial free tie on the pedicle, followed by a transfixion suture ligature distal to the first tie. This secures the suture on the pedicle and prevents development of an ascending hematoma. The pedicle should be carefully inspected for bleeding before cutting the sutures, because once the sutures are cut it will become more difficult to re-grasp the pedicle.

Vaginal oophorectomy can be performed safely if several important steps are taken. First, the location of the ureter must be known and its injury prevented.[159] Several techniques have been described for this. This ideal method of locating and protecting the ureter is by direct palpation of the ureter through the broad ligament. Another technique for identification of the ureter is to place ureteral stents cystoscopically prior to the procedure. These may aid in the tactile identification of the ureter, although their benefit in preventing ureteral injury has not been clearly proven. Second, the surgeon should avoid blind clamping of structures during oopherectomy as this may increase the risk of injury to bowel, as well as hinder the surgeon from knowing if the pedicle had indeed been completely secured.

Despite limitations of visualization from the vaginal approach, transvaginal oophorectomy at the time of hysterectomy can be very successful. Sheth reported on 740 hysterectomies performed with attempted oopherectomy and compared them with 700 hysterectomies without oophorectomy. He was successful in removing the ovaries 94% of the time, without added morbidity.[160]

Selected Difficulties and Complications of Vaginal Hysterectomy

The Massive Leiomyomatous Uterus

The uterus measuring greater than 12 weeks' gestational size presents difficulties for the gynecologist for two reasons.

● First, the uterus is obviously enlarged to the point where it cannot readily be removed through the vagina without morcellation. There are several techniques, including intramyometrial coring, transvaginal myomectomy, or bivalving the uterus. All these techniques require the ligation of the major blood supply to the uterus through the uterine arteries. Once the uterine vessels have been ligated and divided as previously described, we begin the process of morcellation. Once the anterior cul-de-sac has been entered, the cervix can be removed with a scalpel (Fig. 13.29). Tenaculi are used to grasp the posterior side of the uterus and deliver some portion of it into the operative field, walking successive bites of tenaculi cephalad. Using a scalpel or Mayo scissors, downward traction is placed on the tissue within the

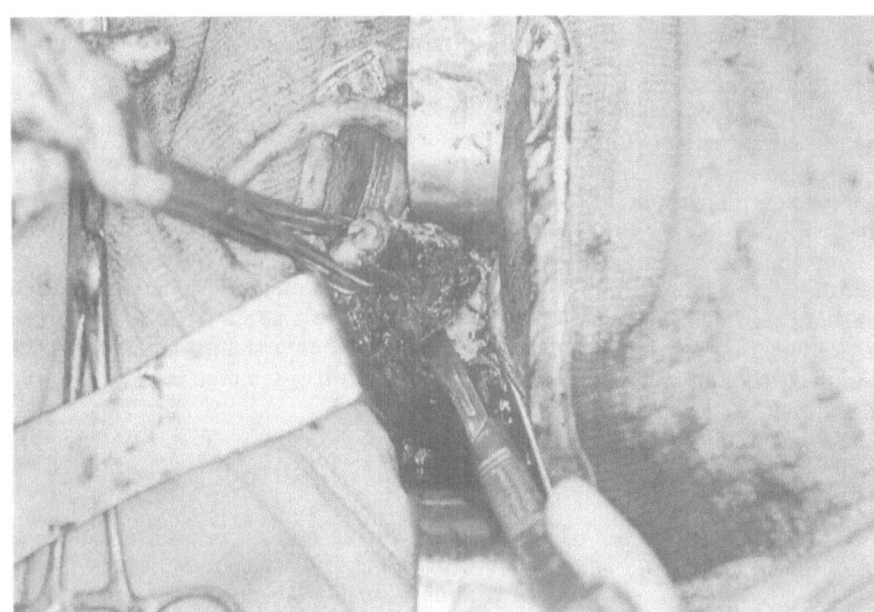

Figure 13.29 Uterine morcellation is performed using a scalpel and tenaculi. Reprinted with permission from Baggish and Karram (2001) Atlas of Pelvic Anatomy and Gynaecologic Surgery. WB Saunders Co., 375.

tenaculum, and this tissue is excised en bloc. The process is repeated until the fundus can be completely delivered. During the procedure, any discrete fibroids which are located may be removed using standard myomectomy techniques. Care should be taken when using this technique that overly aggressive morcellation is not performed, as the scalpel can pass through the fundus and injure hollow viscera if large volumes of material are taken. Use of a long retractor such as a Breisky Navratil will prevent bladder or bowel injury. No matter how tedious, it is better to take several small cones of tissue than one large one (Fig. 13.29). Finally, if the fundus of the uterus can be located, the remaining myometrium can be bivalved and the individual pedicles created as previously described. An alternative to morcellation, especially in patients in which the posterior fundus cannot be delivered, is intramyometrial coring. A circumferential excision into the body of the uterus at or near the isthmus is made using a scalpel or Mayo scissors. This should be wide enough to include the endometrial cavity in the core specimen, but not so wide that the instrument perforates the fundus. Downward traction delivers the cored specimen, eventually turning the uterus "inside out."

- The second problem with enlarged leiomyomatous uteri is enlarged lateral fibroids in the isthmic region of the uterus distorting the normal anatomy which may make it difficult to ligate the uterine vessels with confidence. It is prudent to continue with securing the lateral pedicles until the uterine vessels can be ligated, then proceeding with the morcellation techniques.

A Narrow Vagina, Particularly in the Nulliparous Patient

Uterine decensus is not a prerequisite for a vaginal hysterectomy. The uterine size and degree of mobility of the uterus must also be assessed. In patients for whom the vagina appears unusually narrow, a relaxing episiotomy may be performed to allow more room in the pelvis. Alternately, a Schuchardt incision may be used. This incision is made into the lateral vaginal sulcus and carried down into the perineal body, in much the same location as a sulcal tear following an obstetric forceps delivery. Because the perineal muscles and medial aspects of the levator ani muscle group are incised during this procedure, the surgeon should ensure that normal anatomy is restored following completion of the hysterectomy.

An Apparent Uterine Prolapse

The finding of an apparent uterine prolapse with a very elongated cervix and a uterine corpus high in

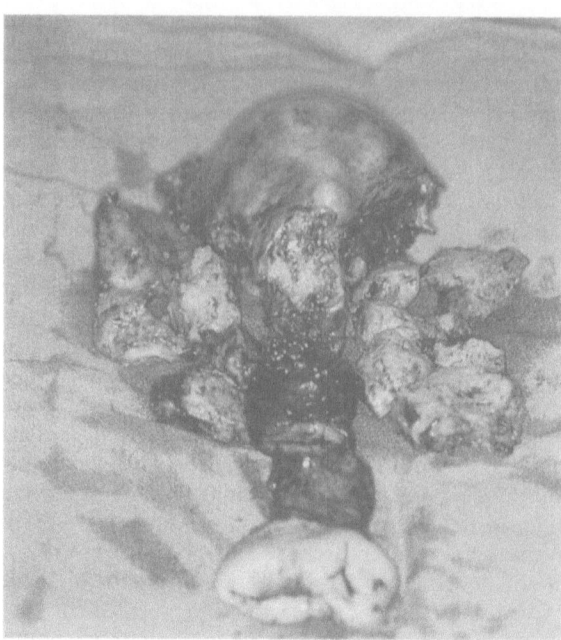

Figure 13.30 A morcellated uterine specimen. It is prudent to take small amounts of tissue repeatedly; no points are gained for the attractiveness of the pathologic specimen. Reprinted with permission from Baggish and Karram (2001) Atlas of Pelvic Anatomy and Gynaecologic Surgery. WB Saunders Co., 375.

the pelvis usually occurs with prolapse at other sites in the pelvis, adding to the possibility of missing the diagnosis preoperatively (Fig. 13.30) If the patient has an elongated cervix and a uterus that is in a fairly normal position, care must be taken to not amputate the cervix prematurely, as this will add to the difficulty of the remaining procedure. Entering the plane between the bladder and cervix, and mobilizing the bladder off the cervix without entering the peritoneal cavity, will enable the surgeon to move clamps along the elongated cervix until the upper portion of the corpus is reached.

A Uterine Prolapse with an Adnexal Mass

Occasionally, an adnexal mass may be missed on preoperative pelvic examination, especially in obese patients. If one is discovered at the time of colpotomy, it and the pelvis should be evaluated. If it is no larger than 3–5 cm in size and the suspicion of malignancy is low, an approach to remove this via the vaginal route may be attempted.

An Obliterated Cul-de-Sac of Douglas

The posterior cul-de-sac can be obliterated as a result of pelvic adhesions, which may lead to injuries to the rectum or small bowel during posterior colpotomy. Careful and meticulous attention to dissection is mandatory. In such cases it may be prudent to enter the anterior cul-de-sac first and then work from above downwards.

An Obliterated Vesico-Uterine Fold

If difficulty is encountered entering the anterior cul-de-sac, dissection should proceed posteriorly, with serial clamping, cutting and ligating. As long as the bladder is adequately dissected off the underlying cervix, entry into the anterior cul-de-sac is not mandatory. If the surgeon proceeds posteriorly until it is possible to pass a finger around the fundus, this may make it easier to expose the anterior peritoneum and avoid bladder injury (Fig. 13.31). The surgeon should be careful to avoid passing lateral to the fundus, as cutting down on the finger will cause the dissection to go lateral, endangering the uterine vessels.

If there is concern for an obliterated vesico-uterine fold, such as from multiple prior cesarean sections, anterior dissection should always be accomplished sharply. Aggressive blunt dissection with traction from a finger may follow a path of least resistance, tearing up and into the bladder.

Accidental Cystotomy

If a cystotomy occurs, it is best to dissect the bladder completely off the uterus before attempting repair. The laceration in the bladder may actually be used to identify the proper plane between bladder and cervix. The vaginal hysterectomy should be completed and hemostasis assured prior to closure of the cystotomy.

Before beginning repair, the extent of injury should be assessed: 5 ml of intravenous indigo carmine dye should be given and cystoscopy performed, with efflux of indigo carmine dye from the ureteric orifices being visualized. Assuming that the ureters and trigone are not involved in the injury, the cystotomy should be closed in two layers using a 3-0 delayed-absorbable suture. It may be advantageous to perform this in an interrupted fashion as the bladder tends to tear easily. One would like to obtain a watertight closure, although this is not always possible. After surgery, the patient should be informed of the cystotomy and the indwelling catheter left in for a minimum of 1 week. A voiding cystourethrogram done before removal of the catheter is helpful in documenting closure.

Accidental Enterotomy

If the small bowel is inadvertently entered during hysterectomy, it can be closed with a simple purse-string suture of absorbable suture if the laceration is small. If the laceration if larger, such that closure may cause narrowing of the bowel lumen, a two-layered closure is advocated. The first layer of a running absorbable suture is followed by a second, imbricating layer of interrupted silk sutures. In such cases, the patient requires nasogastric suction for 4–5 days to keep the bowel deflated and pressure off the surgical site. Laceration of the rectum may be closed in two layers using absorbable suture.

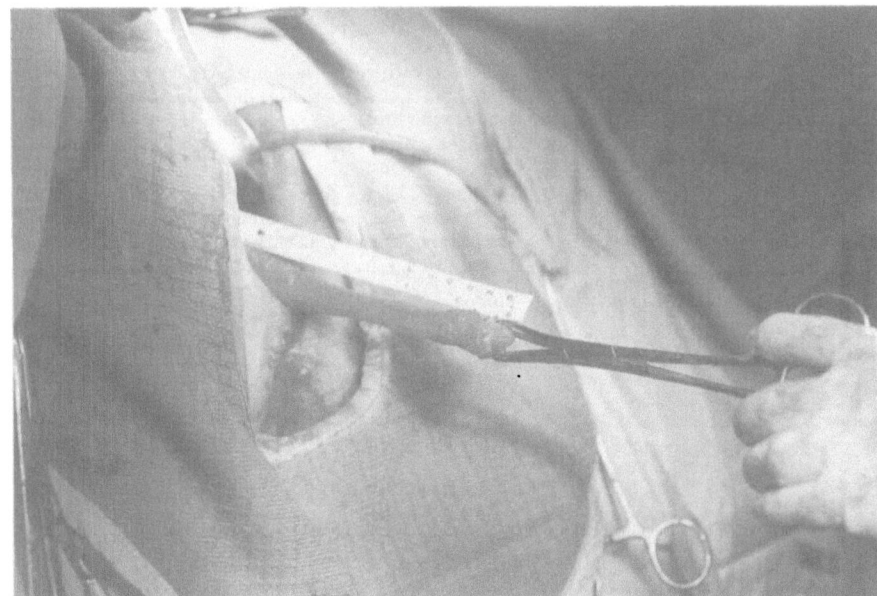

Figure 13.31 An elongated cervix. Before surgery, this condition may be indistinguishable from uterine prolapse. Reprinted with permission from Baggish and Karram (2001) Atlas of Pelvic Anatomy and Gynaecologic Surgery. WB Saunders Co., 371.

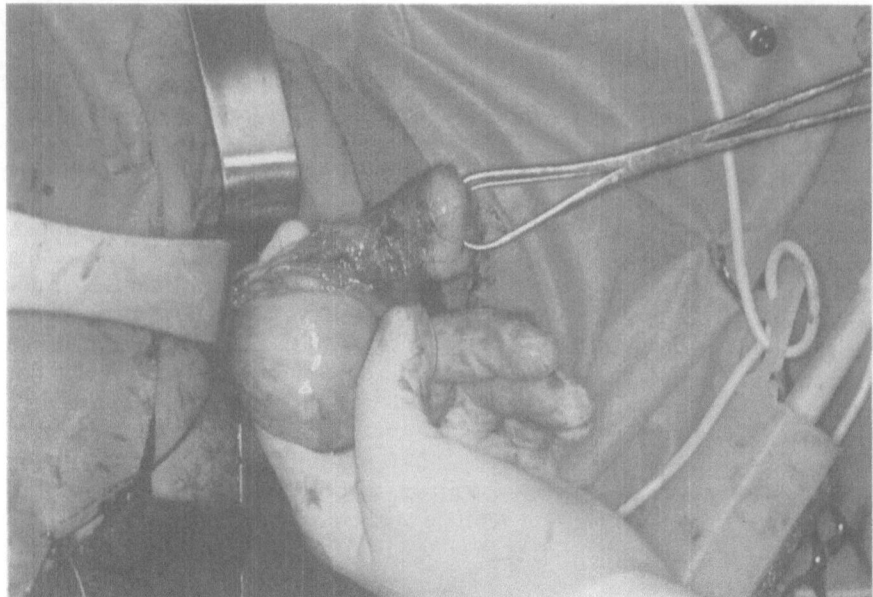

Figure 13.32 Gently passing a finger around the uterine fundus may facilitate entry into the anterior cul-de-sac.

Hemorrhage Due to a Lost Vascular Pedicle

Blood loss can be rapid in such situations and the surgeon should not linger to the point where hemorrhagic shock develops. After several attempts at controlling the bleeding by the vaginal route, it is best to discontinue and proceed abdominally.

Conclusion

Vaginal hysterectomy represents a vital technique for the pelvic surgeon. Safely performing this procedure requires a firm understanding of the anatomy of the pelvis from the vaginal approach. In a field in which many physicians receive the preponderance of their training performing abdominal surgeries, this change in perspective can be likened to driving to a familiar destination from a new direction. Cadaveric dissection should continue throughout the gynecologist's career.

In an era where surgical volume and available teaching cases are decreasing, training programs must continue to aggressively teach the techniques of vaginal hysterectomy. It is hoped that the vaginal hysterectomy does not go the way of the breech delivery.

References

1. Lane FE (1962) Repair of posthysterectomy vaginal vault prolapse. Obstet Gynecol 126: 590–6.

2. Timmons MC, Addison WA, Addison SB, Cavenar MG (1992) Abdominal sacral colpopexy in 163 women with posthysterectomy vaginal vault prolapse and enterocele. J Reprod Med 37: 322–7.

3. Nichols DH (1982) Sacrospinous fixations for massive eversion of the vagina. Am J Obstet Gynecol 142: 901–4.

4. Morley GW, DeLancey JOL (1988) Sacrospinous ligament fixation for eversion of the vagina. Am J Obstet Gynecol 158: 872–81.

5. Mouritsen L, Hansen PT, Kielmann J, Nielsen EL (1987) Results of abdominal levator-muscle repair in urinary stress incontinence. Scand J Urol Nephrol 21: 281–284.

6. Romanzi LJ, Chaikin DC, Blaivas JG (1999) Effect of genital prolapse on voiding. J Urol 161: 581–586.

7. Lemack GE, Zimmern PE (2001) Voiding cystourethrography and magnetic resonance imaging of the lower urinary tract. In: Corcos J, Schick E (ed) The Urinary Sphincter. Marcel Dekker, New York, pp. 407–422.

8. Zeidman EJ, Chiang H, Alarcon A et al. (1989) Suprapubic cystostomy using Lowsley retractor. Urology (Urotech supplement): 11–12.

9. Holley RL, Varner RE, Gleason BP, Apfell LA, Scott S (1996) Sexual function after sacrospinous ligament fixation for vaginal vault prolapse. J Reprod Med 41: 355–8.

10. Birnbaum SJ (1973) Rational therapy for the prolapsed vagina. Am J Obstet Gynecol 115: 411–19.

11. Symmonds RE, Williams TJ, Lee RA, Webb MJ (1981) Posthysterectomy enterocele and vaginal vault prolapse. Am J Obstet Gynecol 140: 852–9.

12. Arthure HGE, Savage D (1957) Uterine prolapse and prolapse of the vaginal vault treated by sacral hysteropexy. J Obstet Gynaecol Br Empire 64: 355–60.

13. Embrey MP (1961) An abdominal sling operation for the repair of enterocele and vault prolapse. J Obstet Gynaecol Brit Emp 68: 471–4.

14. Lane FE (1962) Repair of posthysterectomy vaginal-vault prolapse. Obstet Gynecol 20: 72–7.

15. Amid PK (1997) Classification of biomaterials and their related complication in abdominal wall hernia surgery. Hernia 1: 15–21.

16. Thompson JD (1997) Surgical techniques for pelvic organ prolapse. In: Rock JA, Thompson JD (eds) TeLinde's

Operative Gynaecology, 8th edn. Lippincott-Raven, Philadelphia, pp. 969–78.

17. Richardson D, Scotti R, Ostergard D (1989) Surgical management of uterine prolapse in young women. J Reprod Med 34: 388–92.

18. O'Brien PM, Ibrahim J (1994) Failure of laparoscopic uterine suspension to provide a lasting cure for utero-vaginal prolapse. Br J Obstet Gynaecol 101: 707–8.

19. Benson T, McClellan E (1993) The effect of vaginal dissection on the pudendal nerve. Obstet Gynecol 82: 387–9.

20. Villet R, Morice P, Bech A, Salet-Lizée D, Zafiropulo M (1993) Approche abdominale des rectocele et des elytroceles. Ann Chir 47: 626–30.

21. Cundiff GW, Harris RL, Coates K et al. (1997) Abdominal sacral colpoperineopexy: A new approach for correction of posterior compartment defects and perineal descent associated with vaginal vault prolapse. Am J Obstet Gynecol 177: 1345–55.

22. Baessler K, Stanton SL (2002) Sacrocolpopexy with mesh interposition and colposuspension for vault prolapse, rectocele and stress incontinence. Am J Obstet Gynecol: Submitted.

23. Bump RC, Mattiasson A, Bo K et al. (1996) The standardization of terminology of female pelvic organ prolapse and pelvic floor dysfunction. Am J Obstet Gynecol 175: 10–17.

24. Ross JW (1997) Techniques of laparoscopic repair of total vault eversion after hysterectomy. J Am Assoc Gynecol Laparosc 4: 173–83.

25. Dorsey JH, Sharp HT (1995) Laparoscopic sacral colpopexy and other procedures for prolapse. Clin Obstet Gynaecol 9: 749–56.

26. Valaitis SR, Stanton SL (1994) Sacrocolpopexy: a retrospective study of a clinician's experience. Br J Obstet Gynaecol 101: 518–22.

27. Lindert ACM van, Groenendijk AG, Scholten PC, Heintz APM (1993) Surgical support and suspension of genital prolapse, including preservation of the uterus, using the Gore-Tex soft tissue patch (a preliminary report). Eur J Obstet Gynecol Reprod Biol 50: 133–9.

28. Virtanen H, Hirvonen T, Mäkinen J, Kiilholma P (1994) Outcome of thirty patients who underwent repair of posthysterectomy prolapse of the vaginal vault with abdominal sacral colpopexy. J Am Coll Surg 178: 283–7.

29. Snyder TE, Krantz KE (1991) Abdominal-retroperitoneal sacral colpopexy for the correction of vaginal prolapse. Obstet Gynecol 77: 944–9.

30. Pilsgaard K, Mouritsen L (1999) Follow-up after repair of vaginal vault prolapse with abdominal colposacropexy. Acta Obstet Gynecol Scand 78: 66–70.

31. Baker KR, Beresford JM, Campbell C (1990) Colposacropexy with Prolene mesh. Surg Gynecol Obstet 171: 51–4.

32. Grundsell H, Larsson G (1984) Operative management of vaginal vault prolapse. Br J Obstet Gynaecol 91: 808–11.

33. Addison WA, Livengood CH, Sutton GP, Parker RT (1985) Abdominal sacral colpopexy with Mersilene mesh in the retroperitoneal position in the management of posterectomy vaginal vault prolapse and enterocele. Am J Obstet Gynecol 153: 140–6.

34. Patsner B, Orr JW (1990) Intractable venous sacral hemorrhage: Use of stainless steel thumbtacks to obtain hemostatsis. Am J Obstet Gynecol 162: 452.

35. Randall CL, Nichols DH (1971) Surgical treatment of vaginal inversion. Obstet Gynecol 38: 327–32.

36. Cowan W, Morgan HR (1980) Abdominal sacral colpopexy. Am J Obstet Gynecol 138: 348–50.

37. Creighton SM, Stanton SL (1991) The surgical management of vaginal vault prolapse. Br J Obstet Gynaecol 98: 1150–4.

38. Timmons MC, Addison WA (1997) Mesh erosion after abdominal sacral colpopexy. J Pelvic Surg 3: 75–80.

39. Benson JT, Lucente V, McClellan E (1996) Vaginal versus abdominal reconstructive surgery for the treatment of pelvic support defects: A prospective randomized study with long-term outcome evaluation. Am J Obstet Gynecol 175: 1418–22.

40. Schettini M, Fortunato P, Gallucci M (1999) Abdominal sacral colpopexy with prolene mesh. Int Urogynecol J 10: 295–9.

41. Powell JL, Joseph DB (1999) Abdominal sacral colpopexy for massive genital prolapse and posthysterectomy vaginal vault prolapse. J Gynecol Tech 5: 45–50.

42. Kohli N, Walsh PM, Roat TW, Karram MM (1998) Mesh erosion after abdominal sacrocolpopexy. Obstet Gynecol 92: 999–1004.

43. Imparato E, Aspesi G, Rovetta E, Presti M (1992) Surgical management and prevetnion of vaginal vault prolapse. Surg Gynecol Obstet 175: 233–7.

44. Fedorkow DM, Kalbfleisch RE (1993) Total abdominal hysterectomy at abdominal sacrovaginopexy: A comparative study. Am J Obstet Gynecol 69: 641–3.

45. Patsner B (2000) Mesh erosion into the bladder after abdominal sacral colpopexy. Obstet Gynecol 95: 1029.

46. Drutz HP, Cha LS (1987) Massive genital and vaginal vault prolapse treated by abdominal-vaginal sacropexy with use of Marlex-mesh: Review of literature. Am J Obstet Gynecol 156: 387–92.

47. Soichet S (1970) Surgical correction of total genital prolapse with retention of sexual function. Obstet Gynecol 36: 69–75.

48. Lilford RJ, Johnson N, Batchelor A (1993) Repair of prolapse of a living ligament. Br J Obstet Gynaecol 100: 859–860.

49. Grünberger W, Grünberger V, Wierrani F (1994) Pelvic promontory fixation of the vaginal vault in sixty-two patients with prolapse after hysterectomy. J Am Coll Surg 178: 69–72.

50. Weidner AC, Cundiff GW, Harris RL, Addison WA (1997) Sacral osteomyelitis: An unusual complication of abdominal sacral colpopexy. Obstet Gynecol 90: 689–91.

51. Cranney A, Feibel R, Toye BW, Karsh J (1994) Osteomyelitis subsequent to abdominal-vaginal sacropexy. J Rheumatol 21: 1769–70.

52. Cailleux N, Daragon A, Laine F et al. (1991) Spondylodiscites infectieuses après cure de prolapsus genital: A propos de 5 cas. J Gynecol Obstet Biol Reprod 20: 1074–8.

53. Addison WA, Timmons MC, Wall LL, Livengood CH (1989) Failed abdominal sacral colpopexy: Observations and recommendations. Obstet Gynecol 74: 480–2.

54. Todd JW (1978) Mesh suspension for vaginal prolapse. Int Surg 63: 91–3.

55. Vries MJ De, Dessel THJM van, Drogendijk AC, Haas I de, Huikeshoven FJM (1995) Short-term results and long-term patients' appraisal of abdominal colposacropexy for treatment of genital and vaginal vault prolapse. Eur J Obstet Gynecol Reprod Biol 59: 35–8.

56. Leron E, Stanton SL (2001) Sacrohysteropexy with synthetic mesh for the management of uterovaginal prolapse. Br J Obstet Gynaecol 108: 629–633.

57. Costantini E, Lombi R, Parziani S, Porena M (1998) Colposacropexy with Gore-Tex mesh in marked vaginal and uterovaginal prolapse. Eur Urol 34: 111–117.

58. Banu LF (1997) Synthetic sling for genital prolapse in young women. Int J Gynecol Obstet 57: 57–64.

59. Timmons MC, Addison WA, Addison SB, Cavenar MG (1992) Abdominal sacral colpopexy in 163 women with posthysterectomy vaginal vault prolapse and enterocele. J Reprod Med 37: 323–327.

60. Feldman GB, Birnbaum SJ (1979) Sacral colpopexy for vaginal vault prolapse. Obstet Gynecol 53: 399–401.

61. Kauppila O, Punnonen R, Teisala K (1986) Operative technique for the repair of posthysterectomy vaginal prolapse. Ann Chir Gynaecol 75: 242–4.

62. Maloney JC, Dunton CJ, Smith K (1990) Repair of vaginal vault prolapse with abdominal sacropexy. J Reprod Med 35: 6–10.

63. Brieger GM, Korda AR, Houghton CRS (1996) Abdomino perineal repair of pulsion enterocele. J Obstet Gynaecol Res 22: 151–6.

64. Hardiman PJ, Drutz HP (1996) Sacrospinous vault suspension and abdominal colposacropexy: Success rates and complications. Am J Obstet Gynecol 175: 612–16.

65. Fox SD, Stanton SL (2000) Vault prolapse and rectocele: assessment of repair using sacrocolpopexy with mesh interposition. Br J Obstet Gynaecol 107: 1371–5.

66. Lansman HH (1984) Posthysterectomy vault prolapse: Sacral colpopexy with dura mater graft. Obstet Gynecol 63: 577–82.

67. Traiman P, Luca LA De, Silva AAF et al. (1992) Abdominal colpopexy for complete prolapse of the vagina. Int Surg 77: 91–5.

68. Brubaker L (1995) Sacrocolpopexy and the anterior compartment: Support and function. Am J Obstet Gynecol 173: 1690–6.

69. Lee RA, Symmonds RE (1972) Surgical repair of posthysterectomy vault prolapse. Am J Obstet Gynecol 112: 953–6.

70 Baessler K, Schuessler B (2001) Abdominal sacrocolpopexy: anatomy and function of the posterior compartment. Obstet Gynecol 97: 678–84.

71. Given FT, Muhlendorf IK, Browning GM (1993) Vaginal length and sexual function after colpopexy for complete uterovaginal eversion. Am J Obstet Gynecol 169: 284–8.

72. Varner RE, Plessala KJ, Richter H (1995) Effects of sacrocolposuspension on the lower urinary tract. Am J Obstet Gynecol 173: 1684–9.

73. Speakman CTM, Madden MV, Nicholls RJ, Kamm MA (1991) Lateral ligament division during rectopexy causes constipation but prevents recurrence: results of a prospective randomized study. Br J Surg 78: 1431–3.

74. Zweifel P (1892) Vorlesungen über Klinische Gynäcologie. Hirschwald, Berlin, pp. 407–15.

75. Miller NF (1927) A new method of correcting complete inversion of the vagina. Surg Gynecol Obstet 44: 550–4.

76. Amreich I (1951) Aetiologie und Operation des Scheiden stump prolapses. Wien Klin Wochenschr 65: 74–7.

77. Richter K (1968) [The surgical anatomy of the vaginaefixatio sacrospinalis vaginalis. A contribution to the surgical treatment of vaginal blind pouch prolapse]. Geburtshilfe Frauenheilkd 28(4): 321–7.

78. Randall CL, Nichols DH (1971) Surgical treatment of vaginal inversion. Obstet Gynecol 38(3): 327–32.

79. Richter K, Dargent D (1986) La spinofixation (vaginae fixatio sacrospinalis) dans le traitement du prolapsus du dôme vaginal aprés hystérectomie. [Spinous fixation (vaginae fixatio sacrospinalis) in the treatment of vaginal prolapse after hysterectomy]. J Gynecol Obstet Biol Reprod (Paris) 15(8): 1081–8.

80. Jacquetin B (1995) Cure des prolapsus génito-urinaires: la sacrospinofixation bilatérale. [Urogenital prolapse cure: bilateral sacrospinous fixation]. In: Villet R, Buzelin J-M, Lazorthes F (eds) Les troubles de la statique pelvipérinéale de la femme. Vigot, Paris, pp. 225–33.

81. Jacquetin B, Fatton B (1997) Traitement chirurgical des prolapsus génitaux par voie vaginale.[Surgical treatment of genital prolapse cure by vaginal route.]. Gunaïkeia 2(5): 186–92.

82. Richardson DA, Scotti RJ, Ostergard DR (1989) Surgical management of uterine prolapse in young women. J Reprod Med 34(6): 388–92.

83. Jacquetin B, Fatton B (1996) Résultats et conséquences de l'intervention de Richardson (sacrospino fixation de l'utérus) [Results and consequences of the Richardson operation (sacrospinous uterine fixation).]. 12ème Congrés de la SIFCP, Bordeaux, 29–30 mars 1996.

84. Miyazaki FS (1987) Miya Hook ligature carrier for sacrospinous ligament suspension. Obstet Gynecol 70(2): 286–8.

85. Sharp TR (1993) Sacrospinous suspension made easy. Obstet Gynecol 82(5): 873–5.

86. Veronikis DK, Nichols DH (1997) Ligature carrier specifically designed for transvaginal sacrospinous colpopexy. Obstet Gynecol 89(3): 478–81.

87. Lind LR, Choe J, Bhatia NN (1997) An in-line suturing device to simplify sacrospinous vaginal vault suspension. Obstet Gynecol 89(1): 129–32.

88. Rosenthal C (1998) [On the article by W. Febbraro: Feasibility of bilateral vaginal sacrocolpopexy with a stapler (letter)]. J Gynecol Obstet Biol Reprod (Paris) 27(4): 457–8.

89. Jacquetin B (1998) [Using the Endo Stitch forceps via the vagina: purely by palpation? (letter)]. J Gynecol Obstet Biol Reprod (Paris) 27(2): 213–14.

90. Barksdale PA, Elkins TE, Sanders CK, Jaramillo FE, Gasser RF (1998) An anatomic approach to pelvic hemorrhage during sacrospinous ligament fixation of the vaginal vault. Obstet Gynecol 91(5): 715–18.

91. Verdeja AM, Elkins TE, Odoi A, Gasser R, Lamoutte C (1995) Transvaginal sacrospinous colpopexy: Anatomic landmarks to be aware of to minimize complications. Am J Obstet Gynecol 173: 1468–9.

92. Sze EHM, Karram MM (1997) Transvaginal repair of vault prolapse: a review. Obstet Gynecol 89(3): 466–75.

93. Ohana M (1992) Sacrospinofixation vaginale selon Richter; évaluation des résultats en fonction des modifications techniques à partir d'une étude rétrospective de 150 cas. [Vaginal sacrospinous fixation according to Richter; technical modifications evaluated by results of a retrospective study of 150 cases]. Thesis. Faculté de Medecine de Clermont-Ferrand; Université d'Auvergne.

94. Mansoor A, Ohana M, Jacquetin B (1993) Vaginal sacrospinous colpopexy in the treatment of urogenital prolapse. Abstract, Annual Meeting of IUGA, Nimes, France. Int Urogynecol J 4(5): 253–332.

95. Fernandez-Busserolles M (1997) Les complications douloureuses de la cure de prolapsus génital par voie vaginale exclusive incluant une sacrospinofixation; étude rétrospective de 800 cas. [Painful complications of the genital prolapse cure by vaginal route only, including sacrospinous fixation; retrospective study of 800 cases]. Thesis. Faculté de Medecine de Clermont-Ferrand; Université d'Auvergne.

96. Barksdale PA, Gasser RF, Gauthier CM, Elkins TE, Wall LL (1997) Intraligamentous nerves as a potential source of pain after sacrospinous ligament fixation of the vaginal apex. Int Urogynecol J Pelvic Floor Dysfunct 8(3): 121–5.

97. Fatton B, Grunberg P, Ohana M et al. (1993) Cure de prolapsus chez la femme jeune: la voie abdominale n'a pas d'avantage sur la voie vaginale; à propos d'une étude prospective randomisée. 1. Résultats anatomiques et sexuels [Cure of prolapse in young women: the abdominal route has no advantage over the vaginal route: a prospective randomized study. 1. Anatomical and sexual results.] J Obstet Gynecol 1(1): 66–72.

98. Fatton B (1994) Résultats fonctionnels et notamment sexuels de la cure de prolapsus génital chez 30 femmes de moins de 55 ans: étude par tirage au sort voie abdominale-voie vaginale. [Functional results, particularly sexual, of 30 women (less than 55 years old) prolapse cure: random-

ized study comparing abdominal route versus vaginal route.]. Thesis, Faculté de médecine de Clermont-Ferrand; Université d'Auvergne.

99. Jacquetin B, Fatton B (1998) Surgical management of genital prolapse in young women: a prospective randomized study (abstract). 23rd Meeting of the IUGA, Buenos Aires, 1998. Int Urogynecol J 9(5): 360.

100. Given FT Jr, Muhlendorf IK, Browning GM (1993)Vaginal length and sexual function after colpopexy for complete uterovaginal eversion. Am J Obstet Gynecol 169(2): 284–7.

101. Richter K, Albrich W (1981) Long-term results following fixation of the vagina on the sacrospinal ligament by the vaginal route (vaginaefixatio sacrospinalis vaginalis). Am J Obstet Gynecol 141(7): 811–16.

102. Nichols DH (1982) Sacrospinous fixation for massive eversion of the vagina. Am J Obstet Gynecol 142(7): 901–4.

103. Morley GW, DeLancey JO (1988) Sacrospinous ligament fixation for eversion of the vagina. Am J Obstet Gynecol 158(4): 872–881.

104. Brown WE, Hoffman MS, Bouis PJ, Ingram JM, Hopes SL (1989) Management of vaginal vault prolapse: retrospective comparison of abdominal versus vaginal approach. J Fla Med Assoc 76(2): 249–52.

105. Kettel LM, Hebertson RM (1989) An anatomic evaluation of the sacrospinous ligament colpopexy. Surg Gynecol Obstet 168(4): 318–22.

106. Cruikshank SH, Cox DW (1990) Sacrospinous ligament fixation at the time of transvaginal hysterectomy. Am J Obstet Gynecol 162(6): 1611–15.

107. Monk BJ, Ramp JF, Montz FJ, Febherz TB (1991) Sacrospinous fixation for vaginal vault prolapse. Complications and results. J Gynecol Surg 7: 87–92.

108. Backer MH (1992) Jr. Success with sacrospinous suspension of the prolapsed vaginal vault. Surg Gynecol Obstet 175(5): 419–20.

109. Heinonen PK (1992) Transvaginal sacrospinous colpopexy for vaginal vault and complete genital prolapse in aged women. Acta Obstet Gynecol Scand 71(5): 377–81.

110. Imparato E, Aspesi G, Rovetta E, Presti M (1992) Surgical management and prevention of vaginal vault prolapse. Surg Gynecol Obstet 175: 233–7.

111. Shull BL, Capen CV, Riggs MW, Kuehl TJ (1992) Preoperative and postoperative analysis of site-specific pelvic support defects in 81 women treated with sacrospinous ligament suspension and pelvic reconstruction. Am J Obstet Gynecol 166(6): 1764–8.

112. Kaminski PF, Sorosky JI, Pees RC, Podczaski ES (1993) Correction of massive vaginal prolapse in an older population: a four-year experience at a rural tertiary care center. J Am Geriatr Soc 41(1): 42–4.

113. Carey MP, Slack MC (1994) Transvaginal sacrospinous colpopexy for vault and marked uterovaginal prolapse. Br J Obstet Gynaecol 101(6): 536–40.

114. Holley RL, Varner RE, Gleason BP, Apffel LA, Scott S (1995) Recurrent pelvic support defects after sacrospinous ligament fixation for vaginal vault prolapse. J Amer Coll Surg 180: 444–8.

115. Sauer HA, Klutke CG (1995) Transvaginal sacrospinous ligament fixation for treatment of vaginal prolapse. J Urol 154: 1008–12.

116. Peters WA, Christenson ML (1995) Fixation of the vaginal apex to the coccygeus fascia during repair of vaginal vault eversion with enterocele. Am J Obstet Gynecol 172: 1894–1902.

117. Elkins TE, Hopper JB, Goodfellow K et al. (1995) Initial report of anatomic and clinical comparison of the sacrospinous ligament fixation to the high McCall culdesac plasty for vaginal cuff fixation at hysterectomy for uterine prolapse. J Pelv Surg 1: 12–17.

118. Pasley WW (1995) Sacrospinous suspension: A local practitioner's experience. Am J Obstet Gynecol 173: 440–8.

119. Penalver M, Mekki Y, Lafferty H, Escobar M, Angioli R (1998) Should sacrospinous ligament fixation for the management of pelvic support defects be part of a residency program procedure? The University of Miami experience. Am J Obstet Gynecol 178(2): 326–9.

120. Fatton B, Jacquetin B (1997) Troubles sexuels aprés chirurgie du prolapsus. [Sexual disorders after surgical treatment of genital prolapse.] 7émes Journées Liégeoises de Gynécologie-Obstétrique (abstract). Gunaïkeia 2(2): 58.

121. Holley RL, Varner RE, Gleason BP, Apfell LA, Scott S 1996) Sexual function after sacrospinous ligament fixation for vaginal vault prolapse. J Reprod Med; 41: 355–8.

122. Paraiso MFR, Ballard LA, Walters MD, Lee JC, Mitchinson AR (1996) Pelvic support defects and visceral and sexual function in women treated with sacrospinous ligament suspension and pelvic reconstruction. Am J Obstet Gynecol; 175: 1423–30.

123. Cruikshank SH (1991) Sacrospinous fixation – should this be performed at the time of vaginal hysterectomy? Am J Obstet Gynecol 164: 1072–6.

124. Scotti RJ (1992) Prophylactic sacrospinous fixation discouraged. Am J Obstet Gynecol 166: 1022.

125. Symmonds RE, Pratt JH (1960) Vaginal prolapse following hysterectomy. Am J Obstet Gynecol 79: 899–909.

126. Symmonds RE, Williams TJ, Lee RA, Webb MJ (1981) Posthysterectomy enterocele and vaginal vault prolapse. Am J Obstet Gynecol 140: 852–9.

127. Cruikshank SH (1987) Preventing posthysterectomy vaginal vault prolapse and enterocele during vaginal hysterectomy. Am J Obstet Gynecol 156: 1433–40.

128. M'Call ML (1957) Posterior culdoplasty; Surgical correction of enterocele during vaginal hysterectomy: A preliminary report. Obstet Gynecol 10: 595–602.

129. Sze EHM, Karram MM (1997) Transvaginal repair of vault prolapse A review. Obstet Gynecol 89: 466–75.

130. Webb MJ, Aronson MP, Ferguson LK (1998) Lee RA. Posthysterectomy Vaginal Vault Prolapse: Primary Repair in 693 Patients. Obstet Gynecol 92: 281–5.

131. DeLancey JOL (1992) Anatomic aspects of vaginal eversion after hysterectomy. Am J Obstet Gynecol 166: 1717–24.

132. Gosling JA (1996) The structure of the bladder neck, urethra and pelvic floor in relation to female urinary incontinence. Int Urogynecol J 7: 177–8.

133. Barksdale PA, Elkins TE, Sanders CK, Jaramillo FE, Gasser RF (1998) An anatomical approach to pelvic hemorrhage during sacrospinous ligament fixation of the vaginal vault. Obstet Gynecol 91: 715–18.

134. Inmon WB (1963) Pelvic relaxation and repair including prolapse of the vagina following vaginal hysterectomy. South Med J 56: 577–82.

135. Shull BL, Capen CV, Riggs MW (1993) Kuehl TJ Bilateral attachment of the vaginal cuff to iliococcygeus fascia: An effective method of cuff suspension. Am J Obstet Gynecol 168: 1696–77.

136. Meeks GR, Washburne JF, McGehee RP, Wiser WL (1994) Repair of vaginal vault prolapse by suspension of the vagina to iliococcygeus (prespinous) fascia. Am J Obstet Gynecol 171: 1444–52.

137. Miyazaki FS (1987) Miya hook ligature carrier for sacrospinous ligament suspension. Obstet Gynecol 70: 286–8.

138. Dwyer PL, Carey MP, Rosamilia A (1999) Suture injury to the urinary tract in urethral suspension procedures for stress incontinence. Int J Urogynecol 10: 15–21.

139. Maher CF, Murray CJ, Carey MP, Dwyer PL, Ugoni AM (2001) Iliococcygeus or sacrospinous fixation for vaginal vault prolapse? Obstet Gynecol 98: 40–44.

140. Benson JT, Lucente V, McClellan E (1996) Vaginal versus abdominal reconstructive surgery for the treatment of pelvic support defects; A prospective randomized study with long term outcome evaluation. Am J Obstet Gynecol 175: 1418–22.

141. **Barlow DH**, Cardozo LD, Francis RM et al. (1997) Urogenital ageing and its effect on sexual health in older British women. Br J Obstet Gynaecol 104: 87–91.

142. Given FY, Muhlendorf IK, Browning GM (1993) Vaginal length and sexual function after colpopexy for complete uterovaginal eversion. Am J Obstet Gynecol 169: 284–8.

143. Emge LA, Durfee RB (1966) Pelvic organ prolapse: four thousand years of treatment. Clin Obstet Gynecol 9: 997–1032.

144. Heaney HS (1942) Technique of vaginal hysterectomy. Surg Clin N Amer 22.

145. Introduction VB (1998) the epidemiology of uterine leiomyoma. Baillière's Clin Obstet Gynecol 12: 169–76.

146. Aberdeen Endometrial Ablation Trials Group (1999) A randomized trial of endometrial ablation versus hysterectomy for the treatment of dysfunctional uterine bleeding: outcome at four years. Br J Obstet Gynaecol 106: 360–6.

147. Kovac SR, Cruikshank SH (1993) Successful pregnancies and vaginal deliveries after sacrospinous uterosacral fixation in five of nineteen patients. Am J Obstet Gynecol 168: 1778–83.

148. Langer R, Ron-El R, Neuman M et al. (1988) The value of simultaneous hysterectomy during Burch colpsuspension for urinary stress incontinence. Obstet Gynecol 72: 866–9.

149. Meeks GR, Harris RL (1997) Surgical approach to hysterectomy: abdominal, laparoscopy-assisted or vaginal. Clin Obstet Gynecol 40: 886–94.

150. Dorsey JH, Holtz PM, Griffiths RI, McGrath MM, Steinberg EP (1996) Costs and charges associated with three alternative techniques of hysterectomy. N Engl J Med 335: 476–82.

151. Dorsey JH, Steinberg EP, Hotz PM (1995) Clinical indications for hysterectomy route: patient characteristics or physician preference? Am J Obstet Gynecol 173: 1452–60.

152. Davies A, Vizza E, Bournas N, O'Conner H, Magos A (1998) How to increase the proportion of hysterectomies done vaginally. Am J Obstet Gynecol 179: 1080–12.

153. Richardson RE, Bournas N, Magos AL (1995) Is laparoscopic hysterectomy a waste of time? Lancet 345: 36–41.

154. Summitt RL, Stovall TG, Lipscomb GH, Ling FW (1992) Randomized comparison of Laparoscopically-assisted vaginal hysterectomy with standard vaginal hysterectomy in an outpatient setting. Obstet Gynecol 80: 895–901.

155. Kovac RS (1986) Intramyometrial coring as an adjunct to vaginal hysterectomy. Obstet Gynecol 67: 131–6.

156. Hoffman MS, DeCesare S, Kalter C (1994) Abdominal hysterectomy versus transvaginal morcellation for the removal of enlarged uteri. Am J Obstet Gynecol 171: 309–15.

157. Pelosi MA, Pelosi MA (1998) III. Should uterine size alone require laparoscopic assistance? Vaginal hysterectomy for a 2003-g. uterus. J Laparoendosc Surg Tech A 8: 99–103.

158. Unger JB, Meeks RG (1998) Vaginal hysterectomy in women with history of previous cesarean delivery. Am J Obstet Gynecol 6: 1473–8.

159. Ballard LA, Walters MD (1996) Transvaginal mobilization and removal of ovaries and fallopian tubes after vaginal hysterectomy. Obstet Gynecol 87: 35–9.

160. Sheth SS (1991) The place of oophorectomy at vaginal hysterectomy. Br J Obstet Gynecol 98: 662–6.

14 Posterior Compartment: Rectocele Reconstruction

Margie A. Kahn

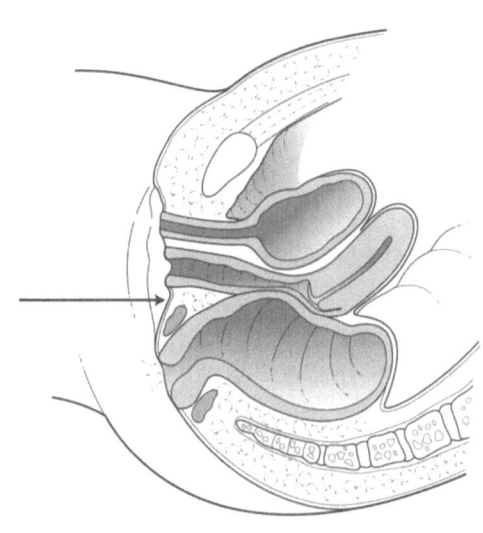

Figure 14.1 Lower vaginal and perineal rectocele. The arrow points to the beginning of the rectovaginal space.

Definition

The posterior vaginal wall prolapses when visceral contents herniate through the "fascia" or fibromuscular posterior wall of the vagina or through a disruption of these fascial attachments to the uterosacral-cardinal ligament complex, levator fascia, or perineal body. Herniation of the rectum is called a rectocele (Fig. 14.1); herniation of peritoneal contents may be called a culdocele, enterocele, peritoneocele, or sigmoidocele, depending on the contents of the hernial sac.

Anatomical Observations

Fascia and Levator Plication

The primary defects occur in the tough, shiny layer of tissue that is interposed between the rectum and the vagina. Often called the endopelvic fascia, vaginal fascia, rectovaginal septum or Denonvillier's fascia, some authors believe that this layer is simply the fibromuscular wall of the vagina.[1-5] In this chapter, we will refer to "fascia" for historical consistency. Most descriptions of vaginal surgical repair refer to plication or reconstitution of this layer. However, it may be unwise to use a tissue with demonstrated incompetence for long-lasting surgical strength. Thus, some techniques reinforce this layer by use of extensive levator plication or artificial mesh[6,7] or cadaveric tissue.[8] A posterior enterocele may also result from herniation of peritoneal contents through a detachment of the rectovaginal fascia to the uterosacral-cardinal ligament complex.[9] Indeed, it may also exist anterior to a normal cul-de-sac.[10] Thus, this type of enterocele constitutes a manifestation of a posterior fascial defect.

Attenuation of the Anterior Rectal Wall and its Plication

Colorectal surgeons have observed that vaginal repair may not correct a ballooning anterior rectal wall and may plicate the excess from inside the rectum – a transanal or endorectal repair.[11]

Symptoms

Vaginal symptoms include awareness of a bulging mass in the vagina, perineal or lower abdominal pressure, slackness at intercourse or dyspareunia, and low back pain that worsens throughout the day and is relieved by lying down. Rectal symptoms include constipation, a feeling of incomplete emptying during defecation, the need to vaginally, rectally, or perineally digitate to effect evacuation, incontinence of feces, pain, and bleeding. Although symptoms of impaired rectal emptying may be present with enterocele, the obstructive nature is questionable. Extrinsic compression of the rectum by the hernia sac may create the sensation of a fecal bolus, even when the rectum is empty.[12] The cause and effect relationship of anorectal symptoms are not always clear because other colorectal disorders can cause similar symptoms[13] and the anatomical findings do not correlate with symptoms.

Signs and Classification

The diagnosis should be made in the unanesthetized patient in the lithotomy, Sims, sitting or standing[14] position with the patient bearing down or straining as if attempting to defecate. Because prolapse is dynamic, ask the patient if the demonstrated prolapse is at its worst.

Rectovaginal examination can help distinguish between rectocele and enterocele by the palpation of a sac dissecting between the rectum and vagina. If the rectum is full of stool, an enema may allow a previously unidentified enterocele to become apparent. However, the physical examination diagnosis is imperfect and may be different from that identified at surgery.

Rectal examination also identifies other causes of impaired defecation or incontinence such as posterior rectocele, intussusception, poor anal sphincter or levator tone, skin tags, and mucosal prolapse.

Grading schemes have been used to quantify the size of the vaginal prolapse. The international standard, the POP-Q (Pelvic Organ Prolapse Quantification)[15] incorporates direct measurements of the degree of vaginal prolapse in relation to the hymen. An adaptation of Baden and Walker's Halfway System,[16] it provides more precise information than the traditional first/second/ third degree or mild/moderate/severe classifications.

Indications for Surgery

Because the symptoms of posterior vaginal wall prolapse are not unique to this condition, it is important to search for other causes of the patient's symptoms:

Constipation

A patient who has one hard bowel movement per week may strain or digitate regardless of the presence of a rectocele. Indeed, if these are the only complaints, they may be entirely resolved by dietary changes alone. Before surgery, bowel habits must be normalized as much as possible by the use of bulking agents such as psyllium and osmotic expanders such as sorbitol or lactulose syrup. Bowel transit studies may be indicated in those in whom bowel frequency and consistency cannot be corrected. These patients are more apt to have postoperative continuation of bowel symptoms;[17] in addition, continued straining at stool may predispose to recurrent prolapse.

Incontinence

Fecal incontinence from rectoceles results from reflex relaxation of the anal sphincter when the rectum is overdistended by stool.[18] However, soiling may be caused by mechanical or neurological anal sphincter abnormalities, anal skin tags, rectal mucosal prolapse, and hemorrhoids. Diarrhea can overwhelm a borderline continence mechanism and may require testing for infection or malabsorption. Further investigation in patients with fecal incontinence should include anorectal physiological and imaging studies.

Bleeding

Rectal bleeding should be evaluated by colonoscopy or barium enema to diagnose malignancy.

Sexual Dysfunction

Sexual problems can be caused by psychological factors, hypo-estrogenism, and partner impotency. The patient and her partner must understand that narrowing a lax genital hiatus may not restore neurological control of the pelvic floor and sexual sensation. Vaginal symptoms attributed to prolapse sometimes resolve with treatment of vulvovaginitis or atrophy.

Surgery is indicated in those women who have a rectocele on physical examination or on imaging studies and whose symptoms, unrelieved by conservative management, are felt to be attributable to the rectocele

Operations

Posterior Colporrhaphy and Perineorrhaphy

Preoperative Preparation

Vaginal estrogen is advised, preferably, at least for 3 months to improve the integrity of the vaginal epithelium. A phosphate enema is given the morning of surgery if the rectal vault is filled with stool. A second-generation cephalosporin is given intravenously preoperatively.

Technique

The patient is positioned in dorsal lithotomy postion as for other vaginal surgery. The labia minora may be sutured laterally to the inner thighs

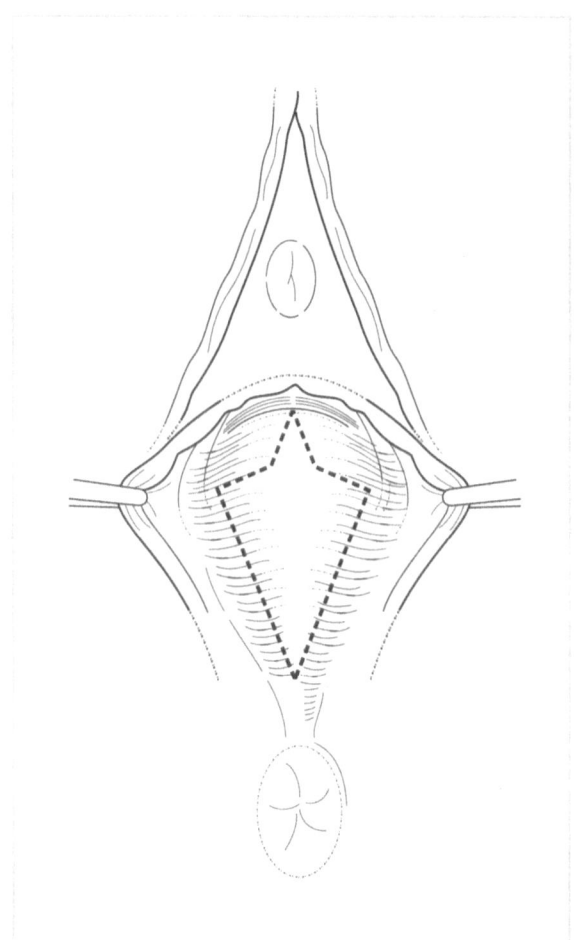

a

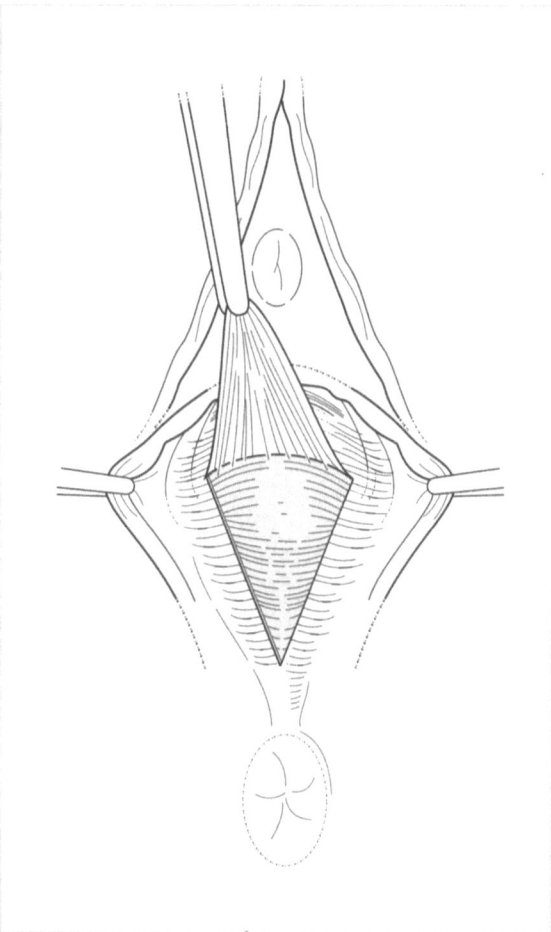

b

Figure 14.2 a,b Diamond-shaped area of the vagina and perineum excised during the perineorrhaphy.

for better exposure. Serial Allis clamps are placed in the midline from the apex to 1–2 cm above the hymen. If a perineorrhaphy is to be performed, the future caliber of the vaginal introitus is estimated by placing Allis clamps bilaterally on the labia minora and approximating them in the midline. The final hiatus should admit three fingerbreadths easily to avoid postoperative constriction. One additional Allis clamp is placed in the midline between the hymen and the anus to mark the inferior extent of the perineorrhaphy. The diamond-shaped piece of vaginal mucosa and perineal skin marked by the four inferior Allises is excised by sharp dissection (Fig. 14.2). A midline incision is made from the apex of the vagina to the top of this diamond. The vaginal mucosa is then freed laterally from the underlying fascia and rectal wall by a combination of blunt and sharp dissection with countertraction on the rectum until the puborectalis portions of the levator ani are reached. At the perineal body, the bulbocavernosus and tranverse perineal muscles are also dissected free of the overlying vagina and perineum. Any enterocele sac or culdocele is obliterated by high concentric purse string sutures. Using 00 or 0 delayed-absorbable sutures, the lateral rectovaginal fascia is plicated in the midline from the apex to the lower portion of the vagina. A finger may be placed in the rectum and curved toward the operator to help identify this tissue and to avoid placing sutures

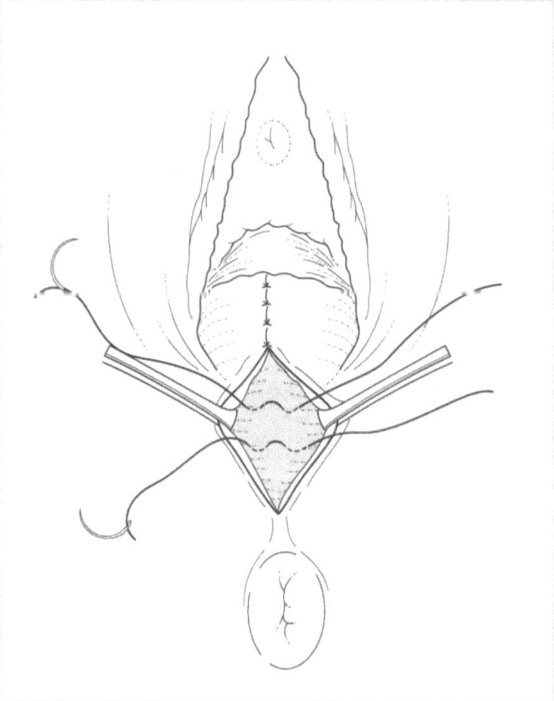

Figure 14.3 Deep perineal sutures that capture bulbocavernosus and transverse perineal muscles.

through the rectum. As the perineal body is approached, deep plication stitches may be placed in the puborectalis portions of the levator ani, taking care to avoid constriction of the vagina. Aggressiveness should be avoided in this part of the operation because it can cause postoperative dyspareunia.[19] Excess vaginal mucosa is trimmed bilaterally and the vaginal incision is closed with a running locked stitch using 00 suture. For the perineorrhaphy, the perineal muscles are approximated with 0 deep sutures and the perineum is reconstituted beginning with the "crown" stitch as in episiotomy repair (Fig. 14.3). The perineal skin is then closed with a subcuticular stitch. No vaginal pack is necessary if adequate hemostasis is obtained. Bladder drainage is usually necessary overnight because the most common immediate postoperative complication is urinary retention due to pain.[20]

Postoperative Management

Patients are discharged with psyllium and sorbitol syrup to keep the stools soft. Sexual activity is not encouraged until after the 6 week check-up. Any vaginal stenosis is treated with dilators and liberal use of vaginal estrogen cream.

Long-Term Results

The operation has long been recognized as a cause of postoperative vaginal scarring, stenosis, and dyspareunia[19,21] in approximately 20–27% of women,[20,22,23] which is greater than that caused by other vaginal operations alone. Most patients experience improvement in bowel symptoms,[17] but many (48–62%) are left with some residual symptoms of impaired bowel emptying.[17,20,23] Prophylactic repair of an asymptomatic rectocele should be discouraged at the time of Burch colposuspension because the rectocele is more likely to recur.[24] At 5 year follow-up, 76% of women were relieved of their vaginal prolapse.[23]

Fascial Defect Repair

In 1993, Cullen Richardson described the directed fascial defect repair.[9] The operation differs from the one above in the fascial plication steps. Rather than universal midline plication, distinct defects are identified as breaks in the smooth, shiny layer of fascia that is identified by its ability to withstand traction by Allises. The most common defect is a low transverse disruption between the fascia and the perineal body. A high transverse defect is often associated with a culdocele. The direction of the reparative suture line conforms to the often irregular or curved shape of the defect as seen in Fig. 14.4a–d. Any residual breaks to be repaired are palpated with a finger in the rectum. Intuitively attractive, this technique has been only minimally evaluated. As with the traditional repair, most patients' rectal emptying improves, but 39–46% experience residual bowel symptoms.[25-27] Although sexual satisfaction improves, 8–46% are left with some dyspareunia.[25-27] It is not known whether repairing these discrete defects maintains adequate strength over time or whether additional plication of fascia or levators improves the longevity of the repair. At 6 month to 2 year follow-up, 77–82%[25-27] were relieved of vaginal prolapse.

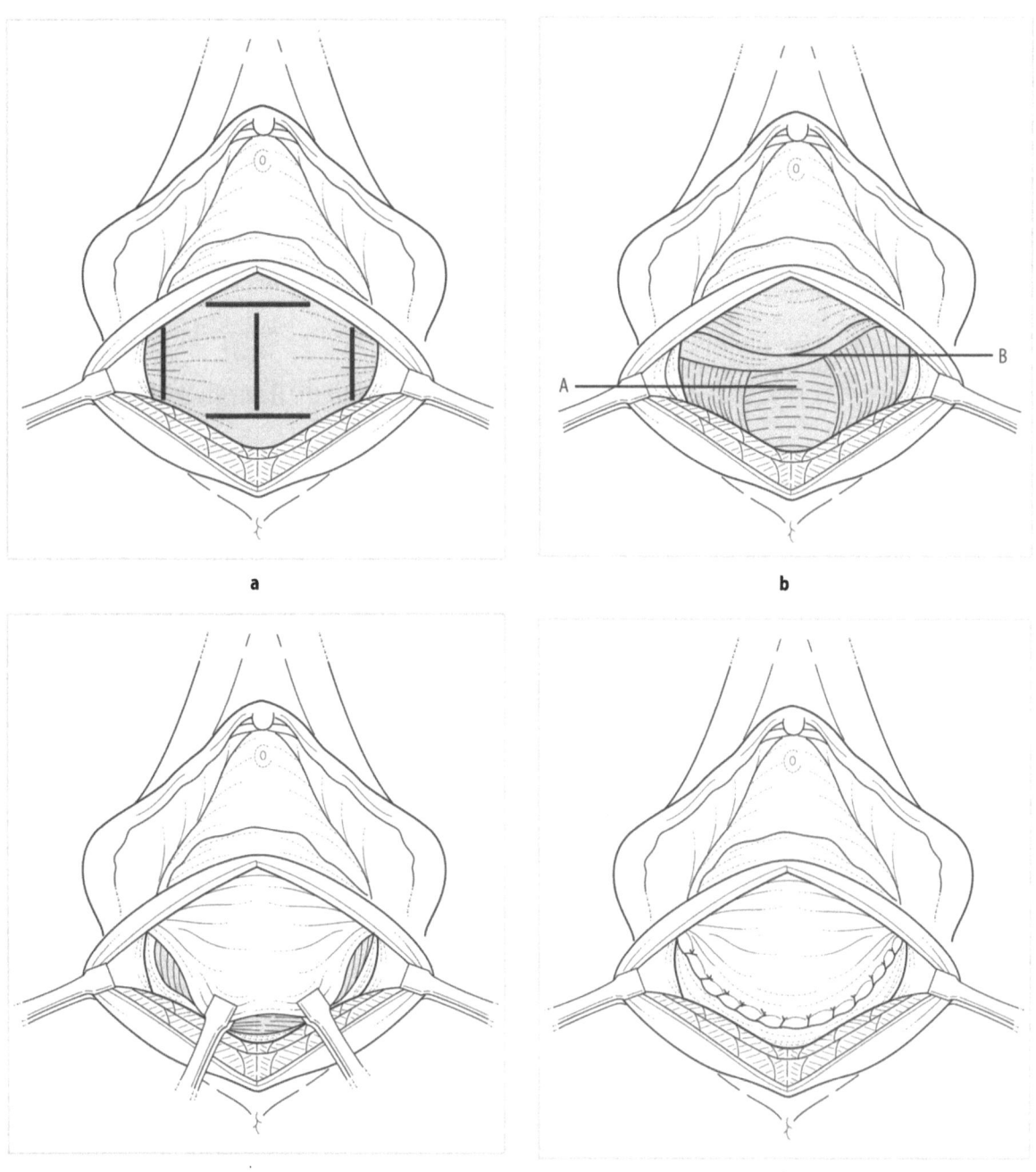

a

b

c

d

Figure 14.4 a Various locations where breaks may occur in the rectovaginal fascia, after dissecting off the vaginal mucosa. **b** Typical low transverse defect. *A*, rectum; *B*, rectovaginal fascia. **c** Fascial edges are approximated and (**d**) sutured together to reconstruct the rectovaginal septum. From Richardson C. The rectovaginal septum revisited: Its relationship to rectocele and its importance in rectocele repair.

Reinforcement of the Rectovaginal Septum by Graft

Techniques that reinforce the rectovaginal septum developed in response to concerns about the intrinisic strength of this tissue.

In 1987, Øster and Astrup[28] described a technique of posterior colporrhaphy without levator plication for large rectoceles in which a dermis graft removed from the thigh is sutured into the rectovaginal space. Fifteen women were followed up for a mean of 2.6 years. Five patients suffered from constipation postoperatively, although the authors state that all 15 were cured of their defecatory and prolapse symptoms. Three patients experienced dyspareunia. Watson et al.[7] described placement of a Marlex mesh via a transperineal approach with levator plication in nine women who digitated to effect evacuation. Postoperatively, eight of the nine were cured of impaired bowel emptying. The mean symptom score for "vaginal lump" improved overall. One patient developed de-novo dyspareunia. Lyons and Winer[6] followed 20 patients following laparoscopic placement of a polyglactin mesh in the rectovaginal space and reported an 80% success rate at 1 year. Unfortunately, they did not define the criteria of success. An early report of cadaveric fascia used in 20 patients has shown promising results at 6 months. However, use of this material for suburethral slings has not been proved to be as satisfactory as with autologous tissue.[29]

Transanal Repair

Technique

The morning of surgery all women receive a phosphate enema. Prophylactic antibiotics of choice are given preoperatively. The patient is place in the prone jackknife position with the buttocks separated by adhesive tape. The anterior rectal mucosa is incised transversely, proximal to the dentate line, and dissected free of the underlying circular muscle to a distance 8–10 cm from the anal verge and extending laterally 180°. The circular muscle is then plicated longitudinally with three or four parallel 0000 polypropylene sutures. The excess mucosa is excised and the defect closed with a running 000 polydioxanone suture. An iodine-soaked gauze roll is placed in the anus and removed the following morning. An intra-urethral catheter avoids the need for subsequent straight catheterization. Discharge is usually after the first bowel movement.

Variations include plicating the rectal wall in two directions,[18,30–33] transversely only,[34–36] longitudinally only,[37] puborectalis plication through the rectum,[30,31,34] or by imbrication of the rectal wall transversely without mucosal dissection.[38,39] Most techniques expose the inner circular muscle, as seen in Fig. 14.5a–e.

Results

As is the case for posterior colporrhaphy, most patients showed symptomatic improvement, but were left with some degree of anorectal complaint. A recent study[35] relates historical data to postoperative improvement. The need for preoperative vaginal or perineal digitation was related to a good result ($p < 0.05$), whereas previous hysterectomy ($p < 0.01$) or the preoperative use of enemas, motor stimulants, or several types of laxatives ($p < 0.05$) was related to a poor outcome. Rectal pain[20] and dyspareunia[40] appear to be less than for the vaginal repair. Vaginal prolapse size is often not evaluated for transanal repair, which may not adequately treat vaginal prolapse.[41]

Combined Vaginal/Transanal Repair

Sullivan et al.[31] originally abandoned the combined approach because of the need for re-operation in 21 of their 28 patients, which led to the development of the totally transanal approach. Recently, Van Dam et al.[42] prospectively studied 74 women who underwent posterior colporrhaphy and transanal repair together. All women had pre- and postoperative defecography with complete resolution of their rectoceles. Postoperatively 50% had marked defecatory disturbances and 18% had mild disturbances.

Summary

Vaginal operations repair the prolapse in 76–82% of women. The small number of prospective studies, varying selection criteria, and variations in technique make comparison difficult. However, postoperatively a large proportion of patients are left with some symptoms of impaired evacuation. Hence, conservative treatment with bulking agents and lactulose or sorbitol syrup are recommended as initial treatment for those with impaired defecation. Those women with fecal incontinence should be referred for anorectal studies. Women with long standing constipation and less than two bowel movements per week will more likely have slow transit constipation and be less likely to benefit from surgery. Dyspareunia remains a complication in 11–46% of patients.[17,20,23,25–27,43]

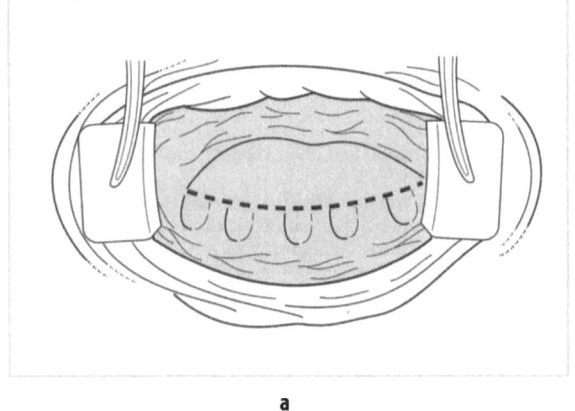

a

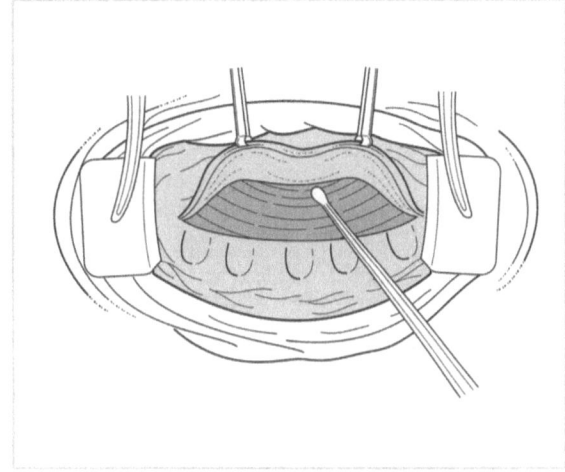

b

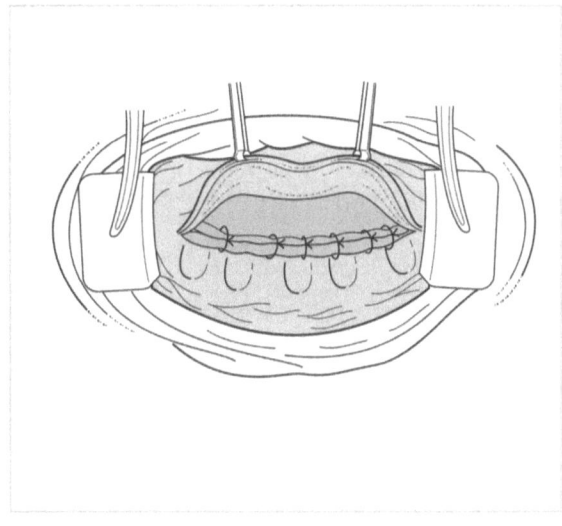

c

d

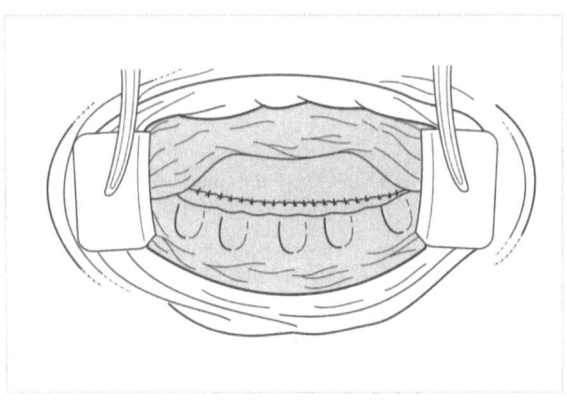

e

Figure 14.5 Transanal repair showing (**a**) the initial incision through the dentate line, (**b**) exposure of the anterior inner circular muscle, (**c**) placement of plication sutures and (**d**) cinching them down, and (**e**) closing the mucosal defect.

Further investigations are needed to identify which patients will most likely benefit from surgery and to compare the risks and benefits of each technique.

References

1. Goff BH (1931) Histological study of the perivaginal fascia in a nullipara. Surg Gynecol Obstet 52: 32–42.
2. Milley PS, Nichols DH (1968) A correlative investigation of the human rectovaginal septum. Anat Rec 163: 443–4.
3. Ricci JV, Lisa JR, Thom CH, Kron WL (1947) The relationship of the vagina to adjacent organs in reconstructive surgery: a histologic study. Am J Surg 74: 387–410.
4. Ricci JV, Thom CH, Kron WL (1948) Cleavage planes in reconstructive vaginal plastic surgery. Am J Surg 76: 354–63.
5. Weber AM, Walters MD (1995) What is vaginal fascia? A U G S Q Rep 13(3).
6. Lyons TL, Winer W (1997) Laparoscopic rectocele repair using polyglactin mesh. J Am Gynecol Laparosc 4: 381–384.
7. Watson SJ, Loder PB, Halligan S et al. (1996) Transperineal repair of symptomatic rectocele with Marlex mesh: a clinical, physiological and radiologic assessment of treatment. J Am Coll Surg 183: 257–61.
8. Kohli N, Karram MM (1998) Use of cadaveric fascia in the treatment of posterior vaginal wall prolapse (abstract). 19th Annual Scientific Meeting of American Urogynecologic Society, 1998, Washington, DC.
9. Richardson CA (1993) The rectovaginal septum revisited. Its relationship to rectocele and its importance in rectocele repair. Clin Obstet Gynecol 36: 976–83.
10. Miklos JR, Kohli N, Lucente V, Saye W (1998) Site-specific fascial defects in the diagnosis and surgical management of enterocele. Am J Obstet Gynecol 179(6): 1418–23.
11. Marks MM (1967) The rectal side of the rectocele. Dis Colon Rectum 10: 387–8.
12. Halligan S, Bartram CI, Hall C, Wingate J (1996) Enterocele revealed by simultaneous evacuation proctography and peritoneography: does defecation block exist? Am J Roetngenol 167: 461–6.
13. Mellgren A, Johansson C, Dolk A et al. (1994) Enterocele demonstrated by defaecography is associated with other pelvic floor disorders. Int J Colorect Dis 9: 121–4.
14. Meigs JV (1947) Enterocele or posterior vaginal hernia. Surg Clin North Am 27: 1226–30.
15. Bump RC, Mattiasson A, Bo K et al. (1996) The standardization of terminology of female pelvic organ prolapse and pelvic floor dysfunction. Am J Obstet Gynecol 175: 10–17.
16. Baden W, Walker T (1992) Surgical Repair of Vaginal Defects. JB Lippincott, Philadelphia.
17. Mellgren A, Anzen BV, Nilsson BY et al. (1995) Results of rectocele repair. A prospective study. Dis Colon Rectum 38: 7–13.
18. Janssen LWM, Dijke CF van (1994) Selection criteria for anterior rectal wall prolapse. Dis Colon Rectum 37: 1100–1107.
19. Goff BH (1928) A practical consideration of the damaged pelvic floor with a technique for its secondary reconstruction. Surg Gynecol Obstet 46: 855–866.
20. Arnold MW, Stewart WR, Aguilar PS (1990) Rectocele repair. Four years' experience. Dis Colon Rectum 33: 684–687.
21. Francis WJA, Jeffcoate TNA (1961) Dyspareunia following vaginal operations. J Obstet Gynaecol Br Comm 68: 1–10.
22. Haase R, Skibsted L (1988) Influence of operations for stress incontinence and/or genital descensus on sexual life. Acta Obstet Gynecol Scand 67: 659–61.
23. Kahn MA, Stanton SL (1997) Posterior colporrhaphy: its effects on bowel and sexual function. Br J Obstet Gynaecol 104: 82–6.
24. Kahn MA, Stanton SL (1997) Letter to the editor. Br J Obstet Gynecol 104: 972–3.
25. Cundiff GW, Weidner AC, Visco AG et al. (1998) An anatomic and functional assessment of the discrete defect rectocele repair. Am J Obstet Gynecol 179(6): 1451–7.
26. Porter WE, Steele A, Walsh P et al. (1999) The anatomic and functional outcomes of defect-specific rectocele repairs. Am J Obstet Gynecol 181(6): 1353–9.
27. Kenton K, Shott S, Brubaker L (1999) Outcome after rectovaginal fascia reattachment for rectocele repair. Am J Obstet Gynecol 180(6): 1360–4.
28. Øster S, Astrup A (1981) A new vaginal operation for recurrent and large rectocele using dermis transplant. Acta Obstet Gynecol Scand 60: 493–5.
29. Soergel T, Heit M (1998) Suburethral slings utilizing rectus abdominus versus donor fascia lata: a retrospective study comparing objective cure rates. AUGS 19th Annual Scientific Meeting, November 1998, P27.
30. Sehapayak S (1985) Transrectal repair of rectocele: an extended armamentarium of colorectal surgeons. A report of 355 cases. Dis Colon Rectum 28: 422–33.
31. Sullivan ES, Leaverton GH, Hardwick CE (1968) Transrectal perineal repair: an adjunct to improved function after anorectal surgery. Dis Colon Rectum 11: 106–14.
32. Khubchandani IT, Sheets JA, Stasik JJ et al. (1983) Endorectal repair of rectocele. Dis Colon Rectum 26: 792–6.
33. Khubchandani IT, Clancy JP, Rosen L et al. (1997) Endorectal repair of rectocele revisited. Br J Surg 84: 89–91.
34. Capps WR (1975) Rectoplasty and perineoplasty for the symptomatic rectocele: a report of fifty cases. Dis Colon Rectum 18: 237–44.
35. Karlbom U, Graf WG, Hilsson S, Pa[o]hlman L et al. (1996) Does surgical repair of a rectocele improve rectal emptying? Dis Colon Rect 39: 1296–1302.
36. Murthy VK, Orkin BA, Smith LE, Glassman LM (1996) Excellent outcome using selective criteria for rectocele repair. Dis Colon Rect 39: 374–8.
37. Sarles JC, Arnoud M, Selezneff I, Olivier S (1989) Endo-rectal repair of rectocele. Int J Colorect Dis 4: 167–71.
38. Block IR (1986) Transrectal repair of rectocele using obliterative suture. Dis Colon Rectum 29: 707–11.
39. Infantino A, Masin A, Melega E et al. (1995) Does surgery resolve outlet obstruction from rectocele? Int J Colorect Dis 10(97): 97–100.
40. Kahn MA, Stanton SL, Kumar DA (1997) Randomized prospective trial of posterior colporrhaphy vs transanal reapir of rectocele: preliminary findings. Int Urogynecol J 8(4): 246.
41. Kahn MA, Stanton SL, Kumar D, Fox SD (1999) Posterior colporrhaphy is superior to the transanal repair for treatment of posterior vaginal wall prolapse. Neurourol Urodynamics 18: 329–30.
42. Dam JH Van, Ginai JH, Gosselink MJ et al. (1997) Role of defecography in predicting clinical outcome of rectocele repair. Dis Colon Rectum 40: 201–7.
43. Siproudhis L, Dautreme S, Ropert A et al. (1993) Dyschezia and rectocele – a marriage of convenience? Physiologic evaluation of the rectocele in a group of 52 women complaining of difficulty in evacuation. Dis Colon Rectum 36: 1030–6.

15 Laparoscopic Repair of Genito-Urinary Prolapse

Tony Smith and Genady Bitman

The early enthusiasm which greeted the first reports of laparoscopic pelvic reconstructive surgery have been tempered by the lack of objective evidence that the laparoscopic approach confers benefit to the patient with speed of recovery and relief of symptoms. In addition the few prospective, randomized studies which have been performed comparing laparoscopic and open surgery have highlighted the new surgical skills required, the additional expense, and the serious complications that may occur.

Reports on laparoscopic treatment of prolapse have been largely descriptive with limited detail about outcome. There is some consensus amongst gynecological surgeons that the laparoscope does enable a clearer visualization of the pelvic anatomy than achieved at open surgery, in which case the challenge for the surgeon is to develop the skills to maximize this benefit. Subjective and objective pre and post-operative assessments are required with long-term follow-up before we can assume that the laparoscopic approach is an advance in pelvic reconstructive surgery.

Indications and Role of Laparoscopic Surgery

Women have an 11% lifetime risk of requiring surgery for uterovaginal prolapse or urinary inconti-

nence.[1] The 29% risk of requiring a repeat procedure may be due to the age-dependent progressive deterioration in support tissues, but may also reflect inadequacies in the techniques of surgical repair. Whether prolapse should be repaired abdominally or vaginally has been debated vigorously throughout this century and is beyond the scope of this chapter. The main role of laparoscopic surgery would seem to be in cases in which the surgeon would normally use the open abdominal approach. If the laparoscopic approach is shown to be beneficial and associated with less perioperative morbidity, comparisons with the vaginal route would then be appropriate.

There are circumstances in which the laparoscopic approach may be more difficult, more hazardous, or contraindicated. Obesity makes all forms of surgery more difficult and adds anesthetic risks. In our view obesity is not a contra-indication and it may well be a relative indication for the laparoscopic approach because of the additional morbidity associated with abdominal wounds in obese patients. Laparoscopic trochar entry carries a risk of visceral injury even when all precautions are taken. This risk is greater when the patient has had previous abdominal surgery, and all patients need to be warned about the potential need for laparotomy. Absolute contraindications are few and mainly relate to anesthetic concerns of using raised intra-abdominal pressure in a patient who has cardio-pulmonary problems. A patient who has had mesh repair of an umbilical hernia represents a challenge that is probably better avoided if possible.

Prolapse in the Anterior Compartment

In 1909 White suggested that a cystocele was best repaired vaginally through two lateral incisions in the anterior vaginal wall through which the endopelvic fascia could be re-attached to the pelvic side wall.[2] Although the anterior repair has been widely adopted for repair of cystocele (more commonly by the technique reported by Kelly in 1913[3]) the problem of coexisting stress incontinence is now viewed to be better treated by a colposuspension.

Many surgeons extend their colposuspension to include a paravaginal repair when a cystocele is present. Given the knowledge that a paravaginal repair does not reliably cure stress incontinence,[4] if an abdominal approach is to be considered for treatment of a cystocele it would be wise to incorporate colposuspension since future surgery in the area will be more difficult. These principles hold for laparoscopic surgery which has abundant reports on colposuspension but no reports on paravaginal repair alone. There are concerns, from the reports on colposuspension, that the incidence of bladder injury is higher than in open surgery and the risk of recurrence may be greater, but results from further well constructed trials is awaited.[5]

Uterine Prolapse

Vaginal hysterectomy is currently more popular than uterine conserving procedures such as the Manchester repair for the surgical management of uterine prolapse. In younger women the laparoscopic approach may confer some advantages, and with increasing concern about preservation of the cervix for support and sexual function the laparoscopic approach may warrant consideration.

Wattiez et al.[6] have described hysterosacropexy which includes opening the vesico-uterine space and the posterior peritoneum between the uterosacral ligaments. A V-shaped Mersilene tape was sutured to both sides of the uterus following fixation to the sacral promontory.

Mangeshikar[7] performed laparoscopic cervicopexy. Mersilene tape was secured to the cervix and after opening the pouch of Douglas peritoneum passed through the broad ligament to the anterior abdominal wall.

At this stage uterine support has only been described in descriptive terms with no outcome data. Our own experience has been largely confined to the management of procidentia by laparoscopic hysterosacropexy combined with paravaginal repair. It would be interesting to compare this procedure with vaginal hysterectomy and pelvic floor repair in a well constructed trial.

Prolapse in the Posterior Compartment; Vaginal Vault, Enterocele, and Rectocele

In the view of the author, laparoscopic sacrocolpopexy is the procedure which represents the most significant advance in pelvic reconstructive surgery. The laparoscopic view of the rectovaginal

space enables dissection down to the level of the pelvic floor and the attachment of supporting mesh along the full length of the vagina. This means that a total laparoscopic approach may be employed without recourse to vaginal repair.

Technique

The technique described here has been developed over the last 9 years.

The patient is catheterized using an 18F Foley catheter. Pneumoperitoneum is established and a steep Trendelenberg position employed. A 10 mm subumbilical port is used for the laparoscope and left lateral 5 mm and right lateral 10 mm ports introduced. Any adhesions are divided to allow free access to the vagina and sacrum. The peritoneum is opened over the vaginal vault which is elevated by a plastic "bowel sizer" (designed for sizing the bowel lumen prior to a stapling anastamosis). The bladder may be adherent to the apex of the vaginal vault, so care is needed to avoid bladder injury. The rectovaginal space is developed by sharp and blunt dissection. Adhesions may be dense when previous surgery has been performed and a bowel sizer may also be placed in the rectum to aid dissection. A piece of polypropylene mesh (Ethicon Ltd, UK) is tailored from a larger piece to fit the needs of the patient. The mesh is introduced through the 10 mm port and placed in between the vagina and the rectum. The mesh is secured to the vagina with a minimum of five 1-0 prolene sutures with extracorporeal knot tying.

The sacral promontory is exposed and the peritoneum over it opened. The peritoneum is opened to the right of the bowel towards the hollow of the sacrum enough to mobilize sufficient peritoneum to cover the mesh after it has been secured to the sacrum. The mesh is now secured to the sacrum. Staples, tacks, or sutures may be employed with equal benefit; suturing is cheaper, but takes longer. The vagina should be elevated from below when it is attached to the sacrum but must not be placed under tension. The mesh is then covered with peritoneum to prevent herniation under it or bowel adhesions.

Results

Prolapse of the posterior compartment, particularly vaginal vault prolapse, rarely occurs in isolation. In addition to the anatomical deformity there is often functional disturbance in relation to bladder, bowel, and coitus. The literature of laparoscopic surgery displays many of the failings of previous publications in this area with lack of clarity of description of pre- and postoperative anatomy, little detail of changes in function and perioperative morbidity.

In 1993 Vancaillie and Butler[8] first described the laparoscopic repair of enterocele. The peritoneum of the enterocele sac was excised and the space reinforced with sutures in the endopelvic fascia of the uterosacral ligaments and anterior rectal wall. In a series of 18 women, 16 had "satisfactory follow-up" 3–16 months later.

Nezhat et al.[9] first described laparoscopic sacrocolpopexy. In one of the 16 cases reported laparotomy was required to stop bleeding from presacral veins. A Gore-Tex (WL Gore, USA) patch was sutured to the vaginal apex and the anterior surface of the third and fourth sacral vertebrae. Anterior and posterior vaginal repair was also performed. Complete relief of symptoms was reported at follow-up ranging from 3 to 40 months.

In an attempt to reduce the risk of hemorrhage from the presacral vessels, Carey et al.[10] used a 5mm tacker to secure the mesh to the sacrum. In a series of 11 cases, one laparotomy was performed because of dense intra-abdominal adhesions. Polypropylene mesh was attached to the upper two-thirds of the posterior vaginal wall and the upper third of the anterior vaginal wall. At follow up ranging from 6 months to 2 years no recurrent prolapse was observed and no patient required further surgery.

The difficulties in operating laparoscopically deep in the pelvis may be overcome by combining vaginal and laparoscopic surgery. Miklos et al.[11] used a combined approach in 17 women for repair of enterocele. Through the laparoscope the uterosacral ligaments were re-secured to the vaginal apex with sutures from the level of the ischial spines and the rectocele repair completed vaginally. At follow up ranging from 1 to 17 months all patients were said to be satisfied, although asymptomatic vaginal vault descent was reported in two cases.

Since 1993 we have used the laparoscopic sacrocolpopexy primarily for vaginal vault prolapse. The procedure has evolved from initially reproducing the open procedure, attaching the mesh to the vaginal apex, to securing the mesh to the full length of the posterior vaginal wall. In 1995 we published the results of the first 29 cases.[12] One case required laparotomy because of difficulty entering the retropubic space for colposuspension. No cases have required transfusion, and no women have had to return to theatre in the postoperative period. We have now reviewed 39 cases at least 4 years after surgery. Two recurrences of vault prolapse have occurred in patients in whom the apex alone was attached to the mesh. One has had a repeat laparoscopic sacrocolpopexy re-using the mesh still secured to the sacrum. Recurrence of posterior vaginal wall prolapse occurred in 18 cases, although

not all were symptomatic. The attachment of mesh to the full length of the posterior vaginal wall should prevent this problem. For some cases we introduced the mesh vaginally and then picked up the mesh laparoscopically. Although this approach ensures full-length support to the posterior vaginal wall, we found that 1 in 4 cases required some mesh trimming vaginally at follow up. We have only seen mesh erosion in 1 case in well over 100 total laparoscopic cases. Stress incontinence is often present preoperatively and may present de novo postoperatively. In 11 women stress incontinence was a problem postoperatively compared to 20 preoperatively. Clearly, the laparoscopic approach does not appear to have found new solutions to all of the problems which can occur after this type of surgery.

Complications

In laparoscopic pelvic reconstructive surgery there are some complications that represent risks inherent in the technique of laparoscopy. There is no method of entirely removing the risk of bowel injury on insertion of the primary trochar. The risk of such injury is greater when the patient has had previous abdominal surgery, as is often the case in reconstructive surgery. The risk of bladder injury at colposuspension appears to be greater than reported from open surgery, although it is acknowledged that this may be part of the learning process and may therefore diminish as the technique and training is improved.

Cost

Most analyses indicate that laparoscopic surgery is more expensive than open surgery. The equipment and additional operating room time are the main reasons for this. No analyses include the costs of managing recurrence; no figures are available for this. Until reliable data is available on the quality of life changes after laparoscopic surgery compared to open surgery it will be impossible to analyze patient benefit and cost meaningfully. The study of patient perception of pain relief and satisfaction with outcome after bladder neck surgery indicates that surgeons may not be as successful as they thought in improving quality of life for their patients.[13] Further study into surgical approaches which may influence this are therefore important.

Conclusions

Laparoscopic pelvic reconstructive surgery has the potential to advance this neglected specialty by providing better visualization and access to the pelvic support structures and reducing patient morbidity. Having demonstrated that such surgery is possible, the challenge now is to compare this approach critically with conventional surgery in well-constructed trials.

References

1. Olsen A, Smith V, Bergstrom J, Colling J, Clark A (1997) Epidemiology of surgically managed pelvic organ prolapse and urinary incontinence. Obstet Gynaecol 89(4): 501–6.
2. White GR (1909) Cystocoele: A radical cure by suturing lateral sulci of vagina to white line of pelvic fascia. JAMA 53: 1707–11.
3. Kelly HA (1913) Incontinence of urine in women. Urol Cutan Rev 17: 291–3.
4. Colombo M, Milani R, Vitobello D (1996) Maggioni A A randomised comparison of Burch colposuspension and abdominal paravaginal defect repair for female urinary stress incontinence. Am J Obstet Gynaecol 175(1): 78–84.
5. Smith ARB, Stanton SL (1998) Laparoscopic colposuspension. Br J Obstet Gynaecol 105(4): 383–4.
6. Wattiez A, Boughizane S, Alecxandre F et al. (1995) Laparoscopic procedures for stress incontinence and prolapse. Curr Opin Obstet Gynaecol 7: 317–21.
7. Mangeshikar P (1994) Laparoscopic cervicopexy: conservative surgery for uterine prolapse (abstract). European Congress of Gynaecol Endoscopic Surgery, 15–18 June1994, Rome. Gynaecol Endosc 3(suppl 1):16.
8. Vancaillie TG, Butler DJ (1993) Laparoscopic enterocoele repair – description of a new technique. Gynaecol Endosc 2: 211–16.
9. Nezhat CH, Nezhat F, Nezhat C (1994) Laparoscopic sacral colpopexy for vaginal vault prolapse. Obstet Gynecol 84: 885–8.
10. Carey MP, Maher CF, Gilmour DT (1998) Laparoscopic and open sacral promontory fixation for vault and marked uterovaginal prolapse using the 5 mm Origin tacker (abstract). International Continence Society Congress, 17–21 September 1998, Jerusalem.
11. Miklos JR, Kohli N, Lucente V, Saye WB (1998) Site-specific defects in the diagnosis and surgical management of enterocoele. Am J Obstet Gynaecol 179: 1418–23.
12. Mahendran D, Prashar S, Smith ARB, Murphy D (1996) Laparoscopic sacrocolpopexy in the management of vaginal vault prolapse. Gynaecol Endosc 5: 217–22.
13. Black N, Griffiths J, Pope C, Bowling A, Abel P (1997) Impact of surgery for stress incontinence: cohort study. BMJ 315(7121): 1493–8.

16 The Surgical Treatment of Fecal Incontinence and Rectal Prolapse

Sharon G. Gregorcyk and Philip J. Huber, Jr.

Fecal Incontinence

The treatment of fecal incontinence varies with its etiology and severity. Nonsurgical therapy is the first step in almost all cases. An intact and functional anorectal ring of adequate length and an appropriate anorectal angle are very important for continence. The majority of operative procedures for fecal incontinence attempt to restore this anatomy.

In this chapter, we describe the indications and techniques of different operative procedures for incontinence. In a similar manner, we also describe surgical techniques for the treatment of rectal prolapse, as it can be a cause of fecal incontinence. For all the described procedures, preoperative preparation includes a full mechanical bowel preparation with oral and intravenous antibiotics.

Overlapping Sphincteroplasty

A direct repair of the sphincters or sphincteroplasty can be performed when there is a single anatomic defect in the muscles. The majority of injuries are associated with obstetric trauma including episiotomies and are, therefore, located anteriorly.

Other causes of an anatomic defect include trauma, fistulotomy, and sphincterotomy with variable locations.

Overlapping sphincteroplasty is the operation of choice for a single anatomic defect in the sphincter muscles. This procedure may be performed under a general or regional anesthesia with the patient in a prone jackknife position. Exposure in this position may be aided by retracting the buttocks with tape. The surgical scrub of the area for all perineal cases should include a vaginal preparation in women. The operative site is first infiltrated with a local anesthetic with epinephrine solution in a 1 : 150 000 or 1 : 200 000 concentration in order to relax the muscles and improve hemostasis.

A curvilinear incision is made parallel to the outer edge of the external sphincter, extending 180–240° (Fig. 16.1a). Dissection is initiated in the center of the defect and carried out in either direction searching for the retracted edges of the sphincter muscles. A needle tip Bovie cautery is quite useful for this dissection. Once the two ends of the sphincter mechanism are identified, they are dissected away from surrounding tissues for adequate mobilization. Care should be taken to preserve the scar tissue (Fig. 16.1b), as this will be the strength of the repair. Also one must be careful to preserve the branches of the pudendal nerves as they enter into the muscle posterolaterally. In dissecting the sphincter mechanism, mobilization proximally to the levators allows for reconstruction of the entire length of the anorectal ring.

The scar tissue is divided (Fig. 16.1c) in its midline to allow the sphincter mechanism to be overlapped (Fig. 16.1d). Although some surgeons try to identify and repair the internal and external sphincters separately, it is often impossible to separate the two muscles and has not been shown to improve the outcome. The sphincters are maintained in an overlapping manner by placing six mattress sutures of 2-0 Vicryl to anchor the scar tissue from

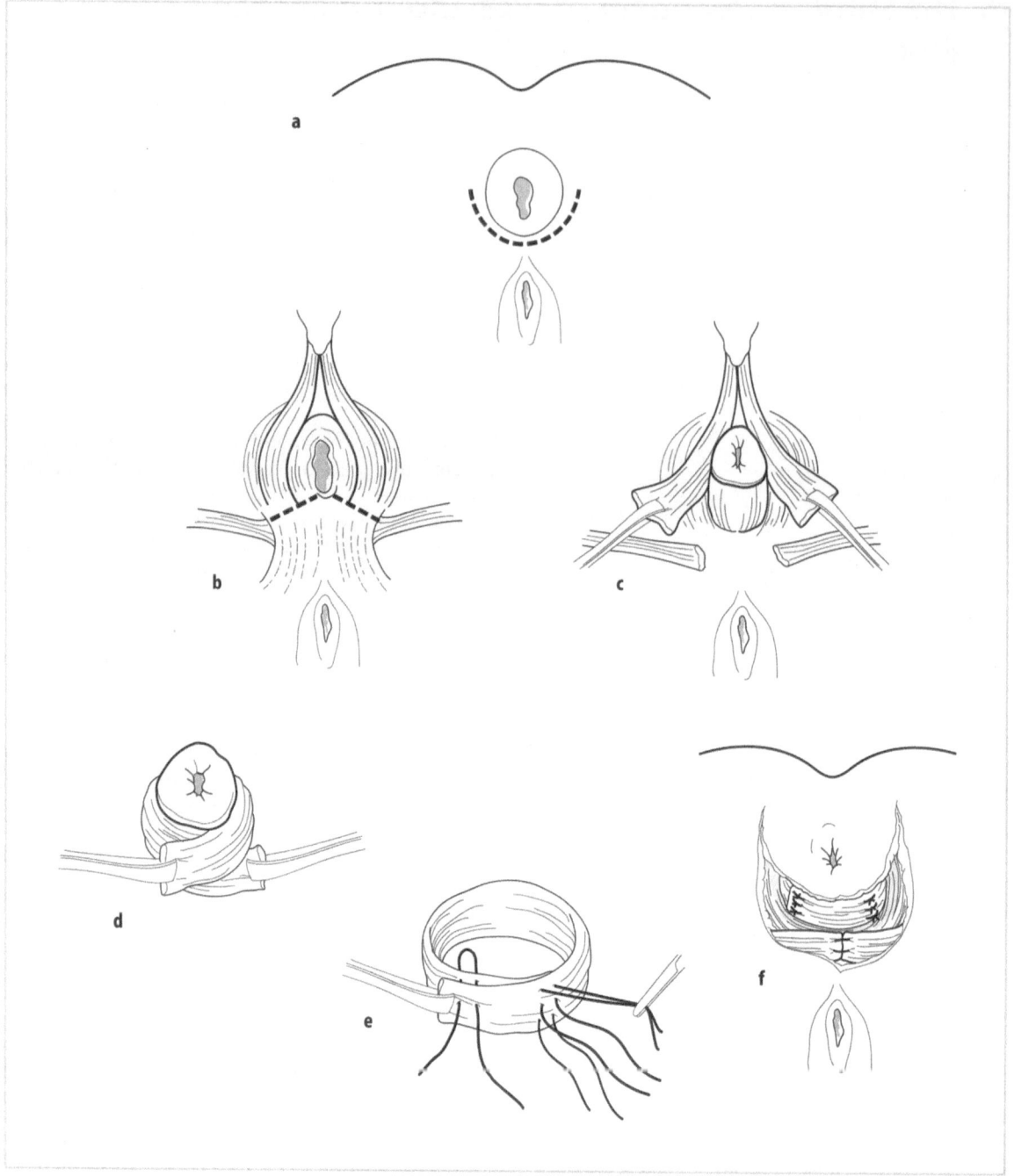

Figure 16.1 Overlapping sphincteroplasty. **a** Curvilinear incision. **b** Scar tissue between retracted sphincter muscles. **c** Mobilization of sphincter muscle with preservation of scar tissue. **d** Overlapping of muscle. **e** Two rows of mattress sutures placed. **f** Superficial transverse perineal muscle reapproximated.

one muscle end to the middle portion of the oppos-ing sphincter muscle (Fig. 16.1e). Once all sutures are in place, they are tied snugly, but not tight, to avoid muscular ischemia.

In women with an anterior repair, the perineal body should be reconstructed. To accomplish this, the transverse perineal muscles, as well as any inter-vening scar tissue, are re-approximated in the midline (Fig. 16.1f). If the vagina is injured during

the anterior dissection, it should be repaired with simple interrupted absorbable sutures.

After assuring meticulous hemostasis and releas-ing all retraction devices, the wound is closed with interrupted 3-0 Vicryl sutures in a Y fashion. The central portion of the wound may be left open or loosely closed. Drains are not usually necessary, but if there is concern over accumulation of fluid, a small drain may be placed.

Postoperatively, the patient is placed on bowel rest and prophylactic perioperative intravenous antibiotics. Different types of bowel confinement have been proposed, including constipating drugs to avoid fecal contamination of the repaired area. A prospective randomized trial by Nessim et al.[1] did not demonstrate any advantage of bowel confinement over a regular diet. Although we do not recommend constipating drugs, we tend to keep the patient on intravenous fluids and nil by mouth for 2–3 days. A diet is then initiated.

Perineal care is aimed at keeping the incision clean and dry, and thus a Foley catheter is in place during most of the hospital stay. Patients are discharged home once they can tolerate a diet. They are instructed on no instrumentation of the anus or vagina and not to soak in a bathtub, as it might promote breakdown of the wound. They are also informed of the high likelihood of a partial breakdown of their wound. With good wound care, however, this does not impact the repair. The wound generally has completely healed within 4–6 weeks.

The majority of authors report a 70–80% success rate for the overlapping sphincteroplasty (Table 16.1). Pudendal neuropathy is the only agreed predictive factor of a poorer outcome.[2-9] Controversy exists as to whether a direct repair is indicated with pudendal neuropathy present. Laurberg et al.[2] reported that 80% of the patients undergoing sphincteroplasty without evidence of neuropathy had an excellent result, compared to only 11% of those patients with neuropathy. On the contrary, Chen et al.[10] noted that all of their patients with an isolated sphincter defect had significant improvement in their incontinence after sphincteroplasty despite having a neuropathy although slightly less than half of the patients actually had an excellent result. They concluded that patients with fecal incontinence and an anatomic sphincter defect should undergo sphincteroplasty, even in the presence of neuropathy, since one can expect a significant improvement in their incontinence with very low morbidity. The authors support this viewpoint. Obviously patient selection must be

taken into account. For example, a patient with a patulous anus and no squeeze would be unlikely to benefit from a sphincteroplasty.

Postanal Repair

For incontinent patients without evidence of sphincter disruption, other repair techniques have been reported. Sir Alan Parks[11] theorized that an adequate anorectal angle was important in the maintenance of continence. He therefore devised an operation to restore this angle in incontinent patients.

Patient position, anesthesia, and local infiltration of epinephrine solution is the same as in the sphincteroplasty. An incision is made posterior to the anus in an inverted V shape (Fig. 16.2a). An intersphincteric plane is developed between the external and internal sphincters (Fig. 16.2b) and continued cephalad until the puborectalis muscle is identified. The pelvic cavity is entered by dividing the rectosacral fascia (Fig. 16.2c), and the levator muscles are exposed after sweeping off the perirectal fat.

The bilateral levator muscles are approximated medially with interrupted 0-Vicryl sutures with the ischiococcygeal muscle being incorporated in the first layer of the repair (Fig. 16.2d). Included in the second layer of the repair is the pubococcygeal muscle (Fig. 16.2e). In tying these sutures, one must be aware of the fact that the muscles will not actually come together, rather the sutures form a type of lattice-work. The final layer approximates the puborectalis muscle (Fig. 16.2f) to further buttress the anorectal angle. Theoretically, this makes the pull of the puborectalis muscle more efficient. The presacral space is drained with a small closed suction drain, which is brought out through a separate stab incision.

In closing the wound, the external sphincter muscles are plicated with interrupted sutures (Fig. 16.2g). At this point some stenosis should be apparent on digital rectal examination. The wound is closed in a Y fashion using absorbable 3-0 sutures

Table 16.1. Sphincteroplasty series

Author	Patients (n)	Age mean (range)	Women (%)	Obstetric (%)	G/E results (%)
Fang (1984)[48]	79	(17–68)	78	88	89
Yoshioka (1989)[49]	27	34 (17–81)	52	70	74
Fleshman (1991)[50]	28	38 (22–75)	100	100	75
Engel (1994)[51]	55	32 (26–52)	100	100	76
Simmang (1994)[52]	14	66 (51–81)	100	79	93
Londono-Schimmer (1994)[53]	128	43 (16–77)	43		
Oliveira (1996)[54,55]	55	48 (27–72)	100	84	71

G, good; E, excellent.

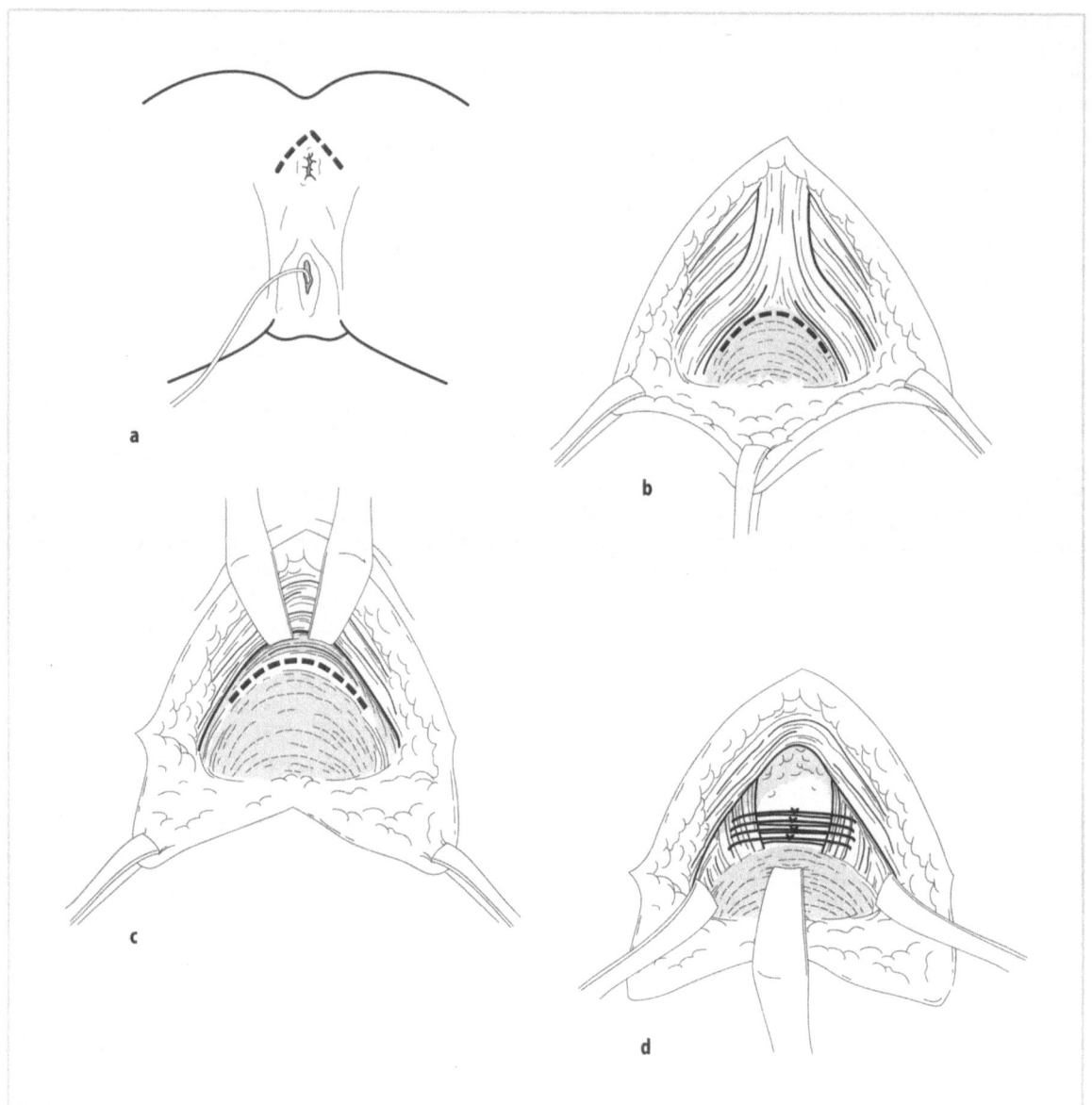

Figure 16.2 Postanal repair. **a** Posterior incision. **b** Development of intersphincteric plane. **c** Divided rectosacral fascia (dotted line). **d** Loose plication of ischiococcygeus muscle. *(Continues opposite)*

in the subcutaneous tissues and a subcuticular stitch for the skin. Postoperative care is essentially the same as that for the overlapping sphincteroplasty.

Looking at multiple series, the success of the Parks postanal repair varies significantly, as seen in Table 16.2. Because of this inconsistency, the postanal repair has not achieved popularity among surgeons in the USA.

Neo-Sphincters

Various procedures have been developed over the years to create a new sphincter mechanism by trans-

Table 16.2. Results of Parks postanal repair

Author	No. of patients	Results (%)		
		Excellent	Good	Poor
Browning et al. (1984)[55]	140	86		14
Henry and Simson (1985)[56]	204	58	12	30
Keighley (1987)[57]	114	32	62	6
Miller et al. (1988)[58]	17	59		41
Womack et al. (1988)[59]	16	88		12
Scheuer et al. (1989)[60]	39	15	54	31
Laurberg et al. (1990)[9]	28	32	43	25

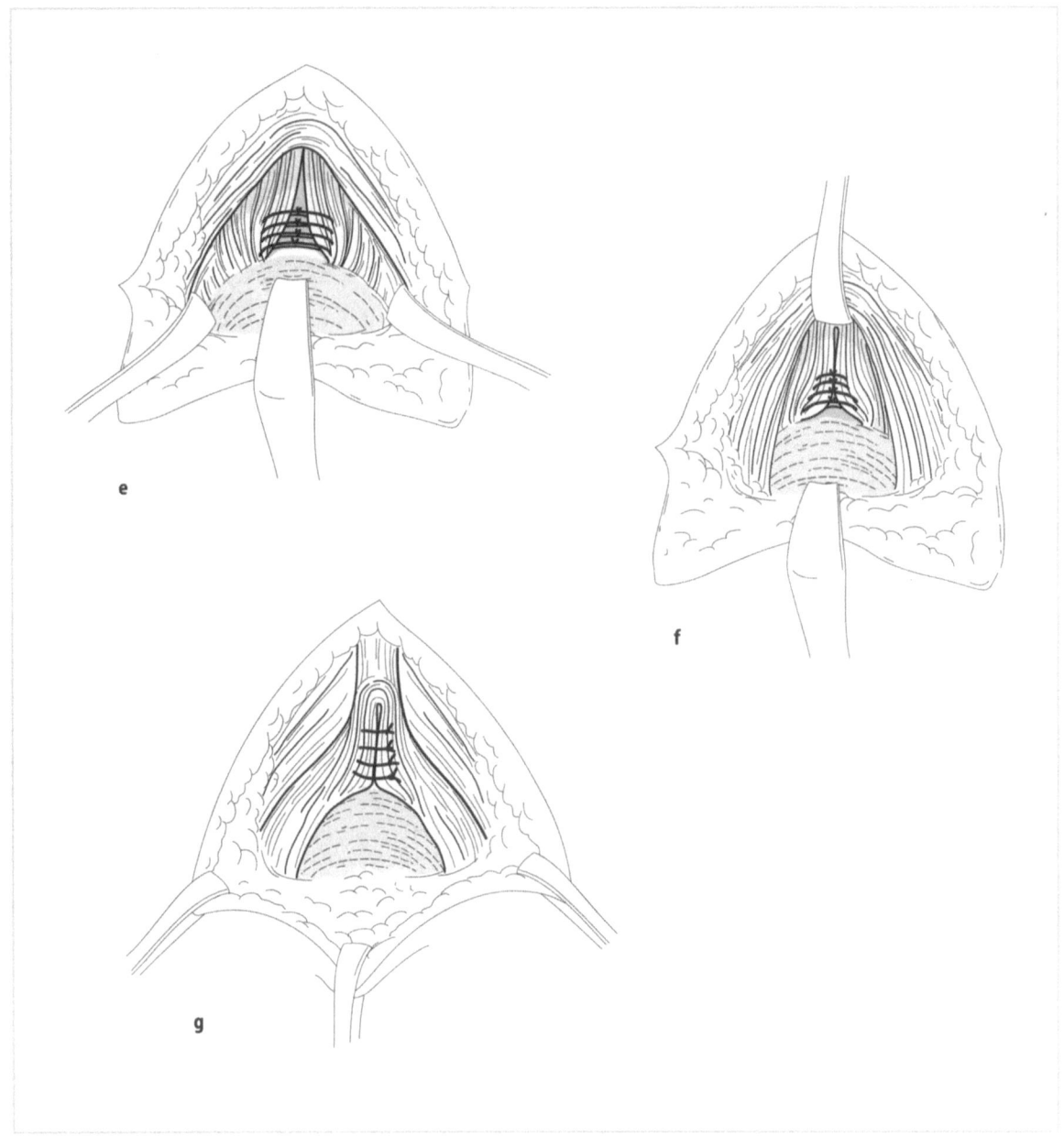

Figure 16.2 e Loose plication of pubococcygeus. **f** Plication of puborectalis muscle. **g** Plication of external sphincter.

position of other muscles. These procedures are much more complex and involved and are, therefore, reserved for patients with severe, disabling incontinence in whom a direct repair is not possible or has failed.

Gracilis Muscle[12-15]

The gracilis muscle runs the length of the thigh from the lower half of the symphysis and pubic arch

to the medial tibia. With the patient in lithotomy position, three small incisions (4 cm) are made starting in the middle of the thigh (Fig. 16.3a) to localize the gracilis muscle belly. The proximal neurovascular bundle lies approximately 12 cm from the origin on the symphysis. Another vascular source connects into the muscle in the distal third–middle junction. This arises from the superficial femoral system and may cause bleeding with mobilization. The proximal neurovascular bundle enters the muscle posterolaterally and must be carefully protected

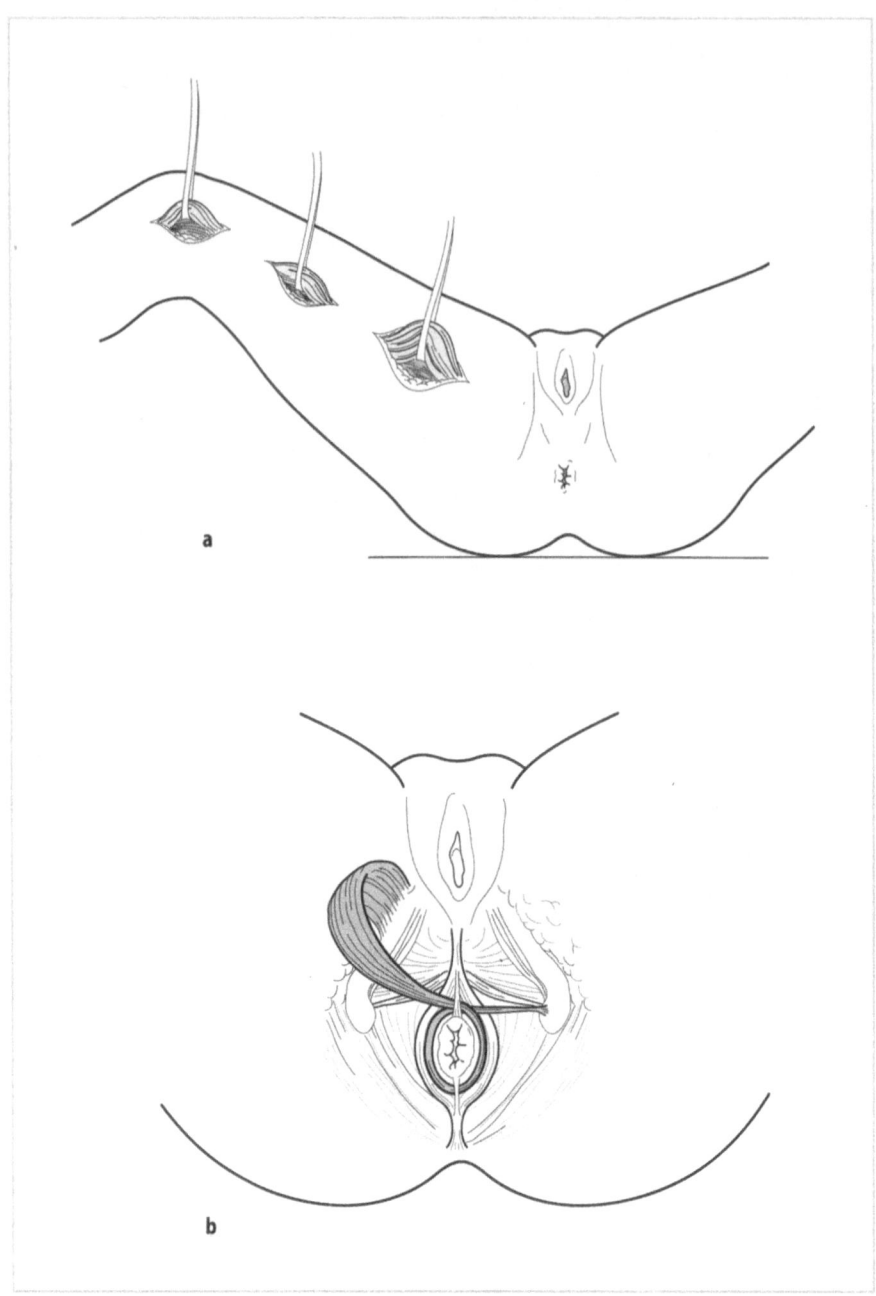

Figure 16.3 Gracilis muscle sling. **a** Gracilis muscle isolation (medial thigh). **b** 360° wrap to contralateral ischial tuberosity.

during mobilization. Complete mobilization of the gracilis to the knee yields the desired length of tendon.

Two lateral perianal incisions are made to create a tunnel around the anal canal deep to the superficial sphincter. A subcutaneous tunnel is made from the medial thigh to the perianal tunnel. The gracilis is passed through the anterior anal tunnel and wrapped 360° back through the anterior tunnel across to the contralateral ischium for fixation with permanent sutures (Fig. 16.3b). The incision to expose the ischium can be a single peri-

anal incision but should not be over the ischium, to avoid pressure on the wound when sitting. The gracilis is pulled snug to create a tight outlet to digital rectal examination. Antibiotic irrigation is used to thoroughly wash out the various tunnels.

A popular technique called "vascular delay" stages mobilization of the gracilis. Ligation of the distal blood supply is performed as a separate procedure 14 days before mobilization and wrap. This permits the muscle to accommodate to the proximal vessel supply.

For the dynamic graciloplasty, electrodes are implanted and sutured proximate to the neural bundle with absorbable sutures. The wires are passed with a ventricular shunt passer in the anterior abdominal wall to a sub-costal pocket where they are connected to a totally implantable stimulator (Itrel 6, Medtronic, Inc., Minneapolis, MN). Postoperatively, electrostimulation is started intermittently and increased every 2 weeks up to 12 weeks postoperatively when the stimulation is continuous.

Gluteus Muscle Transposition[16-18]

Gluteus muscle transposition may be bilateral or unilateral as described here with two distal muscle slips turned back to go around the anus. These slips are either sewn as an overlap of each other or sewn to the contralateral ischium. The concept of using the origin of the gluteus is flawed because length and blood supply restrict muscle slip advancement around the anus. By separating the inferior half of

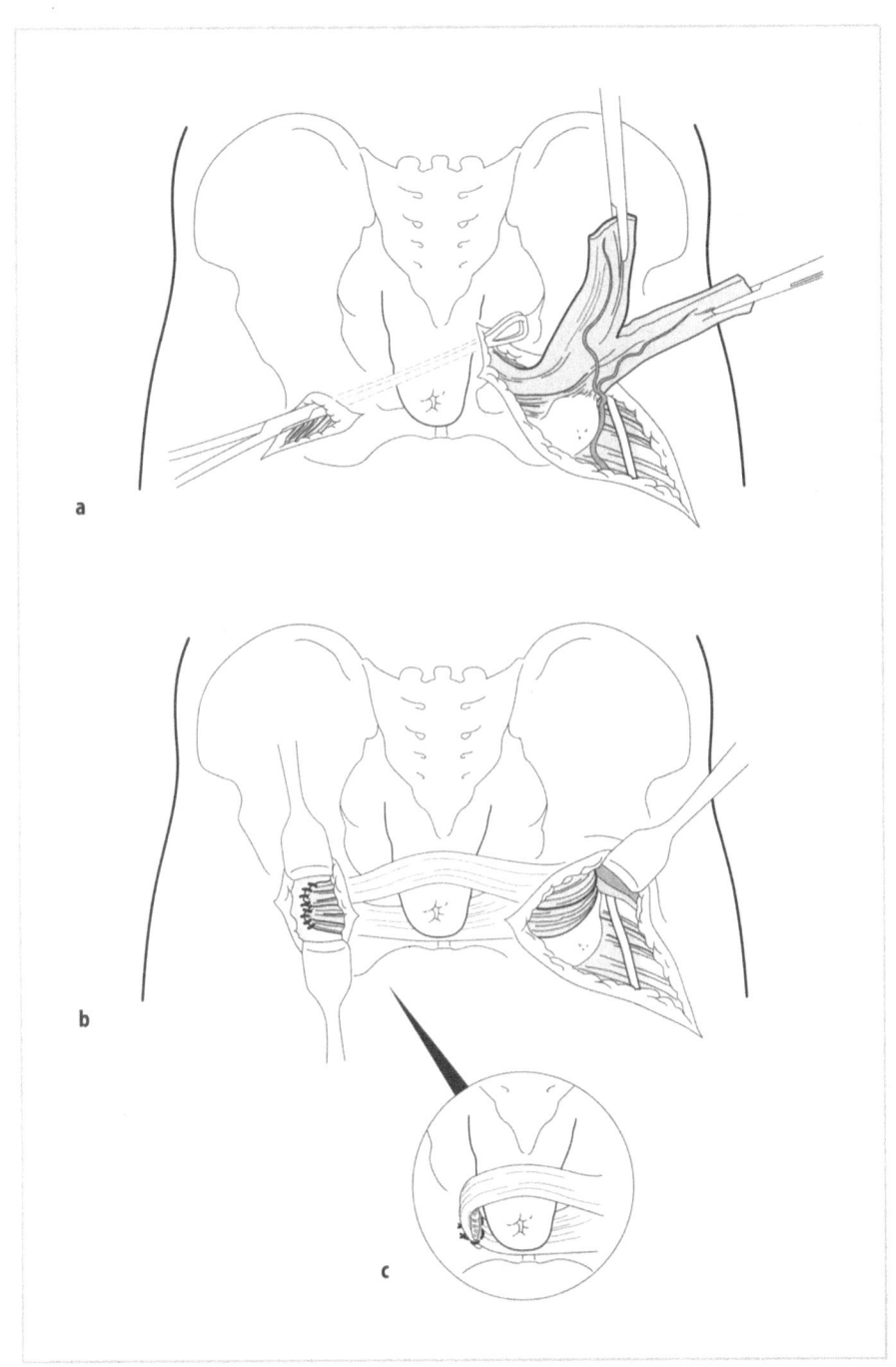

Figure 16.4 Gluteal muscle transposition. **a** Isolation of inferior half of gluteus maximus and its division for two slips to wrap. **b** First option, dependent on length, is to bring slips around anal canal and suture to contralateral ischial tuberosity. **c** Second option is to wrap slips on each other and overlap suture fixation.

the gluteus and mobilizing distally to the insertion on fascia lata, two long muscle slips can be rotated around the anus with adequate length and neurovascular supply.

The skin incision can be a curvilinear lateral incision as depicted (Fig. 16.4a) or an inferior gluteal fold incision. The lateral incision gives excellent visualization; the smaller, more cosmetic buttock fold incision requires lighted angle retractors to mobilize the subcutaneous fat from the gluteal fascia. Skin flaps are created to define the gluteus fascia from the sacral edge to the fascia lata. The inferior half of the gluteus muscle is separated from the superior half and a doppler is used to identify and preserve the superior gluteal neurovascular bundle proximally.

The inferior half of the muscle is sharply excised off the fascia lata and the muscle is carefully lifted off posterior attachments to visualize and protect the sciatic nerve. Once the muscle is elevated, both sciatic nerve and the proximal muscle neurovascular bundle can be visualized. The muscle is divided into two equal slips with occasional bleeders tied with absorbable suture.

A subcutaneous tunnel is developed through the incision around the anus. Care must be taken not to enter the anal canal and to stay a centimeter deep to skin for the perianal wrap. If the plan is to suture the muscle slips to the contralateral ischium (Fig. 16.4b), a counter-incision is made medial (not overlying) to the ischium. If the slips are to be wrapped around the anus and sutured to themselves in overlap fashion, a small, perianal incision is made. The slips must be pulled snugly into the perianal tunnels so that the anal canal is snug to a simple digital examination. Permanent sutures are used to suture the slips to themselves or to the ischium. Two Jackson–Pratt drains are placed under the subcutaneous flaps.

Postoperatively it is imperative to keep the patient from sitting on the rotated flap. Patients can lie on the unaffected side, but they must not put pressure on the flap for 6 weeks to prevent vascular compromise. Jackson–Pratt drains can be pulled when drainage drops to negligible amounts.

Artificial Bowel Sphincter

The artificial bowel sphincter (Acticon) is a device manufactured by American Medical Systems which mimics their artificial urinary sphincter. As of this writing, the device is pending full FDA approval in the USA but is available for humanitarian use. The device consists of a cuff filled with fluid that is implanted around the anus, a reservoir balloon that sits in the prevesical space and a pump device that is implanted in the labia in women and in the scrotum

in men (Fig. 16.5d). When activated, the cuff is filled with fluid, which occludes the anal aperture. To have a bowel movement, the patient pumps the device in the labia or scrotum and the fluid shifts from the cuff to the balloon reservoir, allowing the anal aperture to open so that the patient can defecate. The fluid slowly flows back to the cuff for return of continence. Current indications define patients with severe fecal incontinence who are not amenable to a direct repair and have failed medical management.

As this is a foreign body implant, the bowel preparation should be meticulous.

The procedure is performed with the patient in a modified lithotomy position under general or spinal anesthesia. Proctoscopy is performed to suction out any effluent and the rectum is irrigated with betadine. The rectum is packed with a betadine-soaked vaginal pack.

Two different approaches can be used on the perineum. The first involves making bilateral incisions 4 cm from the anus in a curvilinear fashion. Dissection is carried proximally into the ischiorectal space. Using blunt finger dissection, a circumferential track is developed around the posterior and anterior anus to connect the incisions. Care must be taken in women to avoid injuring the vagina. A second approach, which is now preferred by most surgeons, is to make one single incision anteriorly to allow the dissection to extend more proximally. Once at the desired level, the circumferential dissection is performed through this single incision.

Sizers are provided to help determine the appropriate size cuff. Once the size has been determined, the scrub nurse prepares the cuff with a radio-opaque filling solution. A balloon is selected (the 91–100 cmH_2O and 101–110 cmH_2O sizes are the most popular) and is filled with the appropriate solution. The cuff, which has been freed of all bubbles and emptied, is then passed circumferentially around the anus with the tubing ending up on the patient's left side in right-handed patients and the right side in left-handed patients (Fig. 16.5a). The tab is secured to the cuff to hold it in place. Caution is continually exercised to prevent air from entering the system.

Simultaneously, a second team can approach the retropubic space through a suprapubic transverse incision. The rectus fascia is divided, and the linea alba separated in the midline to expose the prevesical space which is bluntly enlarged to accommodate the balloon. The balloon will rest on the same side as the tubing from the cuff. A plane is bluntly dissected from this wound below Scarpa's fascia into the ipsilateral labia or scrotum for placement of the pump (Fig. 16.5b). A large Hegar dilator is useful for this purpose. The tubing from below can be passed to the incision above using the metal passer tracking lateral to the dissected pocket in the subcutaneous tissue.

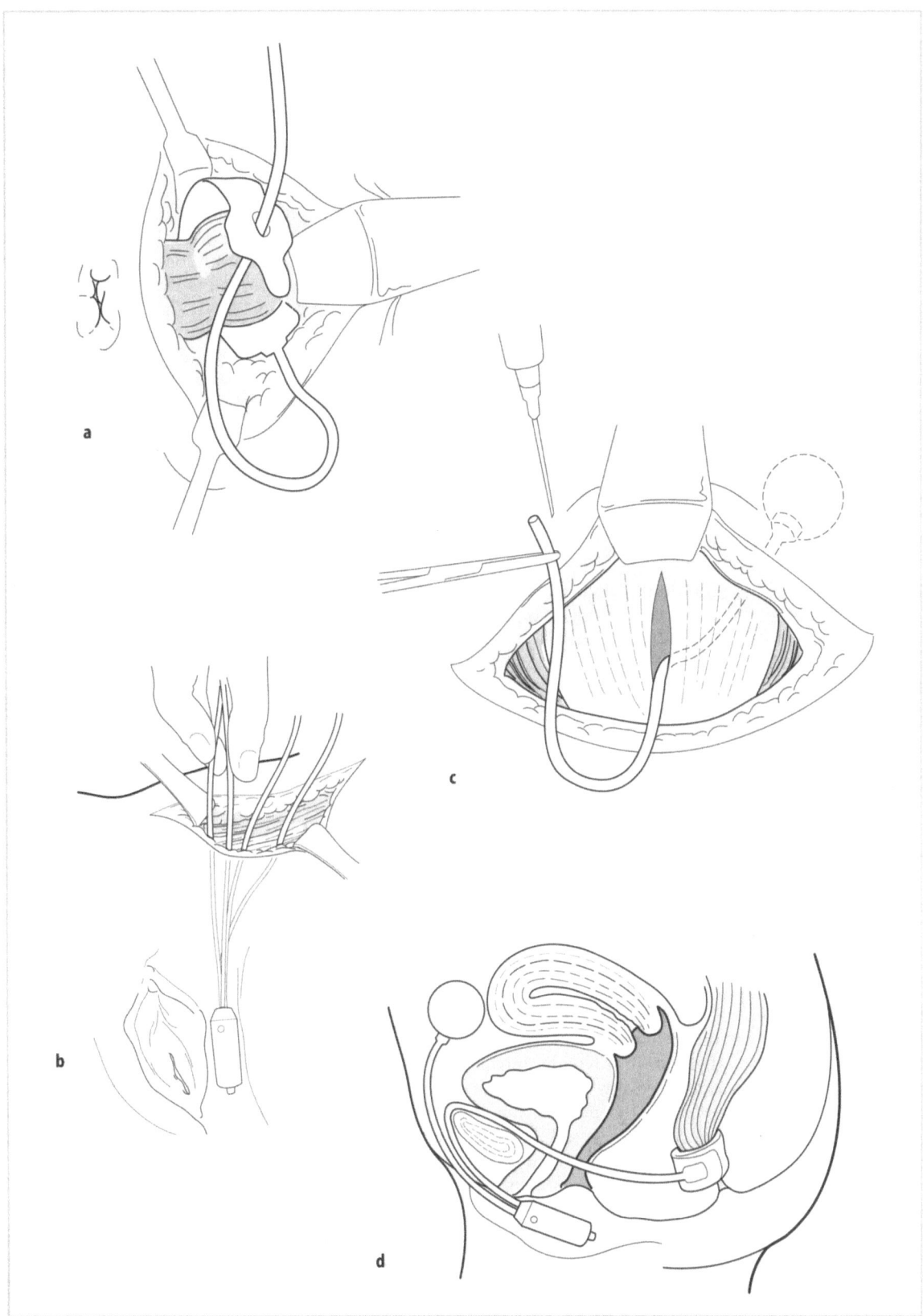

Figure 16.5 Technique of artificial bowel sphincter. **a** Cuff passed around anal canal. Dissection shown here was done with bilateral vertical incisions. Single transverse anterior incision preferred. **b** Pump placed through the suprapubic incision into previously dissected pocket in labia. **c** Balloon placed in retropubic space and refilled with 40 ml of solution. **d** All components connected and device deactivated at end of case.

The balloon containing 55 ml of filling solution is then brought on to the field. A temporary connector is placed between the tubing from the balloon and the tubing of the cuff and 1 minute is allowed for the cuff to pressurize. The tubings are then reclamped, separated, and the remaining amount of fluid in the balloon is measured to determine the fluid remaining in the cuff. A recommended minimum of 5 ml should remain in the cuff. The balloon is refilled with 40 ml of filling solution and placed in the retropubic space (Fig. 16.5c). The pump device is prepared and placed into the labia or scrotum with the deactivation button facing medially (Fig. 16.5b). A 3-0 suture is placed between the two limbs of tubing down in the pocket to prevent migration of the pump. All tubing is then cut to appropriate length and connected to its color-coded match so that both the balloon and the cuff tubing are connected to the pump tubing.

Throughout the procedure, irrigation of wounds with antibiotic solution is recommended. The suprapubic incision is closed in its appropriate layers with the tubing remaining above the fascia. The perineal incision is also closed in multiple layers with absorbable sutures in an attempt to create more than one layer between the skin and the device and to prevent migration of the device distally. The skin edges are closed with a Vicryl subcuticular stitch. Although the anus can be gently digitalized, a complete digital rectal examination is not recommended with the cuff inflated at this time.

The cuff is then emptied utilizing the pump and the system is deactivated. With the cuff now deflated, a digital rectal examination may be performed to feel for the integrity of the rectal wall. Proctoscopy is recommended to remove the rectal packing and to visualize the lumen for any obvious defects. A dressing is applied to the abdominal incision and the perineal incision should be heavily coated with antibiotic ointment per protocol and a dressing applied.

Postoperatively, the patient is kept nil-by-mouth for 2–4 days to help delay their first bowel movement. The Foley catheter is left in place for the majority of the hospitalization in a female. Intravenous antibiotics are continued for 48 hours and antibiotic ointment is kept on the perineal incisions. As soon as the patient has a bowel movement they are encouraged to immediately wash off the perineum, pat it dry, and apply antibiotic ointment to the incision site. This should be done after every bowel movement and at least three times a day. After 4–5 days the patient is discharged home on a regular diet with meticulous perineal wound care. The patient is to abstain from sex and nothing should be placed per rectum. Patients are instructed not to soak in a bathtub, to prevent maceration of the per-

ineal incision. Close patient follow-up is necessary, looking for any signs of infection. The device is activated after 6 weeks, if all the incisions are well healed.

The FDA protocol for the artificial bowel sphincter closed at the end of 1999 with 105 patients enrolled. Analysis of that data is currently pending. The largest published series is 24 patients by Lehur et al. from France, Spain, and Belgium.[19] Seven of the patients had to have their device explanted for reasons such as infection, but four were successfully reimplanted. The authors note that with experience the explant rate decreased. At the end of the study approximately 75% of the patients were highly satisfied with the artificial device. This success rate is comparable to previous studies[20,21] on the artificial bowel sphincter with all authors agreeing that with experience the complications are decreasing and the success rate increasing. In time, the artificial bowel sphincter will likely be preferred over other neo-sphincter procedures in most cases.

Other Procedures

Thiersch Procedure

Thiersch originally described this procedure in 1895 for the treatment of rectal procidentia or prolapse. The simple palliative procedure consisted of encircling the anal orifice with a silver wire. Since that time, the procedure has had many modifications and has been proposed for the treatment not only of rectal prolapse, but of incontinence as well. Although it does provide a static barrier to the passage of stools and in fact can lead to impaction, it offers no voluntary control and is a poor barrier for liquid feces or flatus. Its only utility is in poor risk patients as it may be performed with a local anesthetic.

The procedure consists of two curvilinear incisions made beyond the outer edge of the external sphincter, either bilaterally or left posteriorly and right anteriorly (Fig. 16.6a). The ischiorectal space is reached on both sides by blunt dissection and a tunnel is developed circumferentially. Materials that have been used for the encirclement have included fascia tendon, Teflon tubes, nylon and polyester tapes, and Dacron-impregnated silastic sheets. Once the material is passed circumferentially, the sling is tightened to fit snugly around the anal canal (Fig. 16.6b) and the ends are overlapped and secured by some means, such as suturing or stapling with a TA 30 device (Fig. 16.6c). The wounds are closed in layers with absorbable suture.

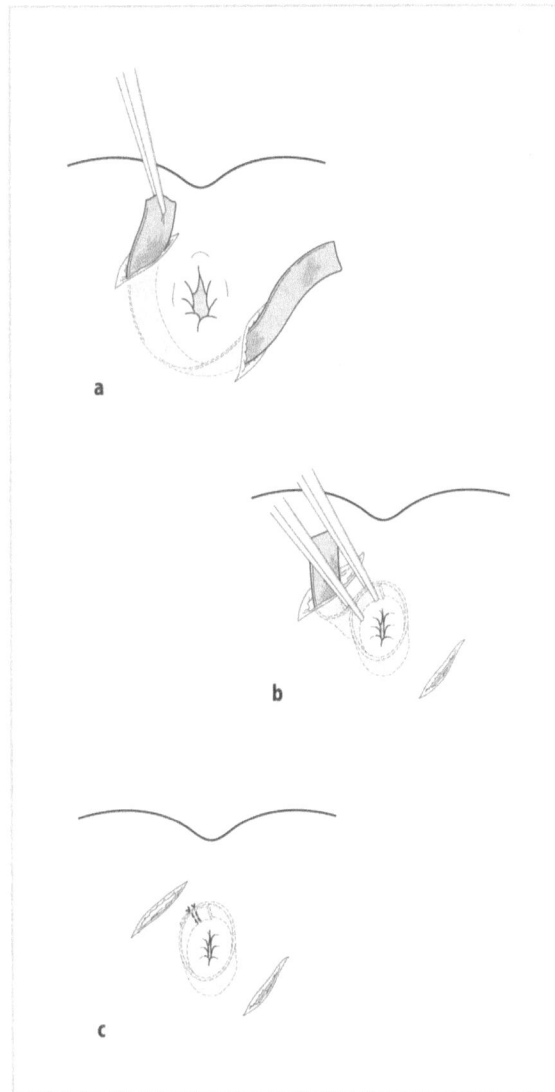

Figure 16.6 Thiersch procedure. **a** Through two 1cm incisions a tunnel deep to the superficial exterior sphincter is created to pass this Dacron-reinforced silastic band. **b** Overlap of the silastic band is tested so that anus is snug to an examining finger. **c** Suture fixation of the overlapping band permits the "collar" to be deep to the skin and away from the skin incisions.

Antegrade Irrigation

The antegrade continence enema technique, also known as ACE, was first described by Malone et al. in 1990[22] and involved creating a continent stoma utilizing the appendix. Through a created small appendicostomy enemas are administered to empty the colon and rectum, thus preventing fecal incontinence. A modification of the technique allows for creation of a neo-appendix from a tubularized cecal flap as an alternative in patients who have previously undergone an appendectomy. The ACE procedure has been utilized in patients with neurological lesions, as well as those with complex anal sphincter lesions not amenable to direct repair. The washout procedure with enemas is inconvenient for most people and can cause abdominal pain. The authors do not recommend the technique routinely but feel there are possible selected circumstances where it might be appropriate.

Stoma Creation

The creation of a stoma remains a viable option for the treatment of fecal incontinence. It is usually reserved for those patients who have failed all other forms of treatment. However, some patients may simply prefer it to the aforementioned procedures. An end-colostomy is the most common form of diversion, although a loop ileostomy is acceptable. For some patients a colostomy is their best option and significantly improves their quality of life. In no way should this be regarded as a treatment failure.

Rectal Prolapse

There are many procedures for the treatment of rectal prolapse. In evaluating the patient, a barium enema is useful. Combined with flexible sigmoidoscopy, it allows assessment for other disease processes, such as neoplasm, inflammatory bowel disease, or diverticula, and assessment of the redundancy of the sigmoid. A transit study may be useful in constipated patients to determine if colectomy would be beneficial. The patient's age and health status must be taken into account in selecting the appropriate surgery.

The procedures for rectal prolapse are broadly divided into abdominal procedures and perineal procedures. Whether the abdominal or perineal approach is selected depends largely on surgeon's preference. Controversy abounds regarding which approach is more effective. The authors defer to the individual surgeon's preference.

Patients with incontinence associated with their prolapse should be counseled that the primary goal of the procedure is to correct the rectal prolapse and incontinence may not improve. If their incontinence persists after correction of their prolapse, a subsequent procedure can be performed for that problem.

Abdominal Procedures for Rectal Prolapse

Sigmoidectomy with Rectopexy

This popular technique is performed under general anesthesia in a modified lithotomy position. The abdomen may be opened via a midline or transverse incision, or a laparoscopically assisted approach is an option. Once the abdomen has been entered, the descending colon and sigmoid are mobilized followed by mobilization of the rectum down to the levator muscles. The upper portions of the lateral stalks are divided.

The redundant sigmoid is then resected, leaving the rectum intact for its reservoir capacity. A colorectal anastomosis is performed using any standard technique of the surgeon's preference. The rectopexy can then be performed in a number of ways. Our preference is to pull the freed rectum up into the abdomen and then suture the lateral stalks to the presacral fascia with a nonabsorbable suture. The cul-de-sac can be obliterated anteriorly by suturing the peritoneum down to the rectum.

Postoperatively, all the abdominal cases are managed the same. A nasogastric tube is not needed. A diet may be started early and progressed as tolerated with resolution of the ileus.

Sigmoidectomy with rectopexy has low recurrence rates of 0% to 9% with low morbidity (Table 16.3). Huber et al.[23] showed a decline in incontinence from 67% to 23%. Studies[23,24] demonstrated an improvement in constipation making this an appealing approach in constipated patients with prolapse.

Rectopexy

Rectopexy alone without resection or use of mesh has also been utilized. The rectum is mobilized as previously described and either nonabsorbable sutures or strips of fascia lata are used to secure the rectum to the presacral fascia. More recently, with the advancement of laparoscopic surgery, it is possible to perform this entire procedure laparoscopically. Recurrence rates and morbidity are low (Table 16.3) and improvement in continence from 36% preoperatively to 74% postoperatively has been noted.[25]

Ripstein Procedure

The Ripstein procedure was developed by Ripstein and Lanter based on their theory that a rectal prolapse is an intussusception that occurs when the rectum loses its attachment and becomes a straight tube. They felt, therefore, that if they could prevent the straightening of the rectum by keeping it fixed to the sacral curve, rectal prolapse would not occur. The first successful material they utilized was fascia lata but they later used Teflon mesh and subsequently Marlex and Gore-Tex mesh.

Table 16.3. Results of procedures for rectal prolapse

Author	No. of patients	Recurrence rate (%)	Mortality rate(%)	Morbidity rate (%)
Sigmoid resection and rectopexy				
Goldberg et al. (1980)[61]	130	0	1	11.7
Watts et al. (1985)[62]	102	1.9	0	4
Husa et al. (1988)[24]	48	9	2.1	0
Rectopexy alone				
Loygue et al. (1971)[63]	140	3.6	1.4	1.4
Blatchford et al. (1989)[25]	42	2	0	20
Ripstein procedure/anterior sling				
Ripstein (1972)[64]	289	0	0.3	–
Gordon and Hoexter (1978)[27 a]	1111	2.3	–	16.6
Holmstrom et al. (1986)[65]	97	4.1	2.8	3.7
Roberts et al. (1988)[28]	135	9.6	0.7	52
Ivalon sponge operation/posterior sling				
Morgan et al. (1972)[66]	150	3.2	2.6	3
Stewart (1972)[67]	41	7.3	0	29
Atkinson and Taylor (1984)[68]	40	10	0	3
Yoshioka et al. (1989)[33]	165	1.5	0	19
Perineal proctosigmoidectomy				
Altemeier et al. (1971)[69]	106	3	0	24
Williams et al. (1992)[35]	114	11	0	12
Johansen et al. (1993)[36]	20	0	5	5

[a] Collected series.

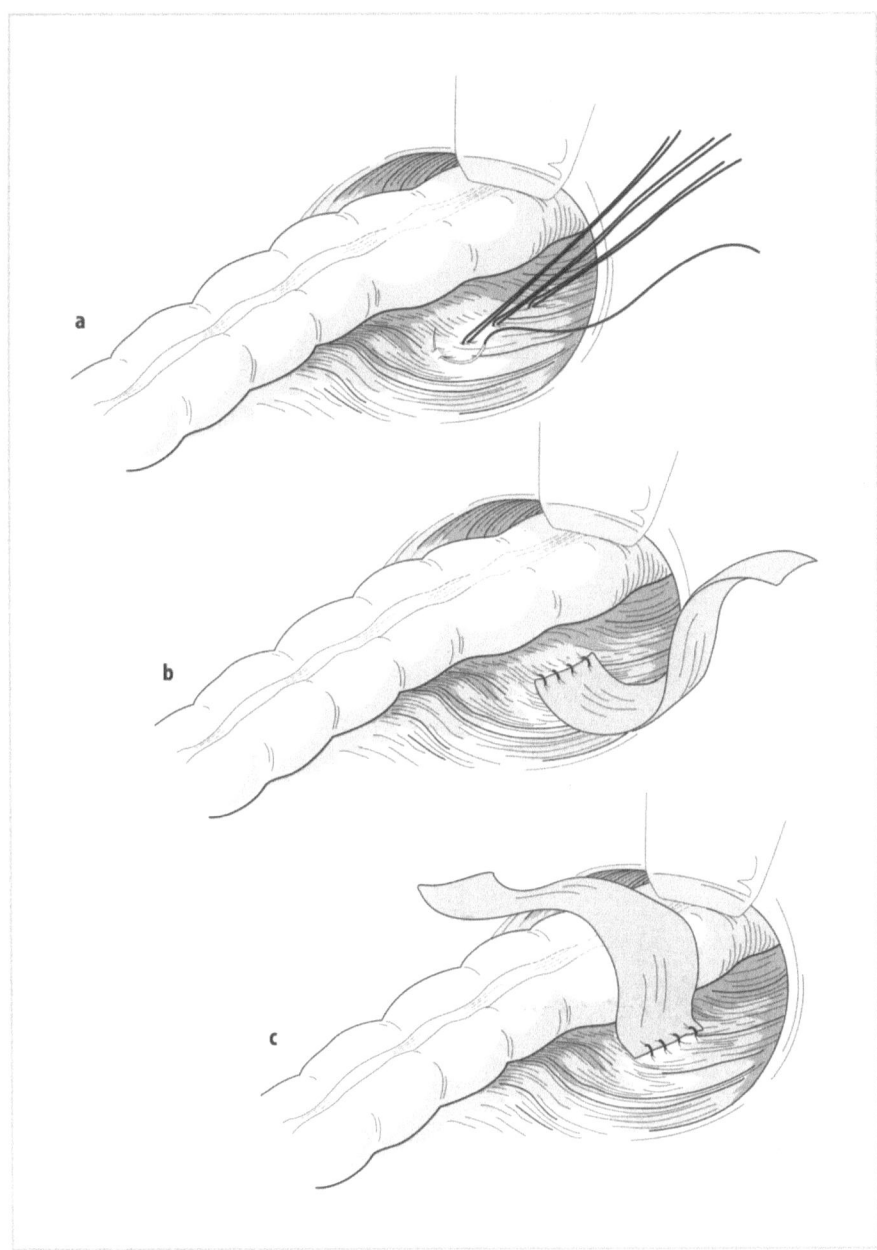

Figure 16.7 Ripstein repair. **a** Sutures placed into periosteum on right side. **b** Mesh sutured to periosteum. **c** mesh wrapped anterior around rectum. *(Continues overleaf)*

The abdomen is entered and dissection is initiated on either side of the rectosigmoid. The rectum is fully mobilized posteriorly down to the tip of the coccyx, and the upper portion of the lateral stalks are divided. A 5 cm band of rectangular mesh is then placed around the rectum at the level of the peritoneal reflection. The free ends are oriented posteriorly and are sutured to the presacral fascia approximately 5 cm below the promontory (Fig. 16.7a,b). Nonabsorbable sutures are utilized and are best placed 1 cm from the midline to help avoid presacral vessels.

The rectum is then pulled upward and the upper and lower borders of the mesh are sutured to the rectum with nonabsorbable sutures taking care to not go full thickness on the bowel (Fig. 16.7d). If the mesh is too tight, it may cause problems ranging from constipation to obstruction. The appropriate amount of tightness should still allow one to two fingers to pass between the bowel and sacral fascia. The mesh is then covered by suturing the peritoneal defect with a running absorbable suture.

The recurrence rate with the Ripstein procedure is only 0–9.6% (Table 16.3) and Tjandra et al.[26] noted a 50% improvement in fecal incontinence. Unfortunately, with the Ripstein procedure there was a high complication rate associated with the mesh.[27–30] These complications included fecal impaction, pre-

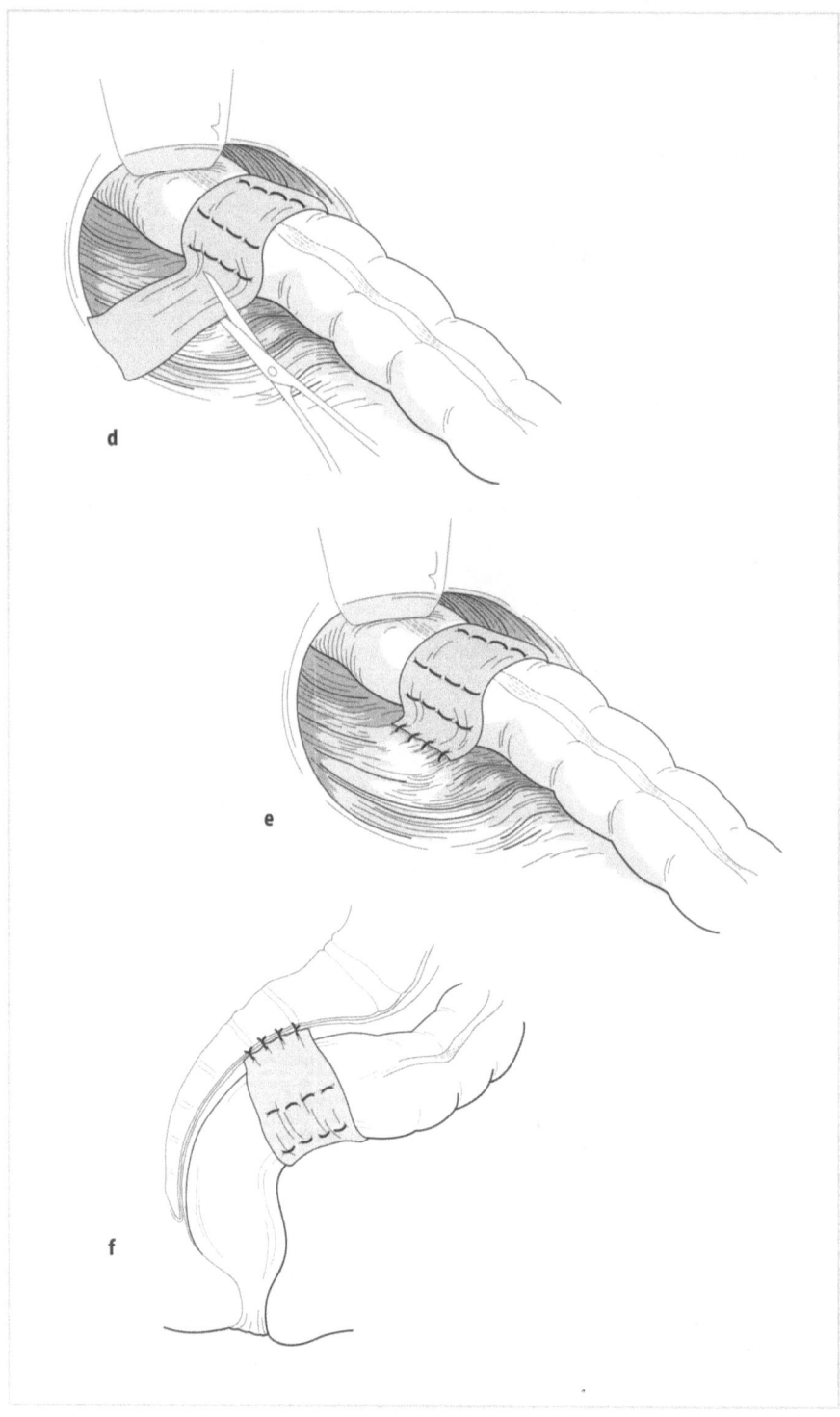

Figure 16.7 d Rectum pulled up and mesh sutured to rectal wall; excess mesh trimmed. **e** Mesh sutured to periosteum on left side. **f** Lateral view.

sacral hemorrhage, stricture, pelvic abscess, small-bowel obstruction, impotence, and fistulas. In one study these complications led to a 4.1% re-operation rate.[27] Modifications of the Ripstein are numerous. The best-known is the Ivalon sponge wrap.

Ivalon Sponge Wrap

Wells[31] postulated that the complications from the Ripstein procedure could be reduced by placing the sling posterior to the rectum allowing the anterior third of the circumference of the rectum to be free to expand. He utilized a polyvinyl alcohol (Ivalon) sponge and wrapped it posteriorly. This procedure has become increasingly popular, especially in the UK. Ripstein himself has adopted this principal, but utilizes Gore-Tex instead.

Once the rectum has been mobilized as in the Ripstein procedure, a rectangular sheet of Ivalon, which has previously been immersed in normal saline to allow it to be pliable, is sutured to the presacral space with nonabsorbable sutures (Fig. 16.8a). The sponge should be placed as distal as possible within the pelvis. The mobilized rectum is then pulled upward removing all redundancy and the lateral edges of the sponge are folded around the rectum leaving the anterior one fourth of the rectum uncovered. The sponge is fastened to the rectum with 3-0 Vicryl sutures at its anterior aspect (Fig. 16.8b). The pelvic peritoneum is closed with a running suture, keeping the sponge in the extraperitoneal space. Various materials have been utilized in place of the Ivalon, including Vicryl or Dexon mesh, which may decrease the incidence of sepsis.[32]

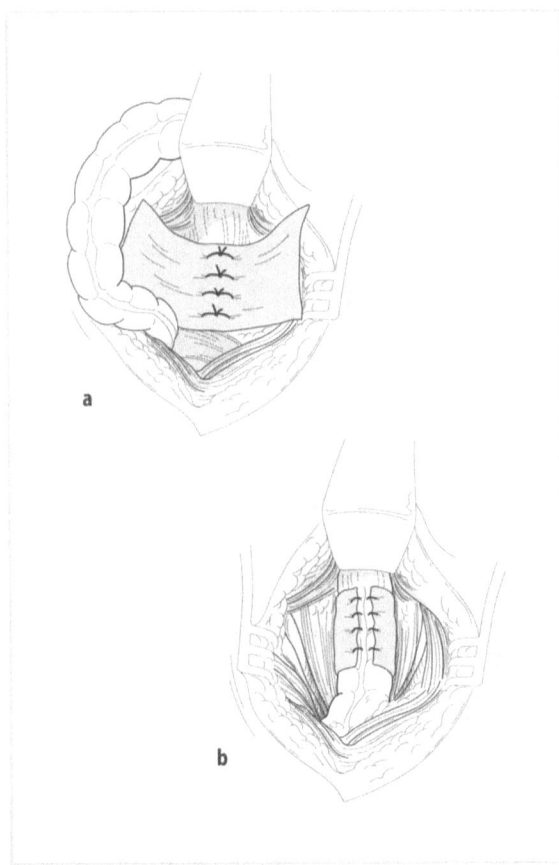

Figure 16.8 Ivalon sponge repair. **a** Ivalon sponge sutured to presacral fascia. **b** Lateral limbs of sponge sutured to anterior aspect of rectum.

The recurrence rates, as with the rest of the abdominal procedures, is low at 1.5–10%. Complications of this posterior sling procedure are actually similar to those of the Ripstein procedure, except that fecal impaction and stricture are not a problem, since the entire circumference of the rectum is not enclosed. Improvement in continence is similar with Yoshioka et al.[33] reporting a decrease in incontinence from 58% to 16%.

Perineal Procedures

Perineal Proctosigmoidectomy

Although frequently referred to as an Altemeier procedure, the perineal proctosigmoidectomy was first described by Mikulicz in 1889. The procedure's obvious appeal is the avoidance of an abdominal operation and also the decrease risk of impotence. The most obvious disadvantage is the loss of the rectal reservoir. Recent studies show low recurrence rates which are comparable to those for abdominal procedures (Table 16.3).

Perineal proctosigmoidectomy may be performed under general or regional anesthesia. The patient may be placed in a variety of positions, including modified lithotomy, prone jackknife, or even a lateral decubitus position. As in the prior perineal surgeries, the operative site is infiltrated with a local anesthetic with epinephrine. The rectum is prolapsed and scored circumferentially with cautery approximately 2 cm proximal to the dentate line (Fig. 16.9a). The incision is carried down through all layers of the rectum, working circumferentially until the proximal segment of the rectum is completely free from this distal edge. During this process, one may place 2-0 Vicryl sutures through the distal segment as stay sutures for easier identification at the time of anastomosis.

Circumferential dissection is continued through the perirectal fat and the anterior wall of the peritoneum is exposed. This is opened and dissection continued proximally. The mesentery is serially clamped (Fig. 16.9b), divided, and ligated as the redundant bowel is pulled through the anus. This is continued until there is no further redundancy in the colon. Great care should be taken with hemostasis as tissues will retract up into the abdomen and then not be easily accessible. The peritoneum may then be closed with Vicryl sutures to aid in preventing herniation into the pelvis. The levator muscles are approximated either posterior or anterior in an attempt to improve continence (Fig. 16.9c).

If the anastomosis is to be hand-sewn, the proximal bowel is sewn in sequence to the distal segment as the pull-through segment is resected

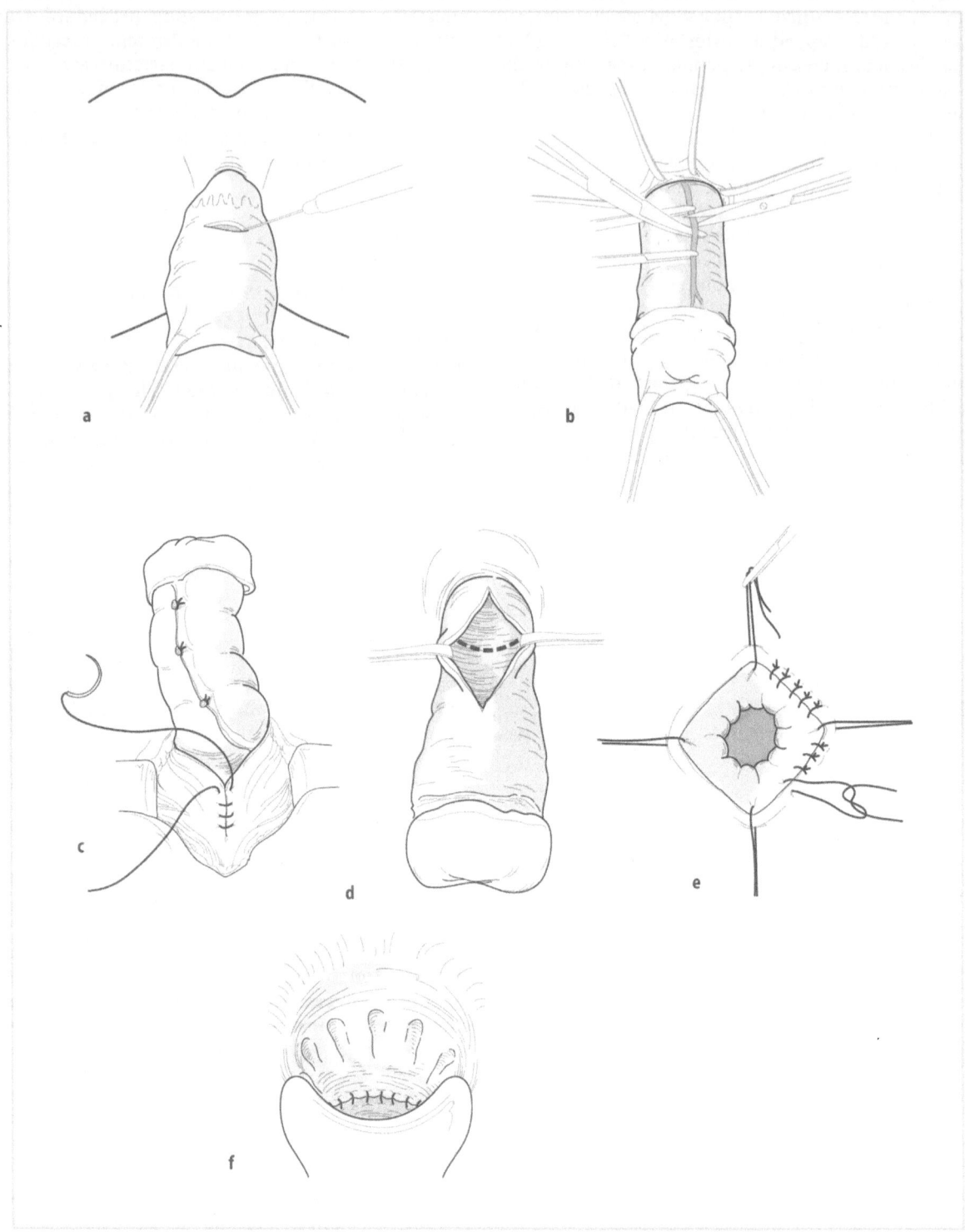

Figure 16.9 Perineal proctosigmoidectomy: **a** The prolapsed segment is incised 2 cm proximal to dentate line. **b** Mesentery of this prolapse is divided between clamps to permit full pulldown of the proplase. **c** Repair of the levators around the pull-through segment can be done anteriorly and/or posteriorly. **d** The prolapsed bowel is transected at the appropriate level. **e** Suture of the prolapsed remnant to the proximal bowel reestablishes bowel continuity. **f** Typically, the finished product retracts into the anal canal.

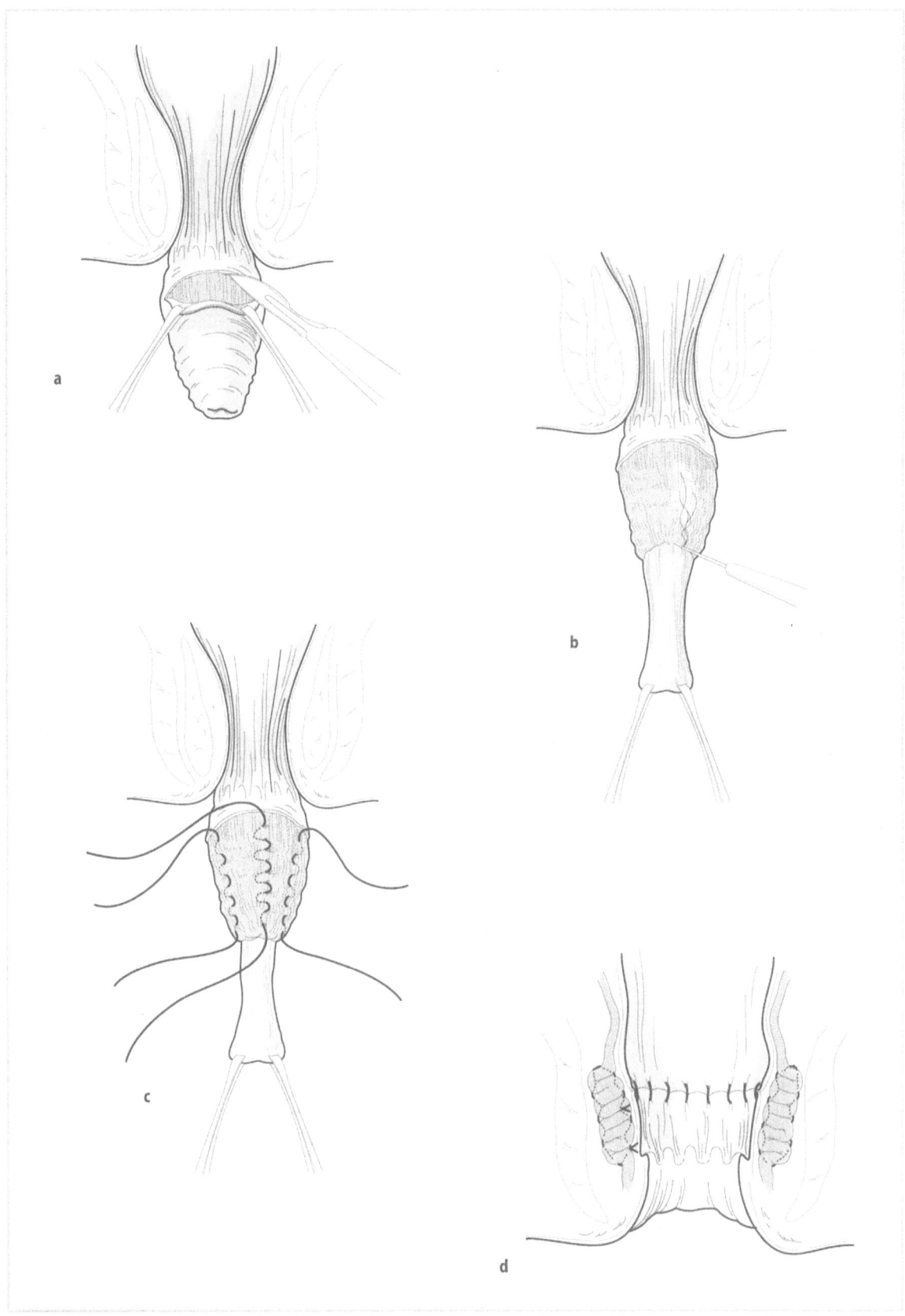

Figure 16.10 Delorme procedure. **a** Incision made circumferential 1 cm proximal to dentate line. **b** Dissection of mucosa from underlying tissue. **c** Plication of muscle. **d** Mucosa re-approximated after excision of excess mucosa.

(Fig. 16.9d,e). If a stapler is used for the anastomosis, the proximal bowel is transected at the desired level and a purse-string is placed. The anvil to the circular end anastomatic stapler is placed into the proximal segment of bowel and the purse-string tied down onto the anvil. A separate purse-string is then placed around the distal segment cuff. The circular stapler is inserted through this distal segment and attached to the anvil. The distal purse-string is tied down to the center shaft. The instrument is then slowly closed and as the anastomosis begins to come together, it is advanced further into the anus before closing the stapler and firing it.

Postoperatively the patient receives intravenous antibiotics for 24 hours and a diet is started as tolerated. Once the patient has adequate oral intake they can be discharged home.

Although some studies had recurrence rates as high as 50%,[34] more recent studies show recurrence rates comparable to abdominal procedures at 0 to 11%[35-38]. Morbidity ranges from 5% to 24% but this includes pneumonia and other things not specific to the procedure. Improvement in incontinence was noted to be 54% by Williams et al.[35] and 90% by Johansen et al.[36].

Delorme Procedure

In 1900 Delorme[39] described a procedure involving stripping the mucosa from the redundant prolapsed rectum and then plicating the denuded muscle wall. This procedure has shown a recent resurgence in popularity.

Patient positioning and anesthesia is the same as for the Altemeier procedure except that the Delorme may be performed under local anesthesia. A dilute epinephrine solution is injected submucosally to aid in hemostasis. A mucosectomy is initiated approximately 1 cm proximal to the dentate line (Fig. 16.10a). This dissection may be carried out with the prolapse either everted or reduced. Metzenbaum scissors or Bovie cautery is used to continue the dissection proximally until there is resistance to further dissection and some tension exists (Fig. 16.10b). The redundant mucosa is excised.

The exposed muscularis is then plicated in a longitudinal manner utilizing 2-0 Vicryl sutures (Fig. 16.10c). The stitches are begun at the most distal area of denuded muscularis and plicating stitches placed continuing proximally on the exposed muscularis. A stitch is placed in all four quadrants with one to two stitches placed in between for a total of 8–12 stitches. After adequate hemostasis is achieved, the sutures are tied down to complete the plication. The proximal mucosa is then anastomosed to the distal mucosa with absorbable sutures (Fig. 16.10d).

The recurrence rate associated with the Delorme procedure has ranged from 5% to 25%.[40-47] Functional results in those studies do not compare to the previous procedures. However, since it can be performed under local anesthesia and is essentially a safe operation, it may be reserved by some for poor-risk patients.

Thiersch Procedure

This procedure has already been described earlier in the chapter and can be utilized both for fecal incontinence and rectal prolapse.

References

1. Nessim A, Wexner SD, Agachan F et al. (1997) Is bowel confinement necessary after anorectal reconstructive surgery? A prospective randomized trial. Dis Colon Rectum 40: A17.
2. Laurberg S, Swash M, Henry MM (1988) Delayed external sphincter repair for obstetric care. Br J Surg 75: 786–8.
3. Wexner SD, Marchetti F, Jagelman D (1991) The role of sphincteroplasty for fecal incontinence reevaluated: a prospective physiologic and functional review. Dis Colon Rectum 34: 22–30.
4. Jacobs PP, Scheuer M, Kuijpers JHC (1990) Obstetric fecal incontinence: role of pelvic floor denervation and results of delayed sphincter repair. Dis Colon Rectum 33: 494–7.
5. Sangwan YP, Coller JA, Barrett RC et al. (1996) Unilateral pudendal neuropathy: impact on outcome of anal sphincter repair. Dis Colon Rectum 39: 686–9.
6. Nikiteas N, Korsgen S, Kumar D et al. (1996) Audit of sphincter repair. Dis Colon Rectum 39: 1164–70.
7. Gilliland R, Altomare DF, Moreira H Jr et al. (1997) Pudendal nerve latencies are predictive of outcome following anterior sphincteroplasty. Dis Colon Rectum 40: A13.
8. Browning GP, Park AG (1983) Post anal repair for neuropathic fecal incontinence: Correlation of clinical result and anal canal pressures. Br J Surg 70: 101–4.
9. Laurberg S, Swash M, Henry MM (1990) Effect of postanal repair on progress of neurogenic damage to the pelvic floor. Br J Surg 77: 519–22.
10. Chen AS-H, Luchtefield MA, Senagore AJ, McKeigan JM, Hoyt C (1998) Pudendal nerve latency: Does it predict outcome of anal sphincter repair? Dis Colon Rectum 41: 1005–9.
11. Parks AG (1975) Anorectal incontinence. Proc R Soc Med 68: 681–90.
12. Pickrell KL, Broadbent TR, Masters FW, Metzger JT (1952) Construction of a rectal sphincter and restoration of anal continence by transplanting the gracilis muscle. Ann Surg 135: 853.
13. Baeten CGMI, Konsten J, Spanns F et al. (1991) Dynamic graciloplasty for fecal incontinence. Lancet 7: 1163–5.
14. Patel J, Shanahah D, Riches DJ et al. (1991) The arterial anatomy and surgical relevance of the human gracilis muscle. J Anat 176: 270–2.
15. Chittenden AS (1930) Reconstruction of the anal sphincter by muscle slips from the glutei. Ann Surg 92: 152–4.
16. Stone HB (1932) Plastic operation for anal incontinence. Arch Surg 24: 120.
17. Henter VR (1982) Construction of a rectal sphincter using the origin of the gluteus maximus muscle. Plast Reconstr Surg 70(1): 82–5.

18. Orgel MG, Kucan JO (1985) A double-split gluteus maximus muscle flap for reconstruction of the rectal sphincter. Plast Reconstr Surg 75(1): 62–6.
19. Lehur PA, Roig JV, Duinslaeger M (1999) Artificial anal sphincter: a prospective clinical and manometric evaluation. 100th Anniversary and Tripartite Meeting of the American Society of Colon and Rectal Surgeons, 1999, Washington, DC.
20. Wong WD, Jensen LL, Bartolo DCC, Rothenberger DA (1996) Artificial anal sphincter. Dis Colon Rectum 39: 1345–51.
21. O'Brien PE, Skinner SA (1999) Restoring control: the artificial bowel sphincter (ABS) in the treatment of anal incontinence (abstract). 100th Anniversary and Tripartite Meeting, 1999, Washington, DC.
22. Malone PS, Rarsley PG, Kiely EM (1990) Preliminary report: the antegrade continence enema. Lancet 336: 1217–18.
23. Huber FT, Stein H, Siewert JR (1995) Functional results after treatment of rectal prolapse with rectopexy and sigmoid resection. World J Surg 19: 138–43.
24. Husa A, Sainio P, Smitten K. (1998)Abdominal rectopexy and sigmoid resection (Frykman-Goldberg) operation for rectal prolapse. Acta Chir Scand 154: 221–4.
25. Blatchford GJ, Perry RE, Thorson AG, Christensen MA (1989) Rectopexy without resection for rectal prolapse. Am J Surg 158: 574–6.
26. Tjandra JJ, Fazio VW, Church JM et al. (1993) Ripstein procedure is an effective treatment for rectal prolapse without constipation. Dis Colon Rectum 36: 501–7.
27. Gordon PH, Hoexter B (1978) Complications of Ripstein procedure. Dis Colon Rectum 21: 277–80.
28. Roberts PL, Schoetz DJ, Coller JA, Veidenheimer MC (1988) Ripstein procedure:Lahey Clinic experience 1963–1985. Arch Surg 123: 554–7.
29. Leenen LPH, Kuijpers JHC (1989) Treatment of complete rectal prolapse with foreign material. Neth J Surg 41: 129–31.
30. Winde G, Reers B, Nottberg H et al. (1993) Clinical and functional results of abdominal rectopexy with absorbable mesh graft for treatment of complete rectal prolapse. Eur J Surg 159: 301–5.
31. Wells C (1959) New operation for rectal prolapse. Proc R Soc Med 52: 602–3.
32. Arndt M, Pircher W (1988) Absorbable mesh in the treatment of rectal prolapse. Int J Colorectal Dis 3: 141–3.
33. Yoshioka K, Heyen F, Keighley MRB (1989) Functional results after abdominal rectopexy for rectal prolapse. Dis Colon Rectum 32: 835–8.
34. Friedman R, Mugga-Sullam M, Freund HR (1983) Experience with the one stage perineal repair of rectal prolapse. Dis Colon Rectum 26: 789–91.
35. Williams JG, Rothenberger DA, Madoff RD, Goldberg SM (1992) Treatment of rectal prolapse in the elderly by perineal rectosigmoidectomy. Dis Colon Rectum 35: 830–4.
36. Johansen OB, Wexner SD, Daniel N, Nogueras JJ, Jagelman DG (1993) Perineal rectosigmoidectomy in the elderly. Dis Colon Rectum 36: 767–72.
37. Gopal FA, Amshel AL, Shonberg IL, Eftaiha M (1984) Rectal procidentia in elderly and debilitated patients. Experience with the Altemeier procedure. Dis Colon Rectum 27: 376–81.
38. Finlay IG, Aitchison M (1991) Perineal excision of the rectum for prolapse in the elderly. Br J Surg 78: 687–9.
39. Delorme E (1900) Sur le traitement des prolapsus du rectum totaux pour l'excision de la muqueuse rectale ou recto-colique. Bull Mem Soc Chir Paris 26: 499–578.
40. Abulafi AM, Sherman IW, Fiddian RV, Rothwell-Jackson RL (1990) Delorme's operation for rectal prolapse. Ann R Coll Surg Engl 72: 382–5.
41. Christiansen J, Kirkegaard P (1981) Delorme's operation for complete rectal prolapse. Br J Surg 68: 537–38.
42. Gunderson AL, Cogbell TH, Landercasper J (1985) Reappraisal of Delorme's procedure for rectal prolapse. Dis Colon Rectum 28: 721–4.
43. Monson JRT, Jones NAG, Vowden P, Brennan TG (1986) Delorme's operation. The first choice in complete rectal prolapse. Ann R Coll Surg Engl 68: 143–6.
44. Henry S, Lechaux JP, Hugier M, Molkhou JM (1987) Treatment of rectal prolapse by Delorme's operation. Int J Colorectal Dis 2: 1249–2.
45. Graf W, Ejerblad S, Krog M, Pahlman L, Gerdin B (1992) Delorme's operation for rectal prolapse in elderly or unfit patients. Eur J Surg 158: 555–7.
46. Tobin SA, Scott IHK (1994) Delorme operation for rectal prolapse. Br J Surg 81: 1681–4.
47. Pulsa SM, Charig JA, Balaji V, Watts A, Thompson MR (1995) Physiological changes after Delorme's procedure for full-thickness rectal prolapse. Br J Surg 82: 1475–8.
48. Fang DT, Nivatvongs S, Vermeulen FD et al. (1984) Overlapping sphincteroplasty for acquired anal incontinence. Dis Colon Rectum 27: 720–2.
49. Yoshioka K, Keighley MRB (1989) Sphincter repair for fecal incontinence. Dis Colon Rectum 32: 39–42.
50. Fleshman JW, Peters WR, Shemesh EI, Fry RD, Kodner IJ (1991) Anal sphincter reconstruction: Anterior overlapping muscle repair. Dis Colon Rectum 34: 739–43.
51. Engel AF, Kamm MA, Sulton AH, Bartram CI, Nicholls RJ (1994) Anterior anal sphincter repair in patients with obstetric trauma. Br J Surg 81: 1231–4.
52. Simmang CL, Birnbaum EH, Kodner IJ et al. (1994) Anal sphincter reconstruction in the elderly: does advancing age affect outcome? Dis Colon Rectum 37: 1065–9.
53. Londono-Schimmer EE, Garcia-Duperly R, Nichols RJ et al. (1994) Overlapping anal sphincter repair for fecal incontinence due to sphincter trauma: Five-year follow up functional results. Int J Colorectal Dis 9: 110–3.
54. Oliveira L, Pfeifer J, Wexner SD (1996) Physiological and clinical outcome of anterior sphincteroplasty. Br J Surg 83: 502–505.
55. Browning GGP, Rutter KRP, Motson RW et al. (1984) Post-anal repair for idiopathic fecal incontinence. Ann R Coll Surg Engl 66 (Suppl): 30–3.
56. Henry MM, Simson JN (1985) Results of postanal repair: A retrospective study. Br J Surg 72 (Suppl): S17–S19.
57. Keighley MRB (1987) Postanal repair. How I do it. Int J Colorect Dis 2: 236–9.
58. Miller R, Bartolo DCC, Locke-Edmunds JC et al. (1988) Prospective study of conservative and operative treatment for fecal incontinence. Br J Surg 75: 101–5.
59. Womack NR, Morrison JF, Williams NS (1988) Prospective study of the effects of postanal repair in neurogenic fecal incontinence. Br J Surg 75: 48–52.
60. Scheuer M, Kuijpers HC, Jacobs pp. (1989) Postanal repair restores anatomy rather than function. Dis Colon Rectum 32: 960–3.
61. Goldberg SM, Gordon PH, Nivatvongs S (1980) Essentials of Anorectal Surgery. JB Lippincott, Philadelphia, p. 248.
62. Watts JD, Rothenberger DA, Buls JG, Gold SM, Nivatvongs S (1985) The management of procidentia: 30 years experience. Dis Colon Rectum 28: 96–102.
63. Loygue J, Hugier M, Malafosse M, Biotois H (1971) Complete prolapse of the rectum: A report on 140 cases treated by rectopexy. Br J Surg 58: 847–8.
64. Ripstein CB (1972) Definitive corrective surgery. Dis Colon Rectum 15: 334–46.
65. Holmstrom B, Broden G, Dolk A (1986) Results of the Ripstein operation in the treatment of rectal prolapse and internal procidentia. Dis Colon Rectum 29: 845–8.
66. Morgan CN, Porter NH (1972) Klugman DJ. Ivalon (polyvinyl alcohol) sponge in the repair of complete rectal prolapse. Br J Surg 59: 841–6.

67. Stewart R (1972) Long-term results of Ivalon wrap operation for complete rectal prolapse. Proc R Soc Med 65: 777–8.
68. Atkinson KG, Taylor DC (1984) Wells procedure for complete rectal prolapse. A 10 year experience. Dis Colon Rectum 27: 96–8.
69. Altemeier WA, Culbertson WR, Schowengerdt CJ, Hunt J (1971) Nineteen years' experience with the one stage perineal repair of rectal prolapse. Ann Surg 173: 993–1006.

17 Perineal Hernia

Saad Juma

Definition and Classification

Numerous synonyms for perineal hernia appear in the literature, including pelvic hernia, ischiorectal hernia, pudendal hernia, and hernia of the cul-de-sac. Perineal hernia is a hernia that occurs through a defect in the pelvic floor. It is different in location from other types of pelvic floor hernias (obturator and sciatic). Anatomically, there are two main types of perineal hernias. Anterior perineal hernia emerges through a defect anterior to the transverse perinei muscle (Fig. 17.1). Posterior perineal hernia occurs through a defect posterior to the transverse perinei muscle and is usually located midway between the rectum and the ischial tuberosity (Fig. 17.1).

Cali et al distinguished between primary perineal hernia and secondary perineal hernia. Primary perineal hernia occurs predominantly in women as a result of the spontaneous development of defect in the muscles of the pelvic floor. An unusually deep cul-de-sac and weakening of the pelvic floor by childbirth, chronic cough, ascites or other causes of increased intraabdominal pressure predispose to this condition. Women develop the condition five times more commonly than men do. Secondary perineal hernia is usually seen following pelvic surgery

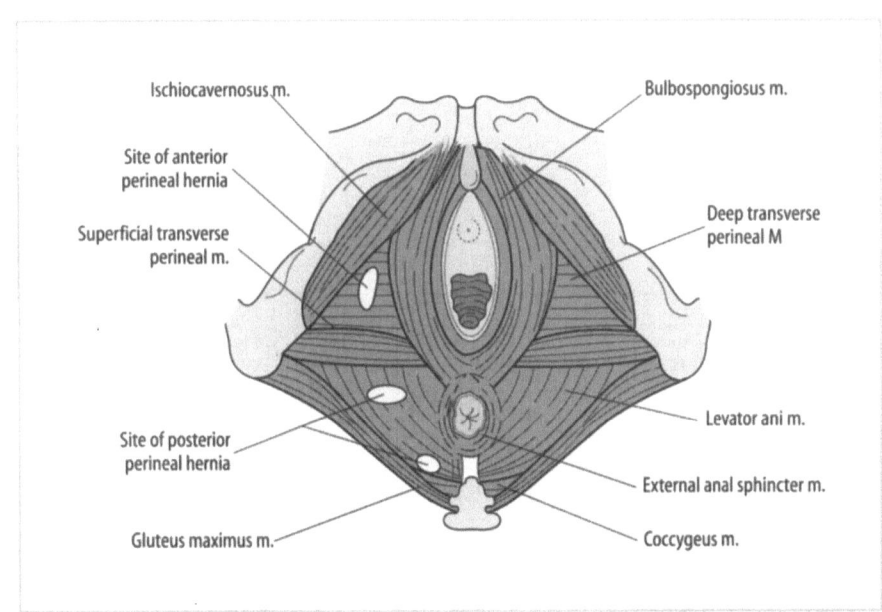

Figure 17.1 Anatomy of anterior and posterior perineal hernia.

including pelvic exenteration, abdominoperineal resection, hysterectomy, and vaginal sling. Perineal hernias are common in canines. Atrophy of the muscles of the pelvic diaphragm, particularly the levator ani muscles has been suggested to be caused by hormonal influences (excess estrogen or androgenic steroids) or by primary neurogenic atrophy in canines. Whether these factors contribute to such hernias in humans is not clear.

Anterior Perineal Hernia

In the literature, anterior perineal hernia has been described under synonyms such as labial hernia, levator hernia, pudendal hernia, or pudendal enterocele. They are exclusively seen in women. Recognized risk factors include aging, multiple prior pelvic surgeries, and general factors such as diabetes and obesity. The hernia represents a descent of the peritoneum or viscera (bladder and small or large intestine) into the labium through a defect in the urogenital diaphragm. The hernia sac emerges through the triangle formed by the transverse perinei muscle posteriorly, the ischiocavernosus muscle laterally and the bulbocavernosus muscle medially.

Clinical Evaluation

Anterior perineal hernia often presents as a mass in the labia (Fig. 17.2). It is usually reducible. In rare instances it may cause difficulty in urination because of the presence of a portion of the bladder within the hernia sac. The hernia has three features:

● it is always in the posterior aspect of the labia

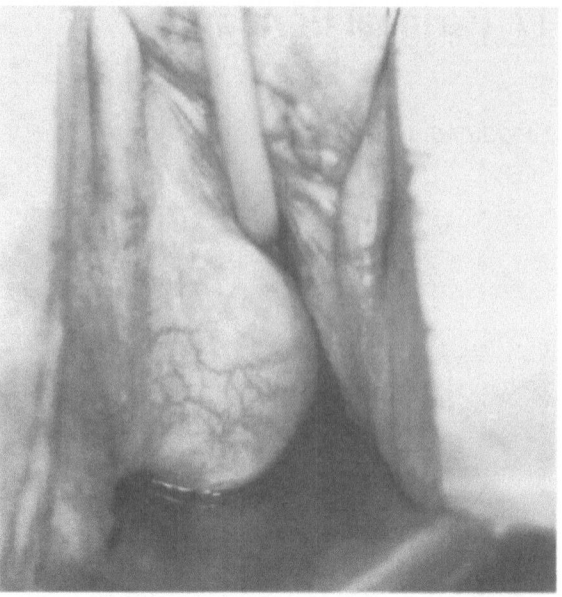

Figure 17.2 Anterior perineal hernia (right labial mass with labia retracted). Reprinted with permission from Brodak P, Juma S, Raz S (1992) Levator hernia. In: J Urol 148(3): 872–73.

● the medial half of the hernia is covered with mucous membrane and the lateral half with integument

● the ordinary signs of hernia are present.

Perineal hernia is a rare cause of labial or vulvar enlargement. Other more common causes of vulvar enlargement should be considered first such as Bartholin's gland cyst, lipoma, or inguinal hernia. Inguinal hernias are reducible but will pass over the pelvic brim, whereas anterior perineal hernia will reduce directly into the pelvis below the pelvic brim. A cystourethrogram may demonstrate an air-filled

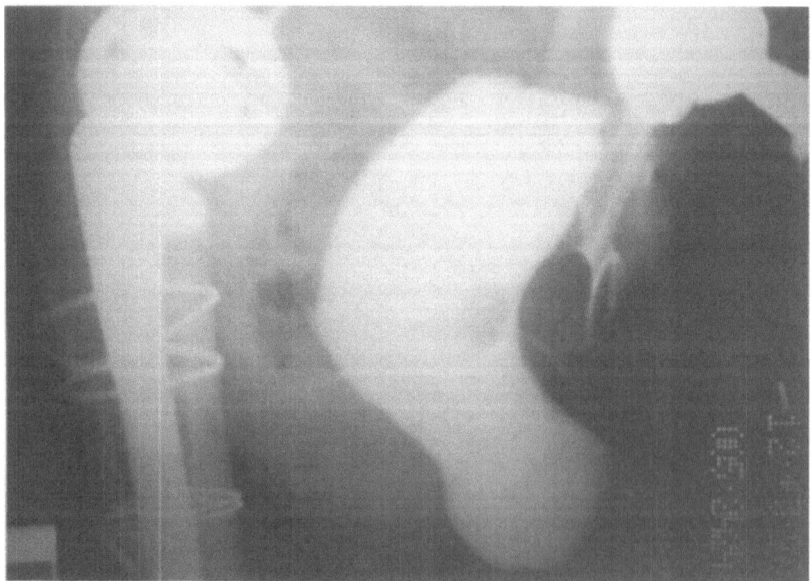

Figure 17.3 Lateral view of a standing cystogram demonstrating a large cystocele descending into the left labia. Reprinted with permission from Zimmern PE, Miyazaki F (1994) Pudendal enterocele with bladder involvement. In: Urology 44(6): 919, with permission from Elsevier Science.

loop of bowel or contrast-filled portion of the bladder below the pelvic brim (Fig. 17.3).

Surgical Management

Though conservative management of anterior perineal hernia may be applied, repair of the hernia is advisable in the absence of any contraindication for surgery. Three approaches for repair of anterior perineal hernia can be considered: translabial, transabdominal, and a combined abdominoperineal approach. The general principles of hernia repair should be used. The hernia sac is dissected from the surrounding tissue until the neck of the sac is identified. The hernia sac is opened and the contents are reduced. A purse-string suture is used to close the neck of the hernia sac. The redundant sac is excised and the defect in the pelvic floor is repaired using nonabsorbable suture.

Translabial Technique

A translabial approach is preferred because of minimal discomfort and disability to the patient. It provides for easy exposure and is most suited for small hernia though high ligation of the hernia sac is more difficult and the risk of recurrence is higher. If the defect of the hernia has easily demarcated margins, a labial approach is warranted. The hernia is exposed through a longitudinal labial incision. The hernia sac is dissected from surrounding tissue and the neck of the hernia sac is exposed. After the hernia sac is opened and the contents are reduced, the edges of urogenital diaphragm are approximated without tension to restore the integrity of the pelvic floor (Fig. 17.4). A mesh or allograft may be used for larger defects, poor quality perineal muscles, and when a primary repair is under tension.

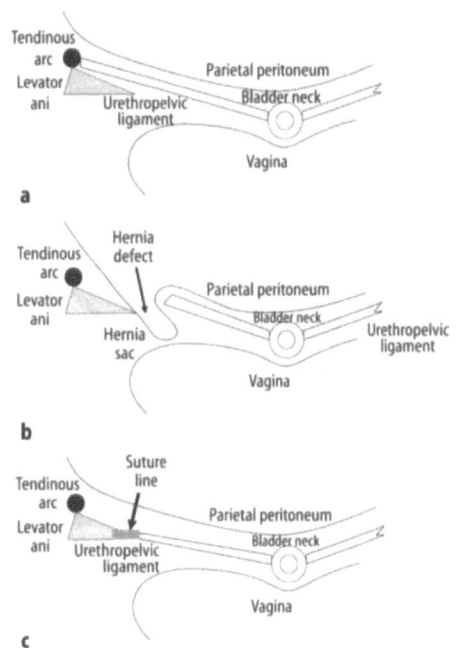

Figure 17.5 a Anterior view of normal female pelvic anatomy. **b** Anterior perineal hernia. **c.** Repair of hernia defect. Reprinted with permission from Brodak P, Juma S, Raz S (1992) Levator hernia. In: J Urol 148(3): 872–73.

Transabdominal and Abdominoperineal Technique

The transabdominal approach and the combined approach offer the best exposure of the hernia defect and its contents and direction. If there are signs of strangulated viscera or the hernia defect margins are indefinite then an abdominal or combined abdominoperineal approach is advisable. The abdomen is entered through a lower midline incision and the abdomen is first explored. The contents of the hernia

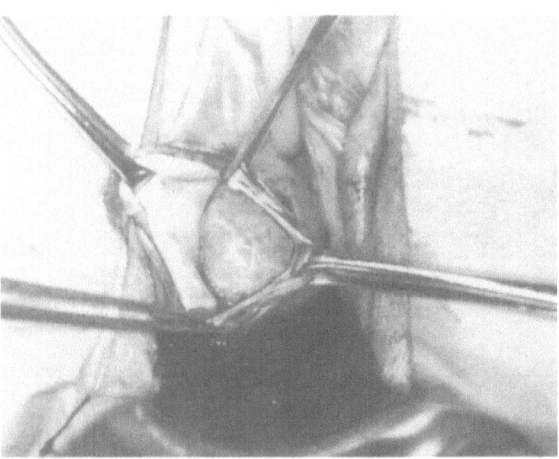

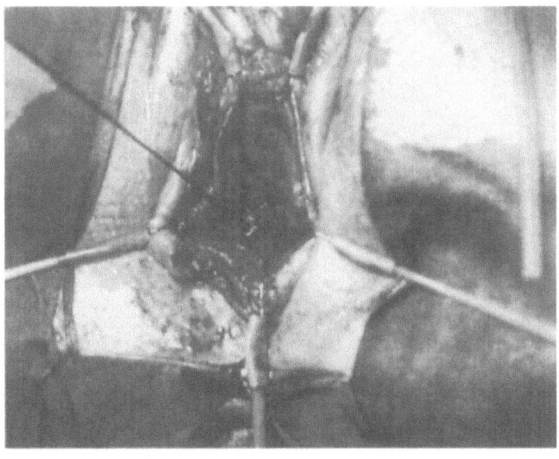

a   b

Figure 17.4 a Posterior perineal hernia sac is isolated, opened, and contents reduced. **b** Hernia repaired by closure of the defect in the urogenital diaphragm. Reprinted with permission from Brodak P, Juma S, Raz S (1992) Levator hernia. In: J Urol 148(3): 872–73.

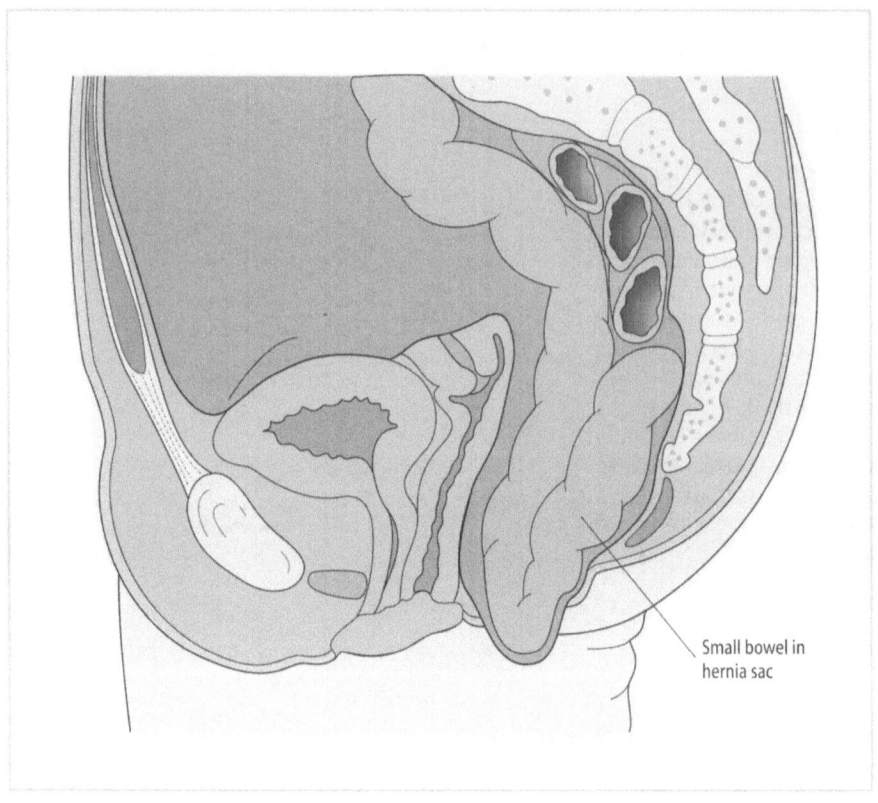

Small bowel in
hernia sac

a

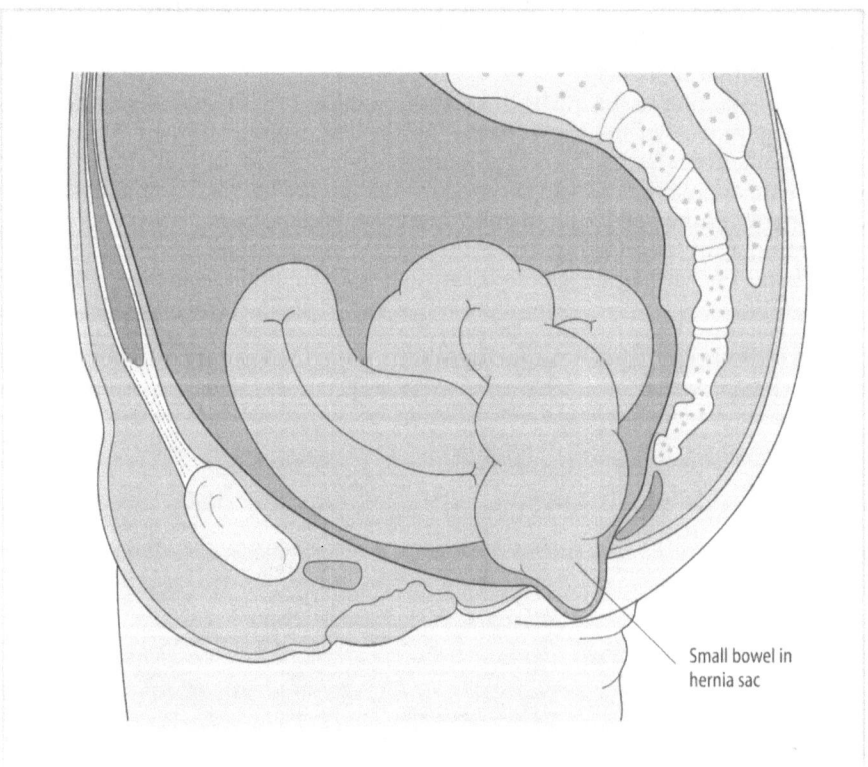

Small bowel in
hernia sac

b

Figure 17.6 Posterior perineal
hernia following abdominoperineal resection (**a**); following pelvic
exenteration (**b**).

sac are reduced and the sac is excised. The edges of the defect in the urogenital diaphragm can be simply approximated by nonabsorbable sutures (Fig. 17.5). If a primary closure of the hernia defect is not possible or satisfactory, an allograft or a synthetic mesh may be used to close the defect. The edges of the graft are sutured to the edges of the defect using non-absorbable sutures. Sacrocolpopexy should be used to anchor the vaginal cuff to the sacral promontory and approximating the anterior rectal wall to the posterior vaginal wall should close the deep cul-de-sac. This reduces the risk of recurrence. Once the defect is repaired, the abdomen is closed. No drains are used, to reduce the risk of infection.

Posterior Perineal Hernia

Posterior perineal hernia occurs through a defect posterior to the transverse perinei muscle and is usually located midway between the rectum and the ischial tuberosity. It may be seen following abdominoperineal resection, pelvic exenteration, and cystourethrectomy and perineal resection of the rectal stump (Fig. 17.6). Although perineal hernia is common after perineal resection, it is rare however, for these hernias to become symptomatic. The incidence of posterior perineal hernia requiring repair is less than 1% after abdominoperineal resection and approximately 3% after pelvic exenteration. However, hernia not requiring repair is much more common and has been reported in 7% after abdominoperineal resection. Leaving the perineal wound partially or completely open appears to be the most significant factor predisposing to hernia formation. Other factors have been postulated to contribute to perineal hernia formation including; coccygectomy, hysterectomy, pelvic radiation, excessive length of small-bowel mesentery, and the large size of the female pelvis.

Clinical Evaluation

Symptoms of posterior perineal hernia include perineal pressure, discomfort or pain, and a bulge in all patients. Small-bowel obstruction and urinary symptoms – usually obstructive voiding symptoms relieved by pressure on the perineum – may also be seen. Stress incontinence has also been reported because of protrusion of the bladder through the hernia. Posterior perineal hernia commonly presents as a mass along the inferior margin of the gluteus maximus muscle. Persistent discharge, threatened perineal skin breakdown, and perineal dehiscence occasionally may be the presenting symptoms. The hernia sac may contain small bowel, omentum, and urinary bladder or may be empty. Strangulation is uncommon because the neck of the hernia sac tends to be wide and the muscular defect is elastic. Rarely, the hernia may rupture and present with bowel prolapse and evisceration.

Plain films of the pelvis may demonstrate posterior perineal hernias as bowel containing fecal material with the buttock's soft tissue contours posterolaterally. A barium enema is recommended to demonstrate the herniated viscus. CT scan directly depicts the location of herniated bowel loops within the ischiorectal fossa adjacent to the anal canal (Fig. 17.7). The loops extend below the level of the levator ani muscle.

Surgical Management

Posterior perineal hernias require repair when they cause distressing symptoms. Various methods of repair have been described, but none is well established. The surgical principles are the same as any other hernia: mobilize the sac, reduce the contents,

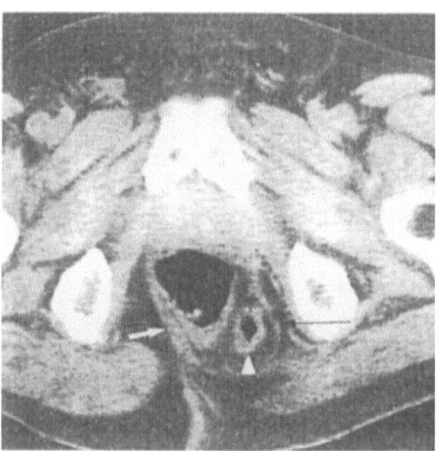

a

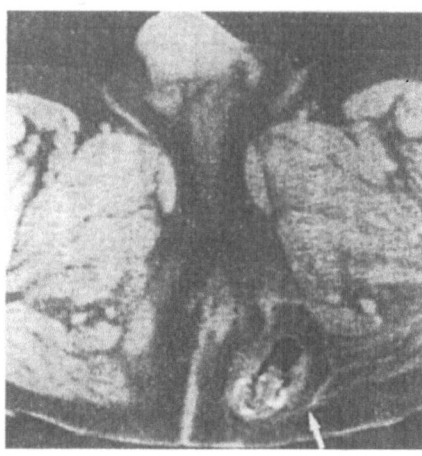

b

Figure 17.7 a CT scan of posterior perineal hernia. **b** CT scan of lower pelvis shows loop of sigmoid colon (arrowhead) surrounded by fat and hernia sac (black arrow) in left ischiorectal fossa adjacent to rectum. More inferior CT scan shows bowel and hernia sac (arrow) extending into subcutaneous tissue of left buttock. Reprinted from Lubat E, Gordon RB, Birnbaum BA, et al (1990) CT diagnosis of posterior perineal hernia. In: AJR 154: 761–62, with permission from the American Roentgen Ray Society.

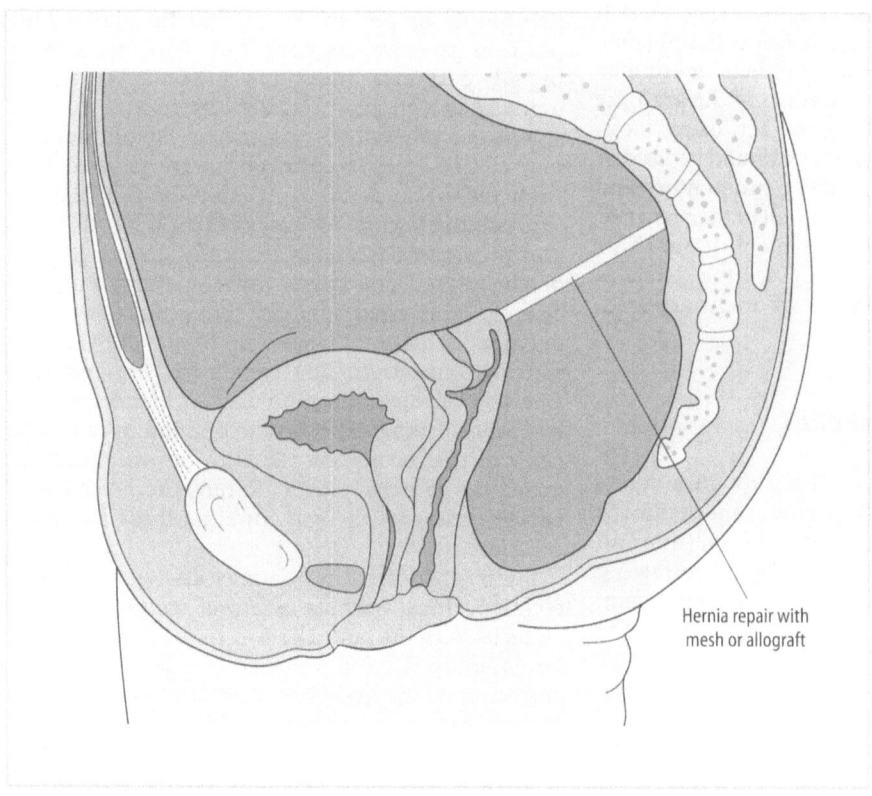

Hernia repair with
mesh or allograft

a

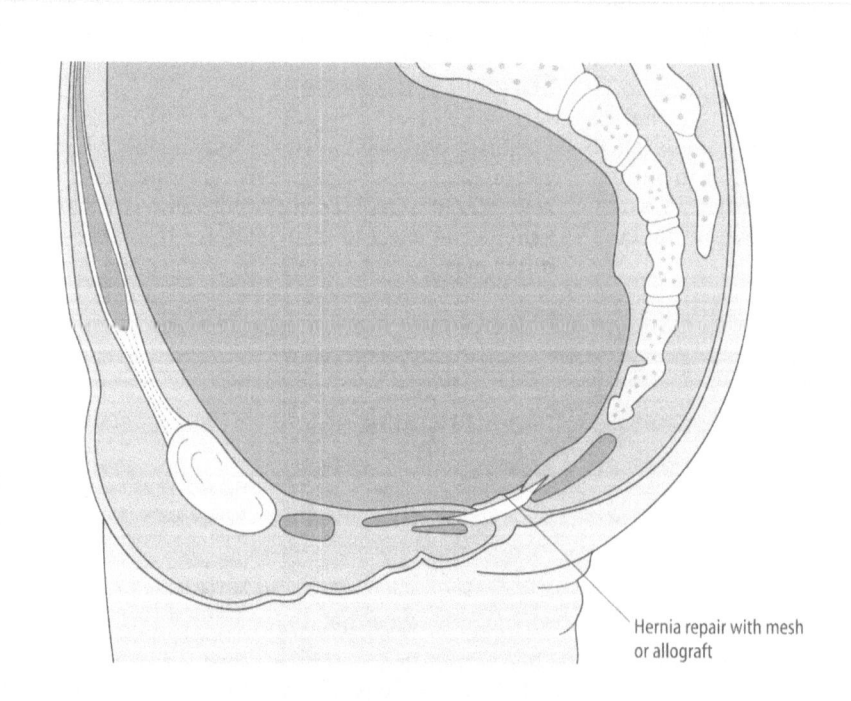

Hernia repair with mesh
or allograft

b

Figure 17.8 a Repair of posterior
perineal hernia with mesh or
allograft. Following abdominoperineal resection. **b** Following
pelvic exenteration.

excise the sac, and repair the defect (Fig. 17.8). The hernia may be repaired via a perineal, abdominal, or abdominoperineal approach.

Transperineal Technique

The simpler perineal approach is attractive because the abdominal cavity is not entered. Nevertheless, exposure is limited and it is difficult to exclude recurrent tumor, mobilize adherent bowel, or repair any injured viscera. The operation is performed under general anesthesia in the prone jackknife position. An elliptical or longitudinal incision is made over the hernia and the hernia sac is dissected from the surrounding tissue. The hernia sac is opened, the contents are reduced and the sac is excised. The levators or most likely the scar tissue can be simply approximated by nonabsorbable sutures. If primary repair is not possible, a graft or mesh is used to cover the defect. The graft is sutured with continuous nylon sutures to the coccyx posteriorly, to the levator ani laterally, and to the vaginal cuff anteriorly to create a new pelvic floor. The repair is reinforced with multiple interrupted sutures. Closed suction drain is inserted in the superficial layer and brought out through a separate stab incision and the skin is closed.

The perineal approach has higher recurrence rate. Recurrent hernia has been reported in 23% of patients following perineal repair and in none following transabdominal or abdominoperineal repair. The incidence of recurrence following simple repair and repair with a mesh is similar (20%). Infection is the major risk factor for recurrence.

Transabdominal Technique

The abdominal approach allows confirmation of the absence of recurrent cancer, and mobilization of bowel under direct vision. A mesh or allograft can be easily attached to the pelvic brim under direct vision, and the risk of injury to other structures is reduced. The abdomen is entered through a lower midline incision and the abdomen is first explored for the possibility of recurrent cancer. Perioperative placement of ureteric catheters will aid in identification of the ureters and avoids injury to them. The contents of the hernia sac are reduced and the sac is excised. The levators can be simply approximated by nonabsorbable sutures. After a radical cancer operation, though, the defect is too large for this to be possible and some additional material is needed to reconstitute the pelvic floor. A synthetic mesh or allograft may be used. Other techniques of repair that appears to provide adequate repair include interposition of the uterus, closure of muscular or fascial flaps from the gluteus muscles, and

closure of the perineal or pelvic fascia. Synthetic mesh is readily available, has adequate strength, and allows ingrowth, which may reduce the chance of infection. The advantage of the human dura as an allograft over synthetic material include equal strength, equal or decreased tissue reaction and rejection, and eventual replacement of the graft by the host's own fibrous connective tissue. If a synthetic mesh or dura graft is used, the edges of the mesh or the graft are sutured to the edges of the pelvic outlet with interrupted non-absorbable sutures. Posteriorly, it is sutured to Waldeyer's fascia and the sacral periosteum at or below the level of S_3. Anteriorly it is sutured to the vagina or the prostatic capsule. The bladder base should be avoided as suturing it may lead to urinary retention. Laterally the mesh or graft is sutured to the fascia and ligaments of the pelvic sidewalls. The attachment should be below the level of the ureters. In exenteration patients where the perineal diaphragm has been previously resected, there is a capacity to obliterate the anterior part of the hernia defect by suturing the mesh to the periosteum of the pubic rami. If the genitourinary structures are present, the pelvic inlet cannot be reached and the mesh must be sutured to the perineal diaphragm. When the perineal wound is contaminated or a mesh repair has failed, mucular flaps of fascia lata, gracilis, rectus abdominis, and gluteus maximus can be used to close the pelvic defect. The technique of gracilis muscle transplantation offers a definite advantage when the hernia occurs in a contaminated perineal wound or when the patient has received adjuvant radiation therapy. Healthy muscle brings improved vascularity to irradiated bed and may effect repair without the need for synthetic material. Closure of the pelvic peritoneum is optional. If a significant dead space is left below the mesh or graft, a large suction drain is placed below the mesh and brought out the abdomen through a separate incision to aid in obliteration of the space.

Abdominoperineal Technique

A combined abdominoperineal approach may provide the best exposure, although it is probably unnecessary except in unusual circumstances. The combined approach allows the advantage of the abdominal repair and the ability to resect the attenuated perineal skin.

References

1. Zimmern PE, Miyazaki F (1994) Pudendal enterocele with bladder involvement. Urology 44(6): 918–21.
2. Cali RL, Pitsch RM, Blatchford GJ, Thorson A, Christensen MA (1992) Rare pelvic floor hernias. Report of a case and review of the literature. Dis Colon Rectum 3: 604–12.

3. Sjollema BE, Haagen AJV, Sluijs FJ Van, Hartman F, Goedegebuure SA (1993) Electromyography of the pelvic diaphragm and anal sphincter in dogs with perineal hernia. Am J Vet Res 54(1): 185–90.

4. Mann FA, Nonneman DJ, Pope ER et al. (1995) Androgen receptors in the pelvic diaphragm muscles of dogs with and without perineal hernia. Am J Vet Res 56(1): 134–39.

5. Thomford NR, Sherman NJ (1969) Primary perineal hernia. Dis Colon Rectum 12(6): 441–3.

6. Brodak P, Juma S (1992) Levator hernia. J Urol 148: 872–3.

7. Anderson WR (1968) Pudendal hernia: unusual cause of labial mass. Obstet Gynecol 32(6): 802–4.

8. Perl JI (1960) Repair of postoperative perineal hernia. J Int Coll Surg 34: 86–92.

9. Lubat E, Gordon RB, Birnbaum BA, Megibow AJ (1990) CT diagnosis of posterior perineal hernia. AJR 154: 761–2.

10. Trackler RT, Koehler PR (1968) The radiographic findings in posterior perineal hernia. Radiology 91: 950–1.

11. Frydman GM, Polgkase AL (1989) Perineal approaches for polypropylene mesh repair of perineal hernia. Aust N Z Surg 59(110): 895–7.

12. Bok-Yan SOJ, Palmer MT (1997) Postoperative perineal hernia. Dis Colon Rectum 40(8): 954–7.

13. Cattell RB, Cunningham RM (1994) Postoperative perineal hernia following resection of the rectum. Surg Clin North Am 24: 679–83.

14. Guzzo CP, Kratzer GL (1963) Late evisceration of small bowel through postoperative perineal hernia after abdomino-perineal resection. Dis Colon Rectum 6: 135–8.

15. Brotschi E, Noe JM, Silen W (1985) Perineal hernia repair after proctectomy; a new approach to repair. Am J Surg 149: 301–5.

16. Beck ED, Fazio VW, Jagelmen DG, Lavery IC, McGonagle BA (1987) Postoperative perineal hernia. Dis Colon Rectum 1: 21–4.

17. Delmore JE, Turner DA, Gershenson DM, Horbelt DV (1987) Perineal hernia repair using human dura. Obstet Gynecol 70(3): 507–8.

18. Bell JG, Weiser EB, Metz P, Hoskins WJ (1980) Gracilis muscle repair of perineal hernia following pelvic exenteration. Obstet Gynecol 56(3): 377–80.

19. Hansen M, Bell JL, Chun JT (1997) Perineal hernia repair using gracilis myocutaneous flap. South Med J 90(1): 75–7.

Part V

Diversion and Bladder Neck Closure

18 Diversion and Bladder Neck Closure

Suzie N. Venn and Tony R. Mundy

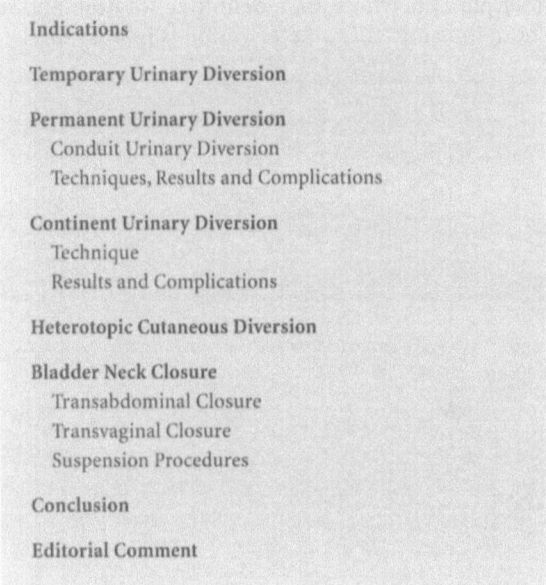
There comes a time, when repeated surgical attempts to restore continence have failed, that a further attempt at reconstruction is not realistic and an alternative must be considered. There are a number of options for diversion, the most simple of these being a urethral catheter. Permanent options are a conduit urinary diversion, heterotopic continent diversion, or bladder neck closure with continent cutaneous diversion. The decision as to, which is best, depends on the patient's condition and wishes. Each option has complications and consequences for the patient.

Indications

Urinary diversion may be required when the urethra is no longer able to maintain continence or because the patient is unable to pass a catheter. The main indications (excluding excision for malignancy) are congenital, neuropathic, and failed stress incontinence surgery. The commonest congenital cause is extrophy-epispadias, usually when reconstruction has failed. Traditionally children with epispadias have been diverted to a ureterosigmoidostomy, but a continent cutaneous diversion should be considered and an ileal or colonic conduit diversion may be appropriate.

Probably the largest group of patients requiring diversion are those with neuropathy, in particular those with spina bifida or spinal injuries. Many patients with neuropathy are temporarily diverted using a urethral or suprapubic catheter, but as problems with the catheter occur a more permanent solution is required.

Some patients with stress incontinence who have under gone repeated operations for incontinence may eventually require diversion. A conduit diversion is the quickest and simplest technique, but many would prefer a continent catheterizable suprapubic stoma connected to their bladder. This group of patients may require bladder neck closure to stop urethral leakage.

Temporary Urinary Diversion

When the urethra is no longer working as a continence mechanism, a urethral catheter is the least invasive surgical option. In a severely debilitated patient, or when any further surgery is refused, this may be the most appropriate option. However, in addition to the social inconvenience of a catheter and an external appliance, long-term catheter complications include infections, stone formation, perforation and malignancy.[1] In addition the patient may still not be dry, as leakage can occur around the catheter, and long-term catheterization is known to worsen this.

The simplest method of urinary diversion away from the urethra is a suprapubic catheter, but in addition to all the catheter complications mentioned above, the patient with a damaged urethra may still leak urethrally. The catheter blocking, or bladder spasm occurring due to the presence of the catheter balloon, will worsen this.

Permanent Urinary Diversion

Permanent diversion away from the urethra either involves diverting the ureters to a conduit, or using the native bladder but closing the bladder neck and forming an alternative conduit to empty the bladder – continent cutaneous diversion. Very occasionally a heterotopic cutaneous diversion may be required.

Conduit Urinary Diversion

The ureters can be brought to the surface as a ureterostomy, but this has a high incidence of stenosis[2] and attachment of a secure drainage bag is difficult to achieve. A simple ureterostomy is for these reasons rarely used as a long-term solution, and will not be discussed further.

The most commonly used conduit is the ileal conduit. This was originally described by Bricker in the 1950s,[3] and gained popularity as it is a relatively simple surgical procedure, with few complications. The ileal conduit is incontinent into a bag on the anterior abdominal wall making it unattractive to some patients, but it is often the best solution in older patients who want a definitive solution and in whom intermittent catheterization is impossible.

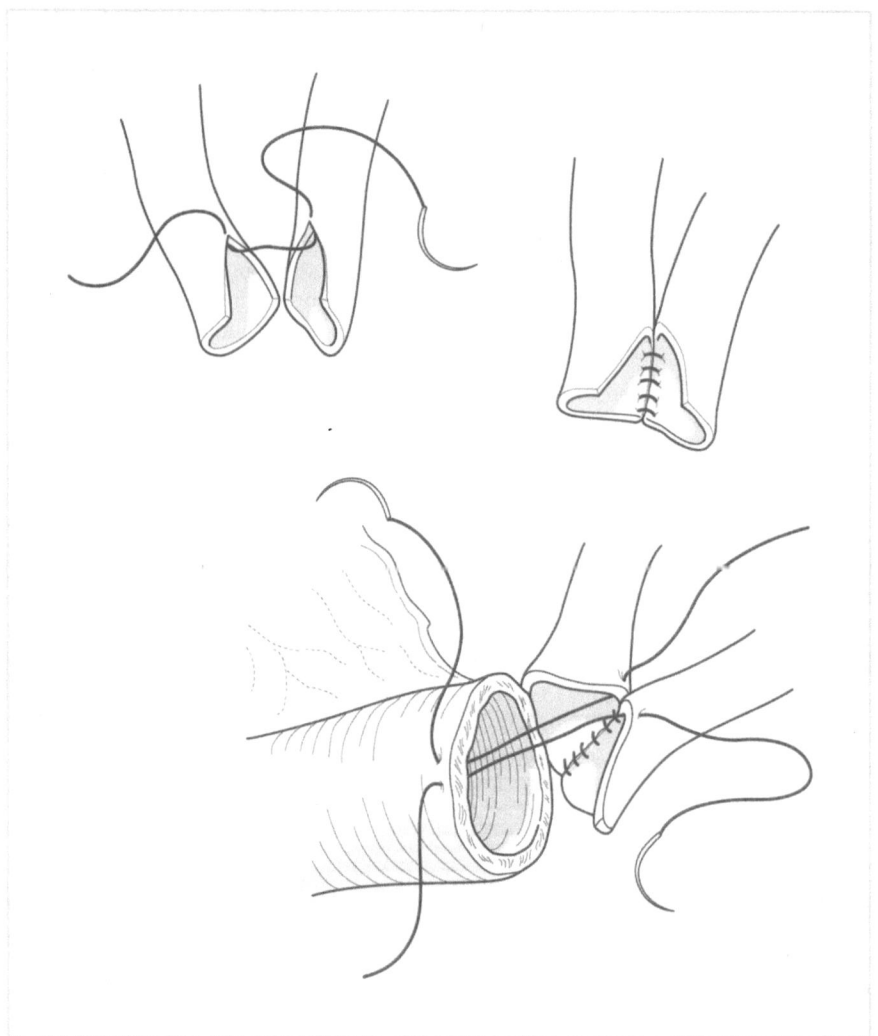

Figure 18.1 Ileal conduit – the ureters are anastomosed to the proximal end of the isolated ileum.

A continent alternative to the ileal conduit is the ureterosigmoidostomy. This was one of the first methods of urinary diversion described[4] and was widely used until the introduction of the ileal conduit. It involves anastomosis of the ureters to the sigmoid colon. The rectosigmoid then acts as a reservoir for urine and the patient voids per rectum. The ureterosigmoidostomy fell from favour because of various complication including pyelonephritis from reflux of feces into the renal pelvis, leading to renal damage; stenosis of the ureterosigmoid junction; metabolic acidosis; incontinence particularly at night; and a substantial risk of developing malignancy at the site of the ureterocolonic anastomosis.[5] Most of these – but obviously not malignant transformation – were due to high intrarectal pressures.

Recently there has been a resurgence of interest in its use following the description of a detubularized rectosigmoid pouch, by the Mainz group.[6] This technique results in lower pressures in the rectosigmoid and thus a lower risk of reflux and pyelonephritis, and improved continence.[6,7] The early results of this relatively straightforward procedure are excellent,

and as it provides a continent diversion without the need for catheterization it is an attractive alternative. The risk of malignancy does remain, however, and the patients must accept this risk and undergo annual sigmoidoscopy to detect this early.

Techniques, Results and Complications

The ileal conduit involves isolating a segment of the distal ileum, attaching the ureters to one end of the bowel and bringing the other end to the surface as a spouted stoma (Figs. 18.1, 18.2). The anastomosis is refluxing, which leads to concern that renal damage might follow. Renal deterioration does occur with long-term use but this is more often due to stenosis at the ureteroileal anastomosis which is reported to occur in 4–8%.[8] In addition obstruction of the conduit is reported at the skin surface in 5–10%[9], and parastomal hernia in a similar percentage. Most of these complications require operative revision.

The operative technique for the Mainz 11 rectosigmoid pouch is shown in Fig. 18.3. The rectum and

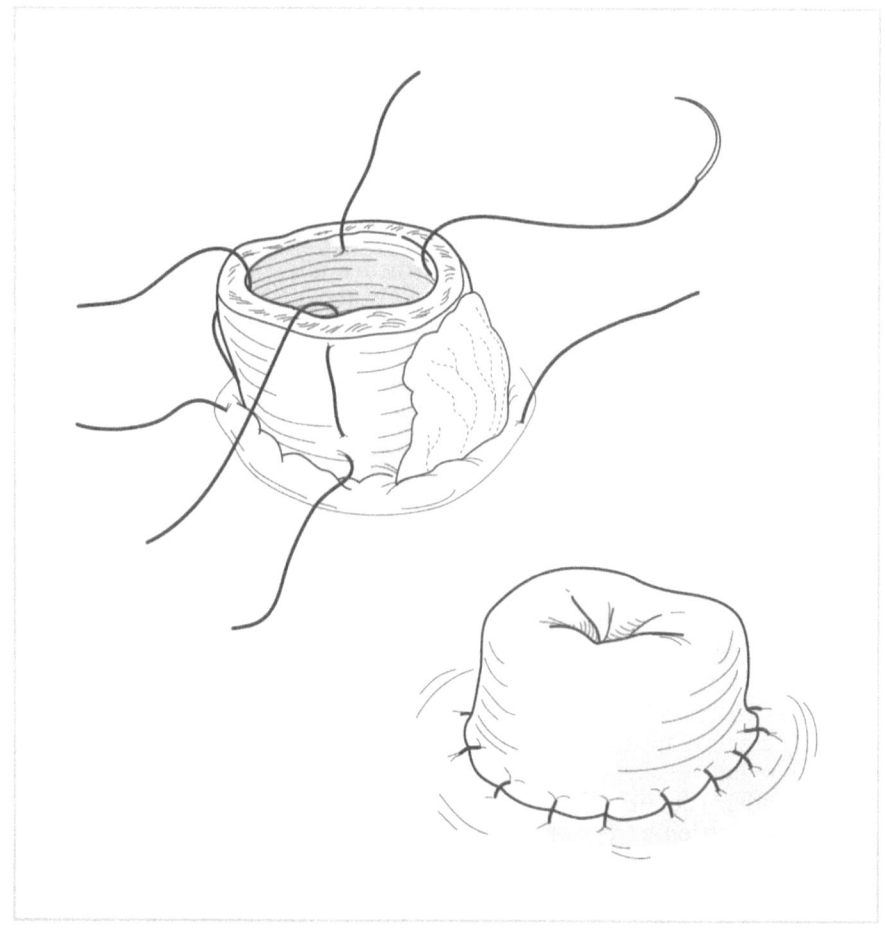

Figure 18.2 Ileal conduit – the distal end of the conduit is brought through the anterior abdominal wall and formed into a spout.

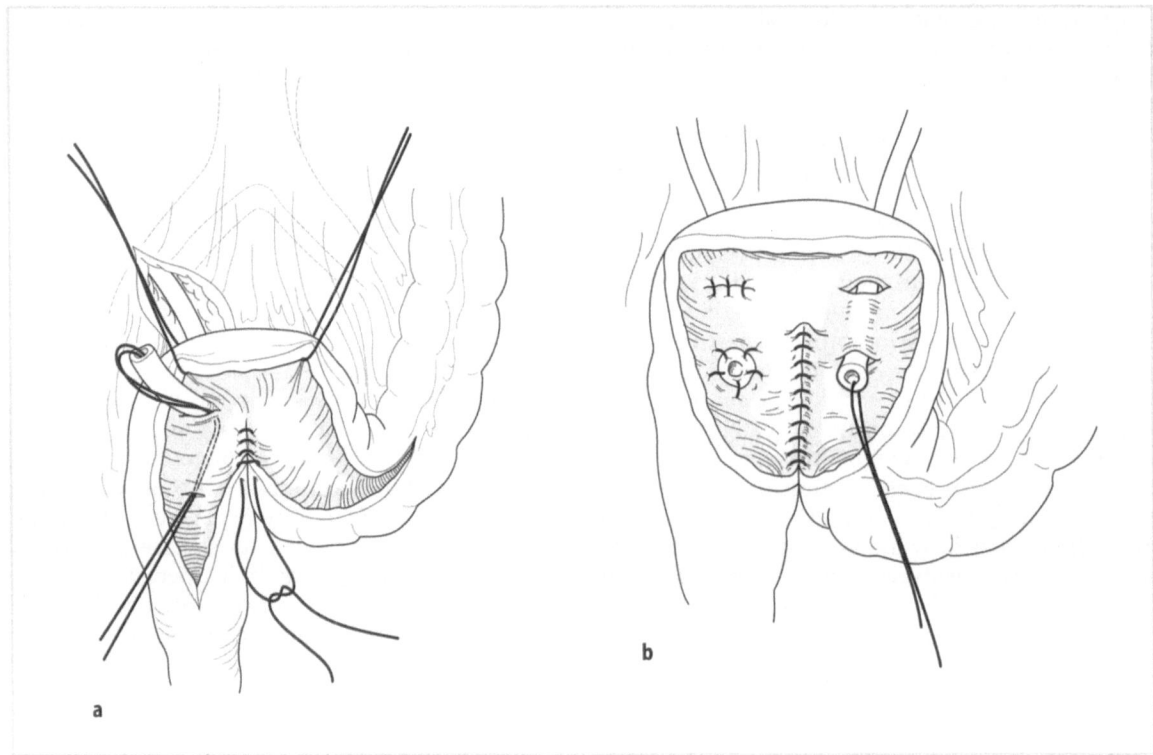

Figure 18.3 Mainz 11 rectosigmoid pouch. **a** The sigmoid colon and rectum are opened and the back wall anastomosed. **b** The ureters are brought forward into the pouch, tunneled under the mucosa and anastomosed.

sigmoid colon are opened on their anterior surface, from the peritoneal reflection proximally so that an inverted U shape can be formed. The back walls are joined and the ureters brought into the pouch and reimplantated using a tunnelled technique. The results of this procedure to date have been excellent, with over 90% continence and no evidence of upper tract damage from reflux.[7] There is no long-term data yet, and the metabolic consequences and malignant risk remain.

Continent Urinary Diversion

In female patients with a destroyed urethra and normal detrusor function the native bladder should be preserved for storage of urine. It is designed for this purpose and avoids the metabolic complications of using the bowel in the urinary tract. With the bladder neck closed, it is necessary to find an alternative method of emptying the bladder. The main indications for continent cutaneous diversion have been discussed previously, but it is only suitable for patients who are motivated to avoid an external appliance.

Technique

Before the bladder can be used in this way it is essential to confirm that it is of adequate capacity, and exclude detrusor instability and poor compliance. If this is not the case then it may be necessary to augment the bladder with an enterocystoplasty. In addition the patient must be motivated and able to perform regular self-catheterization, unless of course the procedure to be performed is simple suprapubic catheterization. If the ability to self-catheterize is in any doubt, an alternative method of diversion should be used.

Mitrofanoff originally described a method of providing continent drainage of the bladder in children with epispadias.[10] He described the use of the appendix, isolated from the bowel, with cecal end brought to the surface as a catheterizable stoma and the opened tip tunneled into the bladder (Fig. 18.4). The tunnelled implantation into the bladder provides a flutter valve continence mechanism through which the patients can catheterize. The use of the appendix has been extended to include its use in a neo-bladder[11] and is known as the "Mitrofanoff principle." When the appendix is unavailable or unsuitable, alternatives include the

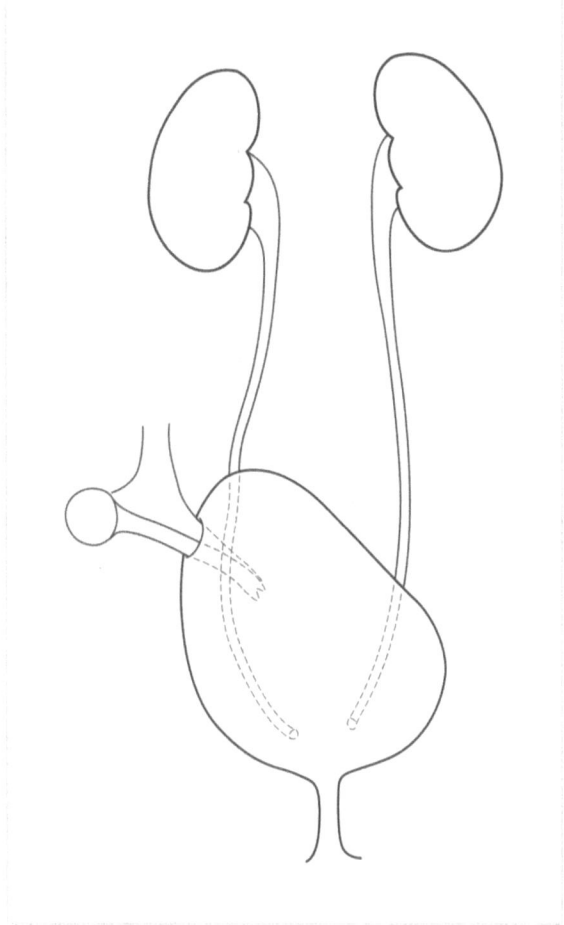

Figure 18.4 Mitrofanoff procedure using the appendix.

ureter,[12] with formation of a transuretero ureterostomy (TUU) (Fig. 18.5), and more recently the Monti
procedure,[13] where a small portion of ileum is isolated and opened longitudinally and closed transversely to form a tube (Fig. 18.6).

Results and Complications

Patients using this method should be dry with the
bladder neck closed. The surgery itself is relatively
straightforward but unfortunately there are a number of complications. The junction of the appendix
to the skin has a high stenosis rate. Various methods
have been described to reduce this, such as a Y–V
skin flap.[14] The other common problem is that the
tunnelled anastomosis to the bladder may allow
reflux, causing incontinence. In summary, one end
leaks and the other stenoses. In fact the reported
revision rate of the Mitrofanoff is a third.[14] Most of
the revisions at the surface are minor procedures,
but inability to catheterize results in an emergency
as a bladder rupture might result. In addition,

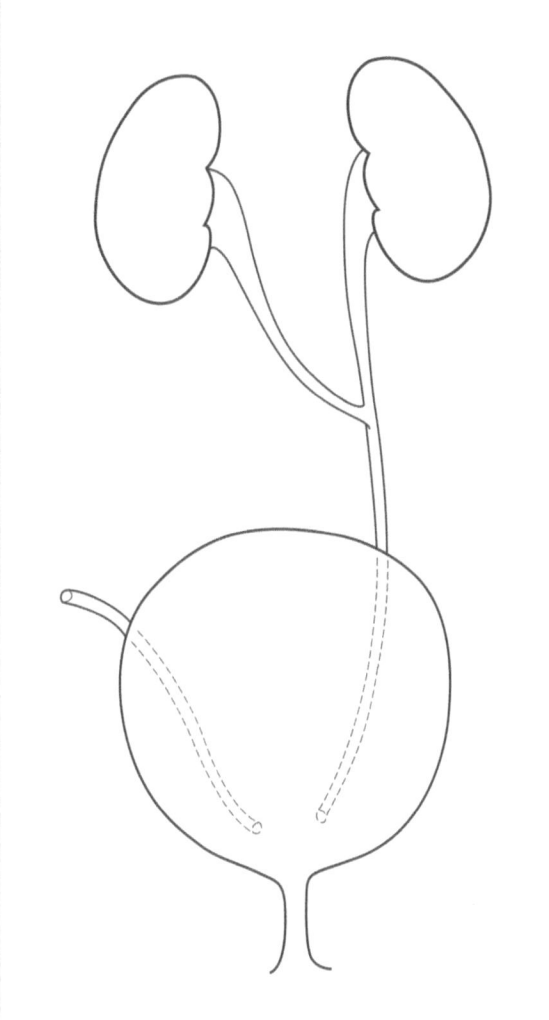

Figure 18.5 Mitrofanoff procedure using the ureter, with a TUU.

catheterization of the closed bladder results in risk
of infection and formation of stones in up to 20% of
patients,[15] presumably due to inefficient emptying of
the bladder from the top.

Heterotopic Cutaneous Diversion

Some patients may have bladders that are unsuitable
for urinary storage, but may still want a continent
diversion. Typically these are patients with neuropathy, due to spina bifida for example, who have
small-capacity, high-pressure bladders. Ideally the
bladder itself should be augmented and then a cutaneous stoma formed, but the body shape of some
patients with spina bifida may make this technically
difficult and a heterotopic cutaneous pouch com
posed entirely of bowel may be more appropriate.

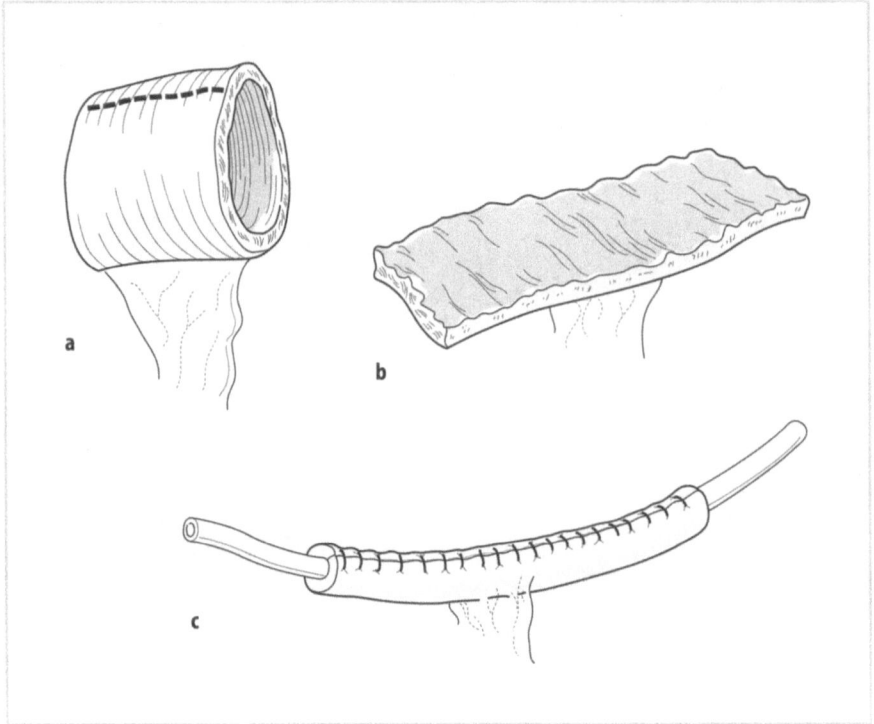

Figure 18.6 Monti procedure. 2 cm of ileum is (**a**) isolated, (**b**) opened transversely, and (**c**) closed longitudinally over a catheter.

There are many techniques of this type, such as the Indiana pouch.[16]

Bladder Neck Closure

The bladder neck needs to be closed when the bladder is to be used as a urinary reservoir but the urethra is incompetent and reconstruction is impossible or impractical. Bladder neck closure seems in theory a relatively simple procedure, but traditional methods are prone to breakdown of the closure and formation of urinary fistula. There are a number of techniques described that can be divided into transabdominal, transvaginal or suspension procedures.

The choice of operation depends in part on the fitness of the patient. Transvaginal closure has a lower morbidity, but higher failure rate.

Transabdominal Closure

To ensure a successful closure at the first operation a transabdominal approach is the most likely to succeed. The methods described are combined vaginal and suprapubic, transvesical, or an extravesical approach. In the combined approach the urethra is mobilized vaginally, the bladder opened, and the urethra brought into the bladder and closed. With the transvesical approach, the urethra is freed suprapubically by dividing the pubourethral ligaments (Fig. 18.7). The extravesical approach is similar, but avoids opening the bladder by invaginating the urethra into the bladder with a purse-string. The distal urethral stump can be excised, and omentum interposed. Success rates using these methods approach 100%[17] and have been shown to be better than transvaginal,[18] but the morbidity from an abdominal operation is obviously higher. If other abdominal procedures are being performed it is undoubtedly the best approach irrespective of morbidity.

Transvaginal Closure

The proponents of a transvaginal approach to closure of the bladder neck cite its lower morbidity, which is particularly relevant in bedridden spinal-injured patients. It may be appropriate to accept the risk of re-operation in an unfit patient for the lower morbidity. The operative technique involves dissecting the urethra from the vagina (Fig. 18.8), invaginating the urethra into the bladder, and closing the defect in the vagina. The success rate of transvaginal closure is approximately 50–70%.[19,20] This is claimed to rise to 90% after one or more further procedures. In addition, longer-term complications (mainly due to the catheter) are reported in a third.[19]

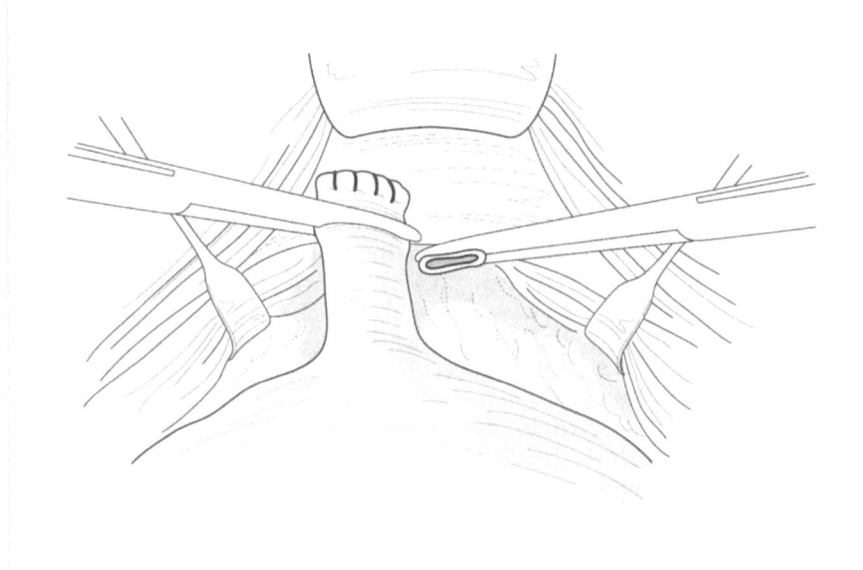

Figure 18.7 Extravesical bladder neck closure.

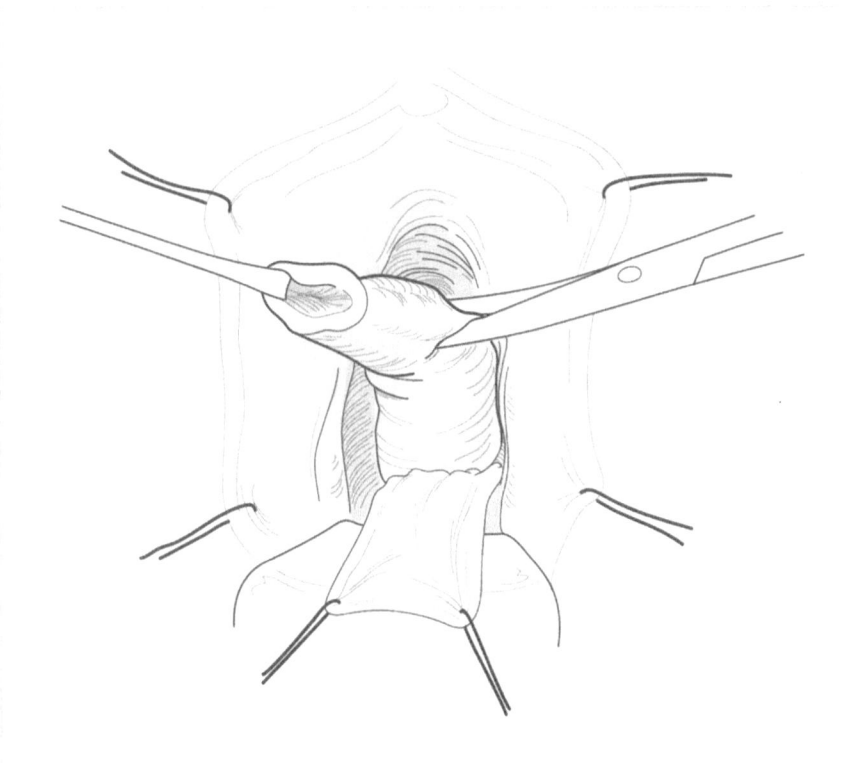

Figure 18.8 Transvaginal bladder neck closure.

Suspension Procedures

A novel approach to bladder neck closure was reported in 1994; this was the use of a tight pubo-vaginal sling to close the urethra.[20] The technique is essentially the same as a standard sling procedure,

but the sling is positioned so the urethra is closed. The initial reports claimed 100% success using clean intermittent self catheterisation (CISC) or a suprapubic catheter to empty the bladder. This technique has the advantage of leaving the urethra available for access if catheterization becomes impossible by the alternative route. However, there have been no further reports in the literature of long-term results.

Conclusion

Numerous methods of urinary diversion are available, and the discussion has been limited to those that have stood the test of time and are currently in common use. Patients in whom diversion may be considered are those with congenital conditions affecting the urethra, with neuropathy affecting the bladder, where long-term use of a urethral catheter has caused destruction of the urethra and with stress incontinence where surgery has failed.

The ileal conduit is the most commonly used permanent diversion, partly due to its simplicity and also because the complications are less than for the alternatives. It has the major disadvantage of being incontinent into a collecting bag. This makes it unattractive, particularly to younger patients. The traditional ureterosigmoidostomy avoids the need to catheterize, but is not reliably continent and has a much higher complication rate, which has discouraged its use. The Mainz 11 modification forming a detubularized pouch has improved the continence rate and reduced the risk of renal damage from reflux, but the risk of malignancy remains. Long-term results are needed before the ureterosigmoidostomy regains widespread popularity.

Continent cutaneous diversion seems a very attractive alternative. The patient is left with a small abdominal stoma, which can be easily concealed, and passes a catheter to empty the bladder when required. The Mitrofanoff principle is used in children, even as a temporary measure when passing a catheter via the urethra is not possible. The large number of published variations attest to the high revision rate of this technique, and the patient must be aware of this. In addition failure to catheterize results in an emergency situation if the bladder neck is closed, so local experienced back up is essential.

Closure of the bladder neck is needed when the urethra fails to maintain continence, even with the urine diverted away. Remarkably little has been published on this historically difficult procedure. The most reliable method is open closure of the bladder neck, with interposition of the omentum. Vaginal closure, with its lower morbidity, may be appropriate in debilitated patients, accepting the risk of failure and the need to re-operate. Suspension procedures seem an attractive alternative leaving access to the bladder, but long-term results have not yet been published following the initial reports. Bladder neck closure is not commonly performed, which may explain the dearth of published results on the subject.

Editorial Comment

There is a dearth of literature on bladder neck closure in women. Continuous urinary incontinence as a late complication of an indwelling urethral catheter for neurogenic bladder can be managed transvaginally with bladder neck closure, suprapubic tube placement, and Martius labial fat pad graft interposition to minimize risk of secondary vesico-vaginal fistula.[21] This technique is appealing in advanced multiple sclerosis patients with neurogenic incontinence, and it is simpler and safer than a supravesical diversion. For the interested reader, the techniques of both abdominal and vaginal bladder neck closure in the female have been extensively described in a recent textbook chapter.[22]

References

1. Woods DR, Bender BS (1989) Long-term urinary tract catheterization. Med Clin North Am 73: 1441–54.
2. Feminella JG, Latimer JK (1971) A retrospective analysis of 70 cases of cutaneous ureterostomy. J Urol 106: 538.
3. Bricker EM (1950) Bladder substitution after pelvic evisceration. Urol Clin North Am 30: 1511–21.
4. Simon J (1852) Ectopia vesica (absence of the anterior walls of the bladder and pubic abdominal parieties); operation for directing the orifices of the ureters into the rectum; temporary success; subsequent death; autopsy. Lancet 2: 568.
5. Mesrobian HG, Kelalis PP, Kramer SA (1988) Long-term follow-up of 103 patients with bladder extrophy. J Urol 139: 719–22.
6. Fisch M, Wammack R, Muller SC, Hohenfellner R (1993) The Mainz pouch 11 (sigma rectum pouch). J Urol 149: 258–63.
7. Fisch M, Hohenfellner R (1996) Urinary diversion. Curr Op Urol 6(3): 136–40.
8. Engel RM (1969) Complications of bilateral uretero-ileal cutaneous urinary diversion. Review of 208 cases. J Urol 101: 508–12.
9. Emott D, Noble MJ, Mebust WK (1985) A comparison of end versus loop stomas for ileal conduit urinary diversion. J Urol 133: 588–90.
10. Mitrofanoff P (1980) Cystomie continente trans-appendiculaire dans le traitement des vessies neurologiques. Chir Pediatr 21: 297–305.
11. Duckett JW, Snyder HM (1986) Continent urinary diversion: variations on the Mitrofanoff principle. J Urol 135: 58–62.
12. Duckett JW, Appendicocolostomy LAH (1993) (and variations) in bladder reconstruction. J Urol 149: 567–9.
13. Sugarman ID, Malone PS, Terry TR et al. (1998) Transversely tubularized ileal segments for the Mitrofanoff or Malone antegrade colonic enema procedures: the Monti principle. Br J Urol 81: 253–6.
14. Woodhouse CR, MacNeily AE (1994) The Mitrofanoff principle: expanding upon a versatile technique. Br J Urol 74: 447–53.
15. Nurse DE, McInerney PD, Thomas PJ, Mundy AR (1996) Stones in entero-cystoplasties. Br J Urol 77: 684–7.
16. Gilchrist RH, Merricks JW et al. (1950) Construction of a substitute bladder and urethra. Surg Gynaecol Obstet 90: 752.
17. Hensle TW, Kirsch AJ, Kennedy WA, Reiley EA (1995) Bladder neck closure in association with continent urinary diversion. J Urol 154: 883–5.

18. Levy JB, Jacobs JA et al. (1994) Combined abdominal and vaginal approach for bladder neck closure and permanent suprapubic tube: urinary diversion in the neurologically impaired woman. J Urol 152: 2081–2.

19. Stower MJ, Massey JA, Feneley RCL (1989) Urethral closure in management of urinary incontinence. Urology 34(5): 246–8.

20. Chancellor MB, Erhard MJ, Kiilholma PJ, Karasick S, Rivas DA (1994) Functional urethral closure with pubovaginal sling for destroyed female urethra after long-term urethral catheterization. Urology 43(4): 499–505.

21. Zimmern P, Hadley R, Leach G, Raz S (1985) Transvaginal closure of the bladder neck and placement of a suprapubic catheter for destroyed urethra after long-term indwelling catheterization. J Urol 134: 554-7.

22. Litwiller S, Zimmern P (1998) Closure of bladder neck in the male and female. In: Graham SD, Jr (ed) Glenn's Urology Surgery, 5th edn. Lippincott-Raven, Philadelphia, pp. 407–14.

Part VI

Fistulae

19 Vesico-vaginal and Urethro-vaginal Fistulae

Paul Hilton

Definition and Classification

A fistula may be defined as an abnormal communication between two or more epithelial surfaces. In the context of gynecology we are concerned primarily with fistulae between the genital tract (vagina, cervix, uterus, or perineum, in decreasing order of frequency) and either the urinary tract (bladder, urethra, or ureter) or the gastrointestinal tract (rectum, colon, anal canal, or small bowel).

Multiple or complex fistulae are common, particularly after attempts at surgical repair. Dual involvement of the bowel and urinary tract is regularly seen, and concurrent involvement of, for example ureter and bladder, or bladder and urethra is often seen in strategically placed or large urinary fistulae. They may also involve an intervening cavity, so the fistulous nature of an inflammatory mass may not be immediately obvious.

Fistulae may be classified into simple cases (where the tissues are healthy and access good) or complicated (where there is tissue loss, scarring, impaired access, involvement of the ureteric orifices, or the presence of coexistent rectovaginal fistula). Urogenital fistulae are also classified, on the basis of anatomical site, into urethral, bladder neck, subsymphysial (a complex form involving circumferential loss of the urethra with fixity to bone), midvaginal, juxta-cervical or vault fistulae, massive fistulae extending from bladder neck to vault, and vesico-uterine or vesico-cervical fistulae. Whereas over 60% of fistulae in developing countries are midvaginal, juxta-cervical or massive (reflecting their obstetric etiology), such cases are relatively rare in western fistula practice; by contrast, 50% of the fistulae managed in the UK are situated in the vaginal vault (reflecting their surgical etiology).[1]

Causes

Congenital fistulae are strictly outside the scope of this chapter, and readers are referred to Chapter 4. The etiology of acquired urogenital fistulae is varied, and may be broadly categorized into obstetric, surgical, radiation, malignant, and miscellaneous causes. In most developing countries over 90% of fistulae are of obstetric etiology, whereas in the UK over 70% follow pelvic surgery (Table 19.1).

Obstetric

The basic physical factors responsible for obstetric fistula development include obstructed labour

Table 19.1. Etiology of uro-genital fistulae in two series, from the north of England (Hilton, unpublished) and southeast Nigeria.[17]

Etiology	NE England (n = 135)		SE Nigeria (n = 2389)	
Obstetric				
Obstructed labor	1		1918	
Cesarean section	2		165	
Ruptured uterus	5		119	
Forceps/ventouse	4			
Breech extraction	1			
Placental abruption	1			
Obstetric subtotal (% of total)	14	(10.4%)	2202	(92.2%)
Surgical				
Abdominal hysterectomy	55		33	
Radical hysterectomy	11			
Urethral diverticulectomy	10			
Colporrhaphy	2		35	
Vaginal hysterectomy	4		25	
TAH and colporrhaphy	1			
TAH and colposuspension	1			
LAVH	1			
Laparoscopic oophorectomy	1			
Cystoplasty and colposuspension	2			
Colposuspension	1			
Sling	1			
Needle suspension	1			
Cervical stumpectomy	1			
Subtrigonal phenol injection	1			
Transurethral resection (tb)	1			
Lithoclast	1			
Panproctocolectomy	1			
Unknown surgery in childhood	1			
Suture to vaginal laceration			12	
Surgical subtotal (% of total)	97	(71.8%)	105	(4.4%)
Radiation	18	(13.3%)	0	(0.0%)
Malignancy	0	(0.0%)	42	(1.8%)
Miscellaneous				
Catheter induced	2			
Foreign body	2			
Trauma	1		11	
Infection			7	
Coital injury	1		22	
Miscellaneous subtotal (% of total)	6	(4.4%)	40	(1.7%)

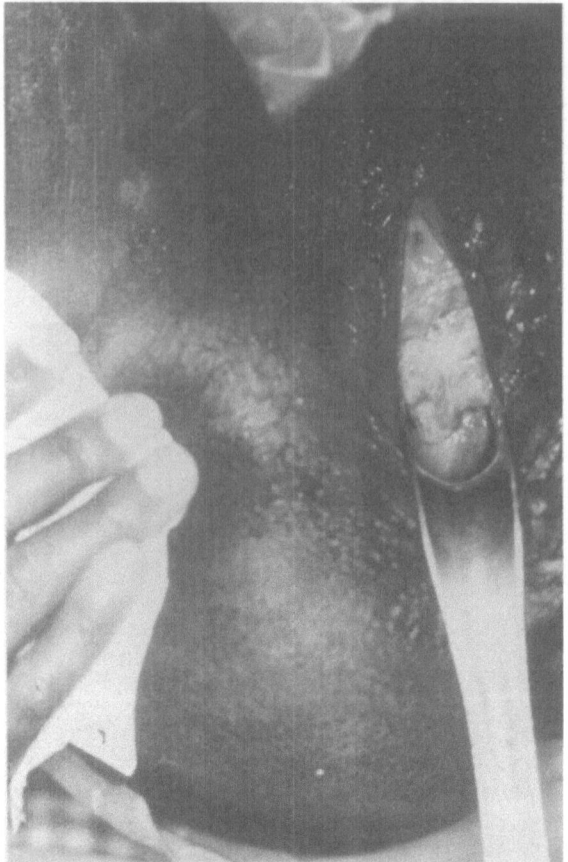

Figure 19.1 Puerperal patient following prolonged obstructed labor. An area of devitalized tissue is seen on the anterior vaginal wall, about to slough with resultant fistula formation. Reprinted with permission from Hilton P (1997) Fistulae. In: Shaw R, Souter W, Stanton S (eds) Gynaecology, 2nd edn. Churchill-Livingstone, London, pp. 779–801.

(Fig. 19.1), accidental injury at the time of cesarean section, forceps delivery, craniotomy, or symphysiotomy, traditional surgical practices including circumcision and gishiri, and complications of criminal abortion.

Tahzib[2,3] reported on the epidemiological determinants of vesico-vaginal fistulae in northern Nigeria. In 84% of cases obstructed labor was the major etiological factor. Thirty-three per cent had undergone gishiri, and in 15% this was felt to be the main etiological factor. Over 50% of patients were under 20 years of age; over 50% were in their first pregnancy, and only 1 in 500 had received any formal education.

Surgical

Genital fistula may occur following a wide range of surgical procedures within the pelvis (Table 19.1). It is often supposed that this complication results from direct injury to the lower urinary tract at the time of operation. Certainly on occasions this may be the case; careless, hurried, or rough surgical technique makes injury to the lower urinary tract much more likely. However of 135 fistulae referred to the author in the UK over the last 10 years, 97 have been associated with pelvic surgery, and 73 followed hysterectomy (Figs 19.2. 19.3); of these only five presented with leakage of urine on the first postoperative day. In other cases compromise to the blood supply may result in tissue necrosis and subsequent leakage; or alternatively a small pelvic hematoma may develop in association with the vaginal vault which subsequently becomes infected and discharges, often with hematuria, 5–10 days later, and incontinence following shortly thereafter.

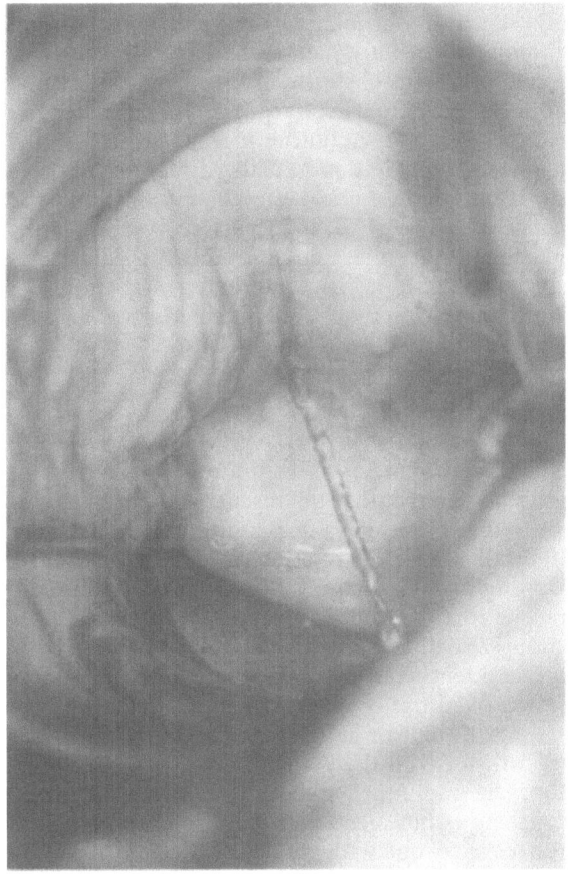

Figure 19.2 Simple post-hysterectomy vesico-vaginal fistula.

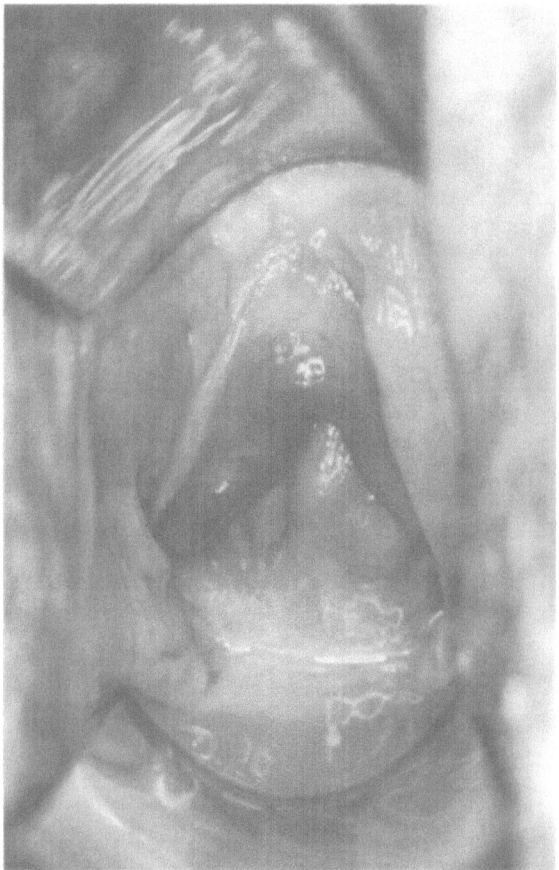

Figure 19.3 Large vesico-vaginal fistula following radical hysterectomy; the right ureteric orifice is seen in the edge of the fistula. Reprinted with permission from Hilton P (1997) Debate: Post-operative urogenital fistulae are best managed by gynaecologists in specialist centres. Br J Urol 80 (suppl) (1): 35–42.

Radiation

Preoperative pelvic irradiation increases the risk of postoperative fistula development, but irradiation itself may be a cause of fistula. The obliterative endarteritis associated with ionizing radiation in therapeutic dosage proceeds over many years and may be etiological in fistula formation long after the primary malignancy has been treated. Of the 18 radiation fistulae in the author's series, the fistula has developed at intervals between 1 and 30 years following radiotherapy.

Malignancy

It is relatively unusual for urothelial tumours to present with fistula formation, other than following surgery or radiotherapy. Carcinoma of cervix, vagina, and rectum are the most common malignancies to present with fistula formation primarily. The development of a fistula may be a distressing part of the terminal phase of malignant disease; it is nevertheless one deserving not simply compassion, but full consideration of the therapeutic or palliative possibilities.

Miscellaneous

Other causes of fistulae in the genital tract include infection (lymphogranuloma venereum, schistosomiasis, tuberculosis, actinomycosis, measles, noma vaginae) and traumatic causes (penetrating trauma, neglected pessary, other foreign bodies, catheter-related injuries, and coital injury) (Fig. 19.4).

Prevalence

The prevalence of genital fistulae obviously varies from country to country and continent to continent as the main causative factors vary. Accurate figures are often impossible to obtain because those areas with the highest overall prevalence are also those with the poorest systems of health data collection. Although the true prevalence in the developing

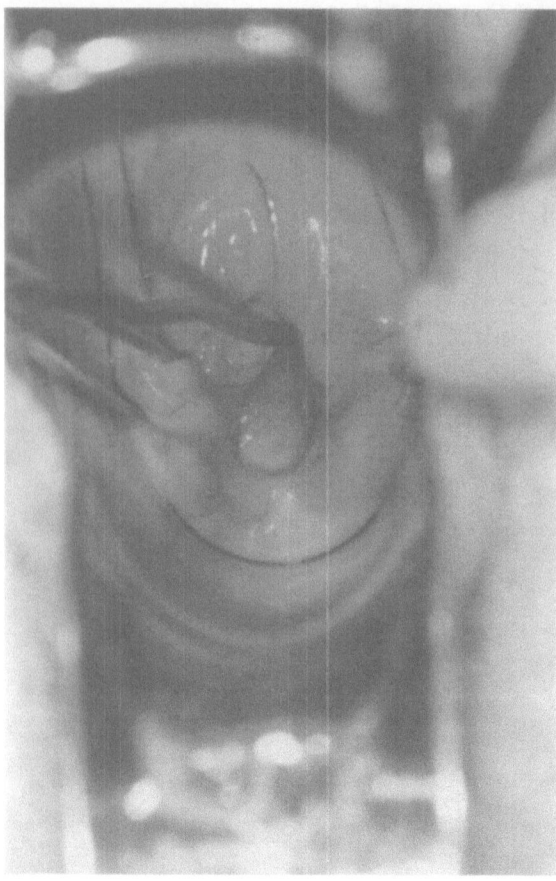

Figure 19.4 Vaginal vault fistula arising following coitus, 8 weeks after abdominal hysterectomy.

world is unknown, particularly high prevalence rates are reported in Nigeria, Ethiopia, Sudan, and Chad. The estimated prevalence in developing countries is 1–2 per 1000 deliveries, with perhaps 50 000–100 000 new cases each year. The units currently existing in these countries of high prevalence nowhere nearly meet the demand, and there are estimated to be perhaps 500 000 untreated cases worldwide.[4]

Recent data from the Regional Health Authority Information Units in England and Wales suggests a national incidence of 120–150 cases per year.[1,5] The best estimate of the post-hysterectomy fistula rate is approximately 1 per 1300 operations (Lawson 1990, personal communication).

Assessment and Investigation

Fistulae between the urinary tract and the female genital tract are characteristically said to present with continuous urinary incontinence, both by day and by night. In patients with large fistulae the volume of leakage may be such that they rarely feel any sensation of bladder fullness, and normal voiding may be infrequent. Where there is extensive tissue loss, as in obstetric fistulae from obstructed labor, or radiation fistulae, this typical history is usually present, the clinical findings gross, and the diagnosis rarely in doubt. With postsurgical fistulae for example, the history may be atypical and the orifice small, elusive, or occasionally completely invisible. Under these circumstances the diagnosis can be much more difficult, and a high index of clinical suspicion must be maintained.

Dye Studies

When the diagnosis is in doubt, it is important firstly to confirm that the discharge is urinary, secondly that the leakage is extraurethral rather than urethral, and thirdly to establish the site of leakage. Although other imaging techniques undoubtedly have a role (see below), carefully conducted dye studies remain the investigation of first choice.

The identification of the site of a fistula is best carried out by the instillation of colored dye (methylene blue or indigo carmine) into the bladder via catheter with the patient in the lithotomy position. The traditional "three swab test" has its limitations and is not recommended. The examination is best carried out with direct inspection; multiple fistulae may be located in this way. If leakage of clear fluid continues after dye instillation a ureteric fistula is likely, and this is most easily confirmed by a "two dye test", using phenazopyridine to stain the renal urine, and methylene blue to stain bladder contents.[6]

Imaging

Excretion Urography

Although intravenous urography is a particularly insensitive investigation in the diagnosis of vesico-vaginal fistula, knowledge of upper urinary tract status may have a significant influence on treatment measures applied, and it should therefore be looked on as an essential investigation for any suspected or confirmed urinary fistula. Compromise to ureteric function is a particularly common finding when a fistula occurs in relation to malignant disease or its treatment (Fig. 19.5).

Cystography

Cystography is not particularly helpful in the basic diagnosis of vesico-vaginal fistulae, and a dye test carried out under direct vision is likely to be more

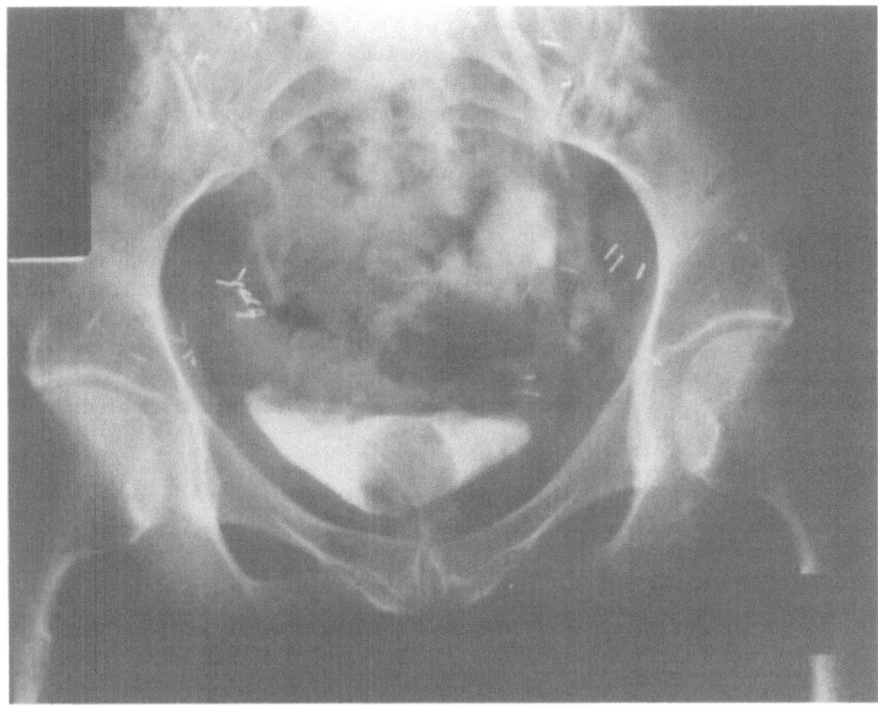

Figure 19.5 Intravenous urogram (with simultaneous cystogram) demonstrating a complex surgical fistula occurring after radical hysterectomy. After further investigation including cystourethroscopy, sigmoidoscopy, barium enema, and retrograde cannulation of the vaginal vault to perform fistulography, the lesion was defined as a uretero-colo-vesico-vaginal fistula.

sensitive. It may however, occasionally be useful in achieving a diagnosis in complex fistulae, or vesico-uterine fistulae, where a lateral view may show the cavity of the uterus filled with radio-opaque dye behind the bladder.

Examination Under Anesthesia

Careful examination, if necessary under anesthetic, may be required to determine the presence of a fistula, and is deemed by several authorities to be an essential preliminary to definitive surgical treatment.[7-10] A malleable silver probe is invaluable for the exploration of the vaginal walls, and tissue forceps or plastic surgical skin hooks are helpful to put tension on the tissues for the identification of small fistulae. It is also important at the time of examination to assess the available access for repair vaginally, and the mobility of the tissues. The decision between the vaginal and abdominal approaches to surgery is thus made; when the vaginal route is chosen, it may be appropriate to select between the more conventional supine lithotomy with a head-down tilt, and the prone (reverse lithotomy) with head-up tilt.[11]

Cystoscopy

It is the author's practice to perform cystourethroscopy in all but the largest defects. The exact level

and position of the fistula should be determined, and its relationship to the ureteric orifices and bladder neck are particularly important. With urethral and bladder neck fistulae the failure to pass a cystoscope or sound may indicate that there has been circumferential loss of the proximal urethra, a circumstance which is of considerable importance in determining the appropriate surgical technique and the likelihood of subsequent urethral incompetence.

The condition of the tissues must be carefully assessed. Persistence of slough means that surgery should be deferred, and this is particularly important in obstetric and postradiation cases. Biopsy from the edge of a fistula should be taken in radiation fistulae, if persistent or recurrent malignancy is suspected. Malignant change has been reported in a long-standing benign fistula, so biopsy should be undertaken where there is any doubt at all about the nature of the tissues.[12]

Management

Immediate Management

Before epithelialization is complete a fistula will tend to close spontaneously, provided that outflow is unobstructed; bypassing the sphincter mechanisms by catheterization may encourage closure. It is worth persisting with this line of management in vesico-vaginal or urethro-vaginal fistulae for 6–8 weeks, because spontaneous closure may occur within this period.[13]

Palliation and Skin Care

During the waiting period from diagnosis to repair incontinence pads should be provided in generous quantities so that patients can continue to function socially to some extent. The vulval skin may be at considerable risk from ammoniacal dermatitis, and liberal use of silicone barrier cream should be encouraged. Topical corticosteroid or estrogen therapy has been advocated by some authors,[9,14] although there is no evidence of benefit.

Counselling

Surgical fistula patients are usually previously healthy individuals who entered hospital for what was expected to be a routine procedure, and end up with symptoms infinitely worse than their initial complaint. Obstetric fistula patients in the developing world are social outcasts. In both situations, therefore, these women are invariably devastated by their situation. It is vital that they understand the nature of the problem, why it has arisen, and the plan for management at all stages. Confident but realistic counseling by the surgeon is essential and the involvement of nursing staff or counselors with experience of fistula patients is also highly desirable. The support given by previously treated sufferers can also be of immense value in maintaining patient morale, especially where a delay prior to definitive treatment is required.

General Principles of Surgical Treatment

Timing of Repair

The timing of surgical repair is perhaps the single most contentious aspect of fistula management.

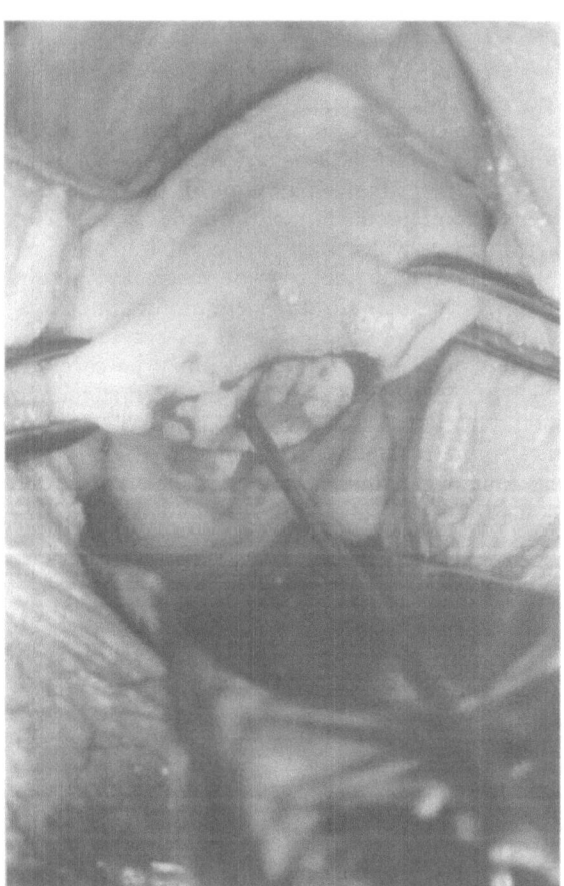
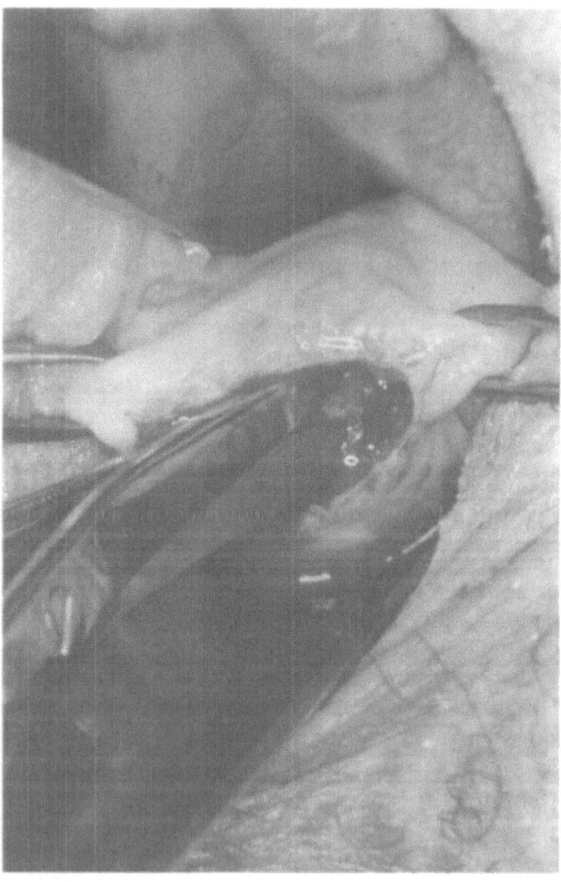

a   b

Figure 19.6 Series of operative photographs demonstrating steps of repair of typical post-hysterectomy vault fistula (same patient as Figure 19.2). **a** Fistula circumcised using #12 scalpel. **b** Sharp dissection around fistula edge. (**c**) Fistula fully mobilized. (**d**) First two sutures of first layer of repair in place lateral to the angles of the repair. (**e**) Second layer completed, sutures catching back of vaginal flaps to close off dead space. (**f**) Final layer of mattress sutures in the vaginal wall. Reprinted with permission from Hilton P (1997) Debate: Post-operative urogenital fistulae are best managed by gynaecologists in specialist centres. Br J Urol 80 (suppl) (1): 35–42.

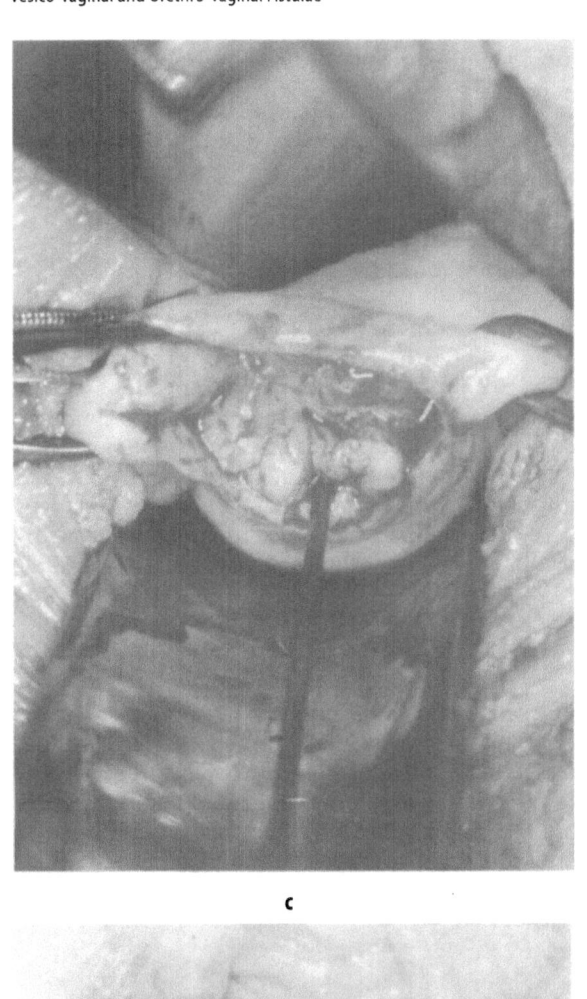

c

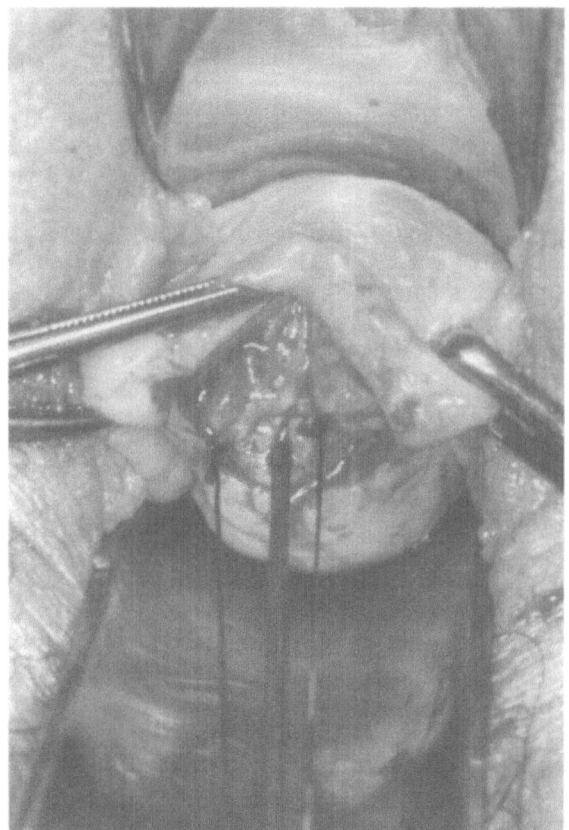

d

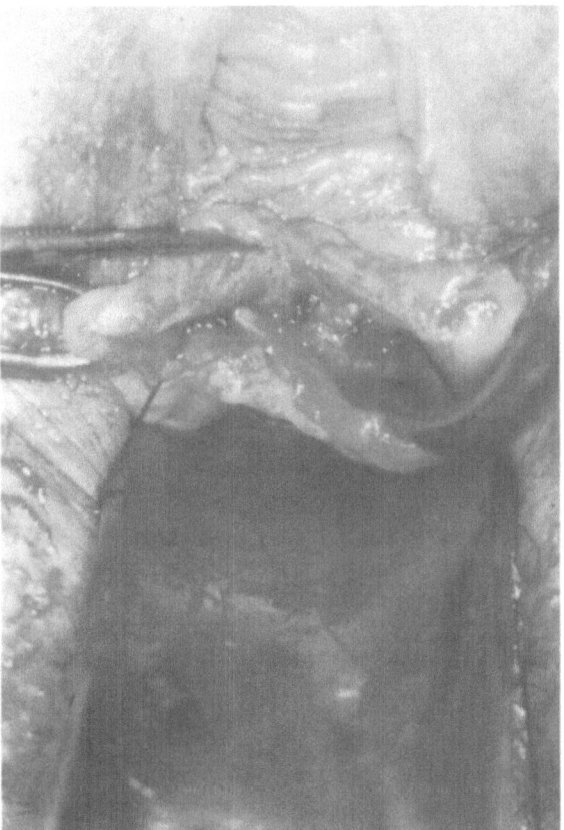

e

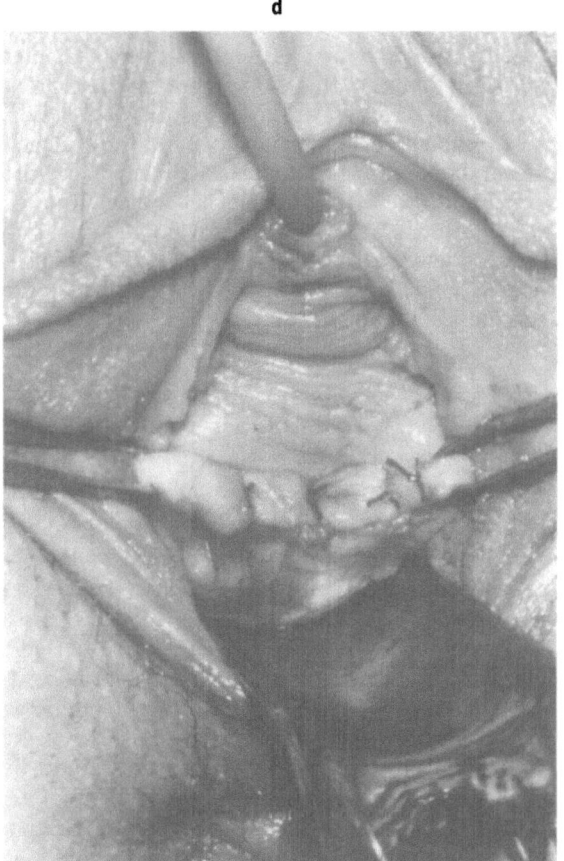

f

Although shortening the waiting period is of both social and psychological benefit to what are always very distressed patients, one must not trade these issues for compromise to surgical success. The benefit of delay is to allow slough to separate, and inflammatory change to resolve. In obstetric cases most authorities suggest that a minimum of 3 months should be allowed to elapse, although Waaldijk has recently advocated surgery as soon as slough is separated.[15] In radiation fistulae it may be necessary to wait 12 months or more.

With surgical fistulae the same principles should apply, and although the extent of sloughing is limited, extravasation of urine into the pelvic tissues inevitably sets up some inflammatory response. Although several authors advocate early repair, again most would agree that 10–12 weeks postoperatively is the earliest appropriate time for repair.

Route of Repair

Surgeons involved in fistula management must be capable of both abdominal and vaginal approaches, and should be prepared to modify their techniques to select that most appropriate to the individual case. Where access is good and the vaginal tissues sufficiently mobile, the vaginal route is usually most appropriate. If access is poor and the fistula cannot be brought down, the abdominal approach should be used. Although such difficulties can sometimes be handled vaginally, where there is concurrent involvement of ureter or bowel in a surgical fistula, an abdominal procedure may be used to advantage.

Overall more surgical fistulae are likely to require an abdominal repair than obstetric fistulae, although in the author's series of cases from the UK, and those reviewed from Nigeria, two-thirds of cases were satisfactorily treated by the vaginal route regardless of etiology.[16,17]

Specific Repair Techniques

Vaginal Procedures

Two main types of closure technique are applied to the repair of urinary fistulae, the classical saucerization technique described by Sims,[18] and the much more commonly used dissection and repair in layers (Fig. 19.6a–f). Sutures must be placed with meticulous accuracy in the bladder wall, care being taken not to penetrate the mucosa, which should be inverted as far as possible. The repair should be started at either end, working towards the midline, so that the least accessible aspects are sutured first. Interrupted sutures are preferred and should be placed approximately 3 mm apart, taking as large a bite of tissue as feasible. Stitches that are too close together, or the use of continuous or purse-string sutures, tend to impair blood supply and interfere with healing.

Dissection and Repair in Layers

With dissection and repair in layers the first layer of sutures in the bladder should invert the edges (Fig. 19.6d); the second adds bulk to the repair by taking a wide bite of bladder wall, but also closes off dead space by catching the back of the vaginal flaps (Fig. 19.6e). After testing the repair a third layer of interrupted mattress sutures is used to evert and close the vaginal wall, consolidating the repair by picking up the underlying bladder wall (Fig. 19.6f).

Saucerization

The saucerization technique involves converting the track into a shallow crater, which is closed without dissection of bladder from vagina using a single row of interrupted sutures. The method is only applicable to small fistulae, and perhaps residual fistulae after closure of a larger defect; in other situations the technique does not allow secure closure without tension.

Vaginal Repair Procedures in Specific Circumstances

The conventional dissection and repair in layers as described above is entirely appropriate for the majority of midvaginal fistulae, although modifications may be necessary in specific circumstances. In juxtacervical fistulae in the anterior fornix vaginal repair may be feasible if the cervix can be drawn down to provide access. Dissection should include mobilization of the bladder from the cervix. The repair must be undertaken transversely to reconstruct the underlying trigone and prevent distortion of the ureteric orifices.

Vault fistulae, particularly those following hysterectomy, can again usually be managed vaginally. The vault is incised transversely and mobilization of the fistula is often aided by deliberate opening of the cul-de-sac.[19] The peritoneal opening does not require to be closed separately, but is incorporated into the vaginal closure.

Where there is substantial urethral loss reconstruction may be undertaken using the method described by Chassar Moir[7] or Hamlin and Nicholson.[20] A strip of anterior vaginal wall is constructed into a tube over a catheter. Plication behind the bladder neck is probably important if continence is to be achieved. The interposition of a labial fat or muscle graft not only fills up the potential dead space, but provides additional bladder neck support and improves continence by reducing scarring between bladder neck and vagina.

Radiation fistulae present particular problems in that the area of devitalized tissue is usually considerably larger than the fistula itself. Mobilization is often impossible and if repair in layers is attempted the flaps are likely to slough; closure by colpocleisis is therefore required. Some have advocated total closure of the vagina although it is preferable to avoid dissection in the devitalized tissue entirely, and to perform a lower partial colpocleisis converting the upper vagina into a diverticulum of the bladder. It is usually necessary to fill the dead space below this with an interposition graft.

Abdominal Procedures

Transvesical Repair

Repair by the abdominal route is indicated when high fistulae are fixed in the vault and inaccessible per vaginam. Transvesical repair has the advantage of being entirely extraperitoneal. It is often helpful to elevate the fistula site by a vaginal pack, and the ureters should be catheterized under direct vision. The technique of closure is similar to that of the transvaginal flap-splitting repair except that for hemostasis the bladder mucosa is closed with a continuous suture.

Transperitoneal repair

It is often said that there is little place for a simple transperitoneal repair, although a combined transperitoneal and transvesical procedure is favoured by urologists and is particularly useful for vesico-uterine fistulae following cesarean section. A midline split is made in the vault of the bladder; this is extended downwards in a racket shape around the fistula. The fistulous track is excised and the vaginal or cervical defect closed in a single layer. The bladder is then closed in two layers.

Interposition Grafting

Several techniques have been described to support fistula repair in different sites. In each case the interposed tissue serves to create an additional layer in the repair, to fill dead space, and to bring in new blood supply to the area. The tissues used include:

- Martius graft – labial fat and bulbocavernosus muscle passed subcutaneously to cover a vaginal repair; this is particularly appropriate to provide additional bulk in a colpocleisis and in urethral and bladder neck fistulae may help to maintain competence of closure mechanisms by reducing scarring.[21]
- Gracilis muscle passed either via the obturator foramen or subcutaneously is used as above.[20]
- Omental pedicle grafts[22,23] may be dissected from the greater curve of the stomach and rotated down into the pelvis on the right gastroepiploic artery; this may be used at any transperitoneal procedure, but has its greatest advantage in postradiation fistulae
- Peritoneal flap graft[9] is an easier way of providing an additional layer at transperitoneal repair procedures, by taking a flap of peritoneum from any available surface, most usually the paravesical area.

Readers wishing further detail of individual operations are referred to operative surgical texts or more specific texts on the subject.[7,10,15,24–26]

Postoperative Management

Fluid Balance

Nursing care of patients who have undergone fistula repair is of critical importance, and obsessional postoperative management may do much to secure success. As a corollary, however, poor nursing may easily undermine what the surgeon has achieved. Strict fluid balance must be kept and a daily fluid intake of at least 3 litres, and output of 100 ml per hour, should be maintained until the urine is clear of blood. Hematuria is more persistent following abdominal than vaginal procedures, and intravenous fluid is therefore likely to be required for longer in this situation.

Bladder Drainage

Continuous bladder drainage in the postoperative period is crucial to success, and where failure occurs after a straightforward repair, it is almost always possible to identify a period during which free drainage was interrupted. Nursing staff should check catheters hourly throughout each day, to confirm free drainage, and check output. Catheters should of course drain into a sterile closed drainage system with a nonreturn valve.[27] In circumstances where supplies of sterile disposables are limited, or where standards of nursing are poor, as in many developing countries, open drainage has been advocated, with good success and low infection rates (Ward 1989, personal communication). Bladder irrigation and suction drainage are no longer recommended.

Views differ as to the ideal type of catheter. The caliber must be sufficient to prevent blockage, although whether the suprapubic or urethral route is used is to a large extent a matter of individual preference. The author's usual practice is to use a "belt and braces" approach of both urethral and suprapubic drainage initially, so that free drainage is still maintained if one becomes blocked. The urethral catheter is removed first, and the suprapubic retained, and used to assess residual volume, until the patient is voiding normally.[27]

The duration of free drainage depends on the fistula type. Following repair of surgical fistulae, 12 days is adequate. With obstetric fistulae up to 21 days' drainage may be appropriate, and following repair of radiation fistulae 21–42 days is required. In any of these situations, it is wise to carry out dye testing (see above) before catheter removal if there is any doubt about the integrity of the repair. Where a persistent leak is identified free drainage should be maintained for 6 weeks.

Mobility and Thromboprophylaxis

The biggest problem in ensuring free catheter drainage lies in preventing kinking or drag on the catheter. Restricting patient mobility in the postoperative period helps with this, and some advocate continuous bed rest during the period of catheter drainage. If this approach is chosen patients should be looked on as being at moderate to high risk for thromboembolism, and prophylaxis must be employed;[28] the author's practice is to use both graduated compression stockings and low-dose subcutaneous heparin starting preoperatively, and continued until fully mobile postoperatively.

Results

It is difficult to compare the results of treatment in different series, because the lesions involved and the techniques of repair vary so greatly. Cure rates should be considered in terms of closure at first operation, and vary from 60% to 98%.[16,17,20,29–37] On average one might anticipate 80% cures, and 10% failures; in the case of obstetric fistulae at least, 10% of patients may suffer from postfistula stress incontinence.

Of the 135 patients in the author's series managed in the UK, 9 (7%) healed without operation, 8 (6%) declined surgery, 1 (with coexistent detrusor instability) was asymptomatic on medical treatment, and 3 (2%) underwent primary urinary diversion. Of the remaining 114 who have undergone repair surgery, 109 (96%) were cured by the first operation.

Of the largely obstetric fistulae from Nigeria reviewed by Hilton and Ward,[17] 87% were cured by a first operation, and 99% eventually successfully anatomically repaired, with less than 1% undergoing urinary diversion.

Prevention

It is estimated by the World Health Organization (WHO) that there are approximately 500 000 maternal deaths per year worldwide, and it is clear that the prevalence of obstetric fistulae is closely related to maternal mortality rates. In recognition of this, WHO established a technical working group to investigate the problems of prevention and management of obstetric fistulae. Their recommendations included:

- the extension of antenatal and intrapartum care
- the transfer of women in prolonged labor for delivery by skilled personnel
- the identification of areas where fistulae are still prevalent, so that resources could be mobilized to deal with fistulae more effectively
- the creation of specialized centers for management, training and research, with a specific aim of treating existing cases within 5 years (WHO 1989).[38]

In addition, it is clear that major social change is required in areas of endemicity. Improvement in the status of women in society, the extension of primary education, deferment of marriage and childbearing, improved nutritional status, and contraceptive services are all vital to the prevention of obstetric fistulae.

In the prevention of fistulae following gynecological surgery, we need to be aware of those factors increasing the likelihood of lower urinary tract injury during surgery and must recognize the limits of our own, and perhaps more importantly our trainees', surgical skills. Staff in training should not be expected to undertake surgery, in cases where risk factors are known to be present, without adequate supervision and support. We should be equally aware of the signs of injury in the postoperative period, and should have standard regimens for the management of patients with voiding difficulty in the postoperative period if bladder overdistension and risk of late damage is to be avoided.

Conclusions

In developing countries over 90% of fistulae are of obstetric origin, and are due to pressure necrosis from prolonged obstructed labor, whereas in the west approximately 75% follow pelvic surgery, and half of these cases are associated with simple abdominal hysterectomy. The best estimate is that vesico-vaginal fistula complicates 1 in 1300 hysterectomies.

Where bladder damage is suspected or fistula confirmed following surgery or childbirth, catheterization should be undertaken and continuous drainage maintained; spontaneous healing may occur up to 8 weeks after the initiating event.

Surgery for urogenital fistulae should be undertaken only by surgeons with the appropriate training and experience, and with the versatility to undertake the most appropriate operation by the most appropriate route. Layered closure with avoidance of tension on the suture lines, good hemostasis, and obliteration of dead space are important technical points for successful closure. Interposition grafting with pedicled fat or muscle may be a useful adjunct in fistula surgery, by providing an additional layer to the repair, filling dead space, bringing new blood supply, and encouraging tissue mobility.

References

1. Hilton P (1995) Sims to SMIS–an historical perspective on vesico-vaginal fistulae. In: The Yearbook of the RCOG. RCOG, London, pp. 7–16.
2. Tahzib F (1983) Epidemiological determinants of vesico-vaginal fistulas. Br J Obstet Gynaecol 90: 387–91.
3. Tahzib F (1985) Vesicovaginal fistula in Nigerian children. Lancet 2(8467): 1291–3.
4. Waaldijk K, Armiya'u Y (1993) The obstetric fistula: a major public health problem still unsolved. Int Urogynecol J 4: 126–8.
5. Hilton P (1997) Debate: Post-operative urogenital fistulae are best managed by gynaecologists in specialist centres. Br J Urol 80 (Suppl)(1): 35–42.
6. Raghavaiah N (1974) Double-dye test to diagnose various types of vaginal fistulas. J Urol 112: 811–12.
7. Chassar Moir J (1967) The Vesico-vaginal Fistula, 2nd edn. Bailliere, London.
8. Lawson J (1978) The management of genito-urinary fistulae. Clin Obstet Gynaecol 6: 209–36.
9. Jonas U, Petri E (1984) Genitourinary fistulae. In: Stanton S (ed) Clinical Gynecologic Urology. CV Mosby, St Louis, pp. 238–55.
10. Lawson J, Hudson C (1987) The management of vesico-vaginal and urethral fistulae. In: Stanton S, Tanagho E (eds) Surgery for female urinary incontinence. Springer, Berlin, pp. 193–209.
11. Lawson J (1967) Injuries to the urinary tract. In: Lawson J, Stewart D (eds) Obstetrics and gynaecology in tropics and developing countries. Edward Arnold, London, pp. 481–522.
12. Hudson C (1968) Malignant change in an obstetric vesico-vaginal fistula. Proc R Soc Med 61: 121–4.
13. Davits R, Miranda S (1991) Conservative treatment of vesico-vaginal fistulas by bladder drainage alone. Br J Urol 68: 155–6.
14. Kelly J (1983) Vesico-vaginal fistulae. In: Studd J (ed) Progress in Obstetrics and Gynaecology. Churchill Livingstone, Edinburgh, pp. 324–33.
15. Waaldijk K (1994) Step-by-step Surgery of Vesico-vaginal Fistulas. Campion, Edinburgh.
16. Hilton P (1997) Fistulae. In: Shaw R, Souter W, Stanton S (eds) Gynaecology, 2nd edn. Churchill-Livingstone, London, pp. 779–801.
17. Hilton P, Ward A (1998) Epidemiological and surgical aspects of urogenital fistulae: A review of 25 years' experience in Nigeria. Int Urogynecol J Pelvic Floor Dysfunct 9: 189–94.
18. Sims J (1852) On the treatment of vesico-vaginal fistula. Am J Med Sci XXIII: 59–82.
19. Lawson J (1972) Vesical fistulae into the vaginal vault. Br J Urol 44(6): 623–31.
20. Hamlin R, Nicholson E (1969) Reconstruction of urethra totally destroyed in labour. Br Med J 2: 147–50.
21. Martius H (1928) Die operative Wiederherstellung der vollkommen fehlenden Harnrohre und des Schiessmuskels derselben. Zbl Gynakol 52: 480.
22. Turner-Warwick R (1976) The use of the omental pedicle graft in urinary tract reconstruction. J Urol 116: 341–7.
23. Kiricuta I, Goldstein A (1972) The repair of extensive vesico-vaginal fistulas with pedicled omentum: a review of 27 cases. J Urol 108: 724–7.
24. Hilton P (2001) Fistula repair. In: Smith R, Priore G Del, Curtin J, Monaghan J (eds) An Atlas of Gynaecological Oncology. Martin Dunitz, London, pp. 187–202.
25. Zacharin R (1988) Obstetric Fistula. Springer, Vienna.
26. Mundy A (1993) Urodynamic and Reconstructive Surgery of the Lower Urinary Tract. Churchill Livingstone, Edinburgh.
27. Hilton P (1987) Catheters and drains. In: Stanton S (ed) Principles of Gynaecological Surgery. Springer, London, pp. 257–83.
28. Thromboembolic Risk Factors (THRIFT) Consensus Group (1992) Risk of and prophylaxis for venous thromboembolism in hospital patients. BMJ 305: 567–74.
29. Chassar Moir J (1973) Vesico-vaginal fistulae as seen in Britain. J Obstet Gynaecol Br Commonw 80(7): 598–602.
30. Turner-Warwick RT, Wynne EJ, Handley-Ashken M (1967) The use of the omental pedicle graft in the repair and reconstruction of the urinary tract. Br J Surg 54(10): 849–53.
31. Hudson C, Hendrickse J, Ward A (1975) An operation for restoration of urinary continence following total loss of the urethra. Br J Obstet Gynaecol 82: 501–4.
32. Goodwin W, Scardino P (1980) Vesicovaginal and uretero-vaginal fistulas: a summary of 25 years of experience. J Urol 123(3): 370–4.
33. O'Conor V (1980) Review of experience with vesicovaginal fistula repair. J Urol 123(3): 367–9.
34. Wein AJ, Malloy TR, Carpiniello VL, Greenberg SH, Murphy JJ (1980) Repair of vesicovaginal fistula by a suprapubic transvesical approach. Surg Gynecol Obstet 150(1): 57–60.
35. Lee R, Symmonds R, Williams T (1988) Current status of genitourinary fistula. Obstet Gynecol 71: 313–19.
36. Patil U, Watyerhouse K, Laungani G (1980) Management of 18 difficult vesico-vaginal and urethro-vaginal fistulas with modified Ingelman-Sundberg and Martius operations. J Urol 123: 653–6.
37. Elkins T, Drescheer C, Martey J, Fort D (1988) Vesicovaginal fistula revisited. J Obstet Gynaecol 71: 97–106.
38. World Health Organisation (1989) The prevention of obstetric fistulae. Report of a technical working group. WHO, Geneva.

20 Ureterovaginal Fistula

Craig V. Comiter, Sandip P. Vasavada, and Shlomo Raz

Definition and Etiology

Assessment and Investigation

Management, Technique of Repair and Results

Summary

Definition and Etiology

A ureterovaginal fistula is an abnormal communication between the ureter and vagina. This condition is rarely congenital, resulting from an ectopic ureteral insertion into the vagina. More often a ureterovaginal fistula is acquired, most commonly resulting from a transmural injury to the ureter sustained during pelvic surgery. Distal ureteral obstruction causes continued urinary extravasation and failure of the ureteral defect to heal. Gynecological surgery is the most common cause of ureterovaginal fistulae, particularly after total abdominal hysterectomy for benign or malignant disease.[1] The ureter is particularly susceptible to injury during pelvic surgery because it courses close to the rectum and the female reproductive organs in the pelvis. In fact, ureteral injury has been reported to occur in 0.5%–1% of all pelvic surgeries,[2] and in 1.4%–2% of patients undergoing radical hysterectomy.[3,4]

When ureteral leakage persists and the urine makes its way to the vaginal cuff, ureterovaginal fistulization results. This serious sequela to ureteral injury and its associated incontinence adversely affects the quality of life for the patient and can provoke extreme anxiety for the surgeon.[5,6] Following pelvic surgery, any unexplained abdominal or flank pain or costovertebral angle tenderness, especially in the presence of a fever, should alert the surgeon to a possible ureteral injury. However, more often than not there are no symptoms of ureteral injury or obstruction before the onset of urinary incontinence. The typical presentation of a ureterovaginal fistula is the sudden occurrence of urinary leakage per vagina 1–4 weeks postoperatively.[5,6] Despite the constant incontinence, the patient is able to void normally as well, as the contralateral ureter (if unaffected) continues to fill the bladder normally.

Assessment and Investigation

Diagnosis may be made by a variety of studies. In a woman with vaginal leakage following pelvic surgery, a double dye test can differentiate between vesicovaginal and ureterovaginal fistulae.[7] The vagina is packed and methylene blue is administered intravenously, while red carmine is instilled intravesically. The vaginal pack will stain red with a vesicovaginal fistula, and blue in the presence of a ureterovaginal fistula. Intravenous urogram (IVU) usually reveals varying degrees of hydroureteronephrosis (Fig. 20.1), and will occasionally show a silent kidney.[8] If IVU fails to demonstrate the fistulous site, retrograde ureteropyelography will frequently show the location and magnitude of the abnormal communication[9] (Figs 20.2, 20.3).

Management, Technique of Repair and Results

The management goals for ureterovaginal fistula are to preserve renal function, to prevent and/or treat urinary sepsis, and to cure the incontinence. Treatment options range from observation, to internal drainage via ureteral stent, to external drainage via percutaneous nephrostomy, to open surgical repair, to nephrectomy. Moreover, there remains controversy regarding the role, if any, of protective nephrostomy drainage and the timing of surgical intervention. Some surgeons advocate immediate surgical repair of the injured ureter as soon as the

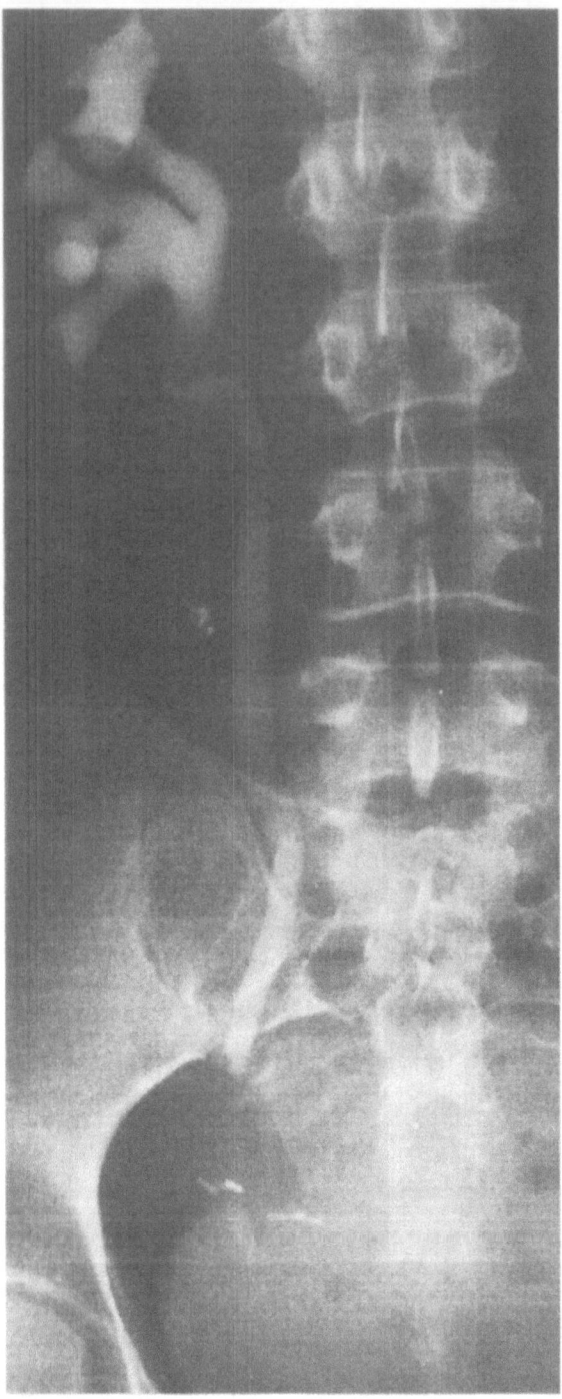

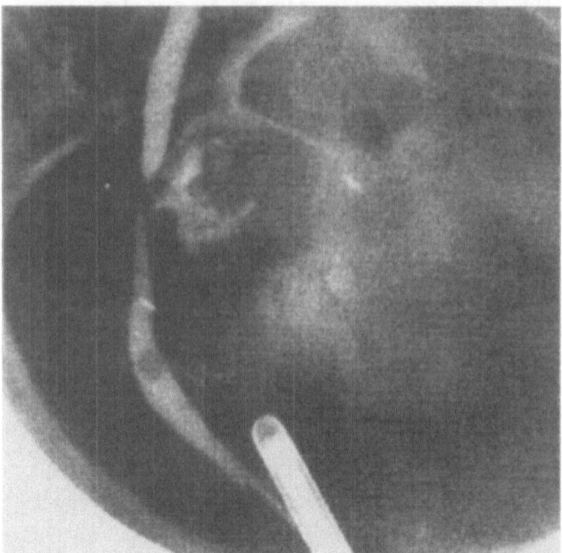

Figure 20.2 Retrograde ureteropyelogram shows the location and severity of ureteral injury. Extravasation of contrast is clearly demonstrated. Reprinted with permission from Patel A, Werthman PE, Fuchs GJ, Barbaric, AL Endoscopic and percutaneous management of ureteral injuries, fistulas, obstruction, and strictures. In: Raz S (ed.), *Female Urology*, 2nd edn. WB Saunders, Philadelphia, 1996, pp. 521–38.

Figure 20.1 Intravenous urogram demonstrating ureteral injury at level of the infundibulopelvic ligament, sustained during transabdominal hysterectomy. Note dilated right ureter above the site of the injury. Reprinted with permission from Patel A, Werthman PE, Fuchs GJ, Barbaric AL: Endoscopic and percutaneous management of ureteral injuries, fistulas, obstruction, and strictures. In: Raz S (ed) *Female Urology*, 2nd edn. WB Saunders, Philadelphia, 1996, pp. 521–38.

Once the diagnosis of ureterovaginal fistula is confirmed, it is crucial that the surgeon define the degree of ureteral obstruction distal to the fistulous site. Any untreated distal obstruction makes spontaneous healing of the fistula extremely unlikely. Ureteral catheterization is recommended in conjunction with retrograde ureteropyelography, for both diagnostic and therapeutic reasons. Inability to pass a ureteral catheter confirms the diagnosis of distal obstruction. If, on the other hand, the surgeon can bypass the fistula with a stent, spontaneous healing is likely with no further treatment.[16–18] The best candidates for nonsurgical management are those with unilateral ureteral injury, documented ureteral continuity, mild to moderate obstruction, and minimal extravasation. Clearly, ureteral stenting should be attempted, as this will better assure a decompressed renal unit while increasing the chance for healing. Conservative management has occasionally succeeded when these radiographic criteria were met, even when ureteral stenting was unsuccessful.[16] In any patient managed nonoperatively, upper tract improvement and resolution of ureteral extravasation must be documented on follow-up evaluation.

Recently, various endourological techniques have been described to improve the likelihood of successful ureteral stenting. Rigid ureteroscopy using low flow irrigation and retrograde passage of a 0.89 mm (0.035 inch) Glide wire across the ureteral defect may be attempted.[18,19] Use of ureteroscopy allows direct vision passage of a wire, and improves the

diagnosis is known.[10–13] Others recommend early upper tract drainage followed by delayed ureteral repair.[14,15] There are also several reports of spontaneous healing of the fistula.[5,13,16]

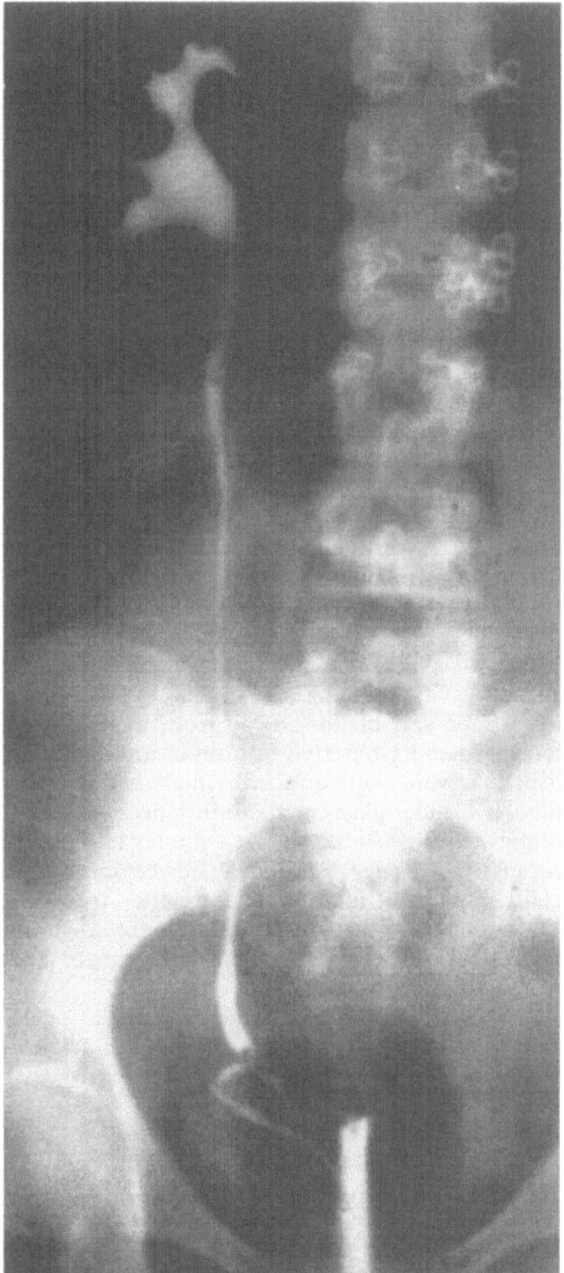

Figure 20.3 Retrograde ureteropyelogram demonstrating ureterovaginal fistula.

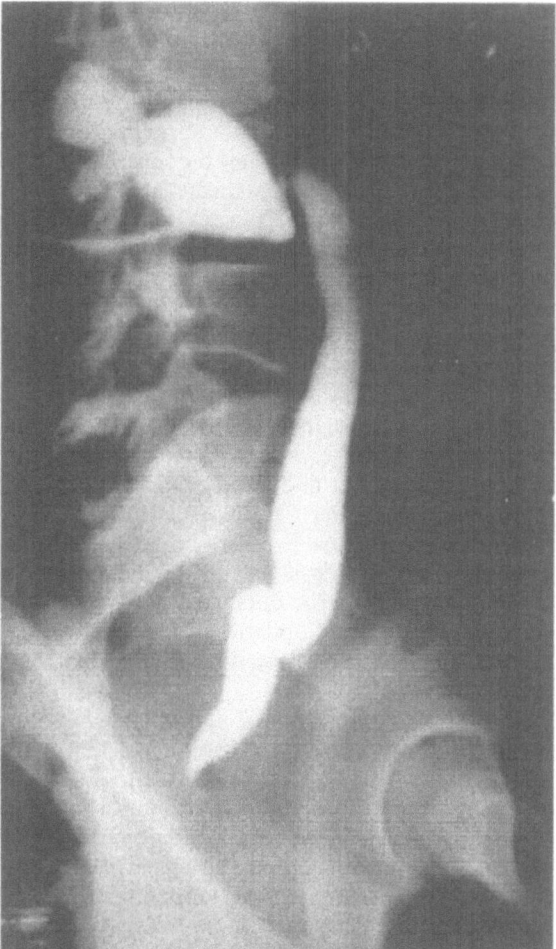

Figure 20.4 Percutaneous nephrostomy was placed for relief of distal ureteral obstruction. Numerous unsuccessful antegrade manipulations resulted in a secondary proximal stenosis. This patient ultimately required Boari flap replacement of the proximal and distal ureter (see Fig. 20.6).

fulcrum at the level of the ureteral orifice, increasing the likelihood of successful stenting.

When retrograde ureteral stenting fails, antegrade percutaneous nephrostomy drainage may be performed under local anesthesia. Placement of a nephrostomy not only relieves obstruction, but also permits access for antegrade ureteral intubation. Percutaneous nephrostomy should clearly be the first option for any patient with an infected collection, or one who is too ill for general anesthesia and retrograde manipulation. Some authors advocate

that a period of observation is warranted after percutaneous nephrostomy, to allow for spontaneous healing of the injured ureter.[20,21] In highly selected individuals, a spontaneous healing rate greater than 50% has been reported following nephrostomy.[20,21]

In most patients, however, prolonged external drainage is undesirable, and elective antegrade stenting is recommended. In cases where antegrade ureteral intubation fails, a combined antegrade-retrograde technique may succeed. After passage of 1–2 antegrade wires, the wire from the bladder is retrieved cystoscopically. With tension applied at both ends of the working wire, sufficient purchase is often provided to permit passage of a retrograde ureteral stent across the fistulous site. When successfully stented, there is a 50–70% chance that the ureterovaginal fistulae will heal without the need for open surgical repair.[18,20–22] Close follow-up is essential, as ureteral stricturing has been reported.[16,22]

If neither antegrade nor retrograde ureteral access is feasible or successful (Fig. 20.4), then open surgical repair is indicated. As with any re-operative procedure, there is controversy regarding the ideal timing of fistula repair. Some surgeons prefer a period of cooling down to allow the inflammation to subside. In such cases, percutaneous nephrostomy is usually performed, for the purpose of draining any infection and for renal protection.[15,23] Others recommend nephrostomy only in cases of azotemia and urosepsis.[5] Simple upper tract drainage will not necessarily stop the incontinence, as some urine will inevitably flow down the ureter and out the vaginal fistulous opening.

Because ureterovaginal fistula can be such a distressing complication, often fostering extreme distress for the patient and anxiety for the surgeon, there has recently been a movement toward early repair of ureterovaginal fistulae. In cases where there is no significant urosepsis, and renal function is relatively preserved, early operative repair may be undertaken.[10–12,21,24] Goodwin and Scardino were the first to show that early repair is feasible with excellent results.[13]

Several principles govern appropriate surgical repair of a ureterovaginal fistula. All abnormal ureter should be sacrificed, little attempt should be made to stay extraperitoneal, continuity should be re-established between a normal ureter and bladder, and adequate drainage must be provided.[11] Occasionally, end-to-end ureteroureterostomy is may be accomplished,[8,9,13] but only in instances of limited inflammation and ureteral loss, so as to permit a tension free-anastomosis. More often than not, ureteroneocystostomy is the preferred repair. Ureteroneocystostomy bypasses the site of injury to the ureter, obviating the need for direct localization by difficult dissection of the injured ureteral segment.[14]

The method of ureteral reimplantation clearly depends on the length of ureteral segment necessary to bypass, which in turn depends on the location of ureteral injury and obstruction, and the degree of ureteral and bladder mobility. Direct ureteroneocystostomy is possible in the majority of cases, often with the aid of psoas bladder hitch to eliminate any anastomotic tension.[6,8,15,25] In the majority of reports, by using sound surgical principles, nearly 100% success may be expected with ureteral reimplantation.[6,8,12,15,25,26] Goodwin and Scardino have recommended the routine use of an antireflux submucosal tunnel in all patients,[13] but others do not feel that antireflux reimplantation is necessary.[1,6] We find that with distal ureteral injuries, a psoas hitch usually suffices to permit a tension-free anastamosis (Fig. 20.5). In cases where the obstructive segment lies more proximally, or when there are multiple sites of obstruction, Boari flap replacement of the distal ureter may be necessary (Fig. 20.6). A Boari flap is also indicated in the presence of a pelvic abscess cavity, enabling the surgeon to anastamose the ureter and bladder away from any infective focus.[5] Falandry reported 14 cases of ureterovaginal fistulae repaired with a cuffed reimplantation with a tubular bladder plasty, with no instances of anastomotic stenosis or leak.[26] More complex methods of reconstruction may occasionally be necessary, especially in cases of high or long ureteral structures. These methods include transureteroureterostomy, renal decensus, renal autotransplantation, or ileo-uretero-cystoplasty.

Nephrectomy or percutaneous ureteral occlusion[27,28] should only be performed as a last resort. Goodwin and Scardino should be credited with

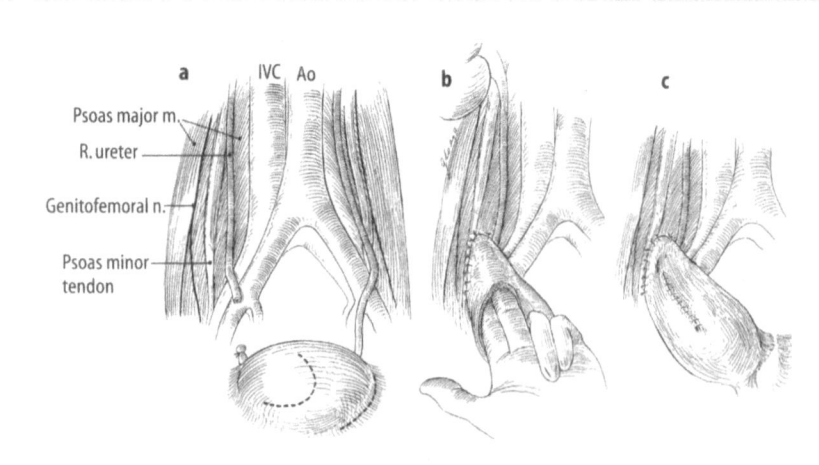

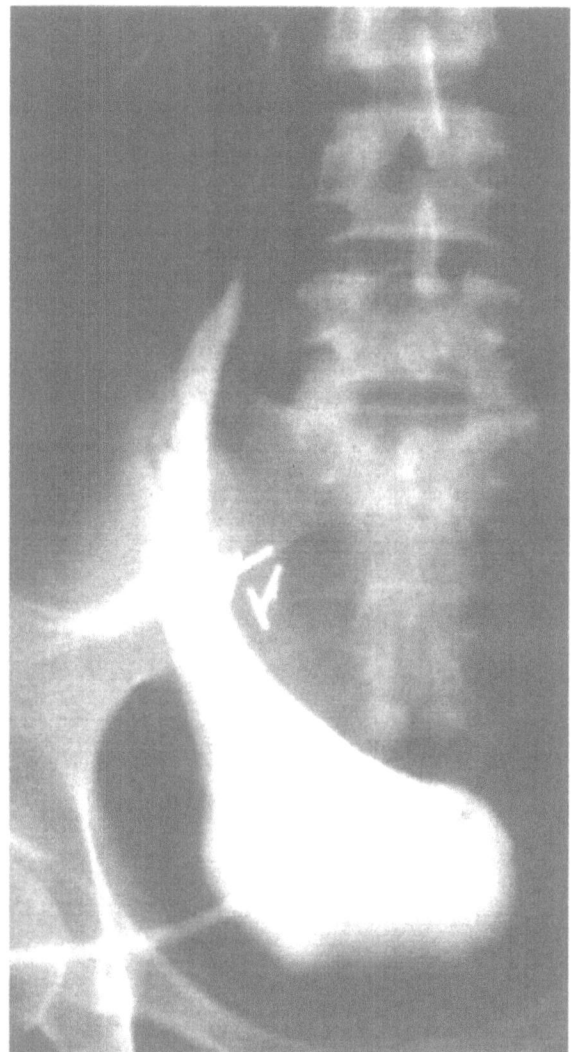

Figure 20.6 In a patient with a ureterovaginal fistula, antegrade manipulation resulted in proximal ureteral stricture. Boari flap ureteral replacement to the proximal ureter solved both problems.

demonstrating that treatments other than nephrectomy can successfully be used to treat ureterovaginal fistula. Lee and Symmonds reported that 48% of patients "required" nephrectomy in their series, the majority of which were performed before 1958,[29] whereas Goodwin and Scardino reported only a 5% nephrectomy rate in their 25 year series culminating in 1980.

Summary

Ureterovaginal fistula is an uncommon complication of pelvic surgery, most frequently occurring after total abdominal hysterectomy and radical hysterectomy. Some degree of distal obstruction in the presence of a transmural injury results in persistence of urinary extravasation, with fistulization to

the vaginal cuff. Urinary incontinence usually presents 1–4 weeks postoperatively, without any prior symptoms. IVU and ureteropyelography will often suffice to demonstrate the location of injury and degree of distal obstruction, both of which are necessary prior to formulating an appropriate treatment plan. Treatment goals should focus on renal preservation, treatment of urosepsis, relief of any obstruction, and alleviation of incontinence.

Given the recent advancements in endourological procedures, retrograde and/or antegrade ureteral stenting is advisable in patients with unilateral injury, only mild to moderate obstruction, minimal extravasation, and some demonstrable ureteral continuity. In patients with complete ureteral obstruction or obstruction with infection, percutaneous nephrostomy is indicated. Definitive surgical repair is necessary for patients in whom ureteral stenting is not possible, and in those who fail conservative therapy. Reimplantation of healthy ureter into a properly mobilized bladder is the procedure of choice. In cases of more proximal ureteral injury, psoas hitch, Boari flap, or even transureteroureterostomy or ileal ureteral replacement may be necessary. Nephrectomy or percutaneous ureteral occlusion should be used only as a last resort.

References

1. Symmonds RE (1976) Ureteral injuries associated with gynecologic surgery: prevention and management. Clin Obstet Gynecol 19: 623.
2. Mattingly RF, Borkowf HI (1978) Acute operative injury to the lower urinary tract. Clin Obst Gynaec 5: 123.
3. Brown RB (1977) Surgical and external ureteric trauma. Aust N Z J Surg 47: 4741.
4. Baltzer J, Kaufmann C, Ober KG, Zander J (1980) Complications in 1,092 radical abdominal hysterectomies with pelvic lymphadenectomies. Geburtshilfe Frauenkeilkd 40: 1.
5. Mandal AK, Sharma SK, Vaidyanathan S, Goswami AK (1990) Ureterovaginal fistula: summary of 18 years' experience. Br J Urol 65: 453.
6. Murphy DM, Grace PA, O'Flynn JD (1982) Ureterovaginal fistula: a report of 12 cases and review of the literature. J Urol 128: 924.
7. Raghavaiah NV (1974) Double-dye test to diagnose various types of vaginal fistulas. J Urol 112: 811.
8. Benchekroun A, Lachkar A, Soumana A et al. (1998) Ureterovaginal fistulas. 45 cases. Ann Urol (Paris) 32: 295.
9. El Ouakdi J, Jlif H, Boujnah B, Ayed M, Zmerli S (1989) Uretero-vaginal fistula. Apropos of 30 cases. J Gynecol Obstet Biol Reprod (Paris) 18: 891.
10. Badenoch DF, Tiptaft RC, Thakar DR, Fowler CG, Blandy, JP (1987) Early repair of accidental injury to the ureter or bladder following gynaecological surgery. Br J Urol 59: 516.
11. Beland G (1977) Early treatment of ureteral injuries found after gynecological surgery. J Urol 118: 25.
12. Witeska A, Kossakowski J, Sadowski A (1989) Early and delayed repair of gynecological ureteral injuries. Wiad Lek 42: 305.
13. Goodwin WE, Scardino PT (1980) Vesicovaginal and ureterovaginal fistulas: a summary of 25 years of experience. J Urol 123: 370.

14. Meirow D, Moriel EZ, Zilberman M, Farkas A (1994) Evaluation and treatment of iatrogenic ureteral injuries during obstetric and gynecologic operations for non-malignant conditions. J Am Coll Surg 178: 144.

15. OnuoraVC, al-Mohalhal S, Youssef AM, Patil, M (1993) Iatrogenic urogenital fistulae. Br J Urol 71: 176.

16. Peterson DD, Lucey DT, Fried FA (1974) Nonsurgical management of ureterovaginal fistula. Urology 4: 677.

17. Kihl B, Nilson AE, Pettersson S (1982) Uretero-neocystostomy in the treatment of postoperative uretero-vaginal fistula. Acta Obstet Gynecol Scand 61: 341.

18. Patel A, Werthman PE, Fuchs GJ, Barbaric AL (1996) Endoscopic and percutaneous management of ureteral injuries, fistulas, obstruction, and strictures. In: Raz S (ed) Female Urology, 2nd ed. W. B.Saunders, Philadelphia, Pa., pp. 521–38.

19. Lingeman JE, Wong MY, Newmark JR (1995) Endoscopic management of total ureteral occlusion and ureterovaginal fistula. J Endourol 9: 391.

20. Lask D, Abarbanel J, Luttwak Z, Manes A, Mukamel E (1995) Changing trends in the management of iatrogenic ureteral injuries. J Urol 154: 1693.

21. Dowling RA, Corriere JN, Sandler CM (1986) Iatrogenic ureteral injury. J Urol 135: 912.

22. Lang EK (1981) Diagnosis and management of ureteral fistulas by percutaneous nephrostomy and antegrade stent catheter. Radiology 1378: 311.

23. Godunov BN, Loran OB, Gazimagomedov GA, Kaprin AD (1997) The diagnosis and treatment of ureterovaginal fistulae. Urol Nefrol (Mosk.) 6: 44.

24. Bennani S, Joual A, El Mrini M, Benjelloun S (1996) Ureterovaginal fistulas. A report of 17 cases. J Gynecol Obstet Biol Reprod (Paris) 25: 56.

25. Server G, Alonso M, Ruiz JL, Osca Garcia JM, Jimenez Cruz, JF (1992) Surgical treatment of uretero-vaginal fistulae caused by gynecologic surgery. Actas Urol Esp 16: 1.

26. Falandry L (1992) Uretero-vaginal fistulas: diagnosis and operative tactics. Apropos of 19 personal cases. J Chir (Paris) 129: 309.

27. Reddy PK, Moore L, Hunter D, Amplatz K (1987) Percutaneous ureteral fulguration: A nonsurgical technique for ureteral occlusion. J Urol 138: 724.

28. Papanicolaou N, Pfister RC, Yoder IC (1985) Percutaneous occlusion of ureteral leaks and fistulae using nondetachable balloons. Urol Radiol 7: 28.

29. Lee RA, Symmonds RE (1971) Ureterovaginal fistula. Am J Obstet Gynecol 109: 1032.

21 Rectovaginal Fistulae

Feza H. Remzi and Tracy L. Hull

Most rectovaginal fistulae are less than 10–20 mm in diameter. Defects less than 5 mm are considered small, those 5–25 mm are considered medium, and those larger than 25 mm are considered large.[4]

Etiology

Most rectovaginal fistulae are acquired. The etiology is secondary to trauma, infection, or inflammation. Congenital abnormalities are rare and will not be discussed here.

A rectovaginal fistula is usually a physically and psychologically debilitating problem for women in all age groups. Discharge of stool and flatus from the vagina may be minimal and tolerable, but most women find this problem disabling and devastating.

Definition and Classification

A *rectovaginal* fistula is an abnormal epithelial-lined communication between the rectum and the vagina. An *anovaginal* fistula is one in which the tract opens at or distal to the dentate line. Most are anovaginal fistula, but for convenience, many authors (including the authors of this chapter) group all under the term rectovaginal fistula. Rectovaginal fistula account for less than 5% of all anal fistulae.[1]

These fistulae can be classified based on location, size, and etiology. When classified by location, they are usually grouped as low, mid, or high fistula depending on anatomic location and relationship to the anus and the rectum.[2,3] In our experience we define low rectovaginal fistulae as those involving the lower third of the vagina and/or anal canal, and the rest as high rectovaginal fistula (Fig. 21.1).

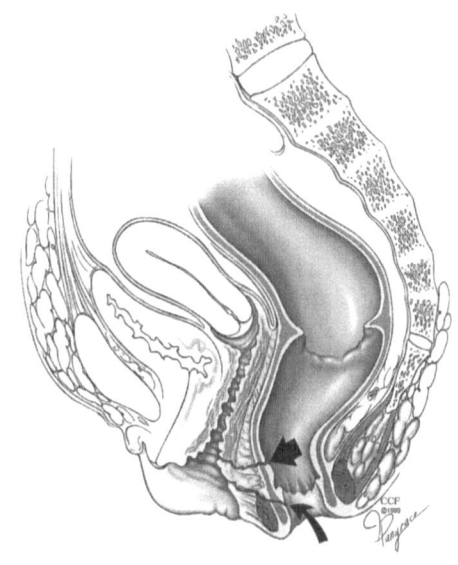

Figure 21.1 Low rectovaginal fistula involve the lower third of the vagina and/or the anal canal. The rest are high rectovaginal fistulae. The figure demonstrates an example of high (wide arrow) and low (thin arrow) rectovaginal fistula. Reprinted with the permission of the Cleveland Clinic Foundation.

The precise incidence of each type of acquired rectovaginal fistula is difficult to determine since most series are small and reflect the referral pattern of the institution. In most institutions, obstetric injuries account for the majority of rectovaginal fistula.[5,6] During vaginal deliveries rectal tears have been reported to occur 5–24% of the time.[7–9] It is difficult to know how many of these result in fistula. Specialized centers, including our own, see a higher rate of rectovaginal fistulae due to Crohn's disease. Other common causes of acquired rectovaginal fistula include irradiation damage, cryptoglandular disease, infections, iatrogenic injury, and malignancy.

Evaluation

Symptomatic fistulae produce varying degree of distress in patients. Some may not even need treatment. Therefore, when considering treatment, physicians must weigh the risks and consequences of treatment with the patient's degree of symptoms. Evaluation starts with a thorough history including careful questions regarding symptoms related to the fistula, bowel habits, and obstetric history. It is important to inquire about other medical problems because these may influence treatment options.

After the history has been completed, a physical examination starts with inspection in the prone jackknife position. Associated skin tags, fissures, anal fistulas, and abscess should raise the suspicion of Crohn's disease. Digital examination should focus on assessing the vagina and anorectum together. Induration in the rectovaginal septum, sphincter tone, and the presence of an anal stricture should be noted. If an adequate examination cannot be performed because of discomfort, the patient should be examined under anesthesia in the operating room. Proctoscopy is performed to evaluate the rectum. This is especially important for patients with Crohn's disease to assess activity and distensibility of the rectum. The site of the fistula (low or high) is noted next. At times, the fistula cannot be found although the patient describes classic symptoms. Examination of the vaginal side may demonstrate darker mucosa at the fistula site. With the patient in the lithotomy position, insufflating the anorectum with air after placing water in the vagina may demonstrate bubbles from the rectal side to the vagina. Rarely, a tampon is placed in the vagina while methylene blue is instilled into the rectum to reveal the tract. If a fistula is present, the tampon will be stained in 15–20 minutes. Occasionally a gastrograffin enema may demonstrate the fistula, but this is rare. If clinical concern of Crohn's disease exists, a colonoscopy and small-bowel series are needed to assess the extent of the disease and exclude the possibility of an enterovaginal fistula.

Incontinence is another issue which may need evaluation preoperatively. If problems with control of stool are found during the history, anal manometry should be considered. Incontinence may be related to destroyed sphincter muscles secondary to Crohn's disease or an obstetric sphincter injury. Incontinence from either of these two reasons will affect the surgical planning and the approach.

Active perianal sepsis will also influence the surgical planning. No definitive successful repair can be done in the face of sepsis. Drainage of the perianal sepsis with insertion of a seton may be needed to control sepsis. Occasionally a diverting stoma may be needed to allow the sepsis to resolve and the surrounding tissue to become soft and supple.

Techniques and Principles of Repair

Rectovaginal fistulae can be repaired transabdominally or via a perineal approach. The type of approach depends on the location, morphology, and etiology of the fistula. The majority of fistulae are repaired via a perineal approach, so in this chapter we concentrate on those approaches.

After a rectovaginal fistula has been identified and the work-up completed, the timing of the surgery is planned. For example, a fistula due to an obstetrical injury may require 3–6 months after the injury to allow the edema, sepsis, and induration to subside. If the surgeon does not wait for this to occur, a successful outcome may be compromised.

Perineal repair of a rectovaginal fistula can be accomplished transanally, transvaginally, or transperineally. Success with all of these approaches has been reported. The choice of the operation depends on the surgeon's training and experience. We usually prefer the transanal approach. This avoids division of the sphincters and allows a repair on the high-pressure side of the fistula (the anorectal side). If there is an accompanying sphincter injury, the transperineal approach is preferred. Repairs are done under general or regional anesthesia. Our patients undergo a full bowel preparation. We give preoperative intravenous antibiotics such as metronidazole and a third generation cephalosporin. Patients have a Foley catheter and pneumatic compression stockings for the operation.

Transanal Technique

There are several types of transanal repairs. Three subgroups of repairs are discussed here: advancement rectal flap, side-to-side flap, and advancement rectal sleeve.

Advancement Rectal Flap

The advancement rectal flap was first described by Noble in 1902,[10] later modified by Laird in 1948[1] and then further modified by Gallagher.[11,12] Patients are placed in the prone jackknife position. Proctoscopy is done to clean any residual fluid. The vagina and perineum are prepared with povidine-iodine. Four to six effacement sutures are placed on the anal verge (Fig. 21.2) A lighted Hill–Ferguson retractor (Electro Surgical, Rochester, NY, USA) is used for optimal exposure. The submucosa is infiltrated with 1 : 100 000 epinephrine to aid in hemostasis and assist in raising the flap. To further clarify the submucosal plane, saline is injected. Saline is used instead of further epinephrine to avoid epinephrine toxicity and help decrease ischemia of the flap. A "smiley face" or curvilinear incision about one-third to one-half circumference of the lumen is created using cutting current with the electrocautery. The incision starts distal to the fistula opening. Using the curvilinear flap avoids ischemia at the corners, which may be seen if a rectangular flap is used. The flap consists of mucosa, submucosa and a few circular muscle fibers of the internal sphincter. Mobilization continues at least 4 cm proximal to the fistula. This allows a viable and tension-free flap to be advanced distally to cover the fistula. After the mobilization is complete, the fistula is next cored out. This can be best achieved by placing a finger in

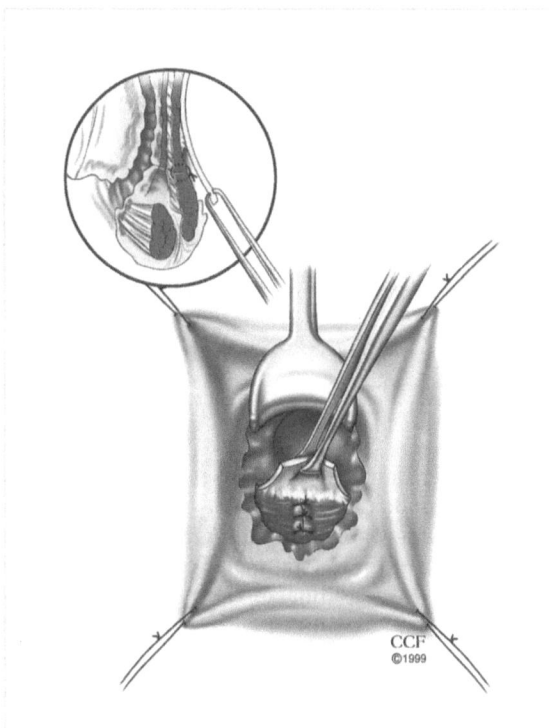

Figure 21.3 After the fistula defect is closed in the muscle, the distal aspect of the flap is trimmed, thus eliminating the area where the fistula traversed the flap. Reprinted with the permission of the Cleveland Clinic Foundation.

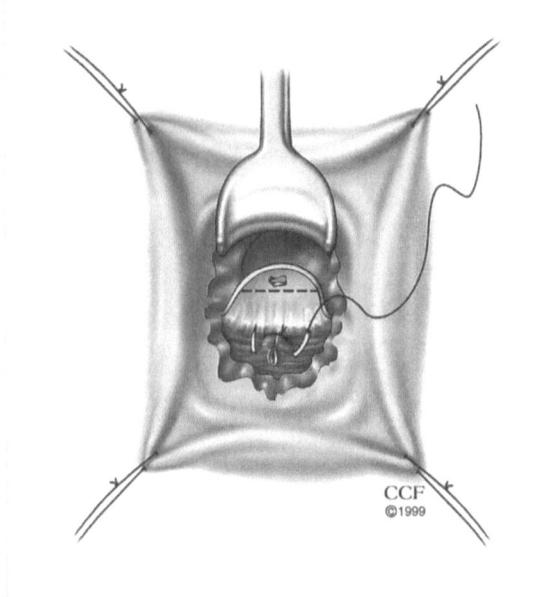

Figure 21.2 For the advancement rectal flap repair, 4–6 effacement sutures are placed on the anal verge to assist in visualization. A semicircular flap of mucosa, submucosa, and a few fibers of the internal sphincter muscle is raised. The fistula is cored out and the defect is closed. Reprinted with the permission of the Cleveland Clinic Foundation.

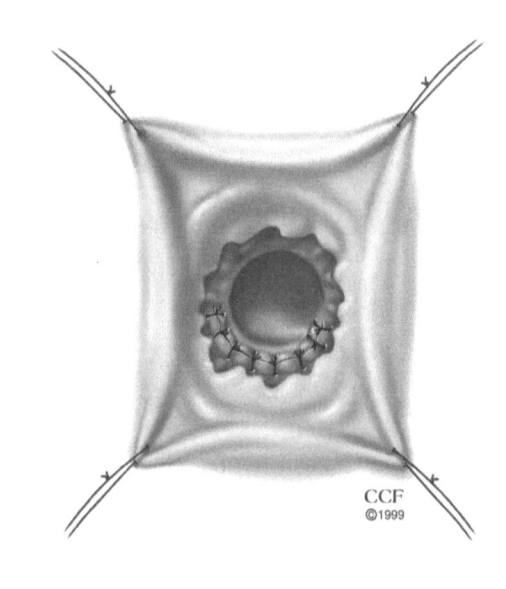

Figure 21.4 The flap is then sutured to the neodentate line with interrupted sutures. Reprinted with the permission of the Cleveland Clinic Foundation.

the vagina and dissecting around the track on to the finger with electrocautery. The vaginal defect is left open, hemostasis is obtained, and the apex of the flap that contains the fistula opening is excised. The defect is closed in two or three layers with 2-0 polyglycolic acid suture on a UR-6 needle (Vicryl; Ethicon, Inc., Somerville, NJ) by placing figure-of eight-sutures. (Figs 21. 2, 21.3) The flap is then sutured to the neodentate line with interrupted 3-0 polyglycolic acid. (Fig. 21.4)

Side-to-Side Flap

Raising a tension-free curvilinear flap can be very difficult or impossible in certain circumstances, for instance when the fistula is 2–5 cm above the dentate line. In these circumstances the defect can be closed in a longitudinal or transverse side-to-side fashion depending on the widest diameter of the internal opening after the excision of the fistula. Figures 21.5 and 21.6 demonstrate this type of flap repair.

Advancement Rectal Sleeve

The advancement rectal sleeve is a complex procedure. This type of repair is reserved for women with severely diseased anal canal mucosa and a normal rectum (such as a fistula from Crohn's disease) or when there is too much tension with a curvilinear flap. This flap involves a 90–100% circumferential mobilization of the anal canal mucosa and submucosa starting distal to the fistula opening. Mobilization continues cephalad above the anorectal ring entering the plane used when doing an Altmeir procedure. When sufficient mobilization has occurred, the fistula is cored out and closed (as described above). The diseased segment is excised and the "sleeve" of tissue is advanced down and sewn to the neodentate line. Usually a temporary ileostomy is used with this type of flap repair (Figs 21.7, 21.8).

Transperineal Technique

The transperineal repair is used when dealing with a rectovaginal fistula associated with a sphincter

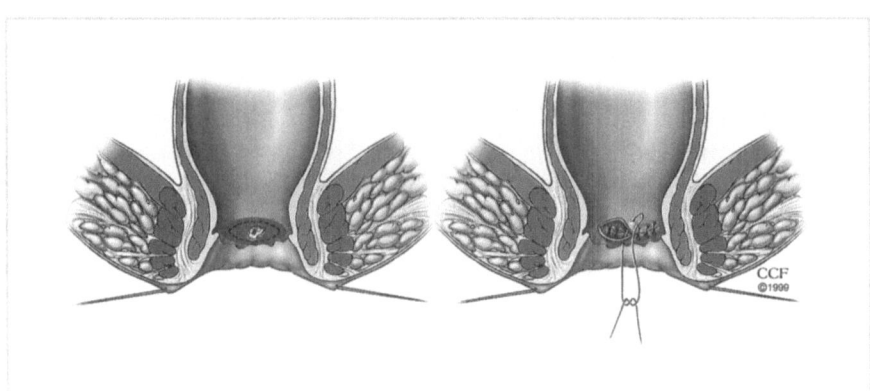

Figure 21.5 When the internal opening of the fistula is widest in the horizontal axis, a side to side flap is chosen. A transverse elliptical excision is made of the fistula. The fistula is cored out and closed. The skin is closed. Reprinted with the permission of the Cleveland Clinic Foundation.

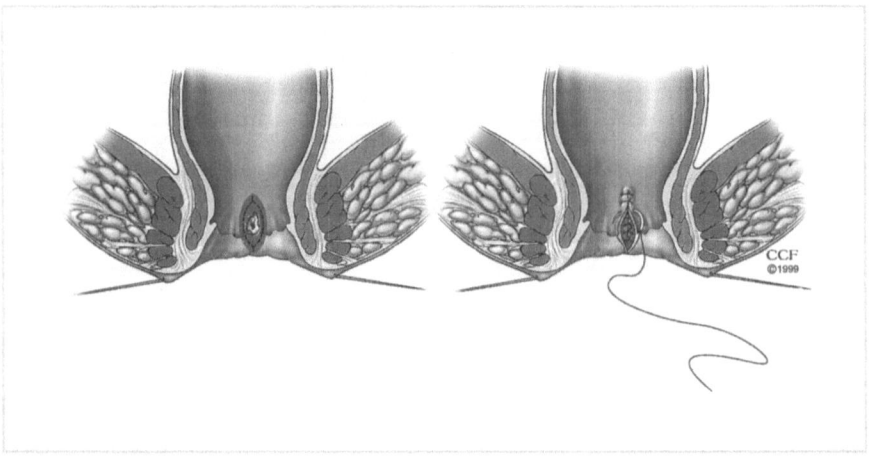

Figure 21.6 When the internal opening is widest in the longitudinal axis or high, another variation of the side to side flap is chosen. A vertical elliptical excision is made of the fistula. The fistula is cored out and closed. The skin is closed. Reprinted with the permission of the Cleveland Clinic Foundation.

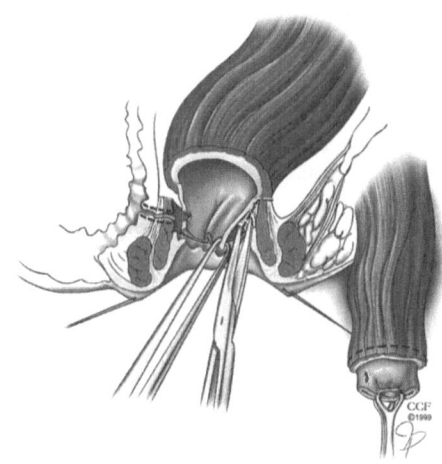

Figure 21.7 If the advancement rectal sleeve flap is chosen, 90–100% circumferential mobilization of the anal canal mucosa and submucosa is first performed. Mobilization continues cephalad above the anorectal ring entering the same plane used when performing an Altmeier procedure. When sufficient mobilization has occurred, the fistula is cored out and closed. The diseased segment is trimmed from the "sleeve" of tissue. Reprinted with the permission of the Cleveland Clinic Foundation.

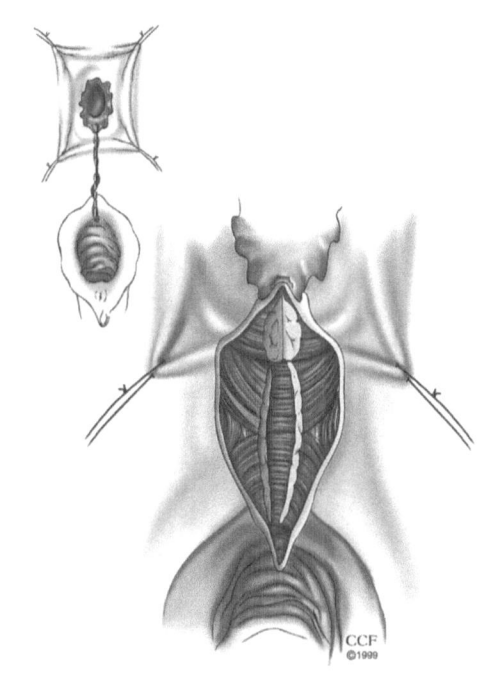

Figure 21.9 With the transperineal technique of rectovaginal fistula closure, the fistula is unroofed. This leaves a defect similar to a fourth-degree obstetric tear. The muscle edges are dissected and the fistula tract debrided or excised. Reprinted with the permission of the Cleveland Clinic Foundation.

injury or incontinence. A probe is placed in the fistula tract and the tissue distal to the probe is incised. This produces a defect similar to a fourth-degree obstetrical tear. The muscle edges are dissected and a layered repair is then performed using an overlapping technique of the sphincter complex. We use mattress sutures of 2-0 PDS suture (Ethicon, Inc., Somerville, NJ) to close the muscle. The skin is closed with 3-0 absorbable suture (Figs 21.9, 21.10).

Transvaginal Technique

The transvaginal technique is not usually used at our institution, but some surgeons prefer this approach. The flap is constructed from vaginal mucosa. The fistula is cored out, closed, and the flap is sutured in place after trimming the diseased portion.[13]

Miscellaneous

Fecal diversion must be considered in certain cases with any of the above repairs. Unfortunately, there are no universally accepted guidelines as to when a stoma should be used. We commonly use fecal diversion in patients with previous multiple repairs, associated major sphincter injury, and complex inflammatory bowel disease cases.

Postoperative management of these repairs depends on the surgeon's preference. We have variation in postoperative care even at our own institution. The senior author's practice consists of postoperative intravenous antibiotics for 2–3 days followed by 5 days of oral antibiotics. Patients are nil-by-mouth for 2 days and then usually discharged on the second

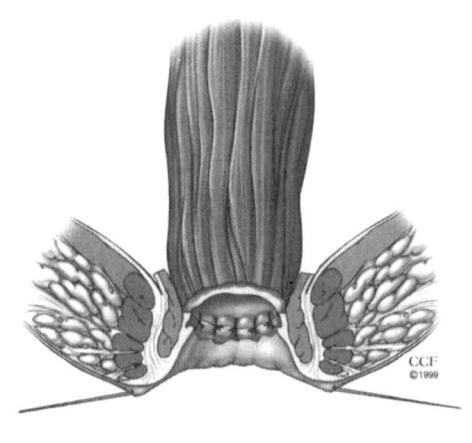

Figure 21.8 The "sleeve" of tissue is advanced down and sutured to the neodentate line. Reprinted with the permission of the Cleveland Clinic Foundation.

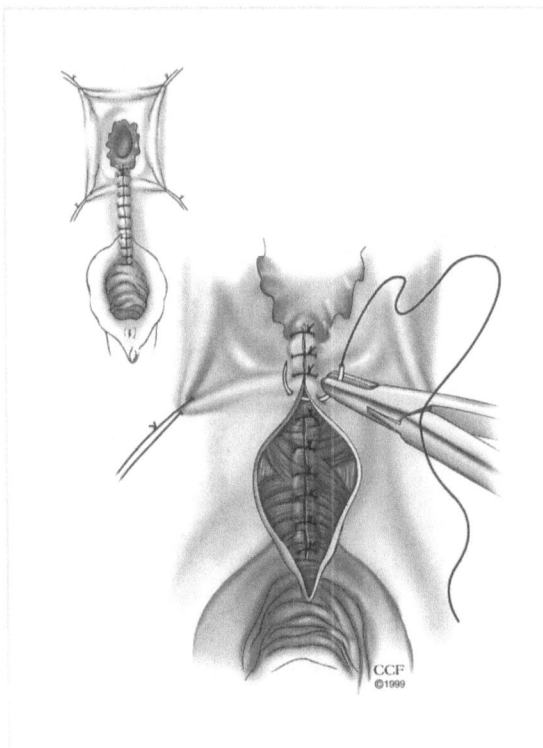

Figure 21.10 The muscles are reapproximated and a layered repair using an overlapping sphincter technique is done if possible. (The figure does not show the overlapping technique but simply an approximation.) The skin is then closed with simple sutures. Reprinted with the permission of the Cleveland Clinic Foundation.

or third postoperative day. Avoiding constipation is important. At discharge, patients are told to take 30 ml (an ounce) orally of mineral oil daily for about 2 weeks along with psyllium supplements to avoid constipation. Should constipation occur, oral laxatives are used.

Results

Excellent results have been reported with each technique described. The mortality is essentially zero and the major morbidity is quite low. The advancement rectal flap is the most common type of repair. Success rates have been reported from 41% to 100%.[14] However, not all authors experience high success rates. Anal sphincter integrity may influence the success rate. In one study advancement rectal flaps were only successful in 50% of patients with a normal preoperative sphincter function and in 33% with abnormal function.[14] This led these authors to recommend a procedure similar to the above described transperineal technique if there was a history of previous repairs or a sphincter defect. Crohn's disease also influences the results. In a study from our institution, 67% of women with Crohn's

disease had healing after initial repair with an advancement rectal flap.[15]

There are not many publications on the side-to-side flap repair. The circumstances which lead to the use of this flap are rare, namely a high, long, and/or wide fistula. In our experience 50% of patients with Crohn's disease and a rectovaginal fistula healed after this procedure.

The advancement rectal sleeve flap is also used under special circumstances. At our institution it is commonly used in women with a scarred anus from Crohn's disease or after an initial failed repair. In women with Crohn's disease 60% healed when this was the primary repair.[15] Other authors have reported healing in case reports using this technique.[16,17]

The transperineal approach achieves success rates of 78–100%.[14] As previously stated, it is important to consider this type of repair if the patient has sphincter compromise.

The transvaginal technique has been reported to be 93% successful.[13] We have no experience with this technique, but it seems to be preferred by gynecologists and in select circumstances of Crohn's disease where anal mobilization would be impossible or rectal disease exists.

Conclusion

Rectovaginal fistulae can be successfully repaired. This chapter has touched on the most popular types of repairs. Initial evaluation is essential to choose the best repair for each individual. Surgeons should be familiar with several types of repairs. Failed repairs should not discourage the surgeon from attempting another repair, as long as the tissue is supple and no sepsis exists.

References

1. Laird DR (1948) Procedures used in the treatment of complicated fistulas. Am J Surg 76: 701–8.
2. Bentley RJ (1973) Abdominal repair of high rectovaginal fistula. J Obstet Gynaecol Br Commonw 80: 364–7.
3. Rosenshein NB, Genadry RR, Woodruff JD (1980) An anatomic classification of rectovaginal septal defects. Am J Obstet Gynecol 137: 439–42.
4. Hull TL, Fazio VW (1996) Rectovaginal fistula in Crohn's disease. In: Phillips RKS, Lunnis PJ (eds) Anal Fistula. Chapman & Hall, London, pp. 143–62.
5. Given FT (1970) Rectovaginal fistula: A review of 20 years' experience in a community hospital. Am J Obstet Gynecol 108: 41–6.
6. Lowery AC, Thorson AG, Rothenberger DA et al. (1988) Repair of simple rectovaginal fistula. Influence of previous repairs. Dis Colon Rectum 31: 676–8.
7. Hibbbard LT (1978) Surgical management of rectovaginal fistulas and complete perineal tears. Am J Obstet Gynecol 130: 139–41.

8. Homsi R, Diakoku NH, Littlejohn J et al. (1994) Episiotomy: Risks of dehiscence and rectovaginal fistula. Obstet Gynecol Surv 49: 803–8.

9. Kozok LJ (1989) Surgical and non-surgical procedures associated with hospital delivery in the United States: 1980–1987. Birth 16: 209–13.

10. Noble GH (1902) A new operation for complete laceration of the perineum designed for the purpose of eliminating danger of infection from the rectum. Trans Am Gynecol Soc 27: 357.

11. Russell TR, Gallagher DM (1977) Low rectovaginal fistulas: Approach and treatment. Am J Surg 134: 13–18.

12. Gallagher DM, Scarborough RA (1962) Repair of low rectovaginal fistula. Dis Colon Rectum 5: 193–5.

13. Bauer JJ, Sher ME, Jaffin J (1991) Transvaginal approach for repair of rectovaginal fistulae complicating Crohn's disease. Ann 213: 151–8.

14. Tsang CBS, Madoff RD, Wong WD et al. (1998) Anal sphincter integrity and function influences outcome in rectovaginal fistula repair. Dis Colon Rectum 41: 1141–6.

15. Hull TL, Fazio VW (1997) Surgical approaches to low anovaginal fistula in Crohn's disease. Am J Surg 173: 95–8.

16. Berman IR (1991) Sleeve advancement anorectoplasty for complicated anorectal\vaginal fistula. Dis Colon Rectum 34: 1032–7.

17. Simmang CL, Lacey SW, Huber PJ Jr (1998) Rectal sleeve advancement: repair of rectovaginal fistula associated with anorectal stricture in Crohn's disease. Dis Colon Rectum 41: 787–9.

22 Diagnosis and Management of Female Urethral Diverticula and Urethrovaginal Fistula

Daniel S. Blander and Philippe E. Zimmern

Urethral Diverticula

Diverticulum of the female urethra (UD) is relatively rare, occurring in less than 6% of the population. Since first reported by Hey in 1805,[1] UD have become more commonly diagnosed due to better understanding of their presentation and to improvements in imaging of the female urethra. But, despite improved ability to diagnose these lesions, surgical repair remains challenging. Maintaining a high index of suspicion for UD and employing meticulous surgical technique in their reconstruction are ways to improve treatment.

Etiology

Two types of UD have been described: congenital and acquired. Congenital UD are considered rare because young patients rarely present with UD.[2] Typically, this type of diverticulum inserts on the anterior surface of the urethra and is thought to be the result of an abortive attempt at urethral duplication.[3] Congenital UD may also be associated with the insertion of an ectopic ureterocele.

Acquired UD probably results from infection of the periurethral glands. Such infection leads to inflammation and obstruction of the ductal system which prevents adequate drainage and encourages formation of an abscess. Eventually, the abscessed gland ruptures into the urethral lumen (Fig. 22.1). Although childbirth has been hypothesized to play a role in the origin of UD, it probably does not. The diagnosis is frequently made in nulliparous women but rarely so in grand multiparous individuals.[4] Other etiologies such as trauma and sexually transmitted diseases have also been hypothesized.[5]

Clinical Presentation

Because of the variable manner in which UD present, the clinician must maintain a high index of suspicion to diagnose them. A typical patient between the ages of 20 to 60 presents with incontinence, urinary tract infection, painful vaginal mass, bladder outlet obstruction, dyspareunia, or postvoid dribbling. Some patients with UD may be asymptomatic. Symptomatically, UD may mimic conditions such as urinary tract infection or interstitial cystitis; however, neither of these conditions produces a painful periurethral mass. Lesions such as urethral tumors, Skene's gland abscess, Gartner's duct cyst, or ectopic ureterocele can mimic closely presentation of a UD.[6]

Several conditions can be associated with UD. Stones may form inside UD,[7] which can often be appreciated as calcifications on KUB radiography or the scout films of voiding cystourethrograms (VCUG). Hematuria is a rare finding with UD and, if

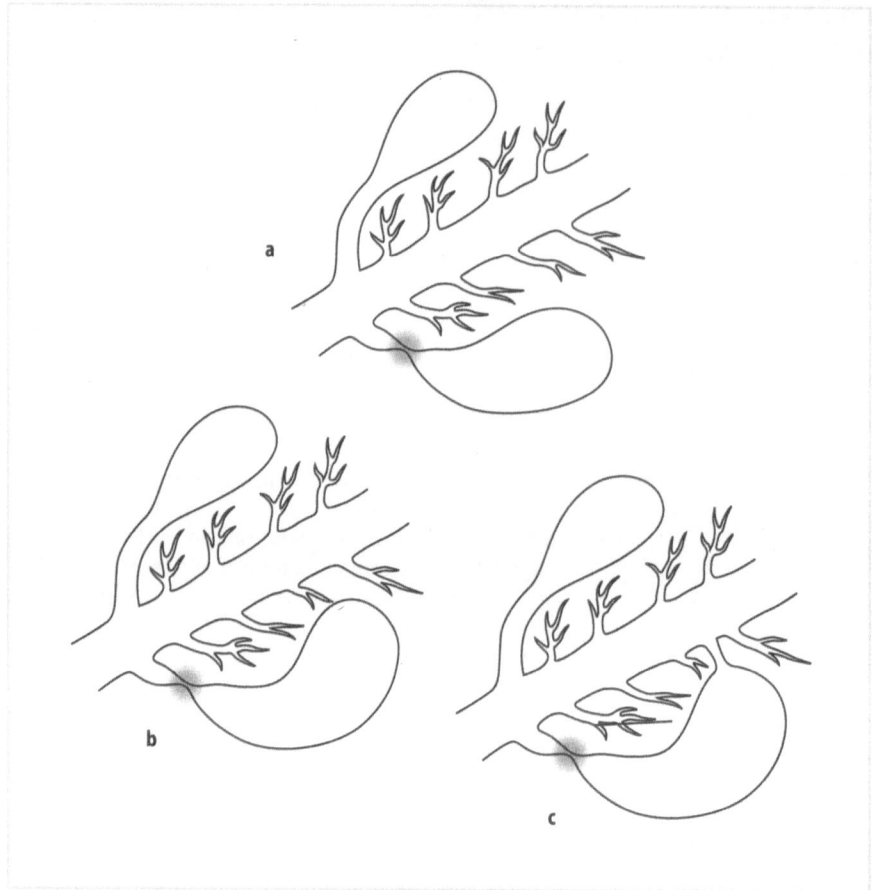

Figure 22.1 a Inflammation of the periurethral ducts can lead to obstruction of that duct. **b** Obstruction of the duct leads to abscess formation in the periurethral gland. **c** The abscess cavity ruptures into the urethral lumen.

found, should raise the concern of an epithelial tumor within the UD.[8,9]

Diagnosis

History and physical examination are the cornerstone of the evaluation of UD. In many cases, purulent drainage can be expressed from the periurethral mass at the time of the physical examination. Urethroscopy with a blunt-ended female cystoscope or flexible cystoscope can be helpful in assessing the level of communication between the UD and urethral lumen, although this connection can not be visualized in all cases.[10]

Imaging

Advances in imaging the female urethra have dramatically improved the ability to detect UD. Diverticula can often be seen during a voiding cystourethrogram (VCUG) or on the post-void film of an intravenous urogram (Fig. 22.2). These examina-

tions depend on a relatively large patent tract between the UD and urethral lumen. Recognizing the limitations of conventional voiding cystourethrography, Davis and Cian[11] developed a double balloon catheter to perform positive pressure urethrography (PPU) of the female urethra. This technique is still considered by some as the "gold standard" for detection of UD.

Recent reports, however, demonstrate the utility of magnetic resonance imaging (MRI) in evaluation of UD. Kim and co-workers[12] report that MRI is more sensitive than either cystoscopy or VCUG in the diagnosis of UD. Neitlich et al.[13] found that MRI was more accurate than PPU in diagnosing UD. Use of an endoluminal coil (eMRI) has been shown to enhance sensitivity of this diagnostic technique, providing excellent anatomic detail of the female urethra, which can be useful in surgical planning[14,15] (Fig. 22.3). Because MRI does not depend on the presence of contrast within a UD for visualization, this technique has even been able to demonstrate UD that do not communicate with the urethral lumen.[16]

Transvaginal ultrasound is also effective in the evaluation of UD.[17] It permits visualization of small

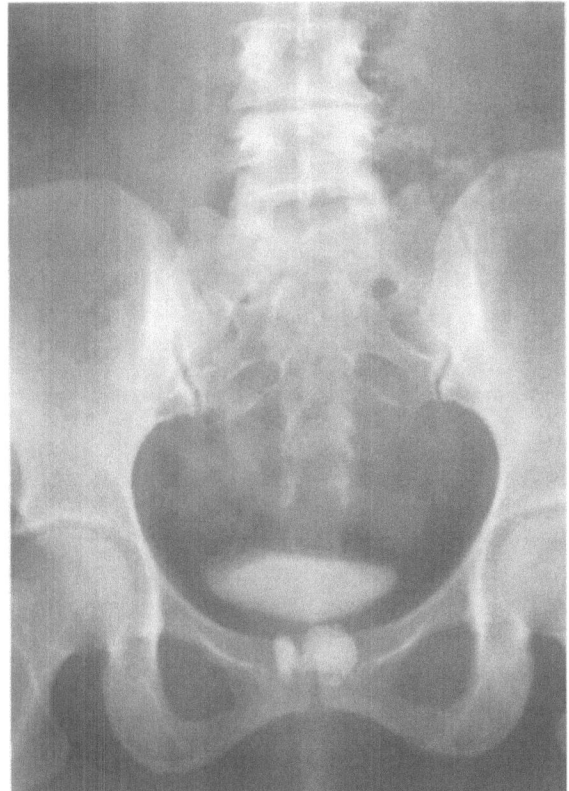

Figure 22.2 Post-void film of an IVU demonstrating a urethral diverticulum.

standing VCUG as the primary radiologic staging procedure for UD and we have found this examination not only sensitive in diagnosing UD, but also very helpful in evaluating patients for concomitant urethral hypermobility. It is essential that patients void during the study and that true lateral views are taken so that the three-dimensional nature of the UD can be appreciated. Endoluminal MRI can be helpful as an adjunctive study in patients whose physical findings do not correlate with the extent of the diverticulum visualized on VCUG or who have had previous surgery for UD.

Urodynamics

Because 50–70% of women with UD present with urinary incontinence,[21,22] proper evaluation of this disorder plays an important role in the workup of UD. A patient complaining of incontinence may have:

- post-void dribbling from spontaneous drainage of the UD between voids
- "pseudoincontinence" or leakage of the diverticular contents with stress maneuvers; or
- concomitant genuine stress incontinence.

Even with exhaustive history taking and careful physical examination, it can be extremely difficult to distinguish among these conditions.

If UD is not the obvious source of incontinence, urodynamic studies may help the clinician decide whether an anti-incontinence procedure should be performed during urethral diverticulectomy. Pre-operative urodynamics may also help identify patients with detrusor instability who may benefit from more aggressive postoperative anticholinergic therapy.

noncommunicating UD and may therefore be helpful in individuals with a normal VCUG.[18] Three-dimensional ultrasound, a new technique, has been shown to provide excellent anatomic detail of the urethra in men and women. This technique may further enhance sensitivity of this imaging modality.[19,20]

Table 22.1 lists the major pros and cons of the various imaging modalities. We generally employ

Table 22.1. Advantages and disadvantages of imaging modalities		
Modality	Advantages	Disadvantages
Voiding cystourethrogram (VCUG)	Inexpensive No special equipment necessary Dynamic study with voiding views	Requires instrumentation of urinary tract May underestimate size and complexity of UD
Positive pressure urethrogram (PPU)	Better sensitivity than VCUG Does not require patient to void	Requires special catheter and trained technician Requires instrumentation of urinary tract Lateral views difficult to obtain
Endoluminal MRI (eMRI)	Provides superb anatomic detail Does not require specially trained technician Visualizes loculations and non-communicating intraurethral wall diverticula Easy to interpret Does not require instrumentation of the urinary tract	Expensive Not universally available
Three-dimensional ultrasound	Provides good anatomic detail Visualizes loculations Does not require instrumentation of the urinary tract	Requires specially trained technician Not universally available Interpretation operator dependent

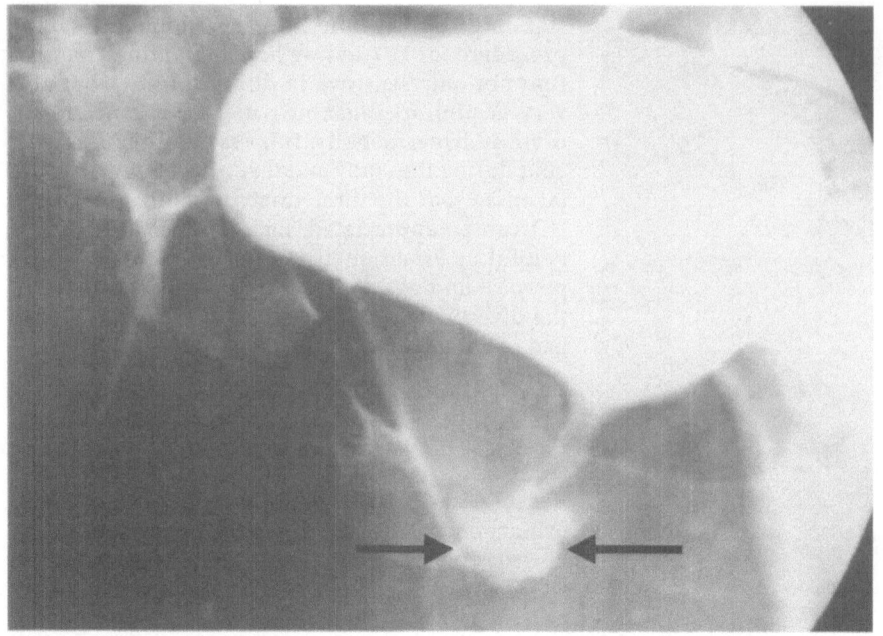

a

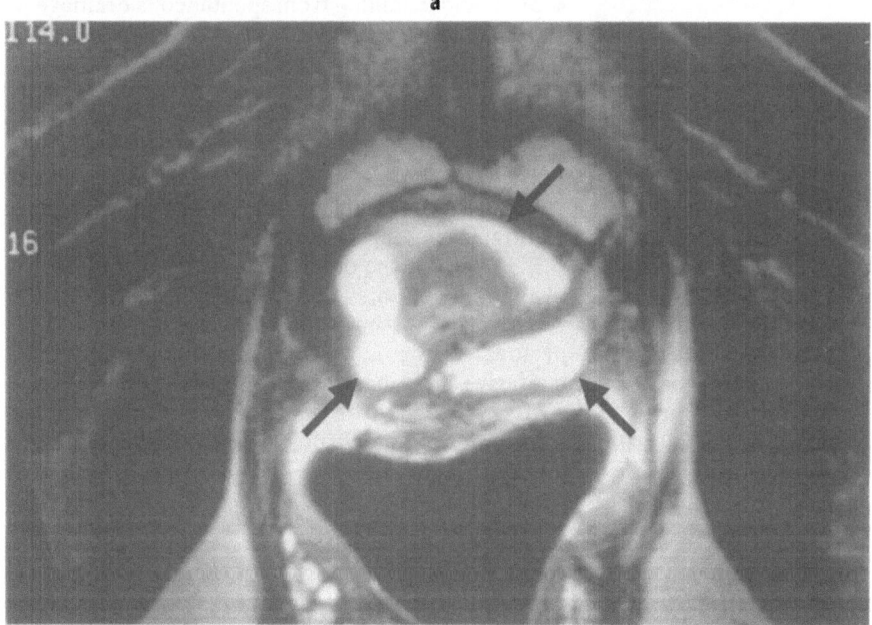

b

Figure 22.3 VCUG (a) and eMRI (b) in a patient with a circumferential UD (arrows). The posterior extent of the diverticulum is not clearly visualized on the VCUG.

Classification

Leach and co-workers[23] propose a comprehensive classification scheme for UD. Their system categorizes UD based on location (L), number (N), size (S), configuration (C1), location of communication (C2), and continence (C3). Because UD vary so significantly in size, configuration, and complexity, this classification system allows precise categorization of UD in order to plan the most effective operative approach and to compare outcomes between series.

A simpler scheme, which categorizes UD type, etiology, and concomitant continence status, has also been proposed.[24]

Repair

The simplest procedure for treating UD was described by Spence and Duckett.[25] This technique involves marsupialization of the diverticulum into the vagina, essentially creating a hypospadiac ure-

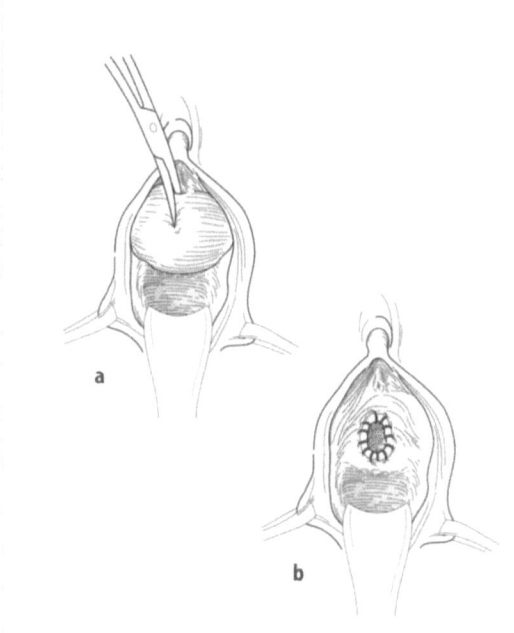

Figure 22.4 Spence–Duckett marsupialization procedure. This procedure is safe only for a distal diverticulum (**a**). The urethra is incised from the meatus to the mouth of the diverticulum (**b**) and the edges of the diverticulum and urethra are spatulated to the vaginal mucosa.

thra (Fig. 22.4). Although this technique is not suited for UD proximal to the continence mechanism, it has been successful in over 90% of cases of distal UD.[26] Miskowiak and Honnens de Lichtenberg[27] described a similar technique in which transurethral incision was used to convert a narrow-mouthed UD into a wide-mouthed diverticulum able to drain more easily. Ellik[28] described a transvaginal incision of proximal UD that employed insertion of oxycel in the diverticulum to induce its "fibrotic assimilation."

Excision of UD has been described as "difficult, irksome, and precarious," and as often being performed in an operative field resembling "a bloody quagmire." (Kropp, 1957). Due to the inherent difficulty of this dissection, many techniques have been described to facilitate transvaginal excision of UD. Originally, Young[29] suggested inserting a sound in the urethra to aid in the definition of the diverticulum during transvaginal incision. Subsequently, many modifications of this procedure were developed. Cook and Pool[30] recommended coiling a catheter within the UD prior to transvaginal excision. Silicon rubber[31] and fibrin[32] have also been used to fill diverticula prior to transvaginal excision.

Transvaginal excision is the preferred procedure for complex or more proximal UD. Transvaginal excision can be performed through semilunar suburethral,[33] vertical midline,[34] laterally based U-flap[35] or inverted U[36] vaginal incisions. Any incision must

allow access to the entire diverticulum so that complete excision can be achieved. And, regardless of approach, it is essential to develop vaginal flaps to allow a tension-free closure in which overlapping suture lines are avoided.

After diverticulum excision, we perform a two-layer closure, using the urethral wall and periurethral fascia, and then a vaginal flap advancement to avoid overlapping suture lines. When a large amount of dead space is created by diverticulectomy or there is a tenuous repair, we interpose a Martius graft before vaginal closure. The graft minimizes the risk of secondary fistula and provides a well-vascularized environment during the initial healing phase.[22,37]

Surgical Technique

The patient may be placed either prone or supine for diverticulectomy. We prefer the high dorsal lithotomy position because it allows us to place a suprapubic tube without repositioning the patient. We use candy cane stirrups. Because these reconstructions can take hours, we carefully pad potential pressure points and use pneumatic compression stockings to help prevent formation of deep venous thrombosis. At the beginning of the procedure, we place a suprapubic catheter using a Lowsley tractor, followed by a urethral Foley catheter to help define the urethral lumen.[36,37] The diverticulum is exposed through a broad-base, inverted U-shaped incision in the anterior vaginal wall. The apex of the incision should be distal to the diverticulum (Fig. 22.5). The flap is then carefully dissected off the diverticulum, leaving the periurethral fascia intact.

Once the flap is developed, a transverse incision is made in the periurethral fascia, exposing the diverticulum. We place many small holding sutures to minimize trauma to the tissues. Meticulous dissection of the diverticulum is then conducted using magnifying loops. The neck of the diverticulum must be carefully isolated (Fig. 22.6). It is often necessary to open the diverticulum to identify the communication with the urethra. The diverticulum is excised at its neck, which leaves a defect in the urethral wall. The diverticular sac should be sent for histologic examination to definitively rule out a neoplastic process. In the case of a horseshoe diverticulum, as much lateral dissection of the diverticulum as possible should be accomplished prior to entering the lumen of the diverticulum. Once the diverticulum is opened, with careful dissection, a plane can be identified medially between the urethral wall and the diverticulum, and the UD can be dissected off the urethra (Fig. 22.7).

A tension-free vertical closure of the urethral wall is then performed using absorbable sutures. Ensuing

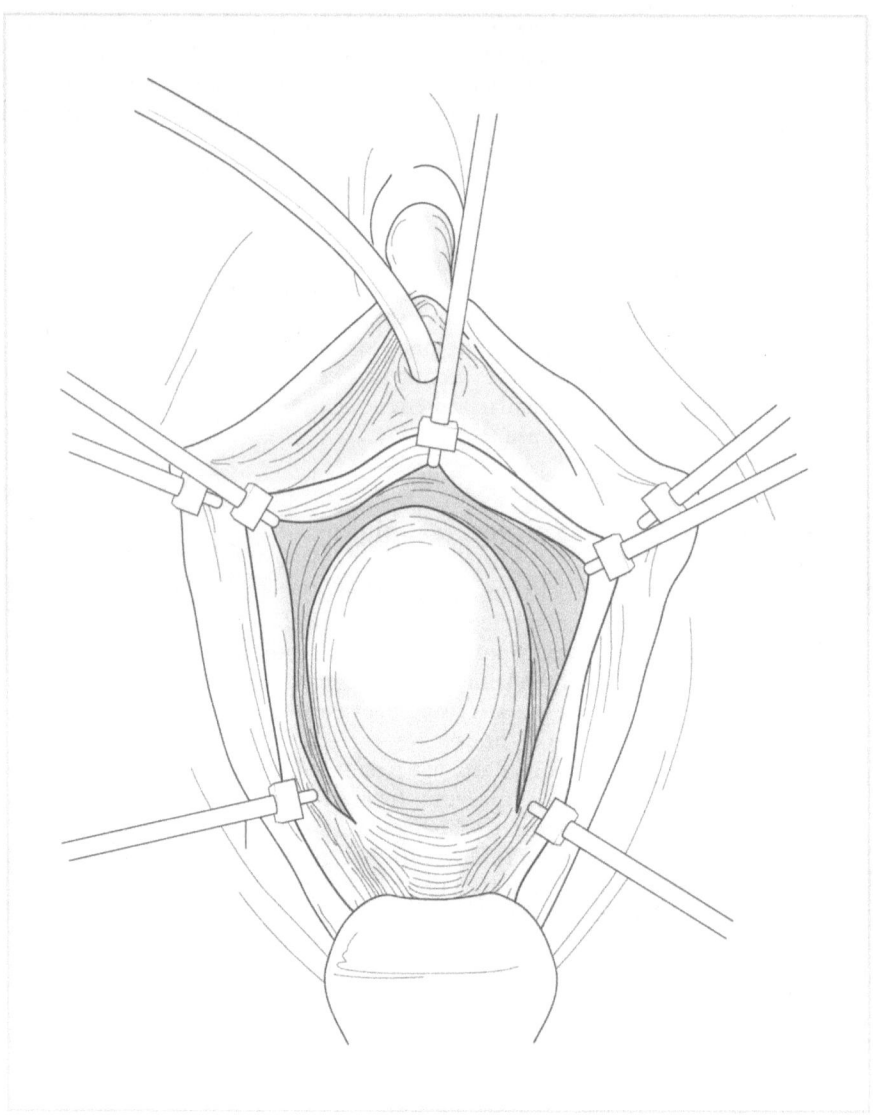

Figure 22.5 Vaginal wall incision for urethral diverticulectomy with hooks from Scott retractor in place.

defects in the urethral wall can be quite large, so it is important to use a small (12–14 French) urethral catheter to facilitate closure of the urethra. After the urethral defect is closed, we place a 5 French catheter along the urethral catheter and infuse saline to ensure the urethral closure is watertight.

The periurethral fascia, when available, is horizontally closed with absorbable sutures. If tissues are of poor quality, or a significant amount of dead space is left after removal of the diverticular cavity, a Martius labial fat pad flap can be interposed between the urethral closure layers and the vaginal wall (Fig. 22.8). Finally, the vaginal wall is closed using a running absorbable suture, and a vaginal pack is placed for 24–48 hours. Use of non-overlapping suture lines minimizes risk of forming postoperative urethrovaginal fistula.

Postoperatively, patients are continued on intravenous antibiotics and aggressive anticholinergic therapy. The suprapubic tube and urethral Foley catheters are left to drainage. Patients are usually discharged on oral antibiotic coverage on postoperative day 1 or 2. A VCUG is performed 10–14 days postoperativley and repeated 2 weeks later if a urethral leak is detected. The suprapubic tube is removed when the VCUG demonstrates no leak and the patient voids with a low postvoid residual. Antibiotic therapy is discontinued after removal of the suprapubic tube.

If simultaneous bladder neck suspension is to be performed, the endopelvic fascia should be perforated and suspension sutures passed prior to dissection of the urethral diverticulum. This minimizes risk of contaminating the retropubic space,[38] although Swierzewski and McGuire[21] reported no complications in 7 patients in whom pubovaginal sling was performed after the excision of a UD. In general, we do not perform concomitant bladder

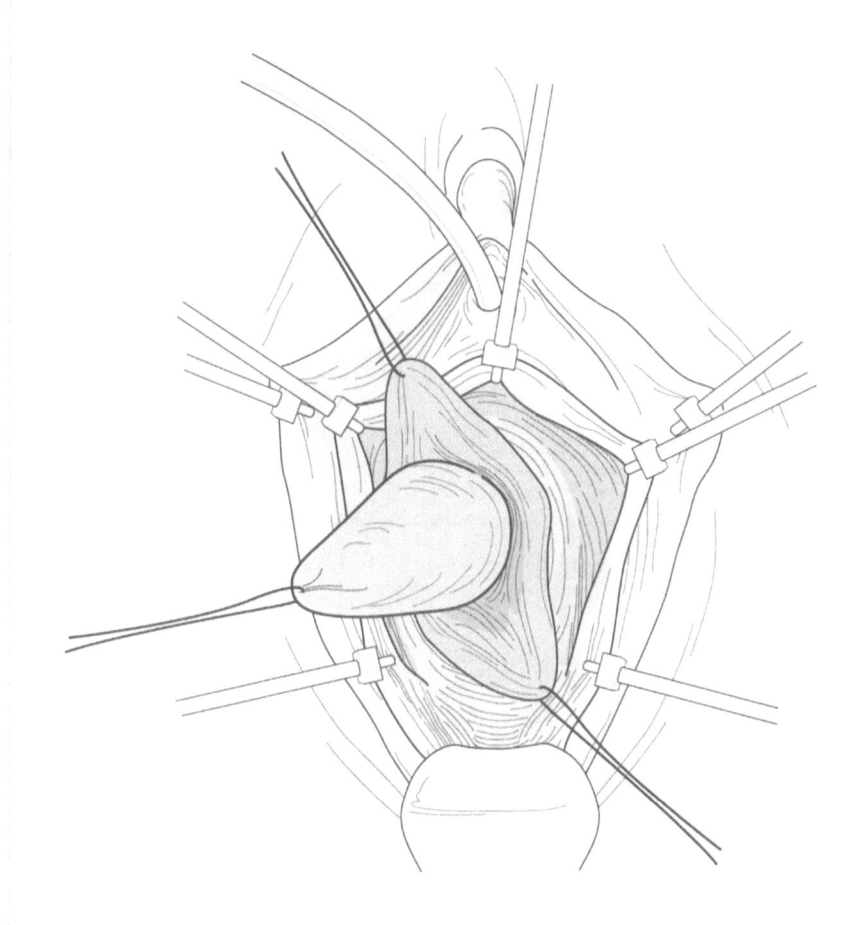

Figure 22.6 Dissection utilizing holding sutures to apply traction on the diverticulum and periurethral fascia.

neck suspension unless the patient has obvious genuine stress incontinence with a large degree of urethral hypermobility. We find it easier to perform this procedure once the patient's vaginal wall has healed from urethral diverticulectomy.

Results

Contemporary series of diverticulectomy demonstrate success rates from 70% to 95%.[22] Using the transvaginal technique described above, Ganabathi and co-workers report a recurrence rate of less than 10%; 86% of patients are cured of their initial complaint. Of patients who underwent a concomitant bladder neck suspension, almost 80% were cured of incontinence. Success rates of over 70% for the treatment of concomitant genuine stress incontinence have been reported with the use of both pubo-vaginal slings[21] and transvaginal bladder neck suspension.[37]

Complications

Postoperative complications after urethral diverticulectomy include urethrovaginal fistula (1–8%; see below), UD recurrence or persistence (1–30%), incontinence from secondary ISD (2–16%), and urethral stricture (0–5%).[22] Recurrence rates should decrease with better-quality preoperative imaging studies. Careful preoperative physical examination to assess hypermobility and performing preoperative urodynamic studies when indicated should limit risk of postoperative incontinence.

Consent

It is essential to obtain informed consent before surgical repair of a UD. Because of the proximity of the diverticulum to the midurethral complex, there is a significant risk of postoperative incontinence. Urethrovaginal fistula and UD recurrence

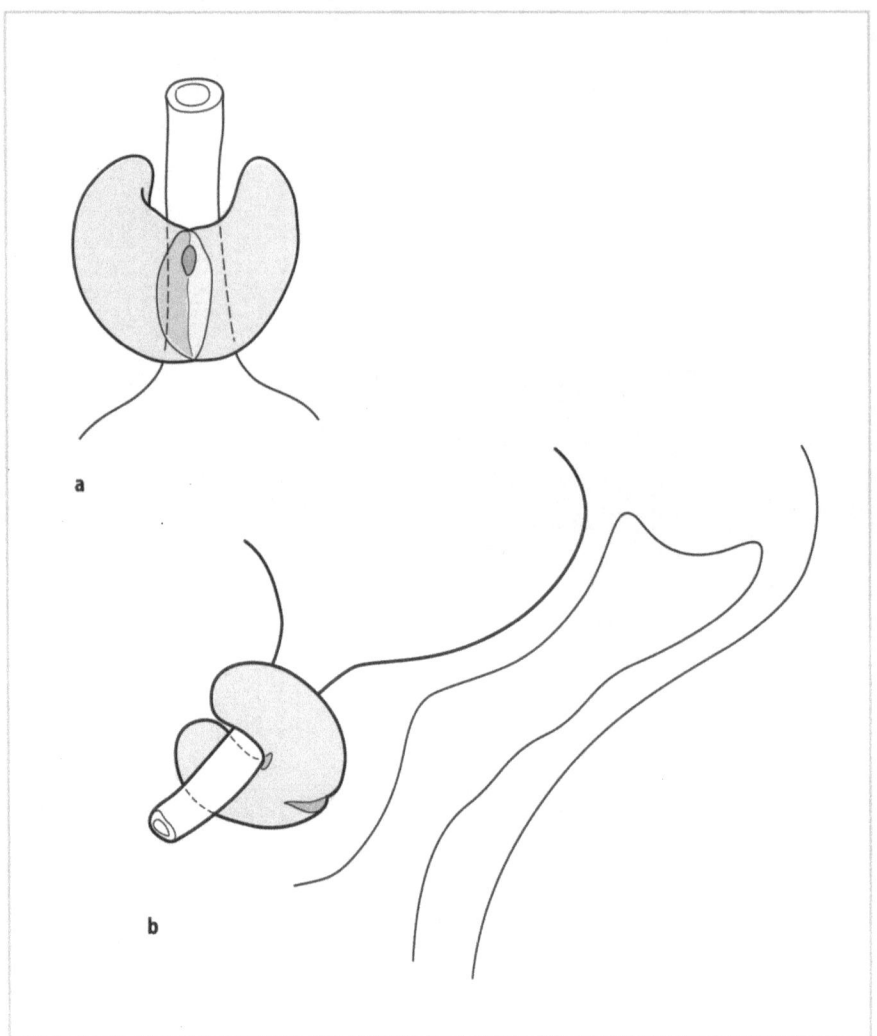

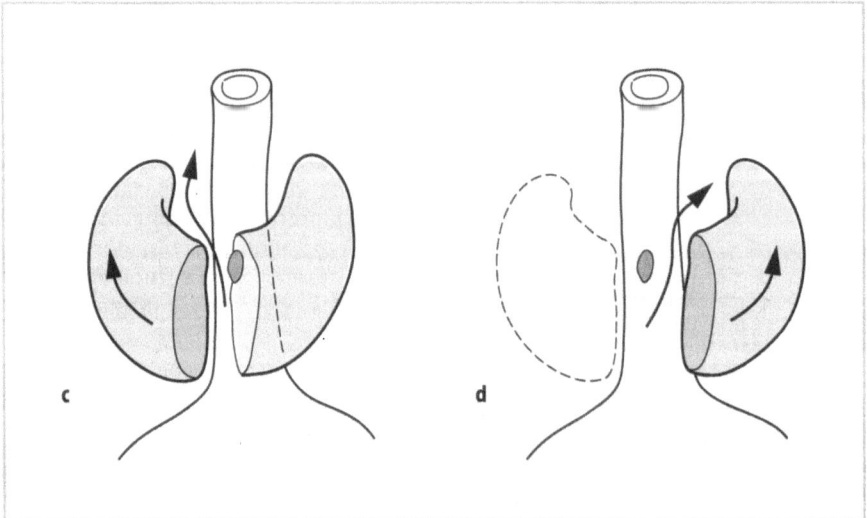

Figure 22.7 AP (**a**) and oblique (**b**) views of a horseshoe diverticulum where the anterior wall of the UD is opened in order to facilitate dissection. The UD is divided in the midline and each "lobe" is dissected off the outer urethral wall (**c,d**).

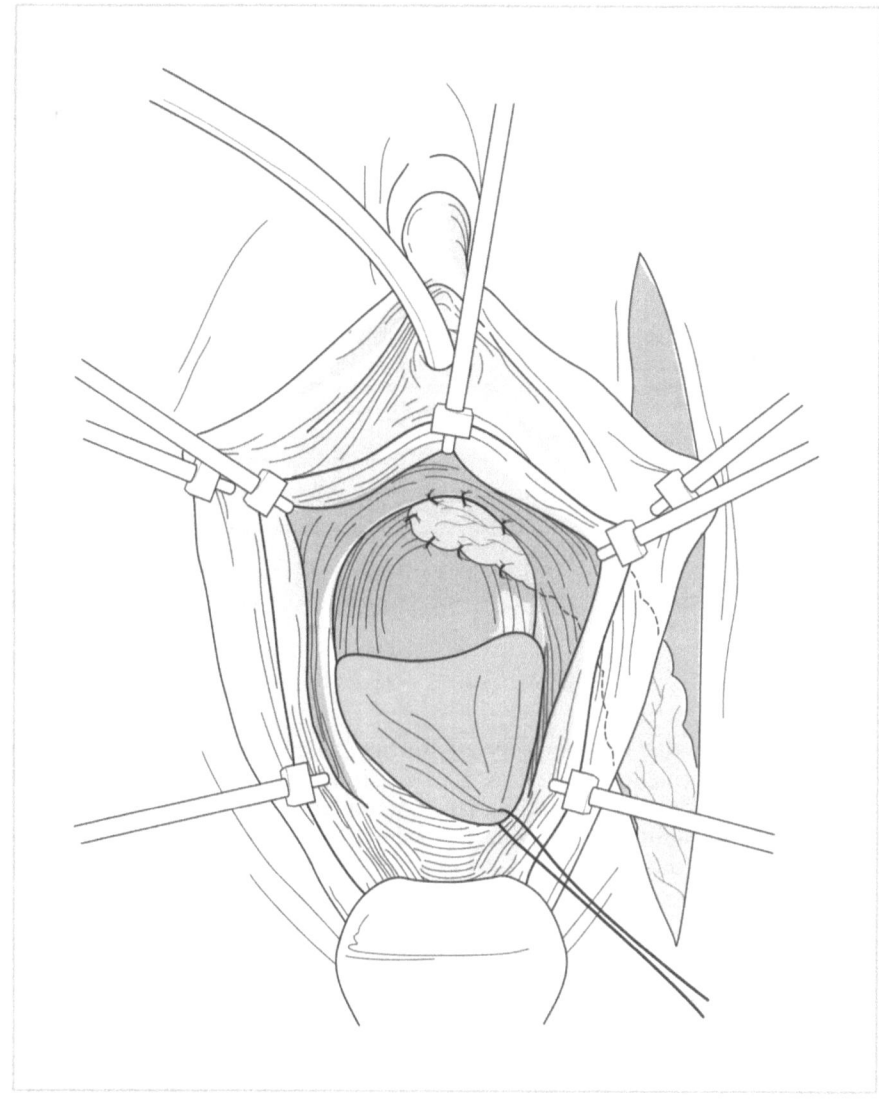

Figure 22.8 Martius flap in situ after diverticulectomy and urethral repair, before vaginal wall closure.

are also possible. Given the significant impact that these conditions can have on her quality of life, a patient must be fully informed of these risks in advance.

Conclusions

The clinician must have a high index of suspicion in order to diagnose urethral diverticula. Improvements in imaging modalities enhance our ability to diagnose and stage UD. With better preoperative staging and meticulous surgical technique, UD can be successfully corrected in many patients.

Urethrovaginal Fistula

Urethrovaginal fistula (UVF) is a rare complication of the repair of UD. In a large contemporary series it occurred in less than 2% of repairs.[22] UVF have also been reported after anterior colporraphy, vaginal hysterectomy, obstetrical trauma, pelvic fracture, vaginal and urethral tumors, and radiation therapy.[39,40]

Presentation

If distal to the continence mechanism, UVF may present with vaginal voiding or split urinary stream,

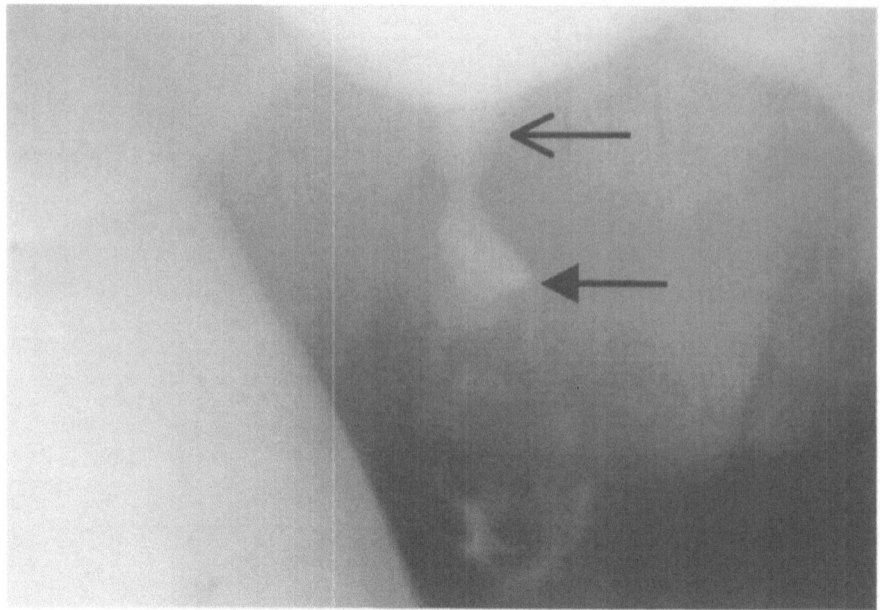

Figure 22.9 Voiding cytourethro-
gram demonstrating a fistula to
the vagina (heavy arrow) arising
from the proximal urethra (light
arrow).

or may be entirely asymptomatic. Proximal UVF may present with stress or continuous incontinence, depending upon the competence of the bladder neck. As a result of previous surgery in many of these patients, the bladder neck may be incompetent, a finding that adds to the complexity of the repair.[41]

Diagnosis

Diagnosis of UVF can be confirmed with careful urethroscopic examination using a short-beaked female cystourethroscope. If the fistula cannot be directly visualized, a speculum may be placed in the vagina to observe spraying into the vagina through the fistula tract. VCUG should also be employed in order to exclude concomitant vesicovaginal fistula and to assess urethral hypermobility on lateral straining and voiding views.[41] (Fig. 22.9)

Repair

Because UVF are generally iatrogenic, tissues should be allowed to maximally recover prior to attempting repair. Traumatic fistulae should not be operated on within 2 months of prior surgery, and in general, it is best to wait at least 1 year to repair UVF in patients who have had radiation to allow maximum revascularization of the tissue.[42]

As in the repair of UD, the simplest form of repair for UVF is urethral marsupialization, but this is only

appropriate for fistulae in the distal portion of the urethra. If the fistula is in the mid or proximal urethra, transvaginal excision with placement of a Martius flap is the preferred procedure.

Surgical Technique

Preoperative antibiotic therapy is recommended. Repair is performed with the patient in high lithotomy position. A suprapubic catheter is placed using a Lowsley tractor. A large, inverted, U-shaped anterior vaginal wall incision should be planned so that the apex of the incision lies just proximal to the fistula tract (Fig. 22.10). Hydrodissection of the vaginal flap with injectable saline is conducted, and the flap is dissected. The fistula tract is then sharply circumscribed and the margins are freed from surrounding scar tissue. Once free, the fistula is closed using a fine, running, absorbable suture. Watertightness of the repair must be verified; then a Martius flap is advanced over the fistula site, followed by advancement of the vaginal wall flap (Fig. 22.11). Antibiotic-soaked gauze is left in the vagina for 24–48 hours. Both the urethral Foley and suprapubic catheters are left to gravity drainage.

On postoperative day 2, the vaginal pack may be removed, and the patient may be discharged on oral antibiotics. The urethral catheter should be removed 10–14 days postoperatively, and a VCUG should be obtained. If there is no urethral extravasation, and the patient voids with no postvoid residual, the suprapubic catheter should be removed. If the

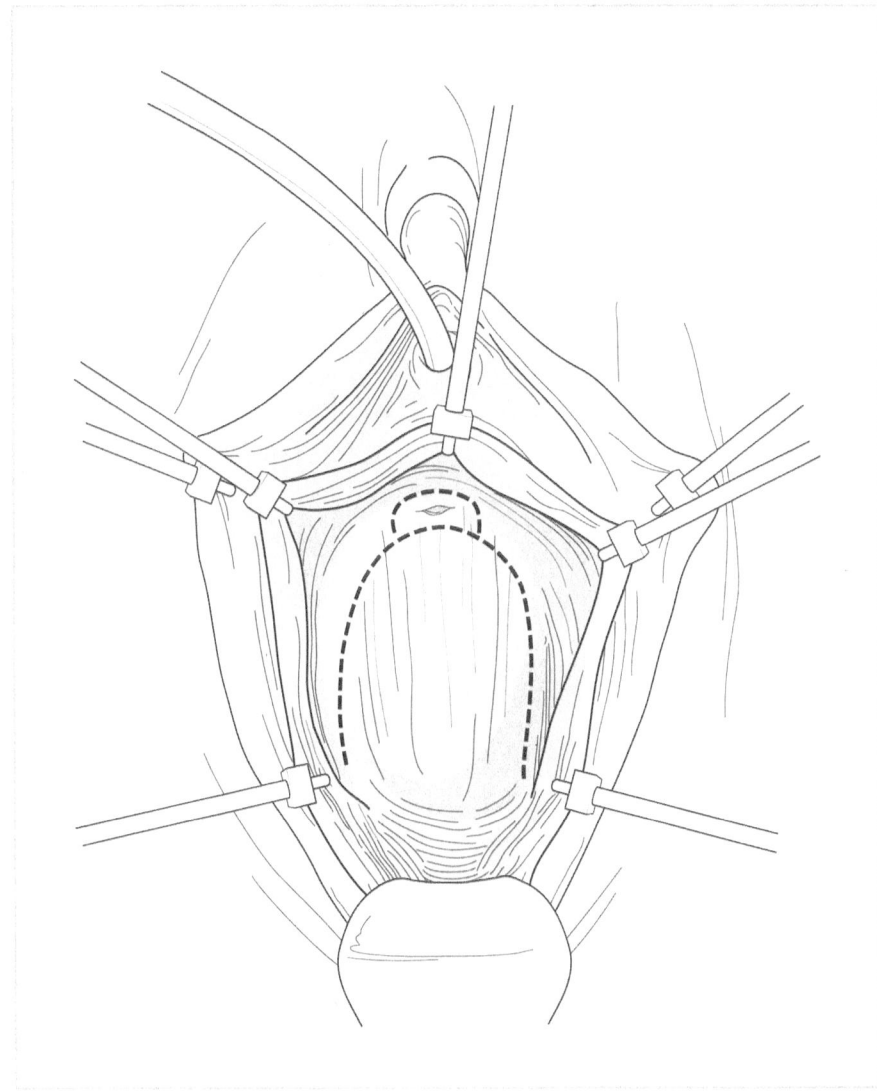

Figure 22.10 Vaginal incision for repair of urethrovaginal fistula. The inverted U-shaped flap will be advanced over fistula site after closure.

suprapubic tube must remain in place, the study should be repeated in 2 weeks.

Results

Given the rarity of this condition, very few large series have been reported in the literature. Patil and co-workers[42] report a 100% success rate in 9 patients undergoing this repair, but 2 patients developed postoperative stress incontinence. In another series, Webster and colleagues report a 100% success rate using a Martius flap, and a failure each time the Martius flap was not implemented. Likewise, Keettel and co-workers[43] report a 100% success rate in a contemporary series of patients in whom Martius flap was used to reinforce fistula repair.

Conclusions

Urethrovaginal fistula is an uncommon complication of the repair of UD. When it is diagnosed, transvaginal urethral reconstruction and a Martius flap interposition can lead to a successful outcome.

References

1. Hey W (1805) Practical Observations in Surgery. J Humphreys, Philadelphia, pp. 303.
2. Davis BL, Robinson DG (1970) Diverticula of the female urethra: assay of 120 cases. J Urol 104: 850–3.
3. Silk MR, Lebowitz JM (1969) Anterior urethral diverticulum. J Urol 101: 66–7.
4. Davis HJ, Telinde RW (1958) Urethral diverticula: an assay of 121 cases. J Urol 80: 34–9.

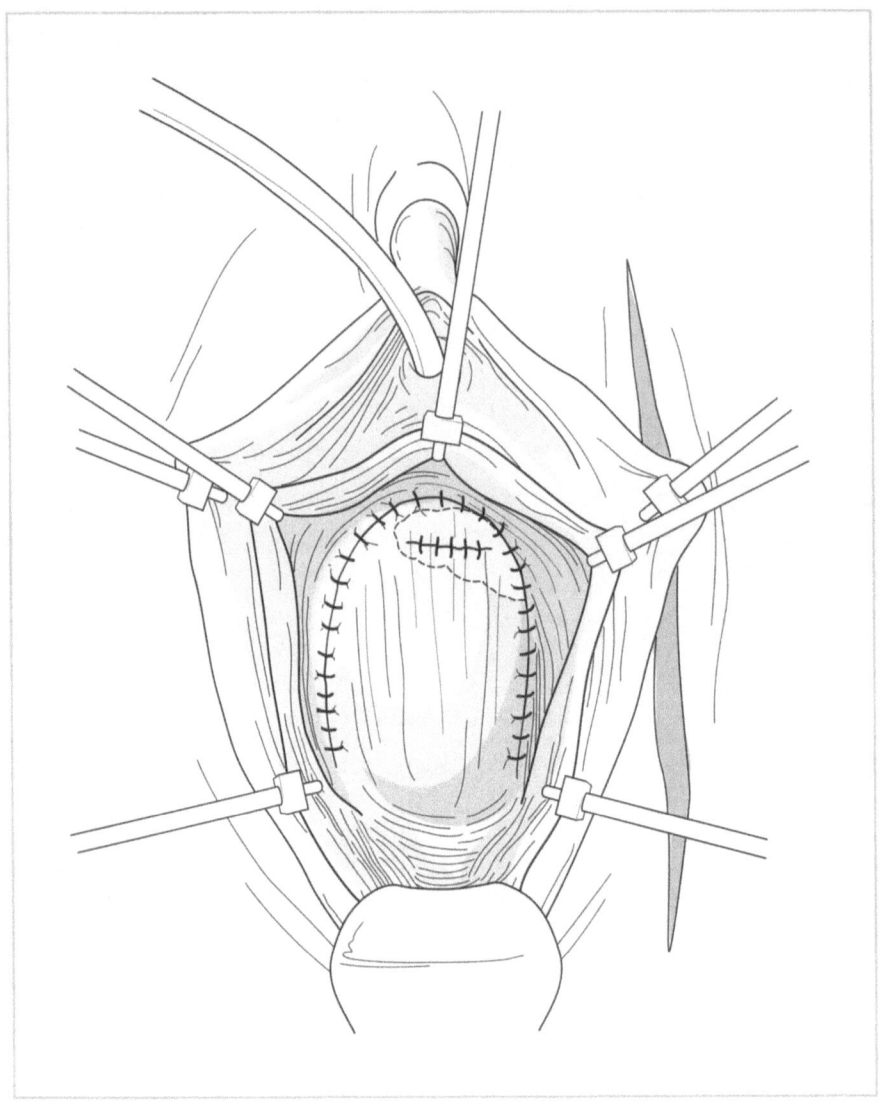

Figure 22.11 Completed fistula closure with Martius labial fat pad interposition before vaginal wall closure.

5. Young GPH, Wahle GR, Raz S (1996) Female urethral diverticulum. In: Raz S (ed) Female Urology W B Saunders, Philadelphia, Pa., pp. 477–89.

6. Dmochowski RR, Ganabathi K, Zimmern PE, Leach GE (1994) Benign female periurethral masses. J Urol 152: 1943–51.

7. Aragona F, Mangano M, Artibani W, Passerini Glazel G (1989) Stone formation in a female urethral diverticulum. Review of the literature. Int J Urol Nephrol 21: 621–5.

8. Wheeler JS, Flanigan RC, Hong HY, Walloch JL (1992) Female urethral diverticula with clear cell adenocarcinoma. J Surg Oncol 49: 66–71.

9. Woodhouse CRJ, Flynn JT, Molland EA, Bland JP (1980) Urethral diverticulum in females. Br J Urol 52: 305–10.

10. Greenberg M, Stone D, Cochran ST et al. (1981) Female urethral diverticula: double-balloon catheter study. Am J Roentgenol 136: 259–64.

11. Davis HJ, Cian LG (1956) Positive pressure urethrography: a new diagnostic method. J Urol 75: 753–7.

12. Kim B, Hricak H, Tanagho EA (1993) Diagnosis of urethral diverticula in women: value of MR imaging. Am J Roentgenol 161: 809–5.

13. Neitlich JD, Foster HE, Glickman MG, Smith RC (1998) Detection of urethral diverticula in women: comparison of a high resolution fast spin echo technique with double balloon urethrography. J Urol 159: 408–10.

14. Nurenberg P, Zimmern PE (1997) Role of MR imaging with transrectal coil in the evaluation of complex urethral abnormalities. Am J Roentgenol 169: 1335–8.

15. Blander DS, Broderick GA, Rovner ES (1999) Magnetic resonance imaging of a "saddle bag" urethral diverticulum. Urology 53: 818–9.

16. Daneshgari F, Zimmern PE, Jacomides L (1999) Magnetic resonance imaging detection of symptomatic non-communicating intraurethral wall diverticula in women. J Urol 161: 1259–62.

17. Mouritsen L, Bernstein I (1996) Vaginal ultrasonography: a diagnostic tool for urethral diverticulum. Acta Obstetricia et Gynecologica Scandinavica. 75(2): 188–90.

18. Siegel CL, Middleton WD, Teefey SA et al. (1998) Sonography of the female urethra. Am J Roentgenol 170: 1269–4.

19. Athansiou S, Khullar V, Boos K, Salvatore S, Cardozo L (1999) Imaging the urethral sphincter with three-dimensional ultrasound. Obstet Gynecol 94: 295–301.

20. Chin JL, McLoughlin RF, Downey DB (1999) Three-dimensional ultrasound and magnetic resonance imaging of pelvic anatomy: potential for complications from minimally invasive procedures. J Endourology 13: 451–9.
21. Swierzewski SJ, McGuire EJ (1993) Pubovaginal sling for treatment of female stress urinary incontinence complicated by urethral diverticulum. J Urol 149: 1012–4.
22. Ganabathi K, Leach GE, Zimmern PE, Dmochowski R (1994) Experience with the management of urethral diverticulum in 63 women. J Urol 152: 1445–52.
23. Leach GE, Sirls LT, Ganabathi K, Zimmern PE (1993) LNSC3: a proposed classification system for female urethral diverticula. Neurourology Urodynamics 12: 523–31.
24. Leng WW, McGuire EJ (1998) Management of female urethral diverticula: a new classification. J Urol 160: 1297–1300.
25. Spence HM, Duckett JW (1970) Diverticulum of the female urethra. J Urol 104: 432–7.
26. Roehrborn C (1988) Long term follow-up study of the marsupialization technique for urethral diverticula in women. Surgery. Gynecol Obstet 167: 191–6.
27. Miskowiak J, Honnens Lichtenberg M de (1989) Transurethral incision of urethral diverticulum in the female. Sandanavian J Urol Nephrol 23: 235–7.
28. Ellik M (1957) Diverticulum of the female urethra: a new method of ablation. J Urol 77: 243–6.
29. Young HH (1938) Treatment of urethral diverticulum. South Med J 31: 1043–7.
30. Cook EN, Pool TL (1949) Urethral diverticulum in the female. J Urol 62: 495.
31. Hirschhorn RC (1964) A new surgical technique for removal of urethral diverticula in the femal patient. J Urol 92: 206–9.
32. O'Connor VJ, Kropp KA (1969) Surgery of the female urethra. In: Glenn JF, Boyce WH (eds) Urologic Surgery. Harper & Row, New York, NY, pp. 572.
33. Sholem SL, Wechsler M, Roberts M (1974) Management of the urethral diverticulum in women: a modified operative technique. J Urol 112(4): 485–6.
34. Judd GE, Marshall JR (1976) Repair of urethral diverticulum or vesicovaginal fistula by vaginal flap technic. Obstet Gynecol 5: 627–9.
35. Appell RA, Suarez BC (1982) Experience with a laterally based vaginal flap approach for urethral diverticulum. J Urol 127(4): 677–8.
36. Leach GE, Schmidbauer CP, Hadley HR et al. (1986) Surgical treatment of female urethral diverticulum. Semin Urol 4: 33.
37. Leach GE, Ganabathi K (1994) Urethral diverticulectomy. Atlas Urol Clin North Am 2: 73–85.
38. Bass JS, Leach GE (1991) Surgical treatment of concomitant urethral diverticulum and stress incontinence. Urol Clin North Am 18: 365–73.
39. Webster GD, Sihelnik SA, Stone AR (1984) Urethrovaginal fistula: a review of the surgical management. J Urol 132: 460–62.
40. Zimmern PE, Schmidbauer CP, Leach GE et al. (1986) Vesicovaginal and urethrovaginal fistulae. Semin Urol 4: 24–29.
41. Leach GE (1991) Urethrovaginal fistula repair with martius labial fat pad graft. Urol Clin North Am 18: 409–13.
42. Patil U, Waterhouse K, Laungani G (1980) Management of 18 difficult vesicovaginal and urethrovaginal fistulas with modified Ingelman-Sundberg and Martius operations. J Urol 123: 653–6.
43. Keettel WC, Sehring FG, deProsse CA, Scott JR (1976) Surgical management of urethrovaginal and vesicovaginal fistulas. Am J Obstet Gynecol 131: 425–31.

Part VII

Neuromodulation

23 Neuromodulation for Idiopathic Detrusor Instability and Urge Incontinence

Daniel S. Elliott and Timothy B. Boone

Most patients presenting with idiopathic bladder instability and urge incontinence are managed by conservative therapy with anticholinergic medication, biofeedback, bladder retraining, and pelvic floor exercises. Bladder instability has a significant impact on the patient's quality of life, and the success rate of conservative therapy has been poor. It has been estimated that 62.5% of surveyed patients with urge incontinence were "not satisfied" with currently available treatments.[1,2]

Because of the inherent limitations of available conservative therapies, there has been a persistent search for more effective therapy to treat idiopathic bladder instability. For several decades now, neurostimulation of the sacral nerve roots has been known to inhibit detrusor contractility and cause external urethral sphincter contraction. Most dysfunctional voiding is associated with an increased activity within the sacral arc reflex that controls the bladder. The therapeutic benefit derived from electrical sacral root stimulation is based on the intrinsic inhibitory action of electrical stimulation.[3] Selective sacral root electrical stimulation of afferent anorectal branches of the pelvic nerve and sensory fibers of the pudendal nerve can thus produce an inhibitory stimulus which interrupts reflex detrusor contractions and thereby decreases or eliminates the effects of detrusor instability and dysfunctional voiding.[4] This physiologic process is the basis for

neuromodulation in patients with refractory urge incontinence. Therefore, the goal of lower urinary tract neurostimulation is to restore the bladder's reservoir function in combination with the capacity for complete voluntary evacuation.[5]

Neuromodulation in the neurologically intact patient with unilateral sacral segmental nerve stimulation by a permanent electrode can potentially offer a nondestructive treatment alternative for individuals whose bladder condition (overactivity or retention) has failed conservative therapy.[4]

Theory and Anatomy of Sacral Nerve Neurostimulation

The sacral dorsal and ventral roots originate from corresponding spinal cord segments (S2–4) extending to the exit of the dura and innervating the pelvis. Each nerve root is separated by an epineural connective-tissue sheath. Each nerve root can be identified by its ventral or dorsal emergence from the spinal cord and also by its configuration with the ventral root passing medially to the dorsal root. At the sacral foramina, the S2–4 ventral and dorsal roots join extradurally and then separate into autonomic and somatic nerve fibers.[5,6] The bladder and the smooth muscle component of the urethra are innervated by autonomic fibers from the pelvic plexus. In contrast, somatic nerve fibers exiting from S2–4 sacral segments form the pudendal nerve. However, a few somatic branches from S2–4 ventral roots run close to the pelvic plexus to innervate the levator ani muscles and the urethral striated rhabdosphincter.[5,6]

In the past, the major limitation of electrostimulation was simultaneous bladder and sphincteric contractions in response to sacral nerve stimulation. The etiology of this problem can be explained by the presence of both somatic and autonomic fibers in sacral ventral roots. This "iatrogenic" detrusor-sphincter dyssynergia impeded complete voiding and so represented a serious clinical problem.[5] Because of this, significant efforts were made by researchers such as Tanagho and Schmidt to identify the sacral ventral root that was the most appropriate location for bladder stimulation. Using microstimulation of the parasympathetic nucleus within the spinal cord, investigations have shown it to be feasible to induce selective bladder contraction without activation of the sphincteric muscle.[5-9] Of the sacral nerve roots, the S3 root is most easily accessible and practical for use with chronic neuromodulation of reflex detrusor activity.[10]

Patient Selection and Evaluation

Patients presenting with a history of refractory urge incontinence who are under consideration for neuromodulation should undergo a baseline diagnostic evaluation. A thorough history and physical examination should be performed focusing on concurrent neurologic and anatomic abnormalities that may be contributing to or the etiology of the voiding dysfunction. Urinalysis, urine cytology, and serum creatinine should be obtained. The patient should complete a voiding diary (2–4 days in duration) focusing on fluid intake, voiding frequency and volume, episodes of urgency and urge incontinence, and number of pads used. All patients should undergo urodynamic evaluation with pressure flow determination. Indications and contraindications for sacral neuromodulation are included in Table 23.1. Patients who meet these criteria, who have failed more conservative therapy modalities, and who are

Table 23.1. Contraindications and indications for sacral nerve neuromodulation.[10,11]

Contraindications	Indications
Pregnancy	Urge/frequency syndromes
Children	Urge incontinence
Stress urinary incontinence	Pelvic pain syndromes
Cerebral vascular accident (<6 months previously)	Urethral pain syndromes
Untreated diabetes mellitus	Idiopathic urinary retention
History of non-compliance	
Known significant psychiatric disturbances	
Sacral dermal lesions or decubitus ulcers at operative site	
Spinal cord injury	
Known neurologic disease process	
Congenital or anatomical sacral abnormalities	
Small bladder capacity (<150 ml)	
Untreated urinary tract infection	

sufficiently bothered by their voiding symptoms should proceed to the percutaneous stimulation test.

Percutaneous Neuromodulation Test

Currently the only method available to determine if a given patient will have an acceptable response to the implantation of a sacral nerve stimulator is to first have the patient undergo a trial percutaneous test stimulation. Under local anesthesia, a spinal needle is placed percutaneously bilaterally into the

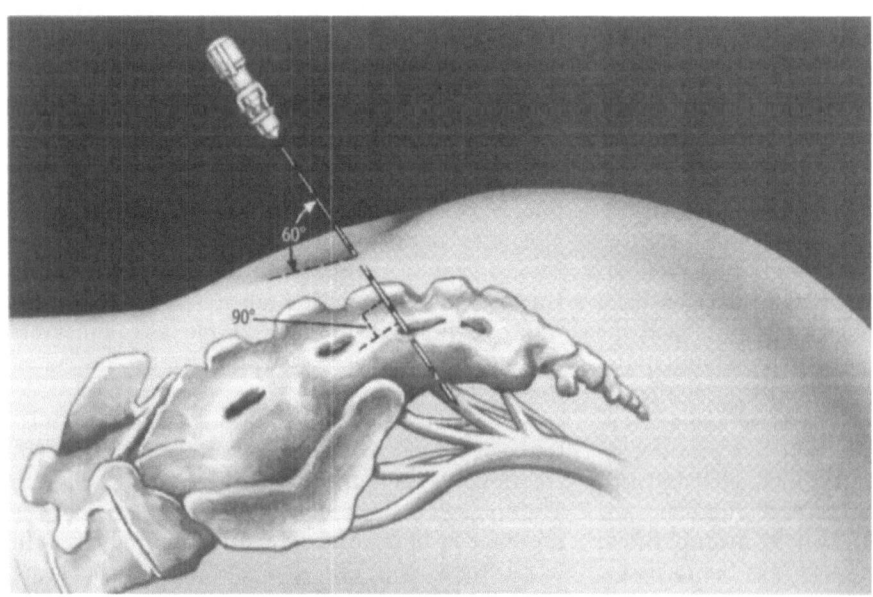

Figure 23.1 Proper location and angle of approach for percutaneous spinal needle approach to S3 foramen. Reproduced with permission from Medtronic Inc.

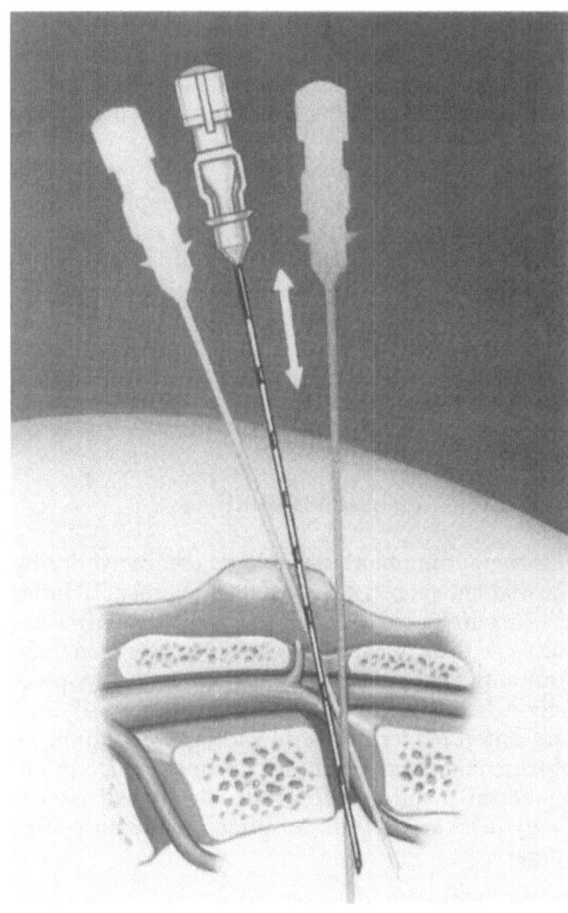

Figure 23.2 Proper location and angle of approach for percutaneous spinal needle approach to S3 foramen. Reproduced with permission from Medtronic Inc.

S3 foramen, which is about one fingerbreadth off the midline at the level of the greater sciatic notch (Figs 23.1. 23.2). Once the spinal needle is positioned near the S3 foramen it is electrically stimulated with an external electrical stimulator (Fig 23.3). To insure proper lead placement in S3, appropriate muscle responses must be seen with electrical stimulation. If the S3 root is stimulated then there should be a contraction of the perineal musculature (bellows) while causing minimal or no foot flexion. A focal great toe contraction may be seen with proper S3 localization. After confirmation that the spinal needle is located near the S3 foramina, a subchronic stimulation wire (3-0 Flexon pacer wire) is then placed through the needle and the spinal needle is removed. The wire is then secured in place on the skin with Tegaderm. The pacer wire should be connected to a pulse generator and should undergo constant and comfortable perineal muscle stimulation for 3–7 days.[1,3,10,11] During this test period, all patients are instructed to keep a voiding diary. They are instructed to maintain a comfortable and noticeable level of electrode stimulation.[12]

If the initial trial is not successful, or if only a partial decrease in symptoms is achieved despite appropriate perineal muscle response, the patient has the option of repeat testing of another nerve root or combination of nerve roots. If there is a >50% decrease in the number of leakage episodes or pads used or a >50% reduction of symptoms then the test is determined to be successful and the patient is a candidate for permanent electrode implantation.[1,3,10,11]

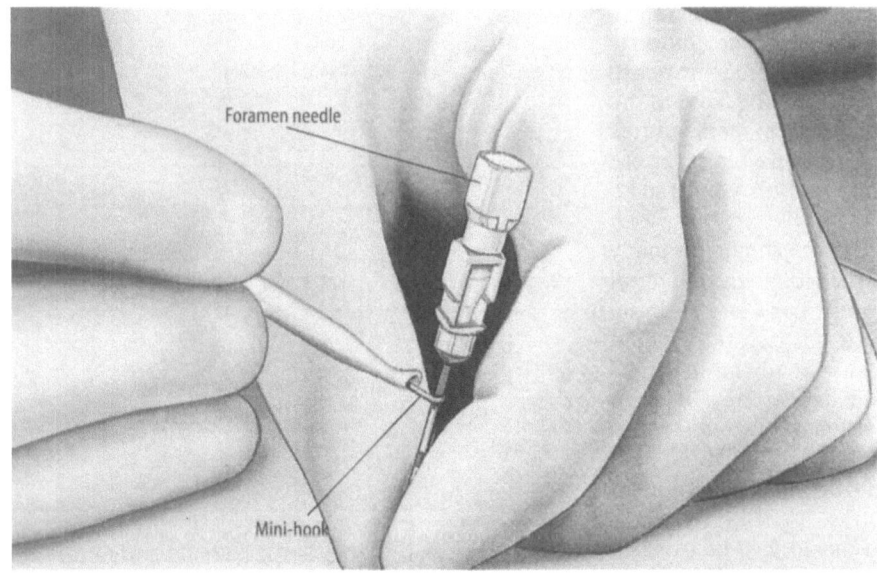

Foramen needle

Mini-hook

Figure 23.3 Test electrical stimulation of spinal needle. Reproduced with permission from Medtronic Inc.

Permanent Surgical Implantation Technique

The permanent electrode implantation is performed under general anesthesia. Prophylactic intravenous antibiotics should be given prior to the incision. The patient should be prepared in the prone position, supported by a laminectomy frame or large padded rolls. This position will facilitate evaluation of perineal muscle responses to the stimulation of each sacral nerve root. The skin overlying the sacrum should be given a full 10 minute betadine scrub. The patient should be draped so as to allow visualization of the anus and perineum. The feet also should be exposed, to allow viewing the motor responses to nerve stimulation during implantation. Before making an incision, the proper sacral foramina are identified using electrical stimulation via an insulated needle.[3,12] A 10 cm midline incision is made over the sacral spinous processes. The upper edge of the gluteus muscle usually marks the level of the S3 foramen. Once the proper nerve root is identified, the test needle is removed and a permanent electrode is inserted into the test needle puncture site.[12] The electrode should be aimed inferolaterally toward the greater trochanter, thus allowing the lead to follow the course of the nerve. The electrode should pass smoothly without any resistance or springback.[3] The proper position should then be tested. The perineum and foot should be observed for appropriate motor responses. It is preferred for the perineal response to be greater than the foot. The electrode should be repositioned if an inappropriate response is seen. An appropriate response should be obtained between 0.5 mA and 2 mA. This will ensure an adequate space between the nerve and the electrode. If a threshold is too low this may indicate the electrode is too close to the nerve and may subsequently cause painful stimulation. Conversely, a high threshold may indicate the electrode is too far from the nerve.[12] Once the ideal muscular response is accomplished, the electrode should be fixed to the posterior sacral periosteum with permanent sutures and a second fixation cuff should be placed more proximally over the electrode and also sutured to the periosteum.[3]

At this point, an incision 7–9 cm should be made three fingerbreadths below the ribs with its lateral most extent along the lateral axillary line running roughly parallel to the iliac crest. Dissection should extend into the subcutaneous fat to the depth of 1 cm in a thin patient and deeper in a heavier patient. The proximal portion of the electrodes should be tunneled subcutaneously toward the ipsilateral flank just cephalad of the iliac crest and exit through the incision site.

The midline sacral incision should then be irrigated copiously with antibiotic solution. Followed by closure of the incision by first closing the fascia with a running 1-0 Vicryl suture followed by an interrupted 1-0 Vicryl suture, with added care to close all dead space thus limiting the chance of a hematoma development.

The electrode should then be appropriately attached to the Itrel generator and implanted into the subcutaneous flank pocket. The subcutaneous pocket should be irrigated with antibiotic solution followed by closure of the subcutaneous fat with an absorbable suture. Care again should be taken so as to eliminate any dead space. Skin can be closed with a running 4-0 Vicryl suture and Tegaderm applied over each incision.

Postoperative Management

Intravenous antibiotics should be continued during the night of surgery then changed to oral antibiotics the morning after surgery. Oral cephalosporins are the usual drug of choice designed to cover skin flora. Antibiotics should be continued for 7–10 days postoperatively. Also, the morning after surgery, a lateral and anteroposterior sacral radiograph should be obtained for documentation of proper electrode and generator position (Fig 23.4). The patient is normally discharged from hospital 24–28 hours after surgery.

Activation and Programming of Implant

Activation of the implant can be initiated during the first several days after surgery. The goal of this early neurostimulation is to confirm the appropriate

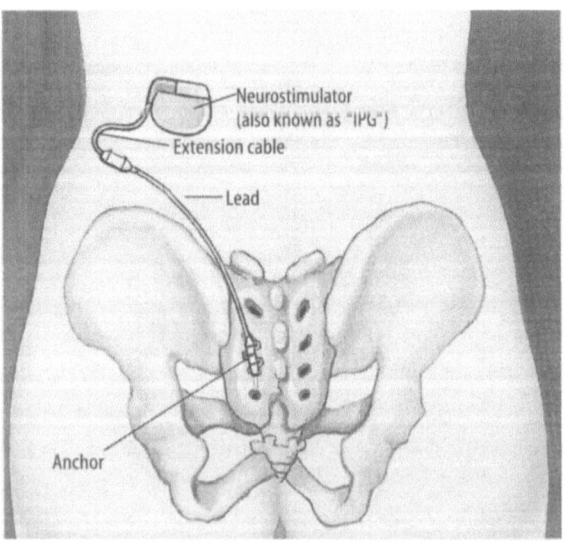

Figure 23.4 Proper position of generator, extension cable, lead, and electrode. Reproduced with permission from Medtronic Inc.

response seen at the time of surgery. Also, a baseline record should be recorded for comparison of future responses. It will take 6–8 weeks after surgery for stabilization of the various stimulation parameters to be established. The patient should be informed that frequent adjustments will most likely be required at 10 days and 3 weeks postoperatively.[3]

Four parameters should be set during the programming of the generator. Final parameters should be:

- *Frequency* set frequency from 5–20 Hz with a pulse width of 200 μs
- *Amplitude* the amplitude should be increased until a maximal muscle contraction, which remains comfortable, is achieved.
- *Pattern* commonly used cycle patterns are: 10 s on–20s off, 15 s on–5 s off, and 0.125 s on–0.325 s off.[3,13,14]

A cycle of 15 s on–5 s off is recommended as the initial cycle of stimulation.[14] Patients should be instructed on varying cycle pattern to achieve comfort level and therapeutic benefit. It is important to remember that there are no set parameters that will provide benefit to all patients. The important feature is to adjust the parameters on the basis of a given patient's symptoms. The ultimate goal is to provide a balance between "on" time and "off" time of stimulation that provides a sufficient therapeutic benefit while remaining within the parameters shown to be safe. Patients should be seen on a scheduled periodic basis to monitor their implant use and to encourage patients to use the implant only as much as necessary to control their symptoms.[14]

Results of Neuromodulation

To date there has been no evidence of chronic neurostimulation causing neurologic deterioration. However, experimental data has suggested that neuronal damage has an increased risk of occur-

ring when neurostimulation is constant rather than intermittent.

Four recent studies have reviewed the long-term results of sacral neuromodulation in neurologically intact individuals.[1,10,11,15] The results are summarized in Table 23.2. A total of 72 patients were enrolled in the studies, all received similar evaluations, and all were initially successfully evaluated with a percutaneous subchronic study. The mean number of incontinence episodes per day was 8.6 preoperatively and decreased to 2.3 postoperatively, a 73% decrease. The number of pads or diapers used per day decreased from 5.9 preoperatively to 1.2 postoperatively, a 72% decrease. Forty-one of the 52 patients (78%) were recorded as having at least a 50% improvement in symptoms after electrical stimulation. In the studies by Schmidt[1] and Bosch[10] the re-operation rates were 11/34 (32%) and 5/18 (27%), respectively. The most common complications were pain at the generator site and at the electrode implant site.

Therapeutic benefit has been consistently the greatest in the patients implanted for the treatment of symptoms related to detrusor instability. Less dramatic results are seen for patients with purely sensory symptoms. Also, patients who preoperatively were shown to have strong sphincteric function, and who had a bladder capacity of > 200 ml before experiencing bladder contractions and significant symptoms, consistently had better results after implantation.[14]

Conclusion

It is clear that the standard treatment regimens for urgency and urge incontinence remain inadequate in treating many patients with detrusor overactivity. Aberrant activity of the pelvic floor and external sphincter may play a significant role in eliciting an urge sensation, more than actual detrusor instabi-lity. Alterations in this "sphincteric instability" with neurostimulation results in inhibition of the

Table 23.2. Comparison of results of sacral neuromodulation for treatment of urge incontinence in patients with detrusor instability

Study	N	Mean follow-up (months)	Incontinence episodes/day		Pads/day		# >50% improved
			Preop	Postop	Preop	Postop	
Schmidt[1]	34	13	9.7	2.6	6.2	1.1	26/34 (76%)
Bosch[10]	18	29	7.5	1.9	6.4	1.6	15/18 (83%)
Hohen[11]	11	13	NR	NR	5.0	1.0	NR
Elabbady[15]	9	3–52	NR	'decreased 50%'	'decreased 50%'	NR	NR
Total/ average	72		8.6	2.3	5.9	1.2	41/52 (79%)

NR, not recorded by investigator.

urge sensation along with subsequent inappropriate initiation of a detrusor contraction.[14]

It is implied in studies by Schmidt et al.[1] that once lower urinary tract dysfunction has been established it is permanent. All 52 patients who underwent inactivation of the sacral nerve stimulator 6 months after implantation had a documented return to baseline symptoms of urge and urge incontinence. This study concluded that sacral nerve stimulation was continuously required to modify the aberrant neuronal activity. Most patients will probably require lifelong neuromodulation in order to derive benefit.

To date there have been no preoperative evaluations which can consistently predict patients who will benefit from neuromodulation.[1,16,17] Urodynamics and voiding diary are important in the preoperative documentation of the severity of the instability and symptoms and serve as a baseline by which the postoperative benefit of neuromodulation can be compared.

A current ~33% revision rate can be expected, and a patient should be counseled about this. With advancement of technology and increased surgical experience, the revision rate is expected to decrease.

Techniques for delivering neuromodulation for the treatment of idiopathic refractory voiding dysfunction are constantly evolving. Future developments may include the introduction of a microchip processor (Advanced Bionics, Sylmar, CA). The microchip may potentially provide a much smaller device for delivering the same degree of neurostimulation. Also, a recent unpublished study by Stoller[18] demonstrated the feasibility of afferent nerve stimulation with electrical stimulation being delivered via needle electrodes inserted approximately 5 cm cephalad from the medial malleolus and just posterior to the margin of the tibia. Electrical stimulation was applied with a similar external pulse generator as used with the InterStim. A total of 90 patients were treated in this manner with a mean follow-up of 5.1 years, of whom 81% demonstrated at least a 50% or greater improvement of voiding symptoms. On the basis of the promising percutaneous results, a minimally invasive peripheral implant device is currently being developed. Though the microchip and the peripheral afferent nerve stimulation device are obviously in their early stages of development, their potential for benefit is real and may potentially improve the ability to successfully treat certain voiding dysfunction.

It is clear that at present a large number of patients have refractory urge incontinence and are not gaining adequate relief of their symptoms with current therapy. Sacral nerve stimulation has proved itself to be safe and effective in treating the symptoms of urge incontinence and, in a carefully selected patient, may serve as the next step in the algorithm in the treatment of idiopathic voiding dysfunction.

Acknowlegments

All figures in this chapter are used by courtesy of Medtronics Corporation, Minneapolis, MN.

References

1. Schmidt R, Jonas U, Oleson K et al. (1999) Sacral nerve stimulation for treatment of refractory urinary urge incontinence. J Urol 162(2): 352–7.
2. National Association for Continence (NAFC) (1996) Consumer Focus '96: A survey of community dwelling incontinent people. National Association for Continence, Spartanburg, SC.
3. Schmidt R (1996) Clinical value of neurostimulation: a urologic viewpoint. In: Raz S (ed) Female Urology, 2nd edn. W.B. Saunders, Philadelphia, pp. 643–55.
4. Bosch R, Groen J (1999) Treatment of refractory urinary incontinence with sacral spinal nerve stimulation in multiple sclerosis patients. Lancet 348(9029): 717–19.
5. Tanagho E, Barrett DM, Abol-Enein H et al. (1998) Surgery for neuropathic bladder. International Consultation on Incontinence, June 1998. World Health Organization, Geneva, Switzerland.
6. Mersdorf A, Schmidt R, Tanagho E (1993) Topographic-anatomical basis of sacral neurostimulation: Neuro-anatomical variations. J Urol 149: 345–49.
7. Haleem AS, Boehm F, Legatt A, Kantrowitz A, Stone B (1993) Sacral root stimulation for controlled micturition: Prevention of detrusor external sphincter dyssnergia by intraoperative identification and selective section of sacral nerve branches. J Urol 149: 1607–12.
8. Rijkhoff N, Wijkstra H, Kerrebroeck P van, Debruyne F (1997) Selective detrusor activation by electrical sacral nerve root stimulation in spinal cord injury. J Urol 157: 1504–8.
9. Tanagho E, Schmidt R (1988) Electrical stimulation in the clinical management of the neurogenic bladder. J Urol 140: 1331–9.
10. Bosch J, Groen J (1995) Sacral (S3) segmental nerve stimulation as a treatment for urge incontinence in patients with detrusor instability: results of chronic electrical stimulation using an implantable neural prosthesis. J Urol 154: 504–7.
11. Hohenfellner M, Schultz-Lampel D, Dahms S, Matzel K, Thuroff J (1998) Bilateral chronic sacral neuromodulation for treatment for lower urinary tract dysfunction. J Urol 160(3): 821–4.
12. Siegel S (1992) Management of voiding dysfunction with an implantable neuroprosthesis. Urol Clin N Am 19: 163.
13. Tanagho E (1992) Urinary incontinence: neurostimulation. In: Benson J (ed) Female Pelvic Floor Disorders, Investigation and Management. W.W. Norton, New York.
14. Schmidt R (1993) Neurostimulation of the bladder and urethra. In: Webster G, Kirby R, King L, Goldwasser B (ed) Reconstructive Urology. Blackwell Scientific Publishers, Boston.
15. Elabbady A, Magdy H, Mostafa E (1994) Neural stimulation for chronic voiding dysfunctions. J Urol 12: 2076–80.
16. Karram M, Bhatia N (1989) Management of coexistint stress and urge urinary incontinence. Obstet Gynecol 73: 4.
17. Diokno A (1995) Epidemiology and psychosocial aspects of incontinence. Urol Clin N Am 22: 481.
18. Stoller M (1999) Afferent nerve stimulation for pelvic floor dysfunction (abstract). International Continence Society, Denver CO, 1999.

Part VIII

Postoperative Management

24 Bladder

Detrusor Instability (Bladder Overactivity)

William H. Turner and Mark C. Slack

Detrusor instability occurring after surgery for stress incontinence or prolapse is diagnosed and treated along standard lines, although it may prove difficult to treat it effectively. It is important in this setting not only because of the crucial role it plays in determining postoperative satisfaction, but also because of the need to counsel patients about it appropriately before stress incontinence or prolapse surgery.

Debate continues about whether stress incontinence or prolapse surgery may lead to detrusor instability, or whether it helps to resolve it. With a large proportion of patients in many referral practices having had previous surgery for stress incontinence or prolapse, or previous hysterectomy, the high prevalence of urgency or urge incontinence in these patients means the issue of whether surgery for stress incontinence or prolapse improves or worsens such symptoms is an important one.

Methodology

A major difficulty with the issue of detrusor instability following surgery for stress incontinence and prolapse relates to the methodology of the studies reported. A fundamental problem is whether to base an assessment on symptoms, objective data (such as urodynamics) or both. The means of evaluating symptoms varies, and a variety of different questionnaires or symptom indices have been used. In some studies the patient reports their own symptoms directly, whereas in others chart review is used to record symptoms, and this probably underestimates problems. In studies which use objective data, the measures used also vary, from uroflowmetry and residual urine estimation to conventional or ambulatory urodynamics. The practical difficulty of getting the consent of patients who have had what they regard as successful surgery to undergo follow-up urodynamics is apparent to anyone who has attempted this. In addition, the lack of sensitivity of conventional urodynamics in the diagnosis of detrusor instability means that it is less of an objective tool than many often appreciate. The lack of sensitivity in diagnosing detrusor instability also contributes to the marked discrepancy often seen between the prevalence of symptoms of bladder overactivity and the urodynamic diagnosis of detrusor instability. Follow-up also varies considerably, from months in some studies to many years in others: the few long-term studies which do exist suggest that a minimum follow-up of 5 years is appropriate before conclusions are drawn about a particular technique[1,2].

All of these factors render comparison of data from the available literature difficult, regardless of the importance of prospective rather than retrospective methodology and the use of randomization in comparative studies. It is with these familiar but major reservations that the following discussion is based.

Definition

Notwithstanding the current controversy about the term "the overactive bladder,"[3] the unstable detrusor is defined by the International Continence Society as

> one that is shown objectively to contract, spontaneously or on provocation, during the filling phase while the patient is attempting to inhibit micturition. The unstable detrusor may be asymptomatic . . . .[4]

In the present context, the asymptomatic nature of detrusor instability is relevant because it may not be apparent subjectively before surgery for stress incontinence or prolapse, but may cause very troublesome symptoms afterwards. Furthermore, unless it has been documented by preoperative urodynamics, its presence postoperatively may be assumed to be a direct consequence of the surgery, when in fact this is not so.

Cause

Debate about the possible neurogenic and myogenic components of detrusor instability continues;[5-8] however, the three clinically defined groups of patients with unstable bladders (those with obstruction, those with neurological disease, and those with neither) remain useful. The cause in the present context is seldom likely to be neurological disease, and the patient with detrusor instability after surgery for stress incontinence or prolapse will either have had clinically undetected detrusor instability preoperatively, or it will result from surgery. The latter group presumably includes patients where

surgery has been complicated by excessive bladder outlet obstruction, and patients where vesicourethral innervation has been damaged by dissection either around the urethra or around the bladder base, be it retropubically or transvaginally.

Postoperative detrusor instability seems not to imply the invariable presence of iatrogenic bladder outlet obstruction.[9] A study of 92 women having colposuspension, 62 of who had stable bladders preoperatively, showed that although detrusor instability resolved in 60% of previously unstable women, it developed in 27% of those who had previously been stable.[10] Pressure-flow studies showed no convincing evidence of postoperative obstruction. The possible role of an open bladder neck in the genesis of symptoms of bladder overactivity has recently been addressed using videourodynamics.[11] This study showed a clear association between the presence of an open bladder neck and such symptoms, but there were obviously other factors involved because the relation was not a constant one.

Significance

The symptoms of the overactive bladder are important after surgery for stress incontinence or prolapse because they have more of an impact on quality of life than those of stress incontinence.[12] The crucial role of these symptoms in determining the outcome of surgery[11] means that the patient who develops bothersome overactive bladder symptoms postoperatively may not only consider the operation a failure, but may also feel worse than she did before surgery. Despite the importance of postoperative symptoms

Table 24.1. Urgency and urge incontinence before and after surgery for stress incontinence

Author	Year	N	Procedure(s)	Follow-up	Urgency (%)		Urge incontinence (%)	
					Preop	Postop	Preop	Postop
Alcalay	1995	109	Burch	5 years	39	20	27	8
		109		At least 10 years	39	29	27	23
Kondo	1998	382	Stamey/Gittes	5–8 years average			53	34
Chaikin	1998	250	Fascial sling	At least 1 year			66	23
		47		At least 5 years			66	31
Hassouna[a]	1999	77	Fascial sling	Average 3.4 years	26	47		
Langer	1988	92	Burch	Average 19 months	55	17	39	13
Raz	1992	206	Raz	Average 15 months	44	17	28	10
Maher	1999	53	Burch	Median 9 months	27	9	19	15
Cardozo	1999	52	Burch	9 months	63	39	46	17
Stanton	1979	50	Burch/anterior repair	6 months			48	22
Brown[a]	1999	65	Burch	3 months	34	57		
Fulford	1999	85	Fascial sling	3 months			69	32
				Median of each series	39	23	44	23

[a] Urgency or urge incontinence.

in determining outcome, it remains unclear whether preoperative symptoms of bladder overactivity will resolve after surgery for stress incontinence or prolapse. Indeed, it has been suggested that preoperative symptoms may not necessarily prejudice the outcome of surgery.[13]

Prevalence

In a community-based survey of noninstitutionalized women over 60 years old, high voiding frequencies (more than eight times per day) were found in 43% of those with a history of surgery for incontinence.[14] This rate is similar to recently reported long-term follow-up data on colposuspension, where urgency and urge incontinence were reported in 32% and 25% of women respectively at 10–20 years,[2] and suggests that symptoms attributable to detrusor instability are common after surgery. As shown in Table 24.1 however, following various procedures for stress incontinence, urgency and urge incontinence typically resolve in about 50% of cases.[1,2,10,11,15–21] Some series however, suggest that both symptoms may become more frequent with longer follow-up.[2,15] Urge incontinence developed de novo in 0–54% of the patients in the series used in Table 24.1. The 3 year results from the pioneer of the tension-free vaginal tape were reported recently: however, no specific comment was made on preoperative or postoperative symptoms of bladder overactivity.[22]

Urodynamics is often done preoperatively, but only done postoperatively in the event of troublesome symptoms, so comparative preoperative and postoperative data are relatively few. However it seems that some women appear to experience denovo detrusor instability after their surgery, although the degree to which this can be accounted for by the lack of sensitivity of conventional urodynamics is unclear. A review of series including nearly 400 women gave a pooled risk of 17% of de-novo instability,[23] and three recent series quote figures of 2%, 8%, and 15%.[2,11,17]

Earlier authors examined whether detrusor instability predicted a poor outcome following surgery for stress incontinence. Two studies showed that in one group of 50 women who had a variety of procedures, the failure rate was 46% in those who were unstable preoperatively compared to 11% in those who were not,[24] whereas in another group of 60 women who had a colposuspension and a bladder neck plication, the "cure" rate was 54% in those who were unstable preoperatively compared to 89% in those who were not.[25] A more recent multicenter audit has produced similar conclusions.[26] Analysis of patients who are regarded or regard themselves as failures often highlights the impact of postoperative detrusor instability. An analysis of patients with

failure after a fascial sling (13% of 112 women) showed that of the 9 who had videourodynamics, none had persistent genuine stress incontinence, but 6 had detrusor instability and only 2 of these were unstable preoperatively.[16]

A recent study of 56 women having colposuspension, which used conventional and ambulatory urodynamics preoperatively and at 3 months post-operatively, showed that although 34% had urgency or urge incontinence preoperatively, none was unstable on conventional urodynamics, whereas 50% of the whole group were unstable on preoperative ambulatory urodynamics.[21] Ambulatory urodynamics identified unstable contractions in 12 patients without symptoms, 11 of whom developed symptoms postoperatively. The postoperative ambulatory studies showed that 70% of the group were unstable, although only 56% had either urgency or urge incontinence. Whether the unstable patients who were asymptomatic at 3 months will become symptomatic subsequently is unknown, and longer follow-up will be of interest.

Presentation and Diagnosis

Troublesome postoperative symptoms of urgency, frequency, or incontinence (either urge-related or without provocation) will lead to reassessment. A frequency–volume chart should ideally have been done preoperatively, and can be compared with a postoperative chart. Vaginal examination will assess pelvic prolapse (and allow comparison with preoperative findings) and pelvic floor contraction strength. Other possible causes of postoperative symptoms are excluded along standard lines (Table 24.2). Some of these are especially relevant in patients initially operated on elsewhere, particularly if the preoperative assessment has been less than ideal.

Urodynamics, optimally with video, will exclude bladder outlet obstruction (BOO) and persistent genuine stress incontinence (GSI), and may confirm detrusor instability, although this may require the use of ambulatory urodynamics. If troublesome symptoms are associated with detrusor instability and BOO, then urethrolysis will be considered (see section by Nitti, below).

Table 24.2. The causes of postoperative symptoms after surgery for stress incontinence and their investigations

Cause	Investigation
Infection	Urine culture
Stone, tumor	Urinalysis
Chronic retention	Ultrasound
Interstitial cystitis	History, cystoscopy, and biopsy

Treatment

Unless BOO seems the likely cause of detrusor instability associated with postoperative symptoms of
urgency, frequency, or urge incontinence, then the
mainstay of treatment is with bladder training,
pelvic floor physiotherapy, and anticholinergics. The
former two modalities are supported by a recent systematic review of the conservative treatment of urge
incontinence.[27] The familiar troublesome side effects
of anticholinergics limit their use on a long-term
basis,[28] although tolterodine and slow-release oxybutynin may have advantages in this respect. Whether the newer options of neuromodulation[29] or
intravesical vanilloid treatment[30] will be helpful
remains to be seen in the light of subsequent data.
Other than urethrolysis, and perhaps neuromodulation, surgical options such as augmentation cystoplasty are unlikely to benefit women who have
troublesome symptoms of detrusor instability after
surgery for stress incontinence or prolapse.

Figure 24.1 shows a treatment algorithm as used
by the authors. The help of a specialist nurse is often
invaluable in this situation, to increase the time
available to the patient, to clarify communication,
and to help with behavioral therapy.

Counselling Before Surgery for Stress Incontinence or Prolapse

Despite the methodological problems with the literature which is available, it seems clear that significant postoperative detrusor instability is a potent
cause of dissatisfaction, and women who have no
symptoms attributable to it before surgery should be

warned that they may occur subsequently. Conversely, although many surgeons might feel instinc-
tively uneasy about operating on a woman with a
significant element of bladder overactivity, the data
available suggest that there is a significant chance
that the problem may become less symptomatic
postoperatively. A balanced discussion of the issue
of detrusor instability and its symptoms to all
women having surgery for stress incontinence is
clearly warranted.

Bladder Outlet Obstruction and Retention

Victor W. Nitti

Surgical procedures for the correction of stress urinary incontinence are designed to restore support to
the urethrovesical junction or improve coaptation of
the urethra in cases of intrinsic sphincter dysfunction. This can be accomplished in a variety of ways
including retropubic cystourethropexy and colposuspension, transvaginal bladder neck suspension
(e.g. needle suspension), and sling procedures. A
potential complication of all these procedures is
iatrogenic outlet obstruction leading to voiding
dysfunction including obstructive symptoms with
partial or total urinary retention or irritative symptoms of frequency, urgency, and urge incontinence.
Postoperative urinary retention and voiding dysfunction may also occur as a result of learned voiding dysfunction and impaired detrusor contractility.
Although most of the discussion in this section
focuses on obstruction, these other causes should
not be overlooked. Patients may also experience

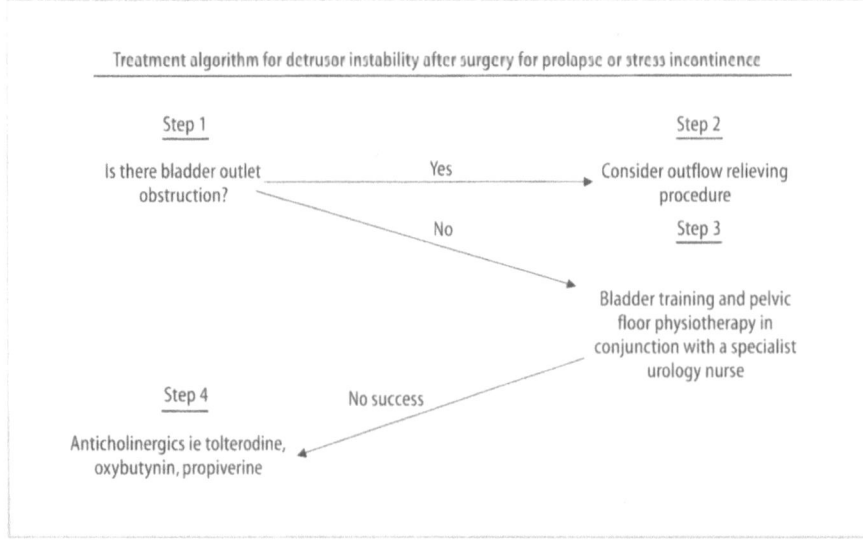

Figure 24.1 Treatment algorithm for detrusor instability after surgery for prolapse or stress incontinence.

detrusor instability without obstruction as a cause of postoperative lower urinary tract symptoms (see previous section on detrusor instability).

The true incidence of obstruction after incontinence surgery is not known. Its estimated incidence varies widely, between 2.5% and 24%.[31-37] Such variation is likely due to a variety of factors including underdiagnosis and incomplete prospective follow-up of patients. Many cases of obstruction may go undiagnosed if obstruction is not severe enough to cause significant retention. For example, it is well known that detrusor instability may occur or persist after incontinence surgery, and in some cases may be due to obstruction. Yet patients are not always evaluated for this. Also some patients will seek second opinions regarding less than optimal surgical outcomes and therefore most series on obstruction after incontinence surgery do not contain the critical denominator of the total number of patients undergoing surgery from which the obstructed patients were derived. A recent meta-analysis of surgical procedures for the treatment of stress incontinence undertaken by the American Urological Association Stress Urinary Incontinence Clinical Guideline Panel showed that the reported incidence of urinary retention greater than 4 weeks postoperative was 5% for retropubic and transvaginal suspensions and 8% for sling procedures (no statistically difference).[38] There was not accurate data to determine the risk of permanent retention, but the panel opinion was that it "generally does not exceed 5%."

Etiology of Postoperative Retention and Voiding Dysfunction

Obstruction

Obstruction after incontinence surgery is usually related to technical factors, i.e. suture or sling placement and tension. When retropubic or transvaginal suspension procedures are performed, sutures placed too medial can cause urethral deviation, kinking, or periurethral scarring. In fact, the original description of the Marshal–Marchetti–Krantz urethropexy described placement of sutures in the lateral urethral wall;[39] however, this was later modified to avoid such placement, reducing the incidence of obstruction.[40] Sutures or slings placed too distally may cause kinking and obstruction at the mid to distal urethral region if the more proximal urethra is not adequately supported. The most common technical problem causing obstruction is excessive tension on sutures or slings causing overcorrection or "hypersuspension" of the bladder neck and proximal urethra. There have been a variety of methods devised to avoid excessive tension at the time of

surgery including intraoperative measurements of tension and the use of spacing devices. However, the most important factor in reducing obstruction has probably been the understanding that operations for stress incontinence work by restoring support, not by changing the resting position of the urethra. Nevertheless clinical obstruction will occur in 1–2% of patients even in the most experienced hands. Some investigators believe that procedures designed to treat stress incontinence work at least partly by causing some degree outlet obstruction. Pope et al. studied 20 women undergoing endoscopic bladder neck suspension with pre- and postoperative urodynamics and found a threefold increase in urethral resistance and almost a doubling of voiding pressure 12 months after surgery.[41]

Obstruction may also be caused by periurethral scarring secondary to sutures placed through the urethral lumen with subsequent extravasation of urine, and fibrosis and scarring caused by the surgical dissection itself.[42] It can also occur as a result of anatomic factors such as a cystocele or other prolapse that was not corrected or occurred postoperatively. Thus it is important to correct all anatomical defects at the time of incontinence surgery.

Learned Voiding Dysfunction

Two types of behavioral problems can result in incomplete emptying or retention after incontinence surgery. One is dysfunctional voiding or pseudodyssynergia where patients "learn" to contract the external urethral sphincter during voiding. This can occur as a result of postoperative pain or detrusor instability. It may be corrected by teaching the patient to relax the voluntary sphincter during voiding, often with the use of biofeedback techniques. A second behavioral problem is voiding by abdominal straining. Many women learn to void by this technique, especially those with stress incontinence who have low outlet resistance. It is not necessarily due to impaired detrusor contractility but may occur simply as a "habit". Since incontinence surgery is designed to resist increases in intraabdominal pressure, voiding by abdominal straining without a detrusor contraction is no longer possible after surgery. If this voiding pattern is identified preoperatively patients should be made aware of it and taught not to use this abdominal straining to void.

Impaired Detrusor Contractility

Women with impaired detrusor contractility are at higher than average risk of developing urinary retention. Even the slightest increase in outlet resistance can alter a delicate balance and prohibit compensatory mechanisms (e.g. abdominal straining, see above) from aiding in the voiding process. Unfortunately, impaired contractility may be difficult to diagnose preoperatively, especially in the women with very low outlet resistance and complete emptying. Incomplete emptying preoperatively, however, should raise a red flag.

Presentation

The most obvious presentation of obstruction after incontinence surgery is inability to void or intermittent retention. Patients may also experience obstructive symptoms including slow or interrupted stream and straining to void. Irritative symptoms of urinary frequency, urgency, and urge incontinence which persist after surgery may also be a sign of obstruction even if emptying is complete. Carr and Webster reviewed the presenting symptoms of 51 women undergoing urethrolysis for voiding dysfunction and obstruction following incontinence surgery and found irritative symptoms in 75%, obstructive symptoms in 61%, de-novo urge incontinence in 55%, need for periodic intermittent catheterization in 40%, persistent retention in 24%, recurrent urinary tract infections in 8%, and painful voiding in 8%.[43] Most series on obstruction after incontinence surgery divide patients into those with retention and those with irritative symptoms.

Diagnosis

The diagnostic evaluation of the patient with voiding dysfunction after incontinence surgery consists of a focused history and physical examination, and in select cases urodynamic, radiographic, and endoscopic studies. The timing of the evaluation is important, as retention and voiding dysfunction are often transient. However, it is often difficult to persuade frustrated women with severe irritative symptoms or retention to be patient. It has been our philosophy to refrain from intervention in the first 3 months after surgery as spontaneous resolution of retention or irritative symptoms often occurs. Between 3 and 6 months evaluation and possible intervention are recommended, depending upon the degree of bother. During this period symptoms may still resolve without intervention, but improvement is less likely than in the first 3 months. After 6 months improvement is unlikely, but some women may elect to continue "watchful waiting." Empirically one would think that a longer delay in intervention is less likely to result in improvement, but we have not found this to be the case.[44]

History

History is a critical part of the evaluation. Specific symptoms and their relationship to incontinence surgery should be assessed. Preoperative voiding history is especially important. For patients with urinary retention, a history of normal voiding and emptying before incontinence surgery is the single most useful piece of information in determining if intervention (e.g. urethrolysis) is indicated.[43,44] Urodynamic data such as uroflow and pressure–flow studies from before incontinence surgery are useful if available. If patients are straining to void (perhaps by habit), they should be instructed to stop this behavior, as incontinence procedures are designed to prevent the flow of urine with abdominal straining. Finally, it is important to determine if the symptom of stress incontinence persists.

Physical Examination

Physical examination may show overcorrection or hypersuspension where the urethra and urethral meatus appear to be pulled up toward the pubic bone and "fixed." The angle of the urethra becomes more vertical than is normal. However, not all obstructed patients will appear to be overcorrected. It is important to assess for cystocele and other forms of prolapse which may cause obstruction (due to a kinking of the urethra). The patient should also be examined for persistent urethral hypermobility and stress incontinence.

Urodynamics

The diagnosis of obstruction in women can be a difficult one to make urodynamically. Absolute urodynamic criteria for obstruction in women have not been defined, although two recently published series have proposed criteria. Nitti et al. defined obstruction videourodynamically as a sustained detrusor contraction of any magnitude associated with reduced flow and radiographic evidence of obstruction between the bladder neck and urethral meatus.[45] Chassagne et al. proposed cutoff values of 15 ml/s or less for maximum flow rate (Q_{max}) combined with a detrusor pressure at Q_{max} of more than 20 cm H_2O to define bladder outlet obstruction in women (sensitivity 74.3%; specificity 91.1%).[46] They defined obstruction clinically (obvious obstruction after incontinence surgery regardless of urodynamic parameters), prospectively evaluated clinically obstructed and control patients with urodynamics, and used receiver operator characteristic (ROC) curve analysis. Although useful, such criteria require that a patient have a demonstrable detrusor contraction during a urodynamic study and 10–64% of women in retention after surgery will not demonstrate such a contraction.[43,44,47] Yet these patients respond well to treatments designed to eliminate obstruction (e.g. urethrolysis). In fact, there appears to be no correlation of any urodynamic parameter with successful urethrolysis.[43,44,47,48] Thus, in the case of the acontractile bladder the diagnosis of obstruction can only be inferred, albeit without certainty, by considering the patient's history of normal voiding and emptying prior to surgery.

Classic high-pressure low-flow voiding dynamics do confirm the diagnosis of obstruction, but are far from a consistent finding. Urodynamics can also yield important information regarding instability, impaired compliance, bladder capacity, and voiding characteristics. Obstruction may be ruled out in the patient who presents with postoperative irritative symptoms. In our experience, videourodynamics offers an advantage over simple urodynamics in this patient population, because of the ability to simultaneously image the bladder outlet.

The utility of urodynamics may be considered as follows:

- For the patient in retention urodynamics can provide valuable information (e.g. detrusor instability or significantly impaired compliance, the later being an absolute indication for intervention) and can confirm a diagnosis of obstruction but should not exclude the patient from urethrolysis, even if there is no contraction or impaired contractility. Urodynamics may also identify learned voiding dysfunction.
- For the patient with irritative symptoms with normal emptying, urodynamics may provide a specific diagnosis and can be helpful in directing therapy, especially if obstruction can be ruled out.

Endoscopy

Endoscopic evaluation of the urethra may show scarring, narrowing, occlusion, kinking, or deviation of the urethra.[48–50] The urethra and bladder should be carefully inspected for eroded sutures or sling material and the presence of a fistula. This is facilitated by the use of a rigid scope with a 0–30° degree lens and little or no beak to allow for complete distention of the urethra.

Radiography

Radiographic imaging may be done independent of videourodynamics. A standing cystogram in the anterior–posterior, oblique, and lateral positions, with and without straining, assesses the degree of bladder and urethral prolapse and displacement or distortion of the bladder. A voiding cysto-urethrogram can assess the bladder, bladder neck, and urethra during voiding to determine narrowing, kinking, or deviation.

Treatment

Treatment for obstruction and retention may be conservative or surgical. Conservative management usually involves the institution of clean intermittent self-catheterization. This may be combined with pharmacotherapy for detrusor instability when necessary. However, it has been our observation that pharmacological therapy for postoperative instability with obstruction is less effective than when used for idiopathic instability and detrusor hyperreflexia. Patients who had severe incontinence before incontinence surgery and who do not have significant detrusor instability are most likely to accept long-term or permanent self-catheterization.

Several surgical procedures have been described to treat postoperative obstruction. These range from simple procedures, such as cutting or loosing suspension sutures or slings, to formal urethrolysis. We have recently had success with pubovaginal sling lysis, simply cutting the sling in the midline via a vaginal approach and freeing it to the endopelvic fascia bilaterally. Simple surgical procedures seem to work in select cases, but no published data are available on large numbers of patients with specific recommendations regarding who are the best candidates. On the other hand, there are several large published series on urethrolysis.[43,44,47,48,50–53]

Urethrolysis may be done by a transvaginal, retropubic, or suprameatal approach. Results appear to be similar for each (Table 24.3). It is effective for both retention and irritative symptoms. All major series included patients felt to be obstructed clinically, regardless of urodynamic findings (see above). There appear to be no consistent preoperative parameters, urodynamic or otherwise, which predict success or failure of urethrolysis. For example, Foster and McGuire[47] found that patients with detrusor instability had a higher rate of failure, but a later study[52] as well as others found this not to be the case. Nitti and Raz[44] found that as the post-void residual increased so did the rate of failure, but others have not confirmed this finding. Carr and Webster found that the only parameter predictive of success was no prior urethrolysis.[43] Failure may be caused by persistent or recurrent obstruction, detrusor instability, impaired detrusor contractility, or learned voiding dysfunction. Continued obstruction may result from recurrent periurethral fibrosis and

Table 24.3. Summary of series on urethrolysis for the treatment of obstruction after incontinence surgery. Success is usually measured in terms of resumption of spontaneous bladder emptying for patients in retention, and resolution symptoms for patients with frequency, urgency and urge incontinence

Study	Number	Type of urethrolysis	Success
Foster and McGuire[47]	48	Transvaginal	65%
Nitti and Raz[44]	42	Transvaginal	71%
Cross et al.[52]	39	Transvaginal	71%
Goldman et al.[53]	32	Transvaginal	84%
Zimmern et al.[51]	13	Transvaginal	92%
Petrou et al.[50]	32	Suprameatal	67%
Webster and Kreder[48]	15	Retropubic	93%
Carr and Webster[43]	54	Mixed	78%

scarring or intrinsic damage to the urethra which has occurred as a result of surgery.

The type of urethrolysis chosen will depend on several factors including patient presentation, type of incontinence procedure performed, failed prior urethrolysis, and surgeon preference. It has been our practice to perform transvaginal urethrolysis as a primary operation, and a retropubic urethrolysis as a secondary operation (e.g. after failed transvaginal surgery). We prefer the transvaginal technique because of its ease and the reduced morbidity and recovery time from avoiding an abdominal procedure. However, there are times when a retropubic approach may be the best primary procedure: for example, when vaginal anatomy precludes a trans-

vaginal approach, in cases where original incontinence surgery was associated with bladder perforation, fistula, or other operative complication, when there is a synthetic sling which must be removed, or in cases where the patient wishes to avoid a vaginal incision. In all types of formal urethrolysis the goal of surgery is to relieve excessive tension and free the urethra from the pubic bone (Fig. 24.2). A description of each approach follows.

Transvaginal Urethrolysis

The most commonly used transvaginal technique was originally described by Leach and Raz.[54] An inverted U incision is made in the anterior vaginal wall with the apex half way between the bladder neck and urethral meatus. Lateral dissection is performed along the glistening surface of the periurethral fascia to the pubic bone. The retropubic space is entered sharply by perforating the attachment of the endopelvic fascia to the obturator fascia (Fig. 24.3a). Sharp and blunt dissection is performed to open the retropubic space on each side. The urethra is then dissected off of the undersurface of the pubic bone. Sharp dissection is usually required here (Fig. 24.3b). The urethra should be completely freed proximally to the bladder neck so that the index finger can be placed between the urethra and the symphysis pubis.

In some cases it may be desirable to resuspend or resupport the urethra after urethrolysis. In the series by Nitti and Raz resuspension by the Raz technique was done routinely and there were no instances of recurrent stress incontinence.[44] When resuspension is not routinely performed recurrent stress incontinence rates between 0 and 19% have been reported.[43,47,52,53] Currently our practice is to perform a resuspension or sling in only select cases, e.g. if the patient has stress incontinence before urethrolysis, or if support structures are severely compromised during urethrolysis.

Sometimes it may be desirable to interpose a Martius labial fat pad flap between the urethra and the pubic to prevent readherence of these structures. We use this in all cases of recurrent transvaginal urethrolysis (after a failed prior urethrolysis) or when scarring is particularly dense. Carr and Webster found that such interposition, even in primary cases, was associated with a more successful outcome and now recommend this as a routine.[43]

In cases where there is associated pelvic prolapse, either cystocele, rectocele, enterocele or uterine prolapse, repair should be performed at the time of urethrolysis.

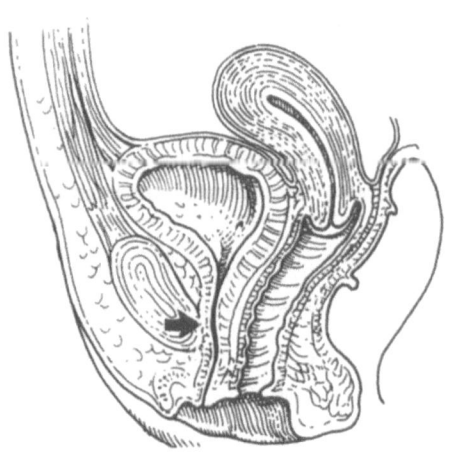

Figure 24.2 Sagittal view showing the urethra fixed to the undersurface of the pubic bone after incontinence surgery (arrow). The urethra should be completely freed by urethrolysis. From Nitti VW, Raz S. Obstruction following anti-incontinence procedures: diagnosis and treatment with transvaginal urethrolysis. *J Urol* 1994; 152: 93–8, with permission.

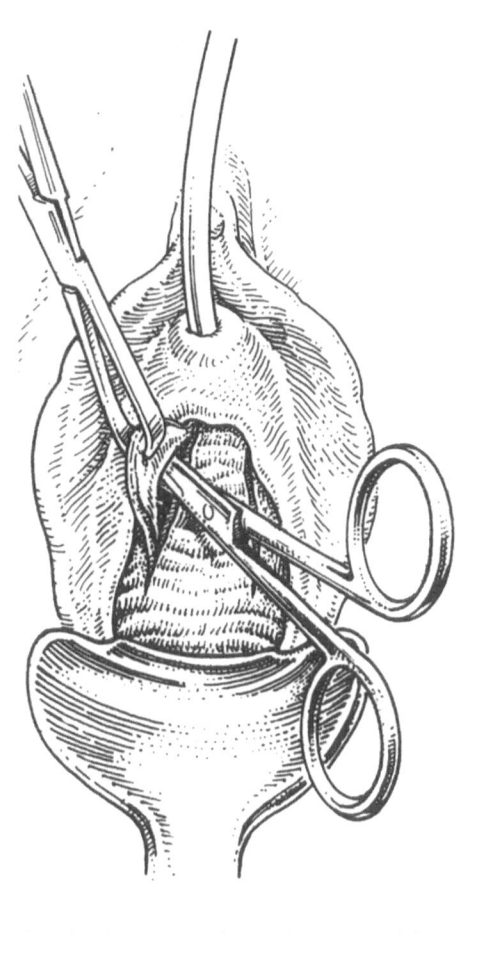

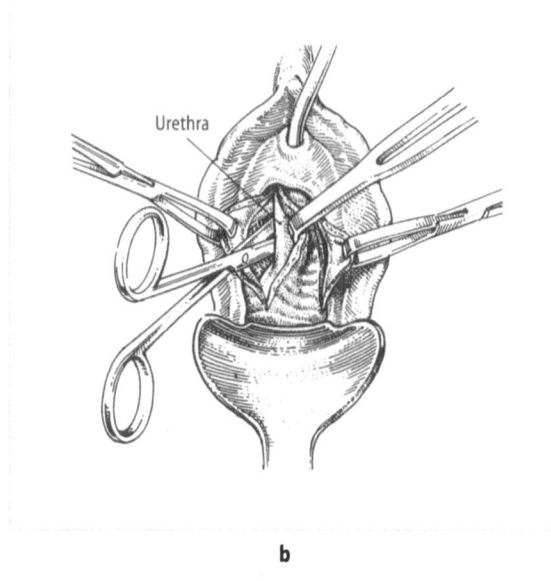

Figure 24.3 Transvaginal urethrolysis. **a** Inverted U incision in the anterior vaginal wall and entrance into the retropubic space. **b** The urethra is sharply dissected off of the undersurface of the pubic bone. The endopelvic fascia, periurethral fascia and vaginal wall are retracted medially to expose the urethra in the retropubic space. From Nitti VW, Raz S. Obstruction following anti-incontinence procedures: diagnosis and treatment with transvaginal urethrolysis. *J Urol* 1994; 152: 93–8, with permission.

Suprameatal Urethrolysis

This alternative transvaginal approach to urethrolysis has been described by Petrou et al.[50] An inverted U incision is made around the urethral meatus (approximately 1 cm away) between the 3 o'clock and 9 o'clock positions. Using sharp dissection, a plane is developed above the urethra. Then with a combination of sharp and blunt dissection the urethra, vesical neck, and bladder are freed from the pubic and pelvic attachments anteriorly and laterally. The index finger may then be passed into the retropubic space, and with a sweeping motion from medial to lateral, further freeing may be performed. If obstruction is caused by a pubovaginal sling, the lateral wings of the sling may be cut. Likewise if the obstruction is caused by suspension sutures, these may be cut. As with transvaginal urethrolysis, a Martius flap may be placed. Petrou et al. reported a 3% recurrent stress incontinence rate.[50]

Retropubic Urethrolysis

The technique of retropubic urethrolysis has been described by Webster and Kreder.[48] It may be accomplished through a Pfannenstiel or low midline incision. After exposing the retropubic space, all prevesical and retropubic adhesions are sharply incised. The object is to restore complete mobility to the anterior vaginal wall, allowing free movement of the vesicourethral unit. The urethra and urethrovesical junction are dissected off the pubic bone, without separating them from the anterior vaginal wall. This is facilitated by the surgeon placing the nondominate hand in the vagina. Some degree of sharp dissection lateral to the urethra is usually required. As a result, one is usually left with a paravaginal defect. This should be repaired by re-approximating the paravaginal fascia to the fascia of the obturator internus along the arcus tendineous . We prefer to place paravaginal sutures and leave them untied until after an omental flap is placed between the pubic bone and the urethra. The omentum fills the dead space and helps to prevent recurrent adhesion. It may be obtained by making a small incision in the peritoneum and if necessary cutting the omentum to create a pedicle flap. Webster and Kreder reported recurrent stress incontinence due to intrinsic sphincter deficiency in 13% of patients.[48]

Summary

Voiding dysfunction and urinary retention may occur after all types of incontinence surgery. They are often transient, but can persist requiring intervention. Obstruction is common among patients with persistent symptoms, especially those with incomplete emptying. However, its diagnosis can be difficult if rigid urodynamic criteria are applied. In cases of unequivocal or presumed obstruction, urethrolysis by a variety of techniques, offers favorable results.

References

1. Kondo A, Kato K, Gotoh M, Narushima M, Saito M (1998) The Stamey and Gittes procedures: long-term followup in relation to incontinence types and patient age. J Urol 160: 756–8.
2. Alcalay M, Monga A, Stanton SL (1995) Burch colposuspension: a 10–20 year follow up. Br J Obstet Gynaecol 102: 740–5.
3. Abrams P, Wein AJ (1999) The overactive bladder and incontinence: definitions and a plea for discussion. Neurourol Urodyn 18: 413–16.
4. Bates CP, Bradley WE, Glen E et al. (1981) Fourth report on the standardisation of terminology of lower urinary tract function. Terminology related to neuromuscular dysfunction of the lower urinary tract. Produced by the International Continence Society. Br J Urol 53: 333–5.
5. Brading AF (1997) A myogenic basis for the overactive bladder. Urology 50: 57–67.
6. Groat WC de (1997) A neurologic basis for the overactive bladder. Urology 50: 36–52.
7. Brading AF, Turner WH (1994) The unstable bladder: towards a common mechanism. Br J Urol 73: 3–8.
8. Turner WH, Brading AF (1997) Smooth muscle of the bladder in the normal and the diseased state: pathophysiology, diagnosis and treatment. Pharm Ther 75: 77–110.
9. Jarvis GJ (1981) Detrusor muscle instability–a complication of surgery? Am J Obstet Gynecol 139: 219.
10. Langer R, Ron-el R, Newman M, Herman A, Caspi E (1988) Detrusor instability following colposuspension for urinary stress incontinence. Br J Obstet Gynaecol 95: 607–10.
11. Fulford SC, Flynn R, Barrington J, Appanna T, Stephenson TP (1999) An assessment of the surgical outcome and urodynamic effects of the pubovaginal sling for stress incontinence and the associated urge syndrome. J Urol 162: 135–7.
12. Lagro-Janssen T, Smits A, Weel C Van (1992) Urinary incontinence in women and the effects on their lives. Scand J Prim Health Care 10: 211–16.

13. Dupont MC, Albo ME, Raz S (1996) Diagnosis of stress urinary incontinence. An overview. Urol Clin N Amer 23: 407–15.
14. Diokno AC, Brown MB, Brock BM, Herzog AR, Normolle DP (1989) Prevalence and outcome of surgery for female incontinence. Urology 33: 285–90.
15. Chaikin DC, Rosenthal J, Blaivas JG (1998) Pubovaginal fascial sling for all types of stress urinary incontinence: long-term analysis. J Urol 160: 1312–16.
16. Hassouna ME, Ghoniem GM (1999) Long-term outcome and quality of life after modified pubovaginal sling for intrinsic sphincteric deficiency. Urology 53: 2872–91.
17. Raz S, Sussman EM, Erickson DB, Bregg KJ, Nitti VW (1992) The Raz bladder neck suspension: results in 206 patients. J Urol 148: 845–50.
18. Maher C, Dwyer P, Carey M, Gilmour D (1999) The Burch colposuspension for recurrent urinary stress incontinence following retropubic continence surgery. Br J Obstet Gynaecol 106: 719–24.
19. Cardozo L, Hextall A, Bailey J, Boos K (1999) Colposuspension after previous failed incontinence surgery: a prospective observational study. Br J Obstet Gynaecol 106: 340–4.
20. Stanton SL, Cardozo LD (1979) A comparison of vaginal and suprapubic surgery in the correction of incontinence due to urethral sphincter incompetence. Br J Urol 51: 497–9.
21. Brown K, Hilton P (1999) The incidence of detrusor instability before and after colposuspension: a study using conventional and ambulatory urodynamic monitoring. BJU Int 84: 961–5.
22. Ulmsten U, Johnson P, Rezapour M (1999) A three-year follow up of tension free vaginal tape for surgical treatment of female stress urinary incontinence. Br J Obstet Gynaecol 106: 345–50.
23. Vierhout ME, Mulder AF (1992) De novo detrusor instability after Burch colposuspension. Acta Obstet Gynecol Scand 71: 414–46.
24. Arnold EP, Webster JR, Loose H et al. (1973) Urodynamics of female incontinence: factors influencing the results of surgery. Am J Obstet Gynecol 117: 805–13.
25. Stanton SL, Cardozo L, Williams JE, Ritchie D, Allan V (1978) Clinical and urodynamic features of failed incontinence surgery in the female. Obstet Gynecol 51: 515–20.
26. Hutchings A, Griffiths J, Black NA (1998) Surgery for stress incontinence: factors associated with a successful outcome. Br J Urol 82: 634–41.
27. Berghmans LCM, Hendriks HJM, de Bie RA et al. (2000) Conservative treatment of urge urinary incontinence in women: a systematic review of randomised clinical trials. BJU Int 85: 254–263.
28. Andersson K-E, Appell R, Cardozo LD et al. (1999) The pharmacological treatment of urinary incontinence. BJU Int 84: 923–47.
29. Bemelmans BLH, Mundy AR, Craggs MD (1999) Neuromodulation by implant for treating lower urinary tract symptoms and dysfunction. Eur Urol 36: 81–91.
30. Chancellor MB, Groat WC de (1999) Intravesical capsaicin and resiniferatoxin therapy: spicing up the ways to treat the overactive bladder. J Urol 162: 3–11.
31. Horbach NS (1991) Suburethral sling procedures. In: Ostergard DE, Bent AE (ed) .Urogynecology and Urodynamics Theory and Practice, 3rd edn. Williams and Wilkins, Baltimore, pp. 413–21.
32. Juma S, Sdrales L (1993) Etiology of urinary retention after bladder neck suspension. J Urol 149: 400A.
33. Spencer JR, O'Conor VJ Jr, Schaeffer AJ (1987) Comparison of endoscopic suspension of the vesical neck with suprapubic vesicourethropexy for treatment of stress urinary incontinence. J Urol 137: 411–15.

34. Mundy AR (1983) A trial comparing the Stamey bladder neck suspension with colposuspension for the treatment of stress incontinence. Br J Urol 55: 687–90.
35. McDuffie RW, Litin RB, Blundon KE (1981) Urethrovesical suspension (Marshall–Marchetti–Krantz). Experience wiuth 204 cases. Amer J Surg 141: 297–8.
36. Cardozo LD, Stanton SL, Williams JE (1979) Detrusor instability following surgery for genuine stress incontinence. Br J Urol 51: 204–210.
37. Rost A, Fiedler U, Fester C (1979) Comparative analysis of the results of suspension-urethroplasty according to Marshall–Marchetti–Krantz and of urethrovesicopexy with adhesive. Urol Int 34: 167–75.
38. Leach GE, Dmochowski RR, Appell RA et al. (1997) Female stress urinary incontinence clinical guidelines panel report on surgical management of female stress urinary incontinence. J Urol 158: 875–80.
39. Marshall VF, Marchetti AA, Krantz KE (1949) The correction of stress incontinence by simple vesicourethral suspension. Surg Gynecol Obstet 88: 509–18.
40. Marchetti AA, Marshall VM, Shultis LD (1957) Simple vesicourethral suspension; a survey. Am J Obstet Gynecol 74: 57–62.
41. Pope AJ, Shaw PJR, Coptcoat MJ et al. (1990) Changes in bladder function following a surgical alteration in outflow resistance. Neurourol Urodynam 9: 503–8.
42. Bass JS, Leach GE (1991) Bladder outlet obstruction in women. Probl Urol 5: 141–54.
43. Carr LK, Webster GD (1997) Voiding dysfunction following incontinence surgery: diagnosis and treatment with retropubic or vaginal urethrolysis. J Urol 157: 821–3.
44. Nitti V, Raz W (1994) Obstruction following anti-incontinence procedures: diagnosis and treatment with transvaginal urethrolysis. J Urol 152: 93–8.
45. Nitti VW, Tu LM, Gitlin J (1999) Diagnosing bladder outlet obstruction in women. J Urol 161: 1535–40.
46. Chassagne S, Bernier PA, Haab F et al. (1998) Proposed cutoff values to define bladder outlet obstruction in women. Urology 51: 408–11.
47. Foster HE, McGuire EJ (1993) Management of urethral obstruction with transvaginal urethrolysis. J Urol 150: 1448–51.
48. Webster GD, Kreder KJ (1990) Voiding dysfunction following cystourethropexy: its evaluation and management. J Urol 144: 670–3.
49. Nitti VW, Raz S (1996) Urinary retention. In: Raz S (ed) Female Urology, 2nd edn. W. B. Saunders, Philadelphia, Pa., pp. 197–213.
50. Petrou SP, Brown JA, Blaivas JG (1999) Suprameatal transvaginal urethrolysis. J Urol 161: 1269–71.
51. Zimmern PE, Hadley HR, Leach GE, Raz S (1987) Female urethral obstruction after Marshall–Marchetti–Krantz operation. J Urol 138: 517–20.
52. Cross CA, Cespedes RD, English SF, McGuire EJ (1998) Transvaginal urethrolysis for urethral obstruction after anti-incontinence surgery. J Urol 159: 1199–201.
53. Goldman HB, Rackley RR, Appell RA (1999) The efficacy of urethrolysis without re-suspension for iatrogenic obstruction. J Urol 161: 196–9.
54. Leach GE, Raz S (1984) Modified Pereyra bladder neck suspension after previously failed anti-incontinence surgery. Urology 23: 359–62.

25 Bowel

Devinder Kumar

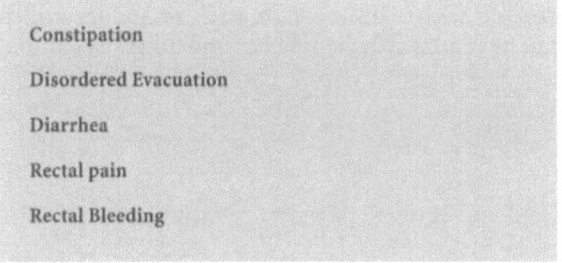

Constipation

Disordered Evacuation

Diarrhea

Rectal pain

Rectal Bleeding

Postoperative bowel symptoms are common following pelvic surgery, especially when operative procedures are performed in the vicinity of pelvic nerves. Most of these symptoms are transient, but when pelvic nerves are damaged, either temporarily or permanently, then the symptoms can be longer lasting or even permanent. Bowel symptoms following pelvic surgery include constipation, disordered evacuation, fecal impaction, diarrhea, anal or rectal pain, and bleeding.

Constipation

This is a relatively common problem following pelvic surgery. In the majority of cases it is due to the effect of anesthetic and analgesic drugs. Prolonged periods of confinement to bed also contribute to the symptom of constipation. This can be managed successfully by commencing the patient on a bulking agent and a mild laxative such as lactulose. It is also important to maintain an adequate oral fluid intake. Early mobilization and adequate pain control are other important prophylactic measures against the development of constipation.

Disordered Evacuation

Defecation following pelvic surgery most commonly is associated with a sensory impairment of the anorectum. The patient loses the urge to defecate and may develop fecal impaction or inability to evacuate. Such cases can be successfully managed with the help of regular use of glycerine suppositories. Occasionally intermittent enemas may be required. The majority of patients developing fecal impaction after pelvic or anorectal surgery are due to inadequate pain control. In these patients there may be associated urinary retention. Adequate analgesia combined with regular use of suppositories or enemas will often result in prompt resolution of such symptoms.

Diarrhea

True diarrhea following pelvic or anorectal surgery is uncommon. The most frequent symptom encountered is frequency of defecation. This is noticed when the compliance or capacity of the rectum is compromised following the surgery. Successful management consists of keeping the stool soft and bulky and the rectum empty with the help of suppositories. In most cases adaptation will occur and the stool frequency will drop to more acceptable levels over a course of 6–9 months when supportive management can be withdrawn.

In patients with true diarrhea, an infective cause must be excluded by stool microscopy and culture. A sigmoidoscopy should be performed to inspect rectal mucosa, looking for evidence of inflammation. The treatment consists of maintaining an adequate fluid and electrolyte balance. If an infective cause is found, then the infection should be treated. When there is no obvious cause, then management with constipating agents such as codeine phosphate or loperamide may be necessary.

Rectal Pain

Anal or rectal pain following pelvic surgery can be due either to the operative procedure itself or to its complications. Whenever possible an appropriate assessment of the expected pain following surgery should be made and remedial measures instituted. These include infiltration of the wound with local anesthetics or a caudal block. Regular use of pain-relieving drugs orally or as patient-controlled analgesia will successfully control postoperative pain in most patients.

Pain secondary to complications of the procedure itself is often due to infection. This must be excluded by careful inspection of the wound or the operation site. If there is evidence for infection then it should be adequately drained and the wound left open. Appropriate antibiotic cover should also be commenced. If evidence for an infective cause is not present on clinical examination, then the help of imaging modalities such as ultrasonography should be sought. It is important to control postoperative pain adequately because the presence of pain will compound other symptoms such as constipation.

Rectal Bleeding

True hemorrhage following pelvic surgery is relatively uncommon. It is usually as a result of a missed bleeding point or venous ooze from the large operative field. The venous ooze will stop spontaneously in most cases. Arterial bleeding accompanied by signs of shock will require re-operation and stoppage of bleeding.

Minor bleeding, either from a suture line or from a pelvic organ such as the urinary bladder due to retraction during the operation, will stop spontaneously and often does not require any specific measures. Suture lines easily accessible from the perineum such as anal or low rectal ones should be dressed with a haemostatic pack or sponge which can be removed 24 hours later under light sedation.

Part IX

Outcome Measures

26 Urinary Incontinence

François Haab, Mouad Nouri, and Calin Ciofu

Stress urinary incontinence (SUI) is a devastating condition that afflicts 20% of women in developing countries. Although many therapeutic options are available to treat SUI, surgery remains the most effective. Recently, the American Urological Association (AUA) published an extensive literature review on surgical treatment for SUI.[1] Its main conclusion was that there is a lack of standardization to measure postoperative outcome. Reported success rates of surgical procedures to treat SUI varied, and much of this variability related to the study methodology selected. More recently, the first International Consultation on Urinary Incontinence reached a similar conclusion concerning the existing literature and therefore proposed clinical and research guidelines on urinary incontinence.[2] It is now clear that evaluation of therapies proposed to correct SUI, including subjective and objective tests, should be extensive.

This chapter reviews and discusses evaluation tools that are already validated and used to assess postoperative outcome after surgery for SUI.

Global Evaluation of Urinary Incontinence

Subjective Tests

Clinical history remains the most common method of assessing patient symptoms. To standardize information reported by patients, some authors have developed very basic questionnaires and scoring systems, the most popular of which is described by Stamey.[3] In this system, scoring varies from no incontinence (score 0) to total incontinence at all times of the day (score 3). However, none of these instruments, including Stamey's, has been tested for validity or reliability.

Recording number and type of pads used to prevent leakage is another way to assess degree of incontinence. However, this information is largely patient dependent. Some dry patients may still use a pad just in case, whereas some patients who leak may not use pads because they prefer to change clothes.

Objective Tests

Objective evaluation of procedures to treat anatomical SUI necessitates use of standardized questionnaires. This was first pointed out in a study published in 1996 by Sirls et al. when they established that study methodology profoundly affects reported outcomes. In this study, only 47% of patients were considered cured according to questionnaire evaluation versus 72% with retrospective chart review.[4] However, cure/dry rates alone do not fully represent potential treatment benefits. Many patients not completely cured for SUI still report substantial improvement or satisfaction. Conversely, some patients report dissatisfaction due to voiding problems or de-novo detrusor instability even when cured for SUI. Therefore, two different types

Table 26.1. Questionnaires used to evaluate symptom and quality of life related to urinary symptoms in women (adapted from reference 5)

Symptom assessment

Urogenital distress inventory (UDI)
King's Health Questionnaire
Symptom Severity Index (SSI)
Bristol Lower Urinary Tract Symptoms (BFLUTS)

Quality of life assessment

Incontinence impact questionnaire (IIQ)
Symptom Impact Index (SSI)
King's Health Questionnaire
Contilife 28

of questionnaire are necessary to adequately describe a patient's condition: one to evaluate symptoms and another to evaluate impact of those symptoms on quality of life.[5]

The validation process for questionnaire development is long and complicated. Any questionnaire must be tested to prove that it measures what is intended and that measurements are reproducible and sensitive to changes over time or intervention.[5] Many questionnaires specific to urinary incontinence have been designed, validated, and translated into different languages[5] (Table 26.1).

Evaluation of SUI

Subjective Tests

Evaluation of SUI can be done subjectively by asking patients to rate efforts that induce urinary leakage from strongest to weakest, e.g. sneezing, practicing sports, coughing, walking, etc. Some authors have attempted to design symptomatic classification of SUI based on findings discovered while taking a history. These classifications usually include three categories: leakage during strong exercise, leakage during intermediate exercise, leakage without exercising[5]. These classifications, even if useful in routine practice, are very subjective and could not be used for clinical studies.

Objective Tests

Evaluation of Urethral Hypermobility

Postoperative evaluation of urethral mobility is crucially important. It should be possible to determine whether recurrence of SUI is due to recurrence of urethral hypermobility or of intrinsic sphincteric deficiency. Urethral position is best evaluated by careful vaginal examination. A cotton swab test has been proposed to objectively quantify the degree of urethral hypermobility.[6] Many authors consider an upward

movement of the urethral axis greater than 30° as indicative of a hypermobile urethra. Therefore, women presenting with SUI and with a cotton swab test showing limited urethral mobility should be suspected of having intrinsic sphincteric deficiency. However, two studies report that the cotton swab test contributed no additional information to the history and simple physical examination.[7] Furthermore, since there is no control of the amount of pressure generated when the patient strains, the test is neither standardized nor reproducible. Several authors have investigated imaging techniques to objectively quantify degree of urethral hypermobility.[8] Lateral films of voiding cystourethrography at rest and during straining can document poor urethral support or persistent urethral hypermobility. However, this technique exposes patients to radiation. Several techniques have been proposed for sonography of the bladder neck, and abnormal rotational descent of the bladder neck from the rest position with cough or Valsalva maneuver can be documented.[9] However, considerable overlap between incontinent and continent women for all anatomical parameters was recorded. All imaging techniques were considered optional tests in the recommendations of the first International Consultation on Urinary Incontinence.[2]

Pad Test

An objective method to detect and quantify urine loss is essential during evaluation of patients with urinary incontinence. Quantification of urine loss in incontinent women by means of pad weighing is widely used in clinical practice, and various forms of perineal pad testing have been proposed in the literature.[10] The 1 hour pad test recommended by the International Continence Society is frequently used in clinical studies.[11] Though some authors consider the test reproducible and correlated to symptoms, others raise concerns over a low inter- and intra-subject reproducibility rate, which therefore limits the test's usefulness. Other pad tests performed with a fixed bladder volume of 50% or 75% of cystometric capacity have been tested and recommended as more reproducible than the standardized 1 hour test.[12,13] Still other authors contend that only the 24 hour or home pad test mimic patients' ordinary life situations.[14,15] Overall, these tests are difficult to organize and are probably best suited for clinical research.

Urodynamic Testing

Urethral Pressure Profilometry

Urethral pressure profilometry at rest is commonly used to measure urethral sphincter function. However, there is continued controversy concerning reliability and clinical usefulness of urethral closure pressure. [7] Urethral pressure profilometry reflects forces tending to produce opposition at the level of the urethra. Thus, measured urethral pressure is a force, not a pressure.[7] Moreover, pressure measured is significantly influenced by artefacts that depend on the specific technique used. From a clinical standpoint, numerous studies show that maximum urethral closure pressure at rest tends to be lower in stress-incontinent women than in continent women.[16] However, the test has not been correlated with type or severity of urinary incontinence. Therefore, urethral closure pressure cannot be considered a reliable assessment of postoperative outcome.[7]

Valsalva Leak Point Pressure

Valsalva leak point pressure (VLPP) – defined as the lowest total bladder pressure at which urinary leakage occurs during progressive increases in intraabdominal pressure by Valsalva maneuver, and proposed as a urodynamic test to identify intrinsic sphincteric deficiency – could theoretically qualify as an objective test to quantify degree of urethral resistance to leakage.[17] Nitti et al. found strong correlation between subjective degree of urinary incontinence and VLPP.[18] However, its lack of reproducibility and the absence of information regarding intra-individual variations have limited its use in clinical practice.[7]

Evaluation of Postoperative Voiding Disorders

Subjective Evaluation

Evaluation of postoperative voiding disorders is critical because these disorders may be the most distressing symptoms after surgery for stress incontinence. Patient history should include questions regarding the frequency of micturition during day and night, the feeling of urgency, and the number of episodes of urge incontinence. These symptoms are best assessed using validated, self-administered questionnaires, which should be completed by patients before and after surgery. Voiding dysfunction is not easy to characterize in women, even by questionnaires. Questions asked regarding abnormal micturition habits and sensation of incomplete bladder emptying should be as precise as possible.

Objective Evaluation

Frequency–volume charts are essential to objectively document frequency, nocturia, and urgency symptoms.[5] For at least three consecutive days patients are asked to daily record: incontinent episodes, frequency of urination day and night, amount of fluid taken, and sometimes also volume voided. Recently, the International Consultation on Urinary Incontinence proposed three levels of voiding diaries for routine practice and clinical trials.[2] The test should be performed pre- and postoperatively. Frequency–volume charts exhibit test–retest reliability and should be part of systematic evaluations of patients suffering from urinary incontinence.

Uroflowmetry with post-void residual measurements is the only objective test to quantify voiding dysfunction. Although the test is noninvasive and easy to perform, normal values for women are still needed. To consider flow normal, most authors have arbitrarily chosen an Q_{max} value of >15 ml/s. Furthermore, flow value does not determine whether there is bladder outlet obstruction or detrusor muscle weakness. Chassagne et al. have presented data on pressure flow measurements in women for objective diagnosis of bladder outlet obstruction.[19]

Conclusions

Urinary incontinence is a multidimensional syndrome for which medical or surgical therapies often alleviate symptoms but do not cure. Therefore, assessment should include all types of evaluation: questionnaires, objective and subjective tests, and medico-economic evaluation. Better evaluation of our practice will help patients and physicians make treatment decisions.

References

1. Leach GE, Dmochowski RR, Appell RA et al. (1997) Female stress urinary incontinence clinical guidelines panel summary report on surgical management of female stress urinary incontinence. J Urol 158: 875–80.
2. Thuroff J, Norton J, Artibani W, Abrams P, Haab F (1999) Clinical guidelines. In: Abrams P, Khoury S, Wein A (ed) Proceedings of the First International consultation on Urinary Incontinence, Paris, 1999.
3. Stamey TA (1980) Endoscopic suspension of the vesical neck for urinary incontinence in females. Report on 203 consecutive patients. Ann Surg 192: 465–72.
4. Sirls LT, Keoleian CM, Korman HJ, Kirkemo AK (1995) The effect of study methodology on reported success rates of the modified Pereyra bladder neck suspension. J Urol 154: 1732–5.
5. Donovan J, Naughton M, Gotoh M et al. (1999) Symptom and quality of life assessment. In: Abrams P, Khoury S, Wein A (ed) Proceeding of the First International Consultation on Urinary Incontinence, Paris, 1999, pp. 297–330.
6. Bergman A, Mc Carthy TA, Ballard CA, Yannai J (1987) Role of the Q tip test in evaluating stress urinary incontinence. J Reprod Med 32: 273–7.
7. Haab F, Zimmern PE, Leach GE (1996) Female stress urinary incontinence due to intrinsic sphincteric deficiency : recognition and management. J Urol 156: 3–17.

8. Zimmern PE (1991) The role of voiding cystourethrography in the evaluation of the female lower urinary tract. Probl Urol 5: 23–9.
9. Mostwin JL, Yang A, Sanders R, Genadry R (1995) Radiography, sonography and magneric resonance imaging for stress incontinence. Contribution, uses and limitations. Urol Clin North Am 22: 539–42.
10. Kroman-Andersen B, Jakobsen H, Andersen JT (1989) Pad weighing tests : a literature survey on test accuracy and reproducibility. Neurourol Urodyn 8: 237–42.
11. Abrams P, Blaivas JG, Stanton S, Andersen JT (1990) The standardization of terminology of lower urinary tract function recommended by the International Continence Society. Int Urogynecol J 1: 45–48.
12. Jakobsen H, Kromann-Andersen B, Nielsen K, Maegaard E (1993) Pad weighing tests with 50% or 75% bladder filling. Does it matter?. Acta Obstet Scand 72: 377–81.
13. Nygaard I, Zmolek G (1995) Exercice pad testing in continent exercisers : reproducibility and correlation with voided volume, pyridium staining and type of exercise. Neurourol Urodyn 14: 125–9.
14. Rasmussen A, Mouritsen L, Dalgaard A, Frimodt-Moller C (1994) Twenty four hour pad weighing test: reproducibility and dependency of activity level and fluid intake. Neurourol Urodyn 13: 261–5.
15. Versi E, Orrego G, Hardy E et al. (1996) Evaluation of the home pad test in the investigation of female urinary incontinence. Br J Obstet Gynaecol 103: 162–7.
16. Versi E (1990) Discriminant analysis of urethral pressure profilometry data for the diagnosis of genuine stress incontinence. Br J Obstet Gynaecol 97: 251–8.
17. McGuire EJ, Fitzpatrick CC, Wan J et al. (1993) Clinical assessment of urethral sphincter function. J Urol 150: 1452–7.
18. Nitti VW, Coombs AJ (1995) Correlation of Valsalva leak point pressure with subjective degree of stress urinary incontinence in females. J Urol 153: 492A.
19. Chassagne S, Bernier P, Haab F, Roehrborn K, Zimmern PE (1998) Female nomogram for bladder outlet obstruction. Urology 51(3): 408–14.

27 Pelvic Organ Prolapse

E. Ann Gormley

Pelvic organ prolapse is a common problem and may occur to some degree in 50% of parous women. An estimated 10–20% of these women will have symptomatic prolapse and present for repair. Despite the relatively common nature of this problem we know little about the natural history of the disease when left untreated. Although operations are commonly performed to treat the problem, long-term outcome data is lacking.

Procedures

Cystocele Repair

Anterior Colporrhaphy

An anterior colporrhaphy is often combined with other surgical procedures and the results are often reported in conjunction with other procedures. Beck[1] in 1991 reported on a series of 519 patients who underwent anterior colporrhaphy. Postoperative follow up was variable depending on why the surgery was performed, and ranged from 6 weeks to over 5 years. The recurrence rate of anterior vaginal wall prolapse was not reported. Although many surgeons have abandoned this procedure as an anti-incontinence procedure, Beck has advocated it for this purpose. He reported a cure rate for genuine stress incontinence of 93.5% and an 84% cure rate for selected patients with mixed incontinence. Five percent of patients not incontinent preoperatively developed genuine stress incontinence following the procedure and 5% developed detrusor instability or mixed incontinence. The complication rate was 1% exclusive of incontinence.

Cystoceles have also been repaired vaginally by using a variety of types of material to close the defect analogous to inguinal hernia repairs. Nicita[2] used a large hammock-shaped piece of polypropylene mesh to support prolapsed pelvic organs, including cystoceles in 44 patients. The mesh was anchored between the two arcus tendinous muscles and was also fixed in the anteroposterior direction. With a short follow-up, median 13.9 months, no recurrent cystoceles were detected using cystography. One patient had a vaginal erosion necessitating removal of a portion of the mesh. The same patient had persistent dyspareunia.

Others have reported using a fascia lata patch.[3] In a group of 26 patients there was 1 small assymptomatic recurrence with a median 12 month follow-up. Five patients had vaginal mucosa sloughing but none required patch removal.

Complications of anterior colporrhaphy include the immediate complications of bleeding, cystotomy, ureteral injury, and urethrovaginal fistula. Urethrovaginal fistula occurred in 2 of Beck's 519 cases. Long-term complications include voiding dysfunction, dyspareunia, and recurrence. Voiding dysfunction, either incontinence or retention, can be a difficult complication to deal with following an anterior colporrhaphy. Incontinence usually occurs when the patient has unrecognized intrinsic sphincter dysfunction that is unmasked once the prolapse is repaired. Preoperatively the pelvic floor prolapse may have obstructed the urethra or bladder neck, preventing leakage from occurring despite intrinsic sphincter dysfunction. Postoperatively, when the pelvic floor is reconstructed, incontinence occurs. Complete retention or incomplete emptying postoperatively has been attributed to a subclinical voiding dysfunction preoperatively.[4] The dissection of the anterior vaginal wall of the bladder may also theoretically denervate the pelvic nerve branches where they enter the bladder at the trigone causing decreased contraction of the bladder. Preoperative urodynamics, including an assessment of the bladder neck with all prolapse reduced, as well as a pressure–flow study to examine the ability of the bladder to contract, can preoperatively predict those patients who are at risk of developing postoperative incontinence or voiding difficulty. Urodynamics can also be used postoperatively to objectively assess outcome.

Sexual dysfunction, has been reported particularly when anterior colporrhaphy is combined with posterior colporrhaphy.

If synthetic material is used in the repair, sloughing of vaginal tissue or erosion of the synthetic material through the vaginal tissue may occur. Reoperation may be difficult because of scarring and fibrosis, particularly when certain synthetic materials are used.

Paravaginal Repair

Richardson[5] in 1976 described the types and locations of fascial defects involved in the pathogenesis of cystoceles. The paravaginal repair was designed to repair a lateral defect. Richardson performed the procedure either as a primary operation for cystourethrocele with stress incontinence or as a secondary operation in those who had failed prior surgery for stress incontinence or cystourethrocele (or both). A satisfactory result was described as correction of the cystourethrocele, relief of stress incontinence, preservation of normal voiding function, and no postoperative bladder dysfunction. In a series of 800 cases a 95% satisfactory result was obtained.[6]

In another report on 233 patients, Richardson[7] described 10 patients who developed recurrent prolapse. He attributed 4 recurrences to technical errors. One patient had a recurrence of the original defect, 4 patients developed central defects and 1 patient developed a contralateral defect after a unilateral repair of a lateral defect.

Complications of paravaginal repair are uncommon and include complications inherent to any surgical procedure.

Rectocele Repair

Little data has been published on the outcomes of rectocele repair. Ginsberg et al.[8] noted that recurrent rectocele is uncommon. They reviewed 144 patients with a mean follow-up of 15 months (range 8–30 months) and found a recurrence rate of only 2%.

Complications of rectocele repair include urinary retention, rectovaginal fistula, vaginal narrowing, and dyspareunia. The major complication of a rectocele repair is dyspareunia. Francis[9] noted that approximately half of sexually active women had some sexual problems after anterior and posterior colporrhaphy with or without hysterectomy. Fifty-five per cent of the affected patients reported lack of libido or impotence in one or other partner. In some cases these problems predated their surgery. The remaining patients had dyspareunia, shortened or stenotic vaginas, or fear of injury. Other studies have shown improvement in sexual satisfaction following pelvic floor surgery. Haase[10] reported that in a group of women who were sexually active preoperatively that postoperatively 24% experienced improvement in sexual function and only 9% experienced deterioration. The improvement was often attributed to cure of urinary incontinence. Deterioration was always due to dyspareunia in patients who underwent posterior colporrhaphy.

Vaginal Hysterectomy

Vaginal hysterectomy is advocated when there is significant uterine prolapse or when there is significant gynecologic pathology to warrant hysterectomy. In patients with stress incontinence or minimal pelvic relaxation the supportive ligaments of the uterus must be evaluated. If the cervix descends below the level of the hymenal ring with traction applied to a tenaculum on the cervix the supporting ligaments of the uterus are considered inadequate and a hysterectomy should be considered.[11]

When a vaginal hysterectomy is performed as part of a pelvic floor reconstruction the cardinal and uterosacral ligaments are shortened and reattached to the vagina, and the cul-de-sac is obliterated.[12] Despite these maneuvers vaginal prolapse post hysterectomy can occur. The incidence of this varies.

Jenkins[13] reported on 50 patients treated with bilateral uterosacral ligament fixation to the vaginal cuff by the vaginal route. Patients had uterine or vaginal vault prolapse with descent of the cervix or the vaginal vault preoperatively. Concomitant enterocele, cystocele, rectocele, and stress incontinence were repaired at the same time. Patients were evaluated at 1, 2, 6, and 12 months and then yearly. The mean follow-up was 33 (range 6–48) months for the uterine prolapse group and 20 (range 6–38) months for the vaginal vault group. None of the patients had recurrent vaginal vault prolapse. Two patients in the uterine prolapse group had recurrent but asymptomatic cystoceles. The author noted that his report was limited by a small number of patients, a short follow-up, and by the operating surgeon having performed the review. In contrast, Marana[14] reported that when vaginal hysterectomy and anterior and posterior repairs were performed for uterovaginal prolapse there was a high rate of unsuccessful correction of prolapse. When patients were examined an average of 5 years after their surgery, 95.7% of patients had some degree of genital prolapse. Three of 47 evaluable patients had complete vault prolapse. These results were obtained despite fixation of the cardinal ligaments to the lateral walls of the vagina and the uterosacral ligaments to the vaginal apex.

In addition to vaginal prolapse the complications of vaginal hysterectomy include bleeding, infection, bladder injury, and bladder or ureteral fistula.

Enterocele Repair

Although an enterocele can occur before a hysterectomy the majority are seen following a hysterectomy or a bladder suspension when there is anterior displacement of the vagina. The enterocele is a herniation of bowel through a defect at the vaginal apex as a result of widely separated uterosacral ligaments. Most enteroceles that occur after hysterectomy can be repaired vaginally. The goal of surgery is to reduce the hernia, plicate the uterosacral and cardinal ligaments, and provide support for the vaginal vault while maintaining adequate vaginal length. Raz[15] reported in 1997 on a technique that utilized absorbable Dexon mesh to reinforce the repair. The repair was performed in conjunction with a formal cystocele repair or sacrospinous fixation if an anterior prolapse or vault prolapse was present. The technique was considered successful in the short term with only one of 47 patients having a recurrence with a mean follow-up of 14 months.

Raz[16] later reported on the same type of enterocele repair performed with a culdoplasty instead of a sacrospinous fixation. The culdoplasty was performed by suturing the apex of the vagina to the pararectal levator fascia. Two of 75 patients had a recurrence of an enterocele at a mean follow-up of 24 months (range 6–45 months).

The immediate complications of enterocele repair include bleeding, ureteric injury and rectal, bladder, or small-bowel perforation. In the 2 series reported above complications included 1 ureteral injury requiring reimplantation, 1 patient with prolonged pain in the distribution of the pudendal nerve and 2 patients with vaginal shortening. No infections of the absorbable mesh have been reported.

Vaginal Vault Prolapse Repair

The vaginal vault can be suspended in a variety of ways but it is reasonable to divide these repairs into those performed vaginally, such as the sacrospinous fixation, and those performed abdominally, such as an abdominal sacral colpopexy.

Sacrospinous Fixation

Methods that have been advocated to prevent vault prolapse following hysterectomy have included a sacrospinous fixation or a McCall culdoplasty. Although these procedures may help to elevate the apex of the vagina or prevent enterocele formation they do not completely prevent against the development of further prolapse. Colombo et al.[17] performed a retrospective case control study to compare patients who underwent sacrospinous ligament fixation and a control group who underwent a modified McCall culdoplasty during vaginal hysterectomy. Patients were followed for 4–9 years. Prolapse recurrence at any vaginal site was 27% in the sacrospinous suspension group and 15% in the modified McCall culdoplasty group. In the sacrospinous group prolapse occurred 4 months to 5 years (median 1 year) after their initial surgery. The time to recurrence in the culdoplasty group was 2 months to 9 years (median 3 years).

Despite a risk of recurrence, a sacrospinous colpopexy has been shown to result in symptomatic improvement. Hewson[18] reported an initial overall satisfaction rate of approximately 90% and this was maintained at 80% even beyond 4 years.

Complications of a sacrospinalis repair include bleeding, bowel or rectal injury, injury to the sciatic or pudendal nerve, and ureteral injury.

When a sacrospinalis repair is performed in conjunction with a transvaginal needle suspension a 33% recurrent prolapse rate has been reported. Sze et al.[19] performed a modification of the Pereyra procedure and a sacrospinous ligament fixation on 54 women with pelvic organ prolapse and coexisting or potential stress incontinence. The control group consisted of 21 women who did not have incontinence and had undergone a sacrospinous ligament fixation. All women underwent anterior or posterior colpoperineorrhaphies and vaginal enterocele repairs when indicated. Patients were followed with an objective evaluation for an average follow up of 24 months (range 3–72 months). Eighteen subjects (33%) developed recurrent symptomatic prolapse whereas only 4 (19%) of the controls developed recurrent prolapse. Although there was no statistical significance between the two groups the authors believe that the recurrence rate in the sacrospinous ligament fixation group and transvaginal needle suspension is clinically important.

The factors responsible for this have been postulated to include an inherent weakness in the woman's tissue, neuropathy, or an anatomic distortion created by the two procedures. When these two procedures are combined the vagina is pulled in two directions, which alters the normal vaginal axis.

Abdominal Sacral Colpopexy

A transabdominal approach is often advocated in patients with recurrent vaginal vault prolapse. It is also used when the surgeon feels that access via the vagina is limited. In order to preserve vaginal function by restoring the normal anatomic axis of the vagina, many surgeons have advocated the use of indirect fixation with a graft which can be autologous or synthetic. Snyder and Krantz[20] retrospectively reviewed 147 patients undergoing abdominal sacral copopexy with either dacron or Gore-Tex grafts. The follow-up ranged from 1 month to 17 years (mean 43 months). Of 116 patients with at least 6 month follow-up, 108 patients had a good surgical result with at least 5 year follow-up. The definition of a good result included restoration of a functional vagina in the proper axis and no recurrence of presenting symptoms.

Recently abdominal sacral colpopexy has been performed laparascopically by anchoring the vaginal vault to the fascia of the abdominal muscles. Fedele[21] performed the procedure on 12 women and had a complete anatomic repair in all at a follow-up of 9–28 months. All patients had recovery of sexual function.

An overwhelming concern when a synthetic graft is used is erosion and infection. In Snyder's study 4 of 147 patients had the graft removed because of graft erosion. Only one of the four had recurrence of symptoms.

Timing of Assessment

The length of follow-up will impact on the recurrence rate of pelvic organ prolapse. Very good outcomes are anticipated in the immediate postoperative period. The optimum time to assess recurrence of vault prolapse or the development of a posthysterectomy vault prolapse or enterocele is after at least 5 years and ideally as long as 10 years. Symmonds et al.[22] reported that although 39% of patients developed symptoms of recurrent prolapse after hysterectomy within 2 years, 37% of patients

did not develop symptoms until 10 or more years. Morley and Delancey[23] reported the mean time to development of vault prolapse after vaginal hysterectomy was 8.9 years.

Assessment of Outcome

Physical examination, symptomatic improvement, or quality of life assessment may be used to evaluate surgical outcomes.

Physical findings of pelvic floor prolapse do not necessarily correlate with symptoms in preoperative patients. In a recently published study[24] the prevalence of any prolapse was 30.8%. No significant differences were noted in symptoms between those women who had prolapse and those who did not. If a patient is found postoperatively to have a small assymptomatic prolapse, should it be considered as a recurrence or is it only significant if it is symptomatic? Objective assessment of symptoms may be difficult in pelvic organ prolapse since there are no validated methods of scoring symptoms.

Quality of life assessment is becoming an increasingly important measurement tool in outcome analysis. A number of quality of life tools[25,26] have been developed and validated for incontinence. There are no published, validated quality of life tools for prolapse, but quality of life incontinence surveys have been adapted and used for prolapse.[27] When patients who had combined procedures for both prolapse and stress incontinence were surveyed postoperatively they had a statistically significant improvement in quality of life, although the improvement was not as great as that seen in those treated for incontinence alone.[28] This difference may be attributed to a greater recurrence rate of prolapse than incontinence.

Why Recurrent Prolapse Occurs

Depending on the original procedure performed, a recurrence of pelvic organ prolapse may not actually be a recurrence but may be a previously undetected defect that was not repaired as part of the original procedure. Once one defect is repaired, a second defect may become more obvious. Delancey[29] has described how an initial procedure may disturb the balance of the structural parts and thus predispose to a second defect occurring or cause an already present defect to increase after the initial procedure. Recurrences of vaginal prolapse occur with increasing age, although the actual frequency of this is unknown. Supporting tissue may have been weak to begin with, or it may weaken with continued stress on the tissue, increasing age, and changes that occur with menopause. Factors that contribute to continued stress on the supporting tissue include obesity, heavy lifting, chronic cough, and pregnancy. Poor nutrition and steroids can further contribute to weakness of the supporting tissues. The risk of prolapse also appears to be increased in patients with a first-degree relative affected.[30] Carley et al.[31] recently showed that patients requiring operative correction of pelvic organ prolapse are more likely than controls to have had increased parity, vaginal births, and maternal age at delivery. They are also more likely to have had an epidural at the time of delivery. Welgoss et al.[32] have shown that perineal neuropathy can occur with surgery for pelvic organ prolapse surgery. Using neurophysiological tests they examined 31 patients preoperatively and at a mean follow-up of 32 months (range 12–60 months). Eleven of 31 women developed perineal neuropathy. This was associated with a suboptimal outcome rather than an optimal outcome. The authors concluded that a surgical induced perineal neuropathy might contribute to failed pelvic floor reconstruction. Only 11 patients in this study were deemed to have an "optimum outcome."

Reporting Outcomes of Prolapse Surgery

In an effort to improve the quality of outcomes analysis in surgery for pelvic organ prolapse, a set of general principles that could be used to report outcomes was developed by a group from the American Urogynecology Society and the Society of Gynecologic Surgeons.[33] The consensus of the group was that standardized data should be collected preoperatively and postoperatively. The eight different areas where specific information is needed are summarized below.

Anatomic Changes

A standardized, reliable, validated, and reproducible system should be used. Each element of pelvic and vaginal support should be assessed. The position of examination and the measurement techniques should be standardized.

The pelvic organ prolapse score developed by the International Continence Society is advocated as a system to describe an individual woman's pelvic support.

Population Description

The patient population that undergoes procedures should be characterized. The methods of recruitment used, the inclusion and exclusion criteria, and

the technique of randomization when applicable should be outlined. The statistical justification for the number of patients needed, including a power analysis, should be provided.

Objective Laboratory Testing

When any objective scientific data is used in the assessment of patient's undergoing surgery for pelvic organ prolapse, the technique used to obtain the information and an analysis of how the information affected the outcome of the study should be reported.

Description of Exact Interventions

The operative procedure should be described in detail, including the materials used. The details of short- and long-term routine postoperative care should be specified.

Acute and Chronic Morbidity

Complications arising from the surgical procedure or occurring during the recovery from the surgery should be described. Methods used to prevent morbidity should also be described.

Description of Patient Follow-up

The same standardized assessment should be performed both before and after surgery. Ideally, independent observers using objective measurements should collect the data. The timing of preoperative and postoperative assessments must be specified and the duration of follow-up should be explicit. Whenever possible follow-up should be continued for at least 5 years. An exception to this is acute surgical failures which should be reported early to discourage others from doing the same operation.

Cost

Both direct and indirect costs should be quantified.

Quality of Life

Standardized and validated health-related quality of life instruments should be used as baseline and outcome variables. Domains examined should include, but not be limited to, social, physical, emotional, and sexual functioning.

To date, most published studies have not reported data using these guidelines. However, as these guidelines were published in 1996 it will be a number of years before we start to see 5 year follow-up data reported in this format. One would hope that this type of data is presently being collected and will be published once long-term follow-up is available.

References

1. Beck RP, McCormick S, Nordstrom L (1991) Experience with 519 anterior colporrhaphy procedures (1965-1990). Obstet Gynecol 78: 1011-18.
2. Nicita G (1998) A new operation for genitourinary prolapse. J Urol 160: 741-5.
3. Schlossberg SM, McCammon KA (1999) Fascia lata patch reconstruction of vaginal prolapse. American Urological Association Meeting, 1999, Dallas.
4. Bhatia NN, Bergman A (1986) Use of preoperative uroflowmetry and simultaneous urethrocystometry for predicting risk of prolonged postoperative bladder drainage. Urology 28: 440-5.
5. Richardson AC (1976) A new look at pelvic relaxation. Am J Obstet Gynecol 126: 568-73.
6. Richardson AC (1992) Paravaginal repair. In: Glenn HW (ed) Urogynecologic Surgery. Aspen Publishers, Gaithersburg, pp. 73-80.
7. Richardson AC, Edmonds PB, Williams NL (1981) Treatment of stress urinary incontinence due to paravaginal fascial defect. Obstet Gynecol 57: 357-63.
8. Ginsberg DA, Rovner ES, Raz S (1997) Pelvic floor relaxation; technique and results of repair in 144 patients. American Urological Association Annual Meeting , 1997, New Orleans.
9. Francis WJA, Jeffcoate TNA (1961) Dyspareunia following vaginal operations. Br J Obstet Gynaecol 68: 1-10.
10. Haase P, Skibsted L (1988) Influence of operations for stress incontinence and/or genital descensus on sexual life. Acta Obstet Gynecol Scand 67: 659-61.
11. Delancey JOL (1994) Surgical repair of uterine prolapse and enterocele. In: Kurch ED, McGuire EJ (ed) Female Urology. Co. J.B. Lippincott, Philadelphia, pp. 309-22.
12. Delancey JOL, Strohbehn K, Aronson MP (1998) Comparison of ureteral and cervical descents during vaginal hysterectomy for uterine prolapse. Am J Obstet Gynecol 179: 1405-10.
13. Jenkins van R II (1997) Uterosacral ligament fixation for vaginal vault suspension in uterine and vaginal vault prolapse. Am J Obstet Gynec 177: 1337-43.
14. Marana HR, Andrade JM, Marana RR et al. (1999) Vaginal hysterectomy for correcting genital prolapse. Long -term evaluation. J Reprod Med 44: 529-34.
15. Raz S, Ginsberg DA, Rovner ES (1997) Enterocele: technique and results of repair in 47 patients. American Urological Association Meeting, 1997, New Orleans.
16. Safir MH, Gousse AE, Ginsberg DA, Raz S (1998) A novel culdoplasty for repair of enterocele obviates need for sacrospinous fixation. American Urological Association Meeting, 1998, San Diego.
17. Colombo M, Milani R (1998) Sacrospinous ligament fixation and modified McCall culdoplasty during vaginal hysterectomy for advanced uterovaginal prolapse. Am J Obstet Gynecol 179: 13-20.
18. Hewson AD (1998) Transvaginal sacrospinous colpopexy for posthysterectomy vault prolapse. Aust N Z J Obstet Gynaecol 38: 318-24.
19. Sze EHM, Miklos JR, Partoll L, Roat T, Karram MM (1997) Sacrospinous ligament fixation with transvaginal needle suspension for advanced pelvic organ prolapse and stress incontinence. Obstet Gynecol 89: 94-6.
20. Snyder TE, Krantz KE (1991) Abdominal-retroperitoneal sacral colpopexy for the correction of vaginal prolapse. Obstet Gynecol 77: 944-9.
21. Fedele L, Garsia S, Bianchi S, Albiero A, Dorta M (1998) A new laparoscopic procedure for the correction of vaginal vault prolapse. J Urol 159: 1179-82.
22. Symmonds RE, William TJ, Lee RA, Webb MJ (1981) Posthysterectomy enterocele and vaginal vault prolapse. Am J Obstet Gynecol 140: 852-9.
23. Morley GW, DeLancey JOL (1988) Sacrospinous ligament fixation for eversion of the vagina. Am J Obstet Gynecol 158: 872-88.
24. Samuelsson E, Victor FTA, Tibblin G, Svardsudd KF (1999) Signs of genital prolapse in a Swedish population of women 20-59 years of age and possible related factors. Am J Obstet Gynecol 180: 299-305.
25. Wagner TH, Patrick DL, Bavendam TG, Martin ML, Buesching DP (1996) Quality of life in persons with urinary incontinence: Development of a new measure. Urology 47: 67-72.
26. Raz S, Erickson D (1992) SEAPI QMM incontinence classification system. Neurourol Urodyn 11: 187-99.
27. Ellison LE, Gormley EA (1998) Effect of combined surgery for incontinence and pelvic floor prolapse on quality of life. New England Section American Urological Association Meeting, 1998, Waterville Valley.
28. Gormley EA, Latini JM (1996) Effect of pubovaginal sling on quality of life. American Urological Association Meeting, 1996, Orlando.
29. Delancey JOL (1994) Relationship of prolapse syndromes to symptoms. In: Kurch ED, McGuire EJ (ed) Female Urology. J.B. Lippincott, Philadelphia, pp. 285-98.
30. Chiaffarino F, Chatenoud L, Dindelli M et al. (1999) Reproductive factors, family history, occcupation and risk of urogenital prolapse. Eur J Obstet Gynecol Reprod Biol 82: 63-7
31. Carley ME, Turner RJ, Scott DE, Alexander JM (1999) Obstetric history in women with surgically corrected adult urinary incontinence or pelvic organ prolapse. J Am Assoc Gynecol Laparoscopists 6: 85-9.
32. Welgoss JA, Vogt VY, McClellan EJ, Benson JT (1999) Relationship between surgically induced neuropathy and outcome of pelvic organ prolapse surgery. Int Urogynecol J Pelvic Floor Dysfunct 10: 11-14.
33. Wall LL, Versi E, Norton P, Bump R (1998) Evaluating the outcome of surgery for pelvic organ prolapse. Am J Obstet Gynecol 178: 877-9.

28 Faecal Incontinence

Ann C. Lowry

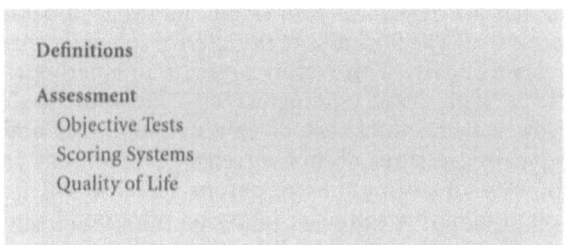
Ideally the measurement of clinical outcomes would include a well-defined clinical entity, appropriate and standardized risk adjustment, and validated objective measures of results. If no objective standard exists, a health status or quality of life instrument might be substituted. Few of these tools exist for fecal incontinence. Measurement of outcomes has not kept pace with the development of new, exciting technology to improve continence.

Definitions

No standardized definition of fecal incontinence exists. Mucus leakage from mucosal or rectal prolapse may be described as incontinence. Some authors separate urge from passive incontinence. *Urge incontinence* is defined as leakage of stool between experiencing the urge to defecate and reaching the bathroom. *Passive incontinence* is loss of stool without any urge to defecate. Although these descriptions fit many patients' histories, the clinical significance is not established. Incontinence of flatus may represent inability to control gas, or lack of concern about its control. How should it be classified?

Further work is clearly needed to clarify and improve the definition and classification of incontinence. Until patients can be accurately classified, comparison of treatment modalities will be somewhat flawed.

Part of the problem is that fecal incontinence is still an incompletely understood entity. Some causes are clear-cut, such as sphincter injury or severe pudendal neuropathy. However, some patients with significant sphincter defects deny incontinence, whereas other patients with normal sphincter anatomy and pudendal nerve latency are severely limited by incontinence. Even with anorectal physiology testing, up to 35% of patients with incontinence remain undiagnosed.[1]

Risk adjustment or severity scoring is a critical component of any clinical evaluation. The lack of accurate risk stratification affects the results of an outcome study.[2] Objective tests are the most straightforward method of risk adjustment. The de Meester score for gastroesophageal reflux relies on pH monitoring data.[3] Blood sugars and glycosolated hemoglobin reflect the level of diabetic control.

Assessment

A number of objective tests exist for fecal incontinence, ranging from digital rectal examination to more sophisticated measures. Digital examination is appealing as a measure for its simplicity and availability, but there is disagreement about its accuracy.[4–8] In one study, digital rectal examination had a sensitivity of 63% for resting tone compared to manometric resting pressure and 84% for external sphincter function when compared to manometric squeeze pressure. The specificity was 57%.[8] Rectal examination was felt to have a role only at the extremes of fecal incontinence. Other investigators found good correlation between the subjective findings on digital examination and manometric measurement of squeeze pressure (correlation coefficient 0.97, $p < 0.05$).[9] However, manometric pressures may not accurately reflect clinical severity. Clinical examination is an important part of patient assessment but by itself is not sufficiently reliable for use in risk stratification.

Objective Tests

The saline continence test measures the ability to retain infused fluid in the rectum. Theoretically it is a good candidate for an objective measure of incontinence. In several studies the median volume of retained fluid was significantly lower in incontinent patients than controls.[9,10] However, there was a notable overlap in values, with 17% of controls retaining less volume than incontinent patients. That degree of overlap limits the utility of the test as a severity measure. A similar test, defecography, has not been found to be helpful in diagnosis or measurement of fecal incontinence.[11]

Manometry is perhaps the most frequently utilized test of sphincter function. Resting pressure largely reflects internal sphincter function and squeeze pressures reflect external sphincter function. Many studies document lower resting and squeeze pressures in incontinent patients compared to controls, but almost all show considerable overlap.[12–16] Up to 40% of incontinent patients have normal manometry values.[17] In addition there is significant variation in values obtained on repeat testing in the same individual.[18]

Pudendal nerve latency (PDNL) is used to assess the function of the peripheral part of the efferent pathway and to diagnose neurogenic incontinence. In one study, prolonged pudendal nerve latency was common in patients with fecal incontinence, but did not correlate with low manometry pressures.[19] The finding was also common in patients complaining of constipation. Whether abnormal PDNL affects patient outcome after sphincteroplasty is controversial. A number of studies suggest that patients with prolonged PDNL do poorly after sphincter repair, whereas others found no relationship.[20–24] Abnormal PDNL does not affect the outcome after biofeedback training.[25]

Anal ultrasound is accurate in identifying sphincter injury.[26–28] External sphincter defects are inversely related to squeeze pressure, whereas internal sphincter defects are associated with significant drops in basal pressure.[29] The thickness of the internal sphincter correlates linearly with resting pressure in elderly patients with intact sphincters and incontinence.[30] However, the thickness of external sphincter and squeeze pressures do not correlate.[28, 31] As many as 10–25% of asymptomatic parous females will be found to have a sphincter injury on ultrasound, and many patients with fecal incontinence have normal sphincter muscles on ultrasound. So, although anal ultrasound is useful in the diagnosis of sphincter injury, the results do not reflect the severity of fecal incontinence.

Scoring Systems

The lack of an objective measure of severity of fecal incontinence led to the development of scoring systems based upon patients' report of symptoms. Numerous systems exist in the literature. The simplest ones grade the patient based on type of incontinence alone; frequency is not included.[32–37] (Table 28.1) These systems are easy to use but do not discriminate between a patient who is incontinent to solid stool once a month and one who is incontinent to solid stool daily. Although none of these systems has been formally tested before and after an intervention, intuitively they seem to sacrifice discriminatory power for simplicity.

A number of more complex systems were then developed. Kelly scores frequency of accidents, frequency of soiling and a subjective assessment of sphincter action.[38] Type of incontinence is not included. Holschneider's scoring system includes stool frequency, stool consistency, soiling, sensibility, pressure profile, squeeze pressure, and adaptation reaction with numerical points of 0–2 assigned to each category.[39] Luniss and colleagues published a system which scores incontinence to solid stool, liquid stool, and flatus as well as ability to withhold stool for more than 15 minutes, difficulty cleaning, and soiling.[40] Numerical values based on frequency

Table 28.1. Simple incontinence scores. Reprinted with permission from Shelton AA, Madoff RD (1997) Defining anal incontinence: Establishing a uniform continence scale. In: Semin colon Rectal Surgery 8(2): 57.

Author	Degree	Definition
Broden et al.[32]	1	No episodes of incontinence
	2	Incontinent to liquid stool
	3	Incontinent to solid stool
Corman[33]	Excellent	No episodes of incontinence
	Good	Continent but may require enemas
	Fair	Incontinent for liquid stool
	Poor	Incontinent for solid stool
Parks[34]	1	Normal
	2	Difficult control of flatus or diarrhea
	3	No control of liquid stool
	4	No control of solid stool
Rainey[35]	A	Continent to solid stool and liquid stool, not necessarily flatus
	B	Incontinent to liquid stool/flatus
	C	Incontinent to solid stool
Rudd[36]	I	Perfect continence
	II	Minor defects, such as incontinence to gas
	III	Still acceptable, minor leakage of feces, and patient wears a pad
	IV	Unsatisfactory; patient wears a pad
	V	Totally unsatisfactory; necessitates a colostomy
Womack[37]	A	Completely continent
	B	Incontinent to flatus
	C	Incontinent to liquid stool/flatus
	D	Completely incontinent

are assigned to the incontinence categories and based on presence or absence of the other symptoms. Pestacori's incontinence score is a summation of points given for type of incontinence and for frequency.[41] The difficulty with these last two systems is that patients with quite different symptoms could obtain the same score. In Luniss's system incontinence to flatus most days is assigned the same numerical value as incontinence to solid stool most days.[40] In Pestacori's system patients with incontinence of flatus at least once a week and patients with incontinence to liquid stool less than once a week receive the same score.[41] That could be appropriate, but there is no data supporting the choice of numerical value.

In the USA, the most frequently used scoring systems are modifications of a system originally proposed by Miller and colleagues.[42] The original system combined the type of incontinence and the frequency with values assigned to each combination. Rothenberger modified it by adding a value for lifestyle alteration which was then included in the summation score[43] (Table 28.2). Jorge and Wexner modified the frequency stratification and added the need to wear a pad[44] (Table 28.3). They also changed the value assigned each combination, but continued the concept of a summation score. Vaizey and colleagues recently published a new scoring system adding the need for constipating medicine and ability to defer defecation to the Wexner score.[45] These authors compared the Pascatori score, the Wexner score, the American Medical Systems score, and their new score to the clinical impressions of two blinded investigators. All the scores correlated with the clinical impressions, which is not surprising as the clinical impressions are undoubtedly based upon similar questions to the scores. In a small number of patients, the scores of all systems changed significantly after an intervention, which is encouraging.

A number of problems exist with all the scoring systems. One concern is the accuracy of the patient information. A part of that problem is the lack of a standardized definition to impart to patients. The known reluctance of patients and providers to discuss fecal incontinence is another aspect of the problem. In one study only 19 of 39 patients with incontinence volunteered the information

to their providers.[10] Other authors report similar experiences.

Imperfect recall and spontaneous variation in severity of symptoms are other aspects of the problem. Although one small study showed good correlation between diary recordings and answers on a questionnaire,[45] several others did not. In one investigation the frequency and type of incontinence reported on a questionnaire differed from the data recorded in a daily diary (R.D. Madoff, personal communication). At least two groups have developed questionnaires to assess fecal incontinence symptoms. One group evaluated reliability, discrimination, validity, and sensitivity of their questionnaire in 36 patients with fecal incontinence.[46] The reliability was high in controls and "acceptable" in the patients. Occurrence of fecal incontinence at all and need to wear a pad were reproducible. However, questions about incontinence to solid stool and ability to differentiate gas from stool, among others, were not reliable. There was good correlation between questionnaire answers and diary recordings for stool frequency and incontinence to gas and loose stool, but not for incontinence to solid stool. The authors concluded that the lack of reliability and validity of questions about incontinence to solid stool is most likely related to spontaneous changes. Fecal incontinence per se and the use of a pad were the only variables recommended for longitudinal studies. However, the results of treatment for fecal incontinence are rarely perfect, so the measure of fecal incontinence per se may not

Table 28.3. Jorge's incontinence score. Reprinted with permission from Jorge JM, Wexner SD (1993) Etiology and management of fecal incontinence. In: Dis Colon Rectum 36(1): 84.

Type	Frequency[a]				
	Never	Rarely	Sometimes	Usually	Always
Solid	0	1	2	3	4
Liquid	0	1	2	3	4
Gas	0	1	2	3	4
Wears pad	0	1	2	3	4
Lifestyle alteration	0	1	2	3	4

[a] 0, perfect; 20, complete incontinence; never = 0 (never); rarely = <1/month; sometimes = <1/week but >1/month; usually = <1/day but >1/week; always = >1/day.

Table 28.2. Rothenberger's incontinence score[a]. Reprinted with permission from Rothenberger DA (1989) Anal incontinence. In: Cameron JD (ed) Current Surgical Therapy. Decker, Philadelphia, PA, 186.

Frequency	Incontinence of gas	Incontinence of liquid	Incontinence of solid	Significantly alters lifestyle
<1/month	1	4	7	10
>1/month but <1/week	2	5	8	11
>1/week	3	6	9	12

[a] The patient's incontinence score is determined by adding points from the above grid. A score of 12 or greater indicates significant incontinence.

be sufficiently sensitive to measure treatment differences. In addition, the use of a pad may be related to anxiety about incontinent episodes as well as frequency of incontinence episodes.

Investigators from the Mayo Clinic also developed a questionnaire to assess symptoms of incontinence.[47] Some items were reliable, but, interestingly, incontinence to solid and loose stool had extremely low kappa values. Whether this reflects difficulty with the wording of the question or spontaneous variation in symptoms is not clear. Although time-consuming for patients, it may be that diary recordings will be necessary for an accurate measurement of severity.

Another concern is the choice of data points. There is general agreement that the frequency and consistency of incontinent episodes should be included. The study by Vaizey and colleagues suggests that the ability to delay defecation or urgency might add discriminatory power to a severity scoring system, but that needs to be tested further.[45] Another possible element is soiling. Perhaps data distinguishing passive and urge continence should be collected. It also seems appropriate that a severity index reflect incontinent episodes as a percentage of the frequency of the patient's bowel movements.

Some scales mix type and frequency with lifestyle issues. Although severity and quality of life are interrelated, they each measure different aspects of incontinence. Ideally severity measures should reflect the extent of pelvic floor or intestinal dysfunction. Quality of life instruments are designed to measure the impact of a given condition on a patient's lifestyle. Although each affects the other, neither is a direct indicator of the other, so they should be measured separately. Identical symptoms affect different patients differently. One patient with incontinence of flatus might be homebound while another considers the symptom insignificant. Inclusion of lifestyle issues in a severity scoring system reduces its accuracy. The two measures are complimentary, however, as patients often modify their lifestyle to reduce the frequency of incontinent episodes. Those changes could not be reflected in a severity scoring system but would be on a quality of life measure.

A final problem common to the existing systems is the arbitrary assignment of numerical values. If a system is to truly reflect severity there must be a factual basis for the score assigned to the type and frequency of incontinence. In addition, two different combinations of type and frequency of incontinence should not be assigned the same value unless data suggests the two are equivalent. For severity systems based upon objective tests the assignment of a score is straightforward. For systems based upon historical information, either patient or physician assessment of relative severity should determine the assignment of numerical values. Ideally physician and patient assessment would agree. In a multicenter study to investigate this issue surgeons and patients were asked to rank 20 combinations of type and frequency of incontinence (e.g. incontinence to solid stool more than once a month but less than once a week).[48] Two scoring systems were developed, one based on patients' rankings and the other on surgeons' rankings. In general the two systems correlated well with each other and a fecal incontinence quality of life scale. However, patients viewed frequent episodes of gas incontinence as more severe than infrequent episodes of incontinence of solid stool. Surgeons ranked those two combinations oppositely. It is therefore possible for a patient to have a different score depending upon which system is used. More work is necessary before well-supported numerical values can be assigned to a severity scoring system. Despite the limitations of historical data, it must be the basis of a severity system for fecal incontinence since no objective measure exists.

An ideal severity index would incorporate a reliable method of data collection, relevant data points, and numerical values based upon data.

Quality of Life

The exclusion of quality of life elements from a scoring system is not intended to minimize the importance of quality of life. Clinicians treating patients with fecal incontinence are well aware of the limiting, sometimes devastating, impact incontinence has on a patient's lifestyle. Traditionally surgeons have focused on mortality and morbidity as the most important outcomes, but for chronic non–life threatening conditions such as fecal incontinence, functional impairment and its impact on patients' lifestyle are more important. The reason to measure quality of life separately is that severity and well-being correlate poorly in many chronic conditions.[49] A given level of dysfunction affects different individuals differently.

Quality of life assessments may be used in surgery for assessing outcomes, comparing treatment options, monitoring and improving the quality of care, selecting patients for surgery, policy decisions, and resource allocation.[50] Given the importance of these applications, it is paramount that the instruments used be valid and reliable. Several approaches to quality of life measures are available: generic instruments that measure global health status, system-specific instruments that focus a body system, and disease-specific instruments that evaluate the impact of a specific condition. These approaches, their strengths and weaknesses are well described in several review articles and texts.[49,51,52]

The SF36 is the global health status instrument used the most frequently in the USA; the General Health Questionnaire and the Nottingham Health Profile are utilized more often in Europe. They are designed to assess overall health status in large populations. In some studies they are reflective of changes related to a specific disease or procedure, but often they are not.

The Gastrointestinal Quality of Life Index (GIQLI) is a validated, reliable instrument designed to assess the impact of gastrointestinal conditions.[53] Two studies are available using the GIQLI to assess patients with fecal incontinence. The GIQLI was used in a study of 325 patients with benign anorectal disorders.[54] The study group included 35 patients with fecal incontinence. The mean GIQLI scores for patients with anal fissure, severe constipation and fecal incontinence were significantly lower than a historical age-matched control group. In a study by Plusa and colleagues, 15 patients completed an incontinence scoring questionnaire, the General Health Questionnaire, and the GIQLI.[55] There was good correlation between results of the General Health Questionnaire and the GIQLI. However, neither the GHQ or the GIQLI correlated with the incontinence score. The authors concluded that the impact of incontinence on lifestyle is complex and not correlated with quality of life, and argued that qualify of life-evaluation must be included in the assessment of treatment. It is also possible that the lack of correlation reflects the lack of sensitivity of a broad instrument to a specific condition. Neither of these studies utilized the GIQLI to assess response to treatment.

Concern that a more specific instrument was necessary led to the development of the Fecal Incontinence Quality of Life measure (FIQL).[56] A panel of experts identified the important domains. Earlier work suggested that the impact of incontinence on sexuality and jobs was important to patients,[57] and these items were included. The instrument was administered with the SF36 to patients with fecal incontinence and a control group. Internal and test–retest reliability was established by repeat administration of the instrument. The instrument passed the requisite psychometric tests. As a validated and reliable instrument, it is now available for use in assessing patients with fecal incontinence.

The measurement of outcomes is critical to appropriately select patients for treatment and treatments for patients, and to improve the quality of care. The viewpoints of both clinicians and patients must be included. In the area of fecal incontinence the measurement of outcomes has not kept pace with the technical advances in treatment. Both severity scoring and quality of life measures are important aspects of outcome measurement. A quality of life instrument for fecal incontinence now exists, but requires more testing; further work must be done to achieve a valid severity scoring system.

References

1. Wexner SD, Jorge JM (1994) Colorectal physiological tests: use or abuse of technology? Eur J Surg 160(3): 167–74.
2. Read TE (1997) Fleshman JW. Outcomes: assessing the effectiveness of fecal incontinence therapy. Semin Colon Rectal Surg 8: 121–5.
3. Klementschitsch P, Meester TR de, Skinner DB, Greep JM (1982) The 24-hour intra-esophageal pH Monitoring Test in the diagnosis of gastroesophageal reflux. Neth J Surg 34(2): 57–62.
4. Kaushal JN, Goldner F (1991) Validation of the digital rectal examination as an estimate of anal sphincter squeeze pressure. Am J Gastroenterol 86(7): 886–7.
5. Felt-Bersma RJ, Klinkenberg-Knol EC, Meuwissen SG (1988) Investigation of anorectal function. Br J Surg 75(1): 53–5.
6. Hallan RI, Marzouk DE, Waldron DJ, Womack NR, Williams NS (1989) Comparison of digital and manometric assessment of anal sphincter function. Br J Surg 76(9): 973–5.
7. Rosen L (1990) Physical examination of the anorectum: A systematic technique. Dis Colon Rectum 33: 439–40.
8. Eckhardt VF, Kanzler G (1993) How reliable is digital rectal examination for evaluation of anal sphincter tone? Int J Colorect Dis 8: 95–7.
9. Read NW, Harford WV, Schmulen AC et al. (1979) A clinical study of patients with fecal incontinence and diarrhea. Gastroenterology 76(4): 747–56.
10. Leigh RJ, Turnberg LA (1982) Faecal incontinence: the unvoiced symptom. Lancet 1(8285): 1349–51.
11. Hiltunen KM, Kolehmainen H, Matikainen M (1994) Does defecography help in diagnosis and clinical decision-making in defecation disorders? Abdom Imaging 19(4): 355–8.
12. Felt-Bersma RJ, Klinkenberg-Knol EC, Meuwissen SG (1990) Anorectal function investigations in incontinent and continent patients. Differences and discriminatory value. Dis Colon Rectum 85(6): 479–85.
13. Rogers J, Henry MM, Misiewicz JJ (1988) Combined sensory and motor deficit in primary neuropathic faecal incontinence. Gut 29(1): 5–9.
14. Rao SS, Patel RS (1997) How useful are manometric tests of anorectal function in the management of defecation disorders? Am J Gastroenterol 92(3): 469–75.
15. Farouk R, Bartolo DC (1993) The clinical contribution of integrated laboratory and ambulatory anorectal physiology assessment in faecal incontinence. Int J Colorectal Dis 8(2): 60–5.
16. Sentovich SM, Blatchford GJ, Rivela LJ et al. (1997) Diagnosing anal sphincter injury with transanal ultrasound and manometry. Dis Colon Rectum 40(12): 1430–4.
17. McHugh SM, Diamant NE (1987) Effect of age, gender, and parity on anal canal pressures. Contribution of impaired anal sphincter function to fecal incontinence. Dig Dis Sci 32(7): 726–36.
18. Pedersen IK, Christiansen J (1989) A study of the physiological variation in anal manometry. Br J Surg 76(1): 69–71.
19. Sangwan YP, Coller JA, Barrett RC et al. (1996) Unilateral pudendal neuropathy. Impact on outcome of anal sphincter repair. Dis Colon Rectum 39(6): 686–9.
20. Tjandra JJ, Sharma BR, McKirdy HC, Lowndes RH, Mansel RE (1994) Anorectal physiological testing in defecatory disorders: a prospective study. Aust N Z J Surg 64(5): 322–6.
21. Laurberg S, Swash M, Henry MM (1988) Delayed external sphincter repair for obstetric tear. Br J Surg 75: 786–8.
22. Jacobs PPM, Scheuer M, Kuipers JHC, Vingerhoets MH (1990) Obstetric fecal incontinence: role of pelvic floor denervation and results of delayed sphincter repair. Dis Colon Rectum 33: 494–7.
23. Ternent CA, Shashidharan M, Flatchford GJ et al. (1997) Transanal ultrasound and anorectal physiology findings affecting continence after sphincteroplasty. Dis Colon Rectum 40(4): 462–7.
24. Nikiteas N, Korsgen S, Kumar D, Keighley MR (1996) Audit of sphincter repair. Factors associated with poor outcome. Dis Colon Rectum 39(10): 1164–70.

25. Jensen LL, Lowry AC (1997) Biofeedback improves functional outcome after sphincteroplasty. Dis Colon Rectum 40(2): 179–200.

26. Law PJ, Kamm MA, Bartram CI (1991) Anal ultrasonography in the investigation of faecal incontinence. Br J Surg 78: 312–4.

27. Cuesta MA, Meijer S, Derksen EJ, Boutkan H, Meuwissen SG (1992) Anal sphincter imaging in fecal incontinence using endosonography. Dis Colon Rectum 35(1): 59–63.

28. Papachrysostomou M, Pye SD, Wild SR, Smith AN (1993) Anal endosonography in asymptomatic subjects. Scand J Gastroenterol 28(6): 551–6.

29. Falk PM, Blatchford GJ, Cali RL, Christensen MA, Thorson AG (1994) Transanal ultrasound and manometry in the evaluation of fecal incontinence. Dis Colon Rectum 37(5): 468–72.

30. Bartram CI, Burnett SJD (1991) Atlas of Anal Endosonography. Butterworth-Heinemann, Oxford.

31. Eckhardt VF, Jung B, Fischer B (1994) Anal endosonography in healthy subjects and patients with isiopathic fecal incontinence. Dis Colon Rectum 37: 235–42.

32. Broden G, Dolk A, Holmstrom B (1988) Recovery of the internal anal sphincter following rectopexy: a possible explanation for continence improvement. Int J Colorectal Dis 3(1): 23–8.

33. Corman ML (1985) Gracilis muscle transposition for anal incontinence: late results. Br J Surg 72 (Suppl): S21–2.

34. Parks AG (1975) Anorectal incontinence. J R Soc Med 68: 28–30.

35. Rainey JB, Donaldson DR, Thomson JP (1990) Postanal repair: which patients derive most benefit? J R Coll Surg Edinb 35(2): 101–5.

36. Rudd WW (1979) The transanal anastomosis: a sphincter-saving operation with improved continence. Dis Colon Rectum 22(2): 102–5.

37. Womack NR, Morrison JF, Williams NS (1988) Prospective study of the effects of postanal repair in neurogenic faecal incontinence. Br J Surg 75(1): 48–52.

38. Kelly JH (1969) Cine radiography in anorectal malformations. J Pediatr Surg 4(5): 538–46.

39. Holschneider AM (1983) Treatment and functional results of anorectal continence in children with imperforate anus. Acta Chir Belg 82(3): 191–204.

40. Luniss PJ, Kamm MA, Phillips RK (1994) Factors affecting continence after surgery for anal fistula. Br J Surg 81: 1382–5.

41. Pescatori M, Anastasio G, Bottini C, Mentasti A (1992) New grading and scoring for anal incontinence. Evaluation of 335 patients. Dis Colon Rectum 35(5): 482–7.

42. Miller R, Bartolo DC, Locke-Edmunds JC, Mortensen NJ (1988) Prospective study of conservative and operative treatment for faecal incontinence. Br J Surg 75(2): 101–5.

43. Rothenberger DA (1989) Anal incontinence. In: Cameron JD (ed) Current Surgical Therapy. Decker, Philadelphia, PA, pp. 185–94.

44. Jorge JM, Wexner SD (1993) Etiology and management of fecal incontinence. Dis Colon Rectum 36(1): 77–97.

45. Vaizey CJ, Carapeti E, Cahill JA, Kamm MA (1999) Prospective comparison of faecal incontinence grading systems. Gut 44(1): 77–80.

46. Osterberg A, Graf W, Karlbom U, Pahlman L (1996) Evaluation of a questionnaire in the assessment of patients with faecal incontinence and constipation. Scand J Gastroenterol 31(6): 575–80.

47. Reilly WT, Talley NJ, Pemberton JH, Zinsmeister AR (2000) Validation of a questionnaire to assess fecal incontinence and associated risk factors: Fecal Incontinence Questionnaire. Dis Colon Rectum 53(4): 146–53.

48. Rockwood TH, Church JM, Fleshman JW et al. (1999) Patient and surgeon ranking of the severity of symptoms associated with fecal incontinence: the fecal incontinence severity index. Dis Colon Rectum 42(12): 1525–32.

49. Guyatt GH, Feeny DH, Patrick DL (1993) Measuring health-related quality of life. Ann Intern Med 118(8): 622–9.

50. O'Boyle CA (1992) Assessment of quality of life in surgery. Br J Surg 79(5): 395–8.

51. Testa MA, Simonson DC (1996) Assesment of quality-of-life outcomes. N Engl J Med 334(13): 835–40.

52. Kane RL (1997) Understanding Health Care Outcomes Research. Aspen Publications, Gaithersburg.

53. Eypasch E, Williams JI, Wood-Dauphinee S et al. (1995) Gastrointestinal Quality of Life Index: development, validation and application of a new instrument. Br J Surg 82(2): 216–22.

54. Sailer M, Bussen D, Debus ES, Fuchs KH, Thiede A (1998) Quality of life in patients with benign anorectal disorders. Br J Surg 85(12): 1716–19.

55. Plusa S, Sharpe A, Read A, Slater B, Varma J (1997) Quality of Life assessment in patients with fecal incontinence. Int J Colorect Dis 12: 124.

56. Rockwood TH, Church JM, Fleshman JW et al. (2000) Fecal Incontinence Quality of Life Scale: quality of life instrument for patients with fecal incontinence. Dis Colon Rectum 7: 9–16.

57. Huppe D, Enck P, Kruskemper G, May B (1992) [Psychosocial aspects of fecal incontinence]. Leber Magen Darm 22(4): 138–42.

58. Shelton AA, Madoff RD (1997) Defining anal incontinence: Establishing a uniform continence scale. Semin Colon Rectal Surg 8(2): 54–60.

Part X

Choice of Surgery

Choice of Surgery for Stress Incontinence

Stuart L. Stanton

In the twentieth century the number of continence procedures for stress incontinence was said to number almost 200. Today, with a better appreciation of the mechanism of continence and incontinence, with evidence-based medicine and audit, there are probably only about 5 procedures of proven effectiveness.

This chapter deals with the correction of stress incontinence due to urethral sphincter incompetence. This term is comparable to genuine stress incontinence. I do not believe in the rather simplistic classification of types I, II, III, and they will not be used. Urethral sphincter incompetence is essentially due to failure of the sphincteric mechanism to withstand the rise in intravasical pressure associated with effort or in worse cases, at rest without effort. Most patients complaining of stress incontinence have some degree of sphincteric incompetence. The role of "hypermobility" is unclear. Recent success with the tension free vaginal tape (TVT) has given insight into an alternative mechanism for the correction of incontinence, namely that bladder neck elevation or support may not be as necessary as previously thought and that midurethral support is equally relevant.

Role of Conservative Treatment

Over the last 10 years, conservative treatment has become increasingly popular, perhaps as patients and surgeons have become more aware and realistic about the objective (rather than the subjective) success of surgery and of its side-effects. In addition, wider exposure of the issue of urinary incontinence has led to greater involvement by physiotherapists and continence advisers who, quite rightly, champion more conservative approaches.

All patients should have the opportunity to discuss with either the surgeon or the continence adviser, the pros and cons of pelvic floor exercises, drugs, and devices.[1,2] However, it must be emphasized that to achieve improvement or success, the patient must remain committed to continuing these treatments. Many do not, and may later seek surgery.

Indications and Contraindications

The *indications* for continence surgery are:

- The complaint of stress incontinence confirmed by urodynamic studies as due to urethral sphincter incompetence.
- Prolapse where urethral sphincter incompetence has been demonstrated on reduction of prolapse.

The *absolute contraindications* to surgery are:

- The physically frail patient for whom surgery would be a risk to life. Even so there may be some patients, surgeons and anaesthetists who would argue otherwise – that surgery would bring an improvement in the quality of life, and they would be prepared to chance the risks.

- The mentally frail patient where surgery may not usefully contribute to the quality of life and where consent would have to take this into account.

The *relative contraindications* to surgery are:

- *Detrusor instability*: A lessened cure rate of urethral sphincter incompetence is found when there is coexistent detrusor instability. Prior management of detrusor instability with bladder retraining and antimuscarinics or the currently effective drug should be used, and the symptoms reviewed after this.
- *Voiding difficulty*: Continence surgery may convert an overt or occult voiding difficulty into retention. These cases are best managed by the selection of an operation least likely to aggravate or initiate voiding difficulties and the decision will be based on the urodynamic and operative characteristics. The place of postoperative intermittent self-catheterisation should be discussed in this context.

Above all, a full discussion on the benefits and alternative options in surgery is always necessary.

Classification of Operations and their Characteristics

Based on medical evidence (either group A or group B) and personal experience, I would regard the operations listed in Table 29.1 as those that are useful and successful. Operations which are less successful, or have significant complications, or are still awaiting adequate randomized control trial evidence on their effectiveness, include the anterior colporrhaphy, endoscopic bladder neck suspension, bone anchor procedures, paravaginal operations, Marshall–Marchetti–Krantz, and laparoscopic colposuspension.

Bulking Agents (see Chapter 5)

These agents are popular and, although they do not have the same success rate as major surgery, they also do not have significant complications. My *indications* for a bulking agent would be:

- mild urethral sphincter incompetence
- as adjunctive to previous continence surgery which has not entirely been corrective
- a patient who is physically unfit for major surgery
- a patient who is between pregnancies.

The *contraindications* to organic substances such as collagen (Contigen) include collagen allergy. The overall contraindications might include autoimmune diseases such as systemic lupus erythematosus.

The technique is without major complication, and can be repeated if it fails. It is a day case/office procedure. Whether the periurethral or transurethral route is better is uncertain. Nager et al.[3] found no difference between the two routes except a higher incidence of urinary retention following the periurethral route.

Tension-free Vaginal Tape

Although the TVT has been universally acclaimed as an innovative and effective procedure to correct urethral sphincter incompetence, the first published report was only in 1996 and careful follow-up is needed to detect the potential complications of erosion or voiding difficulty.

The *indications* include:

- Primary and secondary urethral sphincter incompetence with or without cystourethrocele. If a cystourethrocele is present, an anterior repair may be carried out as well.
- A narrowed or shortened vagina where access is difficult and would exclude other procedures such as a colposuspension.
- As a prophylactic measure in reconstructive surgery for a prolapse when the patient does not complain of stress incontinence but stress incontinence is demonstrable on reduction of prolapse.
- The physically frail patient where a minimally invasive procedure with a swift recovery is ideal.

The *contraindications* include

- a previous urethrovaginal fistula
- coagulation disorders
- anticoagulation therapy.

An obliterated retropubic space following previous surgery such as a Marshall–Marchetti–Krantz procedure needs caution.
There is increasing evidence to show that the TVT is effective for patients with a significant decrease in maximum urethral closure pressure.

Table 29.1. Effective continence procedures	
Vaginal	Suprapubic
Bulking agents	Colposuspension (open)
Tension free vaginal tape (TVT)	Artificial urinary sphincter (AUS)
Sling	

Sling

The sling has been overshadowed by the TVT and it is likely that the mechanisms of action are different. My preference for sling has always been silastic combined with Dacron[4] which is strong and, of course, readily available, but like all inorganic materials it carries a risk of erosion.

The main *indications* for a sling are:

● secondary surgery with reduced maximum urethral closure pressure (MUCP)
● significant vaginal narrowing which precludes other procedures such as colposuspension

The *contraindications* are:

● voiding difficulty
● past radiotherapy if an inorganic sling is chosen.

Colposuspension

Over the past 30 years the colposuspension has been my primary and often secondary method of choice to correct urethral sphincter incompetence. The main modifications have been to use polybutylate-coated polyethylene (Ethibond, Ethicon) sutures in place of polyglycolic acid sutures (Vicryl, Ethicon) and the avoidance of over-tightening bladder neck sutures to minimize the risk of voiding difficulty. More recently, when this operation was combined with a posterior colporrhaphy for rectocele, analysis of our posterior colporrhaphy results have shown that poorer results are obtained when the two operations are combined together, I suspect because the posterior colporrhaphy is carried out after the colposuspension.[5] I therefore prefer to carry out the posterior colporrhaphy first, followed by the colposuspension: this gives greater access to the vagina before it is compromised by the elevation produced by a colposuspension.

In the last 3 years the TVT has gradually replaced the colposuspension in my practice. My *indications* for the colposuspension now are:

● Primary and secondary urethral sphincter incompetence (where the MUCP exceeds 20 cm of water) coexisting with a grade 2 cystourethrocele.
● When other abdominal surgery is performed (e.g. sacrocolpopexy) and it is sensible to use just the suprapubic route.

The vaginal capacity and mobility must be adequate to allow paravaginal tissues to reach the pelvic side wall but without, however, having to approximate to the iliopectineal ligament. Bowstringing of the sutures is, therefore, perfectly acceptable.

Artificial Urinary Sphincter

The place of the artificial sphincter is in primary and secondary reconstructive surgery, but never in primary surgery for urethral sphincter incompetence. Where secondary reconstructive surgery is to be carried out, appropriate conventional surgery must have been tried and failed already and the patient has considered but rejected a urinary diversion. There should be an adequate bladder capacity (of at least 250 ml), normal upper tracts, and absence of chronic urinary tract infection. The patient must have manual dexterity and be sufficiently mentally alert to be able to use the device.

Patient Characteristics

The following patient features are considered when matching the operation to the patient:

● *Raised body mass index (BMI)*: A raised BMI, i.e. a morbidly obese patient, will increase the technical difficulty and intra- and postoperative morbidity. A bulking agent or TVT may be more appropriate than any other procedure.
● *Physical frailty:* A quick operation and relatively pain-free postoperative course is required and a bulking agent or TVT would be suitable.
● *Coexistent prolapse:* Where a suprapubic route is chosen to correct prolapse then a colposuspension or sling would seem appropriate. Conversely, if the vaginal route was preferred, the TVT would be the choice.
● *Voiding difficulty:* Most continence operations impair voiding, some more than others. The bulking agent and TVT are less likely than others to do this.
● *Detrusor instability:* This condition is found after most continence procedures, particularly the colposuspension and least with bulking procedures.
● *Incomplete family:* If the patient is so incontinent between pregnancies that she requires treatment then it is sensible to offer this with an elective cesarean section if she still remains dry at 36 weeks. Any procedure in Table 29.1 may be undertaken.
● *Comorbidity* (e.g. asthma, constipation, chronic cough): These conditions can always raise the intraabdominal pressure and reduce the success of any continence procedure. Preoperative management should try to improve these conditions, and inadequate procedures such as an anterior colporrhaphy or endoscopic bladder neck suspension should be avoided.
● *Active or sporting lifestyle:* Most studies suggest that primary operations have the best chance of

success, and unless the patient has had many operative failures, it is reasonable that she be allowed to continue her lifestyle. However, unnecessary heavy lifting (e.g. furniture or luggage) should be avoided and an anterior colporrhaphy or endoscopic bladder neck suspension is not advised. A colposuspension or sling using unabsorbable materials and sutures or a TVT would be appropriate.

Choice

- I would choose a *bulking agent* where there is mild stress incontinence, physical frailty, incomplete family, and a reluctance to undergo major surgery.
- I would choose a *colposuspension* where a suprapubic approach is required, where there is a grade II or more cystourethrocele and preferably where there is minimum voiding difficulty or detrusor instability. If a posterior colporrhaphy is required I would do this first then proceed to the colposuspension at the same operation.
- I would choose a *TVT* where there was uncomplicated urethral sphincter incompetence, for secondary procedures particularly with a low MUCP (less than 20 cm of water), and where vaginal surgery is required either for reconstructive surgery or other reasons.
- I would choose an *artificial urinary sphincter* where there is recurrent failure of conventional surgery with or without a reduced maximum urethral closure pressure.
- Where there is recurrent failure with significant detrusor instability I would prefer a *clam operation*.

Vaginal Surgery for Stress Urinary Incontinence: Beyond Horizon 2000

Philippe E. Zimmern

> Certainly new surgical procedures should be subject to the same rigorous tests that new drugs undergo before they can be recommended as a suitable treatment for a particular condition ...
> *Fryman* et al. BJU 2000; 85: 46–53.

This quote from a recent article reviewing the treatment and management of benign prostatic obstruction (BPO) should touch all of us who deal with the management of stress urinary incontinence (SUI), which is first and foremost a social and bothersome condition, and secondly, not a life-threatening condition. These simple words remind us of our ethical responsibilities toward patients and toward the progress of our specialty. In the last decade or so, we have witnessed an alarming trend of new surgical procedures driven by the recognition of incontinence as a potential large-scale market (over 50 millions of women in America today) and by the aggressive marketing that resulted from this recognition. This concluding chapter oversees several critical issues on the surgical management of SUI.

Female Stress Urinary Incontinence Clinical Guidelines Panel: More About What We Don't Know

In 1995, at the request of the American Urological Association, a group of experts led by G. Leach reviewed the world literature on the surgical treatment of SUI.[6] After rejecting 92% of over 5000 articles because of incomplete methodology or data acquisition, he and his group published a landmark update in 1997 outlining the durability of the Burch colposuspension (84% cure at 4 years) and of the pubovaginal sling (same performance but in a more complex group of patients having failed at least one prior suspension procedure). The authors acknowledged several obvious flaws, including the definition of cure (one could be cured of SUI but plagued for life with urge incontinence) and the heterogeneity of the needle suspension procedure group.

About What We Think We Know! Ten-Year Follow-up Study ... Has Flaws

In addition to this impressive literature review, Trockman et al. published a long-term follow-up study (mean 9.8 years in 125 patients) of needle suspension, based on questionnaire interviews.[7] Using a strict definition of cure (do you ever leak urine at any time? yes or no), they reported that 20% of patients had no incontinence of any type, and 71% of patients experienced significant improvement in their incontinence. These results led to the conclusion, often since reiterated, that the modified Pereyra bladder neck suspension procedure incorporating periurethral tissues which are inherently weak has poor durability.

But, what were the weaknesses of that report? Several were apparent, including:

- the lack of physical examination to determine if the procedure had really failed with recurrent urethral hypermobility
- the inclusion of 64 patients (36%) who had previous incontinence procedures

- the urge incontinence component, which has been reported in epidemiologic studies as occurring in up to 15–25% of healthy middle-aged (45–65 year old) women.[8]

Thus, considering the preoperative mean age of the group (53.9 years), the 21% incidence of urge incontinence nearly 10 years later should have been no surprise. Certainly, one could take home the message that the high satisfaction rate and low re-operation rate in that study imply that "perfectly dry at all times" may not be such an important goal after all, and that durably "nearly always dry" may be sufficient!

A Sling Is a Sling Is a Sling

Equipped with the above data, and despite lack of long-term data on sling effectiveness and risks, many experts started to recommend the sling as the procedure of choice for all types of SUI.[9,10] In one study emphasizing long-term analysis, only 47 and 20 (of the initial 250 patients) were available for follow-up at 5 and 10 years, respectively, and their specific type of SUI was not even specified. Yet, of those few patients, 31% at 5 years and 41% at 10 years experienced urge incontinence. No report of flow pattern, post-void residual, or questionnaire data was presented to confirm what most other reports on sling outcome have shown, namely obstruction (over-correction) or persistent incontinence (under-correction).[11]

So, is the sling procedure safe, reproducible, and efficacious long-term? Historically, it has been reserved for recurrent incontinence and for patients with severe incontinence secondary to intrinsic sphincteric deficiency, because of its potential complications.[12] Indeed, the very historical fact that the sling has been reserved as a "second line or last resort" procedure suggests that it is not "safe." In addition to doubts about its safety, the reproducibility of the sling procedure has been challenged on the basis of the artistic difficulties that occur in applying "minimal tension" when adjusting the sling position beneath the urethra. These difficulties are highlighted by the consistent rate of permanent urinary retention in all published sling series today (1–10%) and by some comparative pre- versus postoperative urodynamic data that reveal decrease in flow rates despite increase in voiding pressures.[13] Efficacy can also be questioned given the few series beyond 4 years, all of which report high incidence of secondary voiding dysfunction (detrusor instability, incomplete emptying) or persistent/recurrent stress incontinence.[14]

Newer materials (cadaveric tissue, prolene tape) may create a sense of added safety in regulating sling tension, especially when the procedure is performed under local anesthesia. Nevertheless, the obstructive nature of the sling is unquestionable. The adjustment in tension, which is so critical to its outcome, remains an unsettled technical challenge. In the worse case scenario, i.e. complete urinary retention, one could expect that undoing the sling would return patients to their preoperative conditions. But this is not so, according to most recent series, which quote that, in expert hands, satisfactory outcome (defined subjectively most of the time) is achieved in 65–70% of patients. How many times a year do we hear patients – after one or two procedures to correct their SUI, another one or two urethrolysis attempts, and with persistent degrees of mixed incontinence – state that, if they had only known, they would have lived with their one or two pads a day! Have we not all heard this confession once? More than once?

Do No Harm . . . so, What Are We Treating?

Our current procedures derive from our concepts regarding the pathophysiology of SUI. One of them is urethral hypermobility at the time of a stressful maneuver. This occurs when, during a downward motion, the anterior vaginal wall is no longer secured to its lateral pelvic attachments. The question is: which is the real issue, disease in the urethra or lack of support or both? Given the acknowledged, satisfactory, long-term outcome of the Burch suspension,[6] the goal of which is to support the anterior vaginal wall on each side of the bladder neck, and which results in a stable, less mobile urethra, one could conclude that laxity in the vaginal wall is the cause and the urethra merely the unfortunate bystander.

Our own experience with the trans-vaginally performed anterior vaginal wall suspension (AVWS), during which two sets of running sutures (bladder neck and upper vagina) are broadly anchored in the vagina, confirms the merit of restoring proper anterior vaginal wall support to the urethra and bladder base[15,16] to correct SUI secondary to urethral lypermobility. However, two important issues must be raised: durability and effect on voiding parameters. As long as the sutures are placed in the vaginal wall away from the proximal urethra and bladder neck (as learned from the initial complications of the Marshall–Marchetti–Krantz procedure[17]), the voiding pattern will not be altered postoperatively, as the bladder neck remains able to relax and funnel properly. De-novo detrusor instability and the incidence of partial or complete retention following either the Burch procedure[18] or any vaginal wall suspension procedure[19] have been extremely low. Durability is partially dependent on the quality of the vaginal wall tissues, but it is more importantly dependent on the degree of postoperative scarring generated in the retropubic space. Thus, supporting the anterior vaginal wall with procedures having minimal morbidity can be viewed as a legitimate goal so long as sufficient scar forms to reattach the vaginal wall to its original support mechanism.[20]

Another mechanism responsible for SUI is intrinsic sphincteric deficiency (ISD), either alone, as the result of several etiologic factors (prior surgeries, denervation, radiation effect), or in conjunction with urethral hypermobility. Repairing the intrinsic deficit itself is on the horizon, but so far, bulking the deficient area (Teflon, collagen, fat, others), replacing the deficient sphincter by an artificial device, or "obstructing" the urethra proximally (pubovaginal sling) or in its midsection (TVT) have been the main treatment options. The advantages and disadvantages of these different approaches have been well addressed in several chapters of this book. Undoubtedly, it behooves us to refine our clinical staging accuracy of each patient with SUI, so to offer her the most appropriate surgical therapy. In no field of medicine does one treatment work for all.

Lastly, when both conditions (urethral hypermobility and ISD) are present – which, according to VLPP data, has been the belief of some authors for all patients with SUI – the current trend is to lean toward a pubovaginal sling. However, careful analysis of outcome data of Burch or AVWS procedures could immediately dispel this belief. The rate of secondary ISD in any series is very low. Thus, it may be time to distinguish conceptually between "functional ISD" (urethral hypermobility with various degrees of low leak point pressure) and "organic ISD" (when there is true damage of the sphincteric mechanism in an otherwise well-supported urethra). With "functional ISD," the urethra needs support. Once support is restored, sphincteric mechanism will likely return to normal function.

Outcome Measures: Be Practical!

Studies on outcome measures in the field of BPO have been initiated to compare randomized control trials with real-life practical trials. For SUI, several outcome measures such as 24 hour pad test, several day diaries, VLPP (not yet standardized!), and videourodynamic studies are ideally suited for research centers, but totally impractical for everyday practise. So, what is practical, and what would help answer the few critical questions on how well our patients are doing postoperatively?

A minimum inquiry could consist in verifying that the presenting symptoms have been cured, that no new symptoms have developed, that any abnormal anatomical feature has been corrected, and that

no re-operation for SUI occurred in the next 5–10 years. Several questionnaires (some validated more or less extensively) are now available to survey the persistence or disappearance of symptoms. Only short questionnaires (7–10 questions) show long-term patient acceptance. If confirmed by other investigators, our recent study correlating the UDI-6 questionnaire[21] with urodynamic findings of stress and urge incontinence may reduce the preoperative assessment in selected individuals.[22] A simple quality of life questionnaire may also offer a global assessment on how the patient is faring pre- and postoperatively. A flow test with a minimum volume voided of 150 ml and a post-void residual assessment by ultrasound scanning can confirm the repair procedure's lack of interference with the voiding process. Anatomical correction of urethral hypermobility can be verified by physical examination, Q-tip test (for those who can reproducibly perform the test), perineal ultrasound, or a standing voiding cystourethrogram (with lateral views at rest and with straining for those wanting to assess the effect of gravity on urethral position).[23] Pad usage is frequently reported, but, as with diaries, is more difficult to compare between patients. The pad test is seldom used because it is time consuming and does not distinguish between stress and urge components, although it can reliably quantify the degree of urine loss. A validated sexual function questionnaire, currently lacking,[24] will add an important dimension to the postoperative assessment.

Hopefully, the time will soon come when our admonition to "do no harm" prevails – provided that the "do no harm," i.e. "minimally invasive," procedures prove to "do good." Time-honored procedures should continue to be offered until newer techniques, studied in selected centers of excellence, provide short-, mid-, and long-term data to support adoption of different surgical concepts. Patients treated with newer procedures must be properly informed of their choices and of their surgeon's preference and track record with the recommended surgical therapy.

References

1. Wang K (2000) Pad, pants and mechanical devices. In: Stanton SL, Monga A (eds) Clinical Urogynaecology, 2nd edn. Churchill Livingstone, Edinburgh, pp. 583–90.
2. Laycock J (2000) Physiotherapy. In: Stanton SL, Monga A (ed) Clinical Urogynaecology, 2nd edn. Churchill Livingstone, Edinburgh, pp. 591–600.
3. Nager C, Schulz J, Stanton SL (1998) Bulking agents for genuine stress incontinence: short term results and complications in randomised comparison of periurethral and transurethral injections. Int Urogynecol J 10: 76.
4. Chin YK, Stanton SL (1995) A follow up of silastic sling for genuine stress incontinence. Br J Obstet Gynaecol 102: 143–7.

5. Kahn M, Stanton SL (1997) Posterior colporrhaphy, its effects on bowel and sexual function. Br J Obstet Gynaecol 104: 82–6.

6. Leach GE, Dmochowski RR, Appell RA et al. (1997) Female stress urinary incontinence clinical guidelines panel summary report on surgical management of female stress urinary incontinence. J Urol 158: 875.

7. Trockman BA, Leach GE, Hamilton J et al. (1995) Modified pereyra bladder neck suspension: 10-year mean followup using outcomes analysis in 125 patients. J Urol 154: 1841.

8. Burgio KL, Matthews KA, Engel BT (1991) Prevalence, incidence and correlates of urinary incontinence in healthy, middle-aged women. J Urol 146: 1255.

9. Chaikin DC, Rosenthal J, Blaivas JG (1998) Pubovaginal fascial sling for all types of stress incontinence: long-term analysis. J Urol 160: 1312.

10. Morgan TO Jr., Westney OL, McGuire EJ (2000) Pubovaginal sling: 4-year outcome analysis and quality of life assessment. J Urol 163: 1845.

11. Haab F, Trockman BA, Zimmern PE, Leach GE (1997) Results of pubovaginal sling for the treatment of intrinsic sphincteric deficiency determined by questionnaire analysis. J Urol 158: 1738.

12. Haab F, Zimmern PE, Leach GE (1996) Female stress urinary incontinence due to intrinsic sphincteric deficiency: recognition and management. J Urol 156: 3.

13. Fulford SC, Flynn R, Barrington J, Appanna T, Stephenson TP (1999) An assessment of the surgical outcome and urodynamic effects of the pubovaginal sling for stress incontinence and the associated urge syndrome. J Urol 162: 135.

14. Iocca A, Herschorn S (1998) Pubovaginal slings in the treatment of recurrent female stress urinary incontinence. J Urol 159: 46.

15. Dmochowski RR, Zimmern PE, Ganabathi K, Sirls L, Leach GE (1997) Role of the four-corner bladder neck suspension to correct stress incontinence with a mild to moderate cystocele. Urology 49: 35.

16. Lemack GE, Zimmern PE (2000) Questionnaire-based outcome after anterior vaginal wall suspension for stress urinary incontinence. J Urol 163: 73.

17. Zimmern PE, Leach GE, Hadley HR, Raz S (1987) Female urethral obstruction after Marshall–Marchetti–Krantz operation. J Urol 138: 517.

18. Dainer M, Hall CDCJ, Bhatia NN (1998) The Burch procedure: a comprehensive review. Obstet Gynecol Surv 54: 49.

19. Raz S, Stothers L, Young GPH et al. (1996) Vaginal wall sling for anatomical incontinence and intrinsic sphincter dysfunction: efficacy and outcome analysis. J Urol 156: 166.

20. DeLancey JOL, Starr RA (1990) Histology of the connection between the vagina and levator ani muscles. Implications for urinary tract function. J Reprod Med 35: 765.

21. Uebersax JS, Wyman JF, Shumaker SA, McClish DK, Fantl J and the Continence Program for Women Research Group (1995) Short forms to assess life quality and symptom distress for urinary incontinence in women: The incontinence impact questionnaire and the urogenital distress inventory. Neurourol Urodyn 14: 131.

22. Lemack GE, Zimmern PE (1999) Predictability of urodynamic findings based on the Urogenital Distress Inventory questionnaire. Urology 54: 461.

23. Zimmern PE (1991) The role of voiding cystourethrography in the evaluation of the female lower urinary tract. Probl Urol 5: 23.

24. Lemack GE, Zimmern PE (2000) Sexual function after vaginal surgery for stress incontinence: Results of a mailed questionnaire. Urology 56: 223–7.

30 Prolapse

Defect Approach to Pelvic Organ Prolapse Surgery

J. Thomas Benson

Throughout the 1960s and 1970s and into the 1980s, operations for prolapse were primarily colporrhaphies performed vaginally. Greater awareness of multiple defects and increased attention to prolapse recurrence in unrepaired compartments of the pelvic floor have led to more comprehensive operations.

With assistance from interested radiologists, dynamic colpocystoproctography became available,[1] augmenting the appreciation of multiple defects in anterior, apical, and posterior compartments. Over 90% of our patients have defects involving more than one compartment.[2]

Anterior Wall Defects

A clinical site-specific pelvic floor examination, frequently in conjunction with radiologic consultation, determines our surgical repair. The anterior compartment examination focuses on the urethrovesical junction, lateral vaginal sulci, central vaginal wall defects, and transverse defects. The more common anterior vaginal wall defects are paravaginal leading to "traction" or "displacement" cystoceles, with pre-served rugae; the central vaginal epithelium remains attached to the muscularis of the vagina while losing lateral vaginal wall attachment to the arcus tendineus fascia. The central defect leading to cystocele, described as "pulsion" or "distension," is characterized by loss of contact between the central vaginal epithelium and muscularis, allowing bladder herniation. Paravaginal defects may be repaired either abdominally or vaginally; central defects may be repaired with colporrhaphy or grafts. Transverse defects, if superior, are often corrected with the apical repair. Defects at the urethrovesical junction, can be repaired by anterior urethropexy, vaginal needle urethropexy or by sling in patients determined to have intrinsic sphincter deficiency.

Apical Defects

Apical defects, with or without an intact uterus, rarely exist in isolation. The extent of the defect guides the operative procedure. With International Continence Society stage 0–2 uterovaginal prolapse, the uterosacral-cardinal ligament complex can be used to support the vagina because the prolapsing apex is still above the levator plate. Surgical replacement to engender posterior positioning of the apex in response to increased abdominal pressure can be obtained. In more extensive apical defects, the prolapsing tissue falls anterior to the levator plate into the genitourinary hiatus. In this situation, surgical repair requires reconstruction either abdominally with sacral colpopexy or vaginally with sacrospinous fixation.

Posterior Wall Defects

Posterior defects include rectocele, enterocele, and sigmoidocele and are frequently associated with perineal descent. Correction of the bulging does not correlate well with relief of symptoms.[3] Techniques of repair include traditional posterior colporrhaphy, specific defect repair, fascial replacement, rectal wall imbrication, and transanal repair.

Choice of Procedure

Until the late 1980s, our most common operative procedures for correction of multiple defects were vaginal hysterectomy, bilateral sacrospinous ligament vault suspension, vaginal paravaginal repair with permanent monofilament suture, needle urethropexy or autologous sling, McCall culdoplasty, and anterior colporrhaphy. If the abdominal route was chosen, abdominal hysterectomy, Burch urethropexy or autologous sling, Halban culdoplasty, and Macer wedge-type anterior colporrhaphy were performed. Posterior colporrhaphy or Parks-type retro-rectal levatoplasty were performed as indicated for posterior vaginal segment defects and excessive perineal descent.

Selection of either the vaginal or abdominal route was easy if there were masses prohibiting vaginal approach, multiple previous abdominal surgeries, prior inflammatory bowel or pelvic disease, or morbid obesity suggesting the vaginal approach. But because the majority of patients do not have these limiting factors, the choice of approach was unscientific. A prospective, randomized study was conducted between 1989 and 1992 to determine if one approach was superior.[4] Surprisingly, this study demonstrated that the abdominal approach was more effective in treating uterovaginal prolapse than was the vaginal approach, with the probability for optimal surgical outcome twice as great with the abdominal approach. The probability for surgical failure requiring re-operation was twice as great with the vaginal approach.

One possible contributing factor to the greater failure rate with pelvic floor surgery involving the vaginal approach in these patients is the production of neuropathy. As measured by terminal motor latency studies, such neuropathy occurs with vaginal dissection,[5–8] and a relationship between the outcome of pelvic organ prolapse surgery and surgically induced perineal neuropathy has been demonstrated.[9] Since the results of our study comparing surgical approaches showed that the abdominal approach has better efficacy and is not associated with production of neuropathy, our patients with multiple pelvic floor defects who desire preservation of vaginal function, and who do not have factors relatively limiting the abdominal approach, have been operated principally by the abdominal route.

Our re-operation rate in 1989 was 33% in the vaginal group and 16% in the abdominal group. Failures occurred sooner in the vaginal group. The mean time of failure was 11 months in the

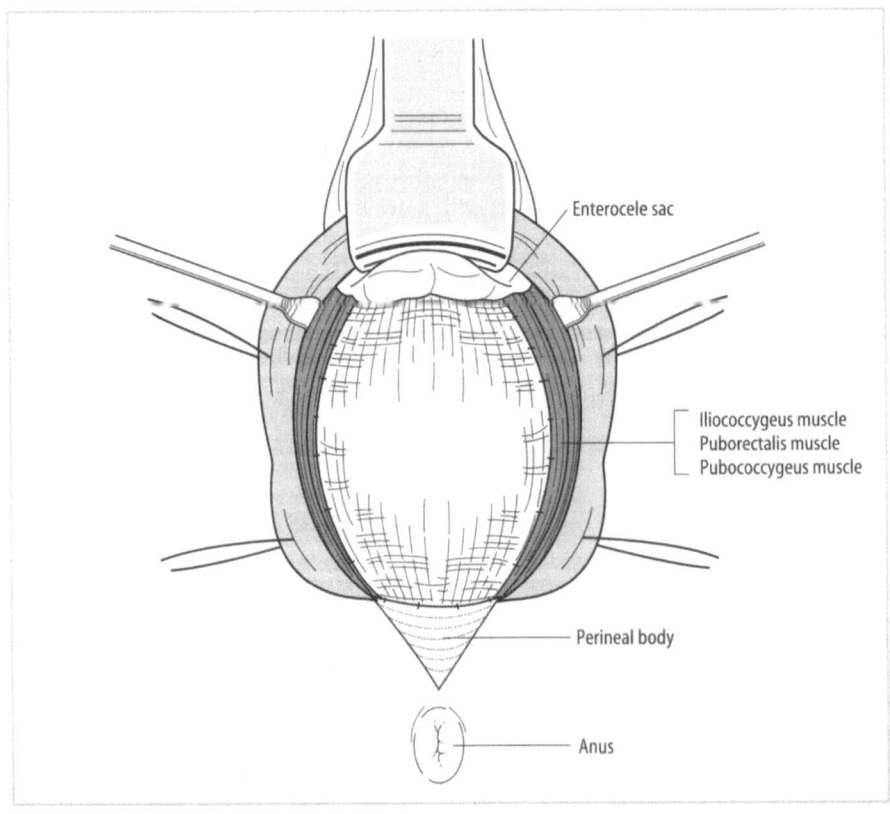

Enterocele sac

Iliococcygeus muscle
Puborectalis muscle
Pubococcygeus muscle

Perineal body

Anus

Figure 30.1 Graft secured to perineal body and lateral graft margins are sutured to the crura of the levator muscles.

vaginal group. The mean time of failure in the abdominal group was 22 months. Failures were predominantly in the anterior compartment (cystocele); rectocele was the second most common indication for re-operation. Since 1992, the majority of the reconstructive pelvic surgeries for both primary and secondary (previously operated) defects have been by the abdominal route, and re-operations have steadily declined. A recent retrospective review of 124 women operated abdominally between January 1997 and May 1998 revealed a single re-operation (1.8%) to date. Of this patient group, 57 had been examined at 1 year postoperatively.[10] Major changes in operative technique of this recent group include the use of cadaveric fascia, and the frequent (102 of the 124 cases) extension of the fascia to the perineum (abdominal sacral colpoperineoplasty) to augment the surgical repair of rectocele and perineal descent.

Technique for our Procedures of Choice

The abdominal sacral colpoperineoplasty is an evolved procedure augmenting the sacral colpoplasty by extending fascial support to the perineal body. The anterior and posterior vaginal wall is reinforced with either fascial tissue or synthetic mesh. The latter has potential for erosion in up to 11% of cases,[11] frequently requiring graft removal. Erosions also occur with donor fascia, but may be handled conservatively without graft removal. Because harvesting and tissue preparation of donor fascia may have significant impact on its strength, the practices of different tissue banks should be reviewed before using this material.

The graft is attached to the perineal body generally by an initial vaginal approach and secured to the perineal body as widely as possible (Fig. 30.1). The vaginal epithelium is mobilized laterally to the level of the pubococcygeus and iliococcygeus, and the graft lateral margins are sutured to the crura of the levator muscles, typically involving a width of 4–5 cm. The apical portion of the graft is then passed through the enterocele sac opening to be retrieved during the abdominal portion of the procedure. The remaining graft is spread widely over the posterior vaginal wall and sutured in place, aided by a vaginally placed lucite stent (Figure 30.2). After attachment to the S2–3 portion of the sacrum, a re-created full-length rectovaginal septum corrects the posterior defects and perineal descent. A second leaf of graft material is placed onto the anterior vaginal wall by sharply dissecting into the vesico-vaginal space. Halban-type vertical sutures close the cul-de-sac and bring the base of it to the graft. After correction of the posterior and apical defects, attention is turned to the retropubic space for anterior compartment defect correction.

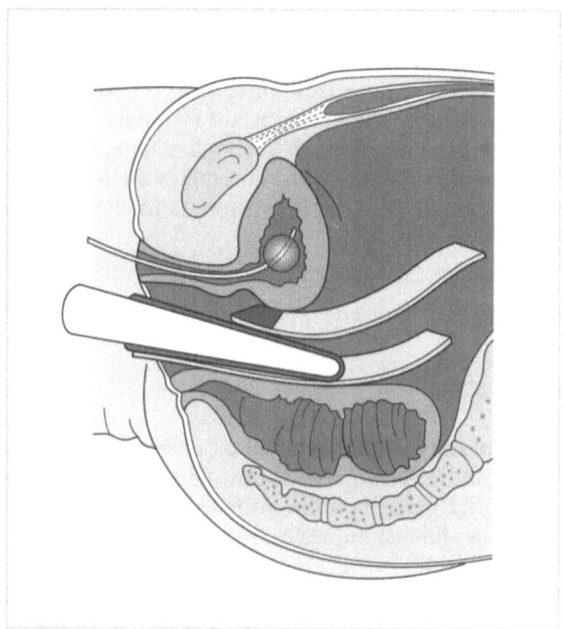

Figure 30.2 Anterior and posterior grafts placed with the aid of a Lucite stent.

Obliterative surgery is also an effective therapy for uterovaginal prolapse. Careful consideration of loss of vaginal function is critical, as perception of body image is just as important to many women as coital capability. Vaginal obliteration may be achieved by colpocleisis, removing the vaginal epithelium and applying successive purse-string sutures, or by colpectomy, removing full-thickness vagina. With either procedure, levator plication with approximation of the muscles to close the genital hiatus to the urethra is performed. These procedures create downward pressure on the urethrovesical junction and are often associated with new onset stress incontinence, thus a supportive procedure for the urethrovesical junction is required. We generally use a needle procedure or a Kelly plication or a sling if intrinsic sphincter deficiency is diagnosed. Frail elderly women with debilitating prolapse problems make up the majority of patients receiving obliterative therapy.

Women who desire uterine preservation for future childbearing and for whom pessary use does not satisfactorily relieve prolapse symptoms are first counseled to complete their childbearing before undergoing reconstructive surgery. Should this option not be acceptable, therapy consists of a modification of a Gilliam procedure. A synthetic strip or fascia is anchored to the posterior isthmic region of the cervix, passed between the leaves of the broad ligament to exit through the internal inguinal ring, and anchored to the anterior rectus sheath. This is combined with a uterosacral plication and perineorrhaphy if necessary.

Summary

This section summarizes our choices for surgery for prolapse today. The one constant is change. Laparoscopic procedures, tension-free vaginal tapes, implantable neuromodulation, and injectables are impacting pelvic floor reconstructive surgery, and evolution of therapies is rapid.

Choice of Surgery for Prolapse

Bob L. Shull

The operative management of pelvic organ prolapse can be accomplished transabdominally, transvaginally, laparoscopically, or by using a combination of routes and techniques. Surgical procedures should be planned following an assessment of the patient's bowel, bladder, and sexual functions, and pelvic support defects, as well as the surgeon's own skills. The ultimate outcome depends on the accuracy of the preoperative diagnosis, the efficacy of surgical skills, the patient's compliance with postoperative instructions, and wound healing. The surgeon is responsible for the diagnosis, surgical skills, and education of the patient regarding postoperative care. Wound healing is a biological phenomenon with maximum wound strength occurring approximately 90–100 days postoperatively. I consider wound healing so important to the ultimate success of the surgical intervention that I frequently use nonabsorbable sutures and regularly instruct patients to minimize increases in intraabdominal pressure for approximately 12 weeks following surgery.

My preference is to treat patients with pelvic organ prolapse by transvaginal surgery and to treat patients with genuine stress urinary incontinence by retropubic surgery. Women may have coexisting pelvic organ prolapse and significant genuine stress urinary incontinence. I would not hesitate to use a combined vaginal and abdominal approach for these women.

Patients with pelvic organ prolapse and the following conditions may be best treated transabdominally:

- bladder exstrophy
- severe orthopedic deformities limiting mobility of legs and hips
- concurrent intra-abdominal pathology requiring an abdominal approach
- vaginal canal so short that elongation is required for intravaginal intercourse
- certain connective tissue disorders
- desire for future childbearing.

DeLancey[12] has described an approach to vaginal support as follows:

- *Level I support:* the cervix or vaginal apex is suspended to the cardinal uterosacral ligaments.
- *Level II support:* the connective tissue supporting the base of bladder, urethrovesical junction, and anterior wall of rectum, is attached to the arcus tendenius fascia pelvis or levator fascia.
- *Level III support:* the distal urethra and distal rectovaginal septum are embryologically different, being derived from the urogenital sinus. Level III is a level of fusion of the underlying connective tissue with the overlying epithelium.

These levels do not account for central or midline defects in the anterior or posterior segments. Midline defects in connective tissue have been traditionally treated by midline plication. I employ the concept of levels of support when planning surgical therapy. For example, level I defects are suspended, level II defects are reattached and/or plicated, and level III defects require some combination of suspension, plication, or reattachment.

My goals in the operating room are to identify the support defects, to determine which defects require suspension, reattachment, or plication, and to use native tissue for the repair. Depending on the patient's bowel, bladder, and sexual function, the operation will be accomplished entirely transvaginally, transabdominally, or by a combination of the two approaches.

The majority of level I support defects are repaired by suspending the pubocervical and rectovaginal fascia to the remnants of uterosacral ligaments. Suspension is performed so that the apex of the fibromuscular tube of the vaginal canal is closed, minimizing the risks of persistent or recurrent apical defects (Figs 30.3–30.6). Level II defects of the anterior segment may or may not be associated with genuine stress urinary incontinence (GSI). In the absence of GSI, I manage these defects transvaginally and in the presence of significant GSI an open retropubic repair works best in my hands. The retropubic repair may be a colposuspension or colposuspension plus paravaginal defect repair. Level III defects of the anterior segment are uncommon; however, level III defects of the posterior segment are commonly seen in parous women. Many gynecologists think these defects of attachment of the distal rectovaginal septum to the perineal body are a consequence of obstetrical trauma which was not well repaired or was well repaired but the repair was not durable. Clinically these women may be asymptomatic, have symptoms of tissue bulging, or describe the trapping of formed stool in the distal rectum. An intraoperative digital rectal examination may help to identify the anatomical defect. Separation of the rectovaginal septum from the perineal body may also be associated with increased mobility of the perineal body.

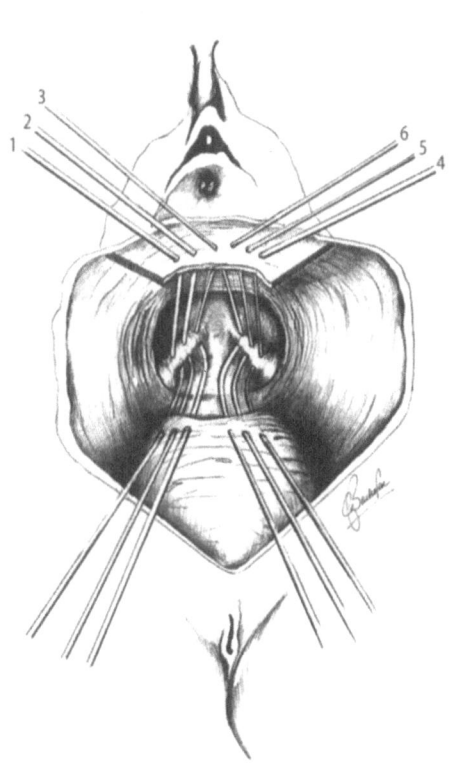

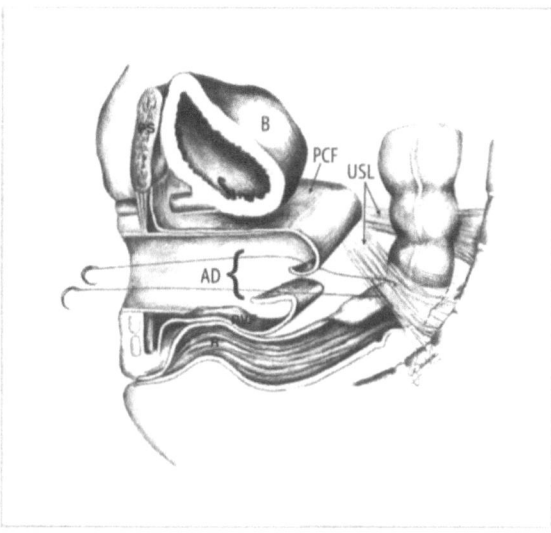

Figure 30.4 The first suture is placed through the transverse (superior) portion of pubocervical and rectovaginal fascia. PCF, pubocervical fascia; USL, uterosacral ligament; B, bladder; AD, apical defect.

Case Studies

Pelvic Organ Prolapse with Cystocele, Uterine Prolapse, Rectocele, and Genuine Stress Urinary Incontinence

A 59 year old woman has a history of pelvic organ prolapse and urinary incontinence with increases in intra-abdominal pressure. She uses three pads per day. She describes pocketing of stool in the distal rectum which requires digital pressure for complete

Figure 30.3 The suspensory sutures are placed through the remnants of uterosacral ligaments bilaterally (as viewed from the vaginal surgeon's perspective: 1–6 refers to the order of the sutures).

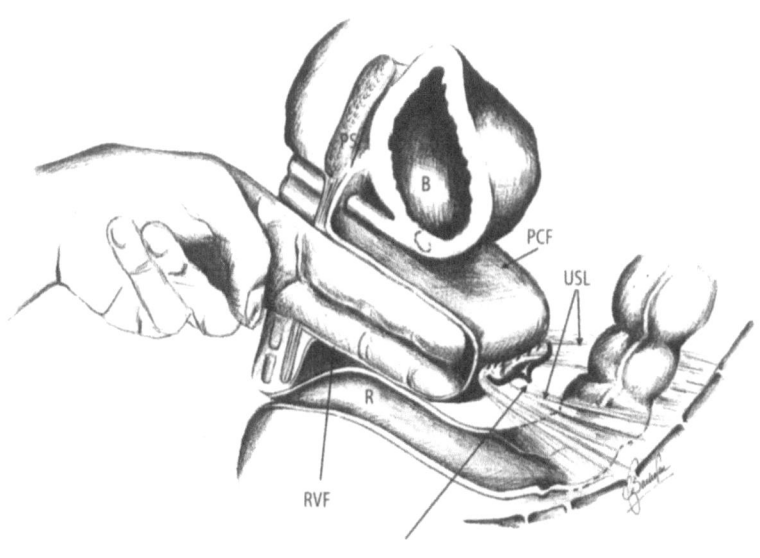

Figure 30.5 The transverse (superior) portion of pubocervical and rectovaginal fascia are used to close the fibromuscular tube of the vagina by suspending them to the uterosacral ligaments.

evacuation. She has intravaginal intercourse twice a week. For the past year she has felt and seen tissue protruding outside the vagina. She has not had any pelvic surgery.

On physical examination the uterus and ovaries are normal size. The pelvic organ prolapse quantification findings are:

Aa 0	Ba +5	C –1
GH 5 cm	PB 3 cm	TVL 10 cm
Ap +1	Bp+3	D –2

Urodynamic tests confirm the diagnosis of genuine stress urinary incontinence. Tests of urethral function are normal.

Discussion

This woman has several separate but related problems: genuine stress urinary incontinence, incomplete rectal evacuation, and pelvic organ prolapse. The pelvic organ prolapse primarily involves the anterior segment but is associated with uterine prolapse and a defect in the posterior segment.

Treatment

My preference is to approach the pelvic organ prolapse transvaginally. First, perform a total vaginal hysterectomy and bilateral salpingo-oophorectomy. The vaginal cuff should be suspended by using the cardinal uterosacral ligament pedicles. These pedicles are tagged early in the operation and secured with 2–3 nonabsorbable sutures. The anterior midline defect is plicated with a braided, nonabsorbable suture. The superior or transverse portion of the pubocervical fascia is then suspended with the series of sutures which have been placed into the uterosacral ligament pedicles. The same sutures are used to grasp the transverse portion of rectovaginal fascia. When the suspensory sutures are tied, the apex of the vagina will be suspended to its normal position and the edges of the fascia anteriorly and posteriorly will be closed. At that point, give the patient intravenous indigo carmine and perform cystoscopy to confirm ureteric patency. Next, trim the anterior epithelium to fit and close the incision with an absorbable suture.

I would perform the rectocele repair by excising a triangular portion of perineal skin, elevating the vaginal epithelium off the rectovaginal septum. An intraoperative digital rectal examination may help identify the fascial defect which is repaired with interrupted delayed absorbable sutures. A perineorrhaphy should be performed to restore the genital hiatus to normal.

Following completion of the vaginal portion of the procedure, reposition the patient on the table to perform a modified Burch colposuspension.

This combination of surgical procedures offers the patient not only an effective, durable therapy of her pelvic organ prolapse, her bowel complaint, and her urinary incontinence, but also the benefits of recovery from primarily a vaginal operation.

Genuine Stress Urinary Incontinence and Rectocele

A 40 year old woman has documented genuine stress urinary incontinence and a posterior segment defect prolapsing outside the hymen. She reports the sensation of stool being trapped in a small pocket in the rectum and must perform digital splinting of the posterior vagina in order to defecate easily. On physical examination she has the following findings:

Aa –1	Ba –1	C –7
GH 4.5 cm	PB 2.5 cm	TVL 9
Ap +2	Bp +2	D –8

There is lateral loss of support for the urethra and urethrovesical junction. The posterior segment defect is associated with increased mobility of the perineal body and apparent separation of the rectovaginal fascia from the perineal body.

Discussion

This woman has two complaints: stress urinary incontinence and a symptomatic rectocele. The best procedure for the urinary incontinence is a retropubic urethropexy, but the rectocele requires a transvaginal approach. My preference is to perform the retropubic repair first. Following the urethropexy, evaluate the complete posterior vaginal segment to determine the extent of the posterior repair. A triangle of tissue is excised from the perineum and the vaginal epithelium is dissected off the rectovaginal fascia and the anterior wall of the rectum. An intraoperative digital rectal examination can be performed to identify the fascial defect. Midline defects are plicated with a series of interrupted sutures and the rectovaginal fascia is then approximated to the perineal body using a series of interrupted sutures. The perineal body is reconstructed using rectovaginal fascia, superficial transverse perineal muscles, and bulbocavernosus muscles. The vaginal repair should correct the "pocket" defect as well as perineal body hypermobility. In some patients the retropubic urethropexy elevates the anterior vaginal segment so significantly that the cul-de-sac is exposed to an increased risk of enterocele formation. The surgeon may choose to extend the posterior dissection to the vaginal apex and reconstruct the entire posterior segment in an effort to minimize the likelihood of enterocele formation.

Enterocele Following Retropubic Urethropexy

A 45 year old women had an abdominal hysterectomy and modified colposuspension performed 2 years ago. There were no complications. She has had normal bladder function with no urinary incontinence. Approximately 15 months after surgery she developed a sense of pelvic pressure and detected tissue protruding outside the vaginal opening. Bowel function is normal. On physical examination she has these findings:

Aa -2	Ba -1	C -1
GH 4.0	B 4.0	TVL 9
Ap -3	Bp +4	D -

Discussion

Support defects in the cul-de-sac and posterior vaginal segment may occur following successful surgery for urinary incontinence. Sling procedures, needle endoscopic procedures, and colposuspensions all elevate the anterior vagina and open the cul-de-sac to increases in intraabdominal pressure. Some authors advocate performance of a prophylactic culdoplasty for all patients at the time of these retropubic procedures for incontinence; however, there are no data to substantiate the success of that approach. A sensible policy is to evaluate the cul-de-sac and posterior segment support carefully pre-operatively and to repair pre-existing defects at the time of the surgical treatment for urinary incontinence. Women who have a hysterectomy performed at the time of the repair for urinary incontinence should also have a culdoplasty performed.

The woman in this vignette is characteristic of women who are cured of urinary incontinence but who acquire an anatomic defect that requires further surgery. The onset of signs and symptoms may occur soon after the colposuspension. In this case, it is appropriate to proceed promptly with surgical correction if the patient prefers.

A transvaginal approach to correct the enterocele as well as the apical prolapse is my choice. Using a longitudinal incision from the vaginal apex to the perineum, the vaginal epithelium is dissected off the underlying hernia sac and rectovaginal fascia. The sac is entered. The remnants of cardinal-uterosacral ligaments are identified and 2–3 nonabsorbable

sutures are sewn into these remnants. The transverse portion of pubocervical fascia is secured with one arm of the suspensory sutures and the transverse portion of rectovaginal fascia is secured with the other arm of the suspensory sutures. When the sutures are tied the pubocervical and rectovaginal fascia will be brought into apposition and suspended from the cardinal uterosacral ligaments. After the suspensory sutures are tied, give the patient intravenous 5 ml of indigo carmine and perform cystoscopy to assess ureteric patency. Tailor the vaginal epithelium and close the incision with an absorbable stitch. Since the genital hiatus is 4.0 cm preoperatively, I would also perform a perineorrhaphy.

Pelvic Organ Prolapse with Apical Enterocele, Cystocele, and Rectocele

A 66 year old woman previously has undergone multiple pelvic surgeries. At age 40, a transabdominal hysterectomy and bilateral salpingo-oophorectomy were performed for benign disease. For approximately 10 years after that surgery she had normal bowel, bladder, and sexual function. At age 55, an abdominal sacrocolpopexy and retropubic urethropexy were performed for vaginal prolapse and genuine stress urinary incontinence. For another 10 years she had normal bowel, bladder, and sexual function and no signs of pelvic organ prolapse. Over the proceeding several years, she has developed progressive symptoms of pelvic organ prolapse and has observed tissue protruding outside the vaginal canal. She has no urinary incontinence, but feels as if she does not empty her bladder completely. Bowel function is satisfactory. Intravaginal intercourse has become difficult because of the prolapsed vaginal tissue.

Her physical findings are as follows:

Aa −2	Ba +4	C +6
GH 3 cm	PB 3 cm	TVL 9 cm
Ap −3	Bp +3	D −

Tests of bladder function are normal and a provoked full bladder stress test is negative.

Discussion

This patient has developed recurrence of pelvic organ prolapse following an abdominal sacrocolpopexy and retropubic urethropexy. Bladder function and bowel function are satisfactory, but intercourse has become a problem because of the prolapse. On physical examination there continues to be good support of the urethra and distal

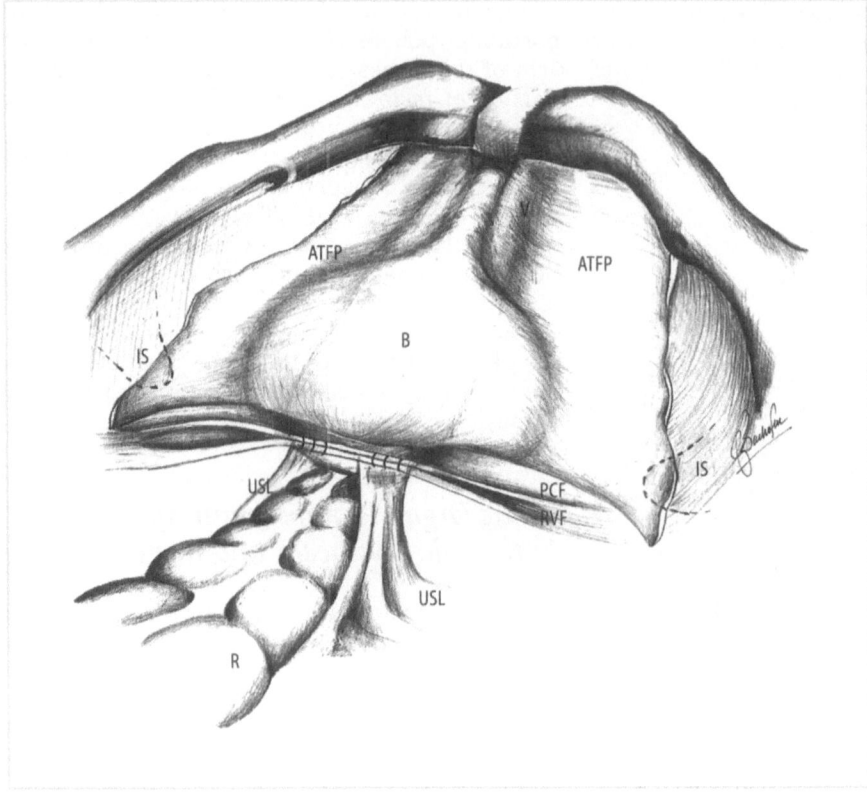

Figure 30.6 An abdominal view of the suspended and closed vaginal apex. ATFP, arcus tendineus fascia pelvis; B, bladder; IS, ischial spine; PCF, pubocervical fascia; PS, pubic symphysis; R, rectum; RVF, rectovaginal fascia; USL, uterosacral ligament; V, vagina.

rectovaginal septum. The base of the bladder, vaginal cuff, cul-de-sac, and upper portion of the rectovaginal septum are prolapsing outside the vaginal canal.

Treatment

Her primary defect is loss of support for the apex. The pubocervical fascia and the rectovaginal fascia are separated at the apex of the vaginal canal resulting in an apical enterocele and vaginal cuff prolapse. Women who have significant pelvic organ prolapse uncommonly have significant adhesions in the hernia sac. Consequently, a transvaginal approach is generally quite straightforward even though the patient has had prior reconstructive surgery.

Use a vertical incision beginning on the anterior segment and extending to the vaginal apex and the posterior segment of the vagina, reflecting the vaginal epithelium away from pubocervical fascia, the hernia sac, and rectovaginal fascia. Enter the hernia sac, identify the remnants of cardinal uterosacral ligaments, and use a series of nonabsorbable sutures to secure the cardinal uterosacral ligaments posterior and medial to the ischial spines. Next, plicate the rectovaginal fascia and pubocervical fascia in the midline using a series of interrupted

nonabsorbable sutures. Following that, incorporate the suspensory sutures in the uterosacral ligament into the superior portion of the rectovaginal and pubocervical fascia. When the suspensory sutures are tied, the rectovaginal and pubocervical fascia will be brought together to close the apex of the vagina and suspend the vaginal canal in the hollow of the sacrum. After the suspensory sutures have been tied, give the patient intravenous indigo carmine and perform cystoscopy to evaluate ureteric patency.

In a woman who has previously had an abdominal sacrocolpopexy, an alternate strategy would be to use the same approach to enter the hernia sac transvaginally. Rather than using remnants of uterosacral ligaments for the suspension, try to identify the graft material which is likely still attached to the sacrum. If the graft material can be identified, it serves as an excellent site for suspension of the apex.

References

1. Kelvin FM, Maglinte DDT, Hornback J, Benson JT (1992) Pelvic prolapse: Assessment with evacuation proctography (defecography). Radiology 184: 547–51.
2. Maglinte DDT, Kelvin FM, Fitzgerald K, Hale DS, Benson JT (1999) Association of compartment defects in pelvic floor dysfunction. AJR 172: 439–44.

3. Kahn MA, Stanton SL (1997) Posterior colporrhaphy: Its effects on bowel and sexual function. Br J Obstet Gynecol 104: 82–6.
4. Benson JT, Lucente V, McClellan E (1996) Vaginal versus abdominal reconstructive surgery for the treatment of pelvic support defects: A prospective randomized study with long-term outcome evaluation. Am J Obstet Gynecol 175: 1418–22.
5. Benson JT, McClellan E (1993) The effect of vaginal dissection on the pudendal nerve. Obstet Gynecol 82: 387–9.
6. Borirakchanyavat S, Aboseif SR, Carroll PR et al. (1997) Continence mechanism of the isolated female urethra: An anatomical study of the intrapelvic somatic nerves. J Urol 158: 822–826.
7. Zivkovic F, Tamussino KI, Ralph G, Schied G, Auer-Grumbach M (1996) Long-term effects of vaginal dissection on the innervation of the striated urethral sphincter. Obstet Gynecol 87: 257–60.

8. Ball TP Jr, Teichman MH, Sharkey FE, Rogenes VJ, Adrian EK Jr (1997) Terminal nerve distribution to the urethra and bladder neck: Consideration in the management of stress urinary incontinence. J Urol 158: 827–29.
9. Welgoss JA, Vogt VY, McClellan EJ, Benson JT (1999) Relationship between surgically induced neuropathy and outcome of pelvic organ prolapse surgery. Int Urogynecol J 10: 11–14.
10. Clark M, Hale D, Benson JT (1999) Cadaveric fascia lata as graft material in sacral colpopexy. Abstract, American Urogynecologic Society Annual Meeting, 1999, San Diego, California.
11. Iglesia CB, Fenner D, Brubaker L (1997) The use of mesh in gynecologic surgery. Int Urogynecol J 8: 105–15.
12. DeLancey JOL (1992) Anatomic aspects of vaginal eversion after hysterectomy. Am J Obstet Gynecol 166: 1717–1728.

31 Anal Incontinence

Cornelius G.M.I. Baeten

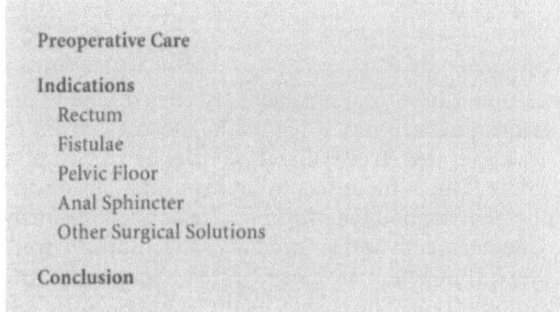

When a patient is incontinent of feces, the first question is whether she should be treated with conservative methods or surgery. Investigations that determine this choice have been discussed in earlier chapters. Indications for surgery exist when there is severe incontinence, when conservative methods (diet, constipating drugs, biofeedback therapy) fail, and when diagnostic tests show that surgical interventions could be useful.

Fecal continence is dependent on several factors, and it is important to consider each of these. For example, it is questionable whether a patient who has a combination of untreatable diarrhea and a sphincter rupture will benefit from a sphincter repair. Surgical interventions for fecal incontinence can be helpful for certain disorders of the rectum, fistulae, pelvic floor, and anal sphincters.

Preoperative Care

In general it is not necessary to give patients a protective colostomy or ileostomy. Only in the case of an intentional opening (low anterior resection) or unintentional perforation of the anorectum is a protective stoma advisable.

Prophylactic antibiotics are advisable, especially when exogenous materials are used (such as artificial sphincters or electrical stimulators).

Preoperative lavage is important in interventions where the bowel has to be opened. In other procedures leakage of lavage fluid through the anus can present a problem during the operation.

Indications

In cases of severe incontinence the results of several assessed tests will indicate whether one or more factors are deficient. When one factor is deficient and this factor can be corrected by an operation, the situation is clear. When there is a problem with more than one factor, the severity of deficiency determines whether a combination of interventions is necessary, or a combination of operation and conservative treatment. The various surgical interventions will be discussed here as if they were single problems leading to fecal incontinence (Table 31.1).

Rectum

Patients with rectocele normally complain of obstructed defecation but sometimes experience leakage of stool and have to go to the toilet frequently. When no facilities are available they experience loss of stool. A rectocele repair – transvaginally, transanally, or a combination of these – is worthwhile.

Rectopexy is indicated for patients with incontinence due to rectal prolapse. The prolapse causes sphincter problems, and in most patients anal pressures are very low. The bad condition of the sphincters is no immediate indication for sphincter surgery, because this might lead to obstruction. The best way to proceed is first to perform a rectopexy. In 40–70% of the cases continence will improve spontaneously.[1-4] If the patient stays incontinent after treatment of the rectal prolapse, because of sphincter damage, this can be an indication to perform a second operation to correct the sphincter.

Table 31.1. Treatment of fecal incontinence

Cause of incontinence	Primary therapy	Secondary therapy	Tertiary therapy
Diarrhea	Constipating drugs		
Pseudo-diarrhea	Laxatives, enemas		
Rectal prolapse	Delorme procedure Rectopexy	Low anterior resection	Colostomy
Rectovaginal fistulae	Fistula closure	Martius graft Graciloplasty	
Pelvic floor insufficiency	Biofeedback therapy	Preanal repair Postanal repair	
Sphincter rupture	Anal repair	Dynamic graciloplasty	
Sphincter agenesis	Dynamic graciloplasty	Artificial bowel sphincter	
Sphincter atrophy	Dynamic graciloplasty Artificial bowel sphincter Sacral nerve stimulation		

The same approach goes for patients with rectal prolapse treated with the Delorme procedure, or rectosigmoidectomy.[5-7] In these cases the adage must be "wait and see." If incontinence due to sphincter damage recovers spontaneously, nothing else needs to be done. In case of permanent damage a sphincter operation at a later date, but never at the same moment as the prolapse correction, will be the right sequence.

Fistulae

Incontinence due to perianal fistulae or rectovaginal fistulae can take place in two ways: loss of stool through the fistulous tract or through the anus, because of sphincter damage.

Sphincter reconstruction when there is sepsis is not advisable. The best sequence of interventions in those cases is to give the patient a protective colostomy and to do an on-table lavage of the distal colon, followed by an operation to correct the fistula. Often this will mean excision of the fistulous tract with closure of the defect and protection of the area with a rectal mucosa advancement flap . When the septic period is over and assessments show sphincter deficiency, the sphincter can be repaired or replaced with a dynamic gracilo-plasty. In the last phase, when tests show acceptable restoration of the sphincter complex, the protective colostomy can be closed.

In cases of Crohn's disease when the anus is completely destroyed, the only solution is a permanent colostomy and an excision of the anorectum.

In cases of recurrence of low rectovaginal fistulae, an interposition of vital tissue can be of help. This can be performed with a Martius graft in which a flap of fat tissue from one labium major is put between the rectum and the back wall of the vagina. A more extensive procedure is a gracilis trans-

position, where vital muscular tissue is placed in the rectovaginal septum. The gracilis muscle is freed in the upper leg from distal to the neurovascular bundle. This bundle has to be kept intact. Here the muscle is flapped backward and led subcutaneously to the perineum and sutured over the anorectal wall, where the defect is closed after excision of the fistulous tract. The defect in the vagina can be left open for drainage.

Pelvic Floor

Incontinence due to pelvic floor denervation seldom reacts to biofeedback therapy. In cases of failure of this treatment it is possible to perform a postanal repair.[8,9] For this operation an incision is made ±5 cm dorsal to the anus. In a plane between internal and external sphincters, the back of the rectum can be reached. On both sides the fibers of the pubo-rectal, pubococcygeal, and ischiococcygeal muscles can be found. These muscles can be sutured together dorsal to the rectum, and finally the external sphincter is plicated. In this way the rectum is pushed forward and upward. The initial results are good, but in long-term follow-up this good effect diminishes and falls below 50%.

In an attempt to improve these results, total pelvic floor repair has been developed. In this case both sides of the sling are sutured in front of the ano-rectum. This preanal repair, in combination with postanal repair, gives better results than postanal repair alone.[10-12]

Anal Sphincter

When incontinence is due to rupture of the anal sphincters, an anal repair is the operation of first choice. The technique has already been described in earlier chapters. Most obstetricians prefer direct end-to-end repair (although this is changing), whereas most colorectal surgeons practice the method described by Parks and perform an overlapping repair.[13-18] There is debate about whether it is meaningful to investigate the quality of the ruptured sphincter. This can be done by EMG of the sphincter remnant or by MRI. MRI gives information about possible atrophy of the ruptured sphincter, and this seems more reliable than information about denervation. A success rate for anal repair is described in 92% of patients without atrophy versus 25% in patients with atrophy of the sphincter.[19] Endosonography is less helpful in determination of atrophy. Very often an anal repair is followed by a preanal repair to create better enforcement of the barrier between anus and vagina.

When incontinence is based on absence of anal sphincters (anal atresia), a failure of anal repair, or severe atrophy of the original sphincter, a new anal repair is not appropriate. The question is how to replace this weak or absent sphincter. The choice is between autologous material or an artificial sphincter.

Autologous replacement by fascia strips is considered obsolete, and the two muscles available for sphincter replacement are the gluteus and gracilis muscle.[20,21] The gluteoplasty is only practiced incidentally, because long-term voluntary contraction is impossible. The same goes for graciloplasty. Recent development shows that the gracilis muscle can be activated by electrical stimulation.[22-24] This stimulation changes the muscle fibers in the gracilis muscle from type II into type I fibers, which are not fatiguable and can contract continuously. The stimulator takes care of the automatic contraction, and it is no longer necessary to contract the muscle consciously. The technique involves a conventional graciloplasty as described in the past, followed by the implant of electrodes and stimulator. The results of this technique are good, and about 75% of patients will experience restoration of continence. In order to defecate, patients switch off the stimulation using a remote control.

In special cases this technique is also employed for patients who need an abdominoperineal resection for low rectal cancer. The bowel can be pulled to the perineum and sutured to the skin. The end of the bowel is then encircled with one or two gracilis muscles that are activated by electrical stimulation.[25-28]

The indications for an artificial bowel sphincter are almost the same as for dynamic graciloplasty. It is the only solution in patients who have no vital and well-innervated gracilis muscles. The artificial bowel sphincter works on the same principle as the artificial urinary sphincter. A cuff is placed around the anus and is filled with fluid from a pressure-regulating balloon. The cuff can be emptied by pressure on a pump, placed in one labium major, which pumps the fluid from the anal cuff to the pressure-regulation balloon. The anus opens, making defecation possible.[29-32] The artificial bowel sphincter technique is not advisable in cases where the risk of infection is high (e.g. patients who have sphincter lesions due to perianal fistulae and sepsis). Patients with almost no tissue between anorectum and vagina have a higher risk of erosions through rectum or vagina, and are better off with the autologous muscle tissue of the dynamic graciloplasty.

Other Surgical Solutions

A very new surgical approach for fecal incontinence is sacral nerve stimulation. The technique is the same as the neuromodulation described for urinary incontinence. Patients with anatomically intact, but very weak sphincters could benefit from this approach.[33-34]

The last solution for intractable fecal incontinence is the creation of a colostomy. When all other methods fail, a colostomy gives the opportunity to transform unmanageable anal incontinence into manageable incontinence at the level of the abdominal wall. This can be a very good solution for patients who are not mobile and are dependent on others for going to the toilet. Stoma care is often possible for these patients, and this approachis a better solution for them than other surgical interventions.

Conclusion

With all surgical interventions to restore fecal incontinence, one has to realize that continence is the result of multiple factors and a "successful" operation for any one of these factors does not automatically mean restoration of continence. It may be necessary to combine surgical and conservative treatments to obtain an acceptable result.

After surgical interventions, one often sees an "overshoot" effect, and development of severe constipation. This is not necessarily due to narrowing of the anal canal. Many patients have constipation for years, leading to prolapse and sphincter problems that in turn lead to incontinence. Treatment of the incontinence allows the original problem of constipation to emerge again. When sphincter restoration leads to fecal impaction, pseudo-diarrhea ironically can give incontinence once more. The solution for this is laxatives and enemas.

References

1. Delamarre JBVM, Gooszen HG, Kruyt RH, Soebhag R, Geesteranus AM (1991) The effect of posterior rectopexy on faecal continence. Dis Colon Rectum 34: 311–16.
2. Tjandra JJ, Fazio VW, Church JM et al. (1993) Ripstein procedure is an effective treatment for rectal prolapse without constipation. Dis Colon Rectum 36: 501–7.
3. Mc Cure JL, Thompson JPS (1991) Clinical and functional results of abdominal rectopexy for complete rectal prolapse. Br J Surg 78: 921–3.
4. Keighley MRB, Fielding JWL, Alexander Williams J (1983) Results of Marlex mesh abdominal rectopexy for rectal prolapse. Br J Surg 70: 229–32.
5. Madoff RD, Williams JG, Wong WD, Rothenberger DA, Goldberg SM (1992) Longterm functional results of colon resection and rectopexy for rectal prolapse. Am J Gastro Ent 87: 101–4.
6. Lechaux JP, Lechaux D, Perez M (1995) Results of Delormes procedure for rectal prolapse. Dis Colon Rectum 38: 301–7.
7. Williams JG, Rothenberger DA, Madoff RD, Goldberg SM (1992) Treatment of rectal prolapse in the elderly by perineal rectosigmoidectomy. Dis Colon Rectum 35: 830–4.
8. Setti Carraro P, Kamm MA, Nicholls RJ (1994) Long-term results of postanal repair for neurogenic faecal incontinence. Br J Surg 160: 637–40.
9. Engel AF, Baal SJ van, Brummelkamp WH (1994) Late result of postanal repair for idiopathic faecal incontinence. Eur J Surg 160: 637–40.
10. Deen KI, Oya M, Ortiz J, Keighley MRB (1993) Randomized trial comparing three forms of pelvic floor repair for neuropathic faecal incontinence. Br J Surg 80: 794–8.
11. Lehur PA, Bruley des Varannes S, Dutre J, Guiberteau-Canfrere V, Galmiche JP, Le Borone J (1995) Pre- and retroanal myoraphy in the treatment of severe anal incontinence. Clinical and manometric results. Ann Chir 49: 621–7.
12. Engel AF, Brummelkamp WH (1994) Secondary surgery after failed postanal or anterior sphincter repair. Int J Colorect Dis 9: 187–90.
13. Briel JW (1998) deBoer LM, Hop WCJ, Schouten WR. Clinical outcome of anterior overlapping external anal sphincter repair with internal anal sphincter imbrication. Dis Colon Rectum 41: 209–14.
14. Oliveira L, Pfeifer J, Wexner SD (1996) Physiological and clinical outcome of anterior sphincteroplasty. Br J Surg 83: 502–5.
15. Engel AF, Kamm MA, Sultan AH, Bartam CI, Nicholls RJ (1994) Anterior anal sphincter repair in patients with obstetric trauma. Br J Surg 81: 1231–4.
16. Yoshioka K, Keighley MR (1989) Sphincter repair for faecal incontinence. Dis Colon Rectum 32: 39–42.
17. Engel AF (1994) vBaal JG, Brummelkamp WH. Late results of anterior sphincter plication. Eur J Surg 160: 641–5.
18. Pinedo G, Vaizey C, Nicholls RJ et al. (1998) The outcome of repeat anal sphincter repair. Colorectal Dis 4: A13.
19. Briel JW, Stoker J, Rociu E et al. (1999) External anal sphincter atrophy on endoanal MRI adversely affects continence after sphinteroplasty. Br J Surg 86(11): 1392–7.
20. Corman ML (1980) Follow up evaluation of gracilis muscle transposition for faecal incontinence. Dis Colon Rectum 23: 552–5.
21. Christiansen J, Ronholt Hansen C, Rasmussen O (1995) Bilateral gluteus maximus transposition for anal incontinence. Br J Surg 82: 903–5.
22. Baeten CGMI, Geerdes BP, Adang EMM et al. (1995) Anal dynamic graciloplasty in the treatment of intractable faecal incontinence. N Engl J Med 332(24): 1600–5.
23. Williams NS, Patel J, George BD, Hallan RI, Watkins ES (1991) Development of an electrically stimulated neo anal sphincter. Lancet 338: 1166–9.
24. Adang E, Engel GL, Rutten B, Geerdes BP, Baeten CGMI (1998) Cost-effectiveness of dynamic graciloplasty in patients with faecal incontinence. Dis Colon Rectum 41(6): 725–33.
25. Baeten CGMI, Rongen MJ (1997) Total anorectal reconstruction; fact or fiction. Swiss Surg 3: 262–5.
26. Geerdes BP, Heineman E, Zoetmulder FAN et al. (1996) De dubbele dynamische gracilisplastiek: alternatief voor het colostoma na een volledig verlies van het anorectum. NtvG 140(14): 773–7.
27. Cavina E (1996) Outcome of restorative perineal graciloplasty with simultaneous excision of the anus and rectum for cancer. Dis Colon Rectum 39: 182–90.
28. Geerdes BP, Zoetmulder FAN, Baeten CGMI (1995) Double dynamic graciloplasty and coloperineal pull-through after abdominoperineal resection. Eur J Cancer 31A(7–8): 1248–52.
29. Christiansen J, Lorentzen M (1989) Implantation of artificial sphincter for anal incontinence. Report of five cases. Dis Colon Rectum 32: 432–6.
30. Lehur P, Michot F, Denis P et al. (1996) Results of artificial sphincter in severe anal incontinence: report of 14 consecutive cases. Dis Colon Rectum 39: 1352–5.
31. Wong WD, Jensen LL, Bartolo DCC, Rothenberger DA (1996) Artificial anal sphincter. Dis Colon Rectum 39: 1345–51.
32. Hajivassiliou CA, Finlay IG (1998) Effect of a novel prosthetic anal neosphincter on human colonic blood flow. Br J Surg 85: 1703–7.
33. Vaizey CJ, Kamm MA, Turner IC, Nicholls RJ, Woloszko J (1997) Sacral nerve stimulation for faecal incontinence: evaluation of short term efficacy and effect on anorectal function. Gastroenterology 112: A842.
34. Matzel KE, Stadelmaier U, Hohenfellner M, Gall FP (1995) Electrical stimulation of sacral spinal nerves for treatment of faecal incontinence. Lancet 346: 1124–7.

Index